Advances in Mental Health and Addiction

Series editor
Masood Zangeneh

More information about this series at http://www.springer.com/series/13393

Edo Shonin • William Van Gordon
Mark D. Griffiths
Editors

Mindfulness and Buddhist-Derived Approaches in Mental Health and Addiction

Springer

Editors
Edo Shonin
Awake to Wisdom
Centre for Meditation and Mindfulness Research
Nottingham, UK

Bodhayati School of Buddhism
Nottingham, UK

Psychology Division, Chaucer Building
Nottingham Trent University
Nottingham, UK

William Van Gordon
Awake to Wisdom
Centre for Meditation and Mindfulness Research
Nottingham, UK

Bodhayati School of Buddhism
Nottingham, UK

Psychology Division, Chaucer Building
Nottingham Trent University
Nottingham, UK

Mark D. Griffiths
Psychology Division, Chaucer Building
Nottingham Trent University
Nottingham, UK

Advances in Mental Health and Addiction
ISBN 978-3-319-22254-7 ISBN 978-3-319-22255-4 (eBook)
DOI 10.1007/978-3-319-22255-4

Library of Congress Control Number: 2015952311

Springer Cham Heidelberg New York Dordrecht London

Printed on acid-free paper

Springer International Publishing AG Switzerland is part of Springer Science+Business Media (www.springer.com)

To Dr. Giulia Cavalli, for her help with introducing people in Italy to the practice of authentic mindful living

E.S.

To the simple monk, Venerable Edo Shonin

W.V.G.

To Fiona, Alyssia, Lucas, and Daniel

M.D.G.

Foreword

In the *Parables of Leadership*, Chan Kim narrates a parable that he first heard as a youth from a Korean master in the temples of Kyung Nam province of Korea. As the parable goes, to prepare his son to succeed him, the king sent the young prince to a renowned master to learn the fundamentals of being a good ruler. The master sent the young prince alone to the local forest and instructed him to return in a year and describe the sounds of the forest. When the young prince returned, the master asked the prince to describe what he heard and the prince replied, "Master, I could hear the cuckoos sing, the leaves rustle, the hummingbirds hum, the crickets chirp, the grass blow, the bees buzz, and the wind whisper and holler." On hearing this, the master sent the young prince back into the forest to listen to the unheard sounds of the forest. The young prince wondered what else there was to hear, but he followed the master's instructions and he began to listen more intently to experience the sounds of the forest. When the young prince returned, the master asked him what more had he heard. The prince replied, "Master, when I listened most closely, I could hear the unheard—the sound of flowers opening, the sound of the sun warming the earth, and the sound of the grass drinking the morning dew," and the master nodded in approval. It was only by cultivating mindfulness that the young prince was able to hear the unheard.

The concept and practice of mindfulness has been in the lexicon of all wisdom traditions in one form or another since the beginning of such traditions. Although individuals in the West have been searching for and/or practicing some form of mindfulness for many years, the practice of mindfulness meditation came into its own in the West when Jon Kabat-Zinn formulated and introduced Mindfulness-Based Stress Reduction (MBSR) about 35 years ago at the University of Massachusetts Medical Center. Mindfulness meditation has slowly gained traction since then and, in the past decade, we have witnessed increasing public and media attention, some favorable and some critical. But what is certain is that mindfulness has taken hold of people's imagination in innumerable fields—medicine, psychology, psychiatry, nursing, occupational therapies, social services, pediatrics, oncology, diabetes, health and wellness, economics, and politics, among many others.

Recent events—wars, medical epidemics, and natural disasters—have heightened our sense of suffering in this world. But suffering has been with us since the beginning of time and there is great need for simple ways by which we can overcome or lessen suffering, regardless of its origins. While we may not be able to overcome the pain associated with various conditions we suffer from, surely we can lessen the suffering that such pain engenders. This quest for finding solutions to our suffering has been embraced by academic and scientific communities in their search for treatments, programs, or regimens that will provide lasting relief. What we need is a resource that informs us of the current status of what we know about these treatments, programs, and regimens, the research evidence that underpins these approaches, and newer approaches that are in development which appear most promising. Fortunately, we now have this resource and we are indebted to the editors of this book for bringing together a stellar group of scientifically and clinically enlightened contributors who have sifted through the growing literature to inform us of the state of the art of mindfulness and its applications.

Mindfulness has always been a difficult term to define in the context of science. Louis Armstrong, a prominent American jazz musician, once observed that, "If you have to ask what jazz is, you will never know." The same could be said of mindfulness. But the notion of experiencing mindfulness to know what it is, as opposed to operationally defining it, is anathema to the scientific mind. Of course, there have been various attempts to define mindfulness, an ill-translated Pāli word *sati*, a relative of the Sanskrit word *smriti*, which is traditionally translated as, "that which is remembered," or recalling to one's mind. In the context of Western science, there does not appear to be much consensus on how it can be defined in a unitary manner. For example, Jon Kabat-Zinn has defined it as "the awareness that emerges through paying attention on purpose, in the present moment, and non-judgmentally to the unfolding of experience moment to moment." The great mindfulness meditation master, Munindra, suggested that in the context of daily life, mindfulness is the ". . . experiencing from moment to moment, living from moment to moment, without clinging, without condemning, without judging, without criticizing—choiceless awareness. . . It should be integrated into our whole life. It is actually an education in how to see, how to hear, how to smell, how to eat, how to drink, how to walk with full awareness."

Over the years, Kabat-Zinn's MBSR became mainstream and a small number of related mindfulness-based interventions (MBIs) emerged. To varying degrees, these MBIs were found to have a positive effect on individuals who had various diseases and disorders—both medical and psychiatric, physical and emotional. Such was the effectiveness of these interventions that they were ruled to be evidence-based, and mindfulness-based treatment guidelines were included by various professional associations in several countries. The first generation of MBIs was uniformly secular in their presentation, often eschewing the spiritual bases of mindfulness meditation practices. The recent advent of the second generation of MBIs has explicitly included other practices, most often Buddhist practices, which place these MBIs squarely in the spiritual realm. While one does not need to be a Buddhist to engage in these MBIs, the developers of these MBIs offer them as being more broad-based and better equipped to produce transformational changes in the practitioners. These MBIs were developed to enable the practitioners to embody the teachings rather than focus on health and wellness as the primary outcomes.

There is natural tension between the secular and spiritual MBI traditions, but it need not be if the essence of both approaches is to be on the journey of life itself. The editors and contributors of this book cover a broad swath of the current mindfulness canvas—from assessment, diagnosis, and treatment to patient engagement in the practices. Taken as a whole, this book paints a very positive picture of the current status of the field and promises even more in the future.

Augusta, GA, USA
2015

Nirbhay N. Singh
Medical College of Georgia
Georgia Regents University

Contents

About the Editors

Venerable Edo Shonin has been a Buddhist monk for 30 years and is Spiritual Director of the international Mahayana Bodhayati School of Buddhism. He has also received the higher ordination in the Theravada Buddhist tradition. He is Research Director of the Awake to Wisdom Centre for Meditation and Mindfulness Research and a research psychologist at the Nottingham Trent University (UK). He sits on the International Advisory Board for the journal *Mindfulness* and is an editorial board member of the *International Journal of Mental Health and Addiction*. He has over 100 academic publications relating to the scientific study of mindfulness and Buddhist practice. He is the author of *The Mindful Warrior: The Path to Wellbeing, Wisdom and Awareness*, and primary editor of the Springer volume on the *Buddhist Foundations of Mindfulness*. He regularly receives invitations to give keynote speeches, lectures, retreats, and workshops at a range of academic and non-academic venues all over the world. He runs the *Meditation Practice and Research Blog* at www.edoshonin.com.

Venerable William Van Gordon has been a Buddhist monk for 10 years and is Operations Director of the international Mahayana Bodhayati School of Buddhism. He has also received the higher ordination in the Theravada Buddhist tradition. He is cofounder of the Awake to Wisdom Centre for Meditation and Mindfulness Research and is a research psychologist based at the Nottingham Trent University (UK). He is currently Principal Investigator on a number of randomized controlled trials investigating the applications of an intervention known as Meditation Awareness Training (MAT) in clinical and occupational settings. He is internationally known for his work and has over 100 academic publications relating to the scientific study of Buddhism and associated meditative approaches. He is co-author of *The Mindful Warrior: The Path to Wellbeing, Wisdom and Awareness*, and a co-editor of the Springer volume on the *Buddhist Foundations of Mindfulness*.

Mark D. Griffiths is a Chartered Psychologist and Professor of Gambling Studies at the Nottingham Trent University and Director of the International Gaming

Research Unit. He has also been carrying out research into mindfulness with Edo Shonin and William Van Gordon. He has published over 500 refereed research papers, four books, 120+ book chapters, and over 1000 other articles. He has served on numerous national and international committees and gambling charities (e.g., National Chair of GamCare, Society for the Study of Gambling, Gamblers Anonymous General Services Board, and National Council on Gambling). He has won 14 national and international awards for his work including the John Rosecrance Prize (1994), CELEJ Prize (1998), Joseph Lister Prize (2004), and the US National Council on Problem Gambling Lifetime Research Award (2012). He also does a lot of freelance journalism and has appeared on over 2500 radio and television programs.

About the Contributors

Jocelyn L. Abrams is a Research Assistant and Research Study Therapist in the Department of Psychiatry and Behavioral Sciences at the University of Texas Health Science Center at Houston. She is a fourth-year doctoral student in the counseling psychology program at the University of Houston. Jocelyn received a B.A. degree in psychology from Binghamton University in 2007 and an M.Ed. degree in counseling from the University of Houston in 2015. Her current research interests are focused upon better understanding cognitive-affective factors related to posttraumatic stress and comorbid conditions, including substance use disorders, in order to ultimately improve treatments for trauma survivors.

Patricia Bloom is a Clinical Associate Professor of Geriatrics at the Icahn Medical School of Mount Sinai, a past Vice Chair of the Brookdale Department of Geriatrics and Palliative Medicine at Mount Sinai Medical Center in New York, NY, and previously the Director of Integrative Health for the Martha Stewart Center for Living at the Mount Sinai Medical Center. Her major interests include integrative health and health promotion, stress reduction, and Mind Body Medicine. A certified teacher of Mindfulness-Based Stress Reduction (MBSR), she teaches MBSR for patients at the Mount Sinai Medical Center in New York NY, conducts stress reduction and mindfulness workshops for professional and workplace groups, is involved in mindfulness research, and lectures widely on integrative medicine and the science of meditation.

Judson A. Brewer is the Director of Research at the Center for Mindfulness and associate professor in medicine and psychiatry at UMass Medical School. He also is adjunct faculty at Yale University and a research affiliate at MIT. A psychiatrist and internationally known expert in mindfulness training for addictions, Brewer has developed and tested novel mindfulness programs for addictions, including both in-person and app-based treatments. He has also studied the underlying neural mechanisms of mindfulness using standard and real-time fMRI and is currently translating these findings into clinical use. He has published numerous peer-reviewed articles and book chapters, presented to the US President's Office of National Drug Control Policy, and been featured on 60 Minutes, at TEDx, in Time magazine (top 100 new health discoveries of 2013), Forbes, Businessweek, NPR, and the BBC among others. He writes a blog for The Huffington Post.

Joanne Cacciatore is an associate professor at Arizona State University and directs the Graduate Certificate in Trauma and Bereavement. Dr. Cacciatore is also the founder of the international nonprofit organizations the MISS Foundation and Center for Loss and Trauma. She earned a doctorate from the University of Nebraska-Lincoln with a focus on traumatic grief and from 2007 to 2015 had published more than 50 peer-reviewed studies in top-tier journals including the Lancet. Her primary area of research is in traumatic grief and death, including epidemiology, culture and ritual, mindfulness- and nature-based approaches, and critical psychiatry. In 2015, she published the text *The World of Bereavement* on death in cultures around the world, and she is currently writing a book on mindfulness and grief for Wisdom Publications. More of her work including a widely read blog can be found at centerforlossandtrauma.com.

José A. Carmona-Torres is a research fellow at the University of Almería (Spain) in the frame of an *Excellence Research Project* (funded by the Regional Ministry of Innovation, Science and Company, Andalusian County). He has been positively evaluated for the figure of *PhD Assistant Lecturer* by The National Agency for Quality Assessment and Accreditation (ANECA) (Government of Spain). In this regard, he is currently a lecturer of Psychopathology, Therapies, and Personality at the University of Almería (Spain). Dr. Carmona-Torres earned a doctoral degree in Psychology with a thesis focused on the application and validation of 3D computer programs applied to clinical psychology. In addition, he has research and applied experience in "experiential therapies" such as Mindfulness and Acceptance and Commitment Therapy (ACT). His research interests also include the study of different spiritual practices (e.g., meditation) and their relationships with mystical or exceptional experiences.

Jesper Dahlgaard has a Ph.D. in stress and evolutionary biology and a master's in positive psychology. He is senior scientist at the Unit of Psychooncology and Health Psychology at Aarhus University. He has more than 15 years of research experience in physical and mental health including clinical trials based on, e.g., gene expression profiles for personalized medicine, Internet-delivered CBT, and mindfulness-based therapy for patients with cancer. He has also worked with positive psychology and mindfulness among college students. In August 2015, he starts in a new position at VIA University College Aarhus, where he will be responsible for a local and international research team investigating mental health and rehabilitation using, e.g., mindfulness-based therapy.

Penelope J. Davis was awarded her doctoral degree from the University of Queensland in Australia and subsequently completed a postdoctoral period in the Department of Psychology at Yale. Since then, she has taught psychology at the University of Sydney, Harvard, and Griffith University in Brisbane, Australia. Her primary research interests include personality, emotion, repression, autobiographical memory, and schizophrenia.

Andrew Day is a Professor in the School of Psychology at Deakin University. Before joining academia, he was employed as a clinical psychologist in South Australia and the UK, having gained his Doctorate in Clinical Psychology from the University of Birmingham and his Master's in Applied Criminological Psychology from the University of London. His primary research interests are focused on the effective rehabilitation of offenders.

Morgan Fish is a student research assistant at The Ohio State University Department of Family Medicine and a recent graduate of economics from the Fisher College of Business. Morgan has her 200-hour yoga teacher certification and teaches vinyasa yoga. Her primary research interests include the use of yoga and meditation in the treatment and prevention of chronic illness. Morgan is pursuing an MD degree, through which she hopes to apply her research to the treatment of patients.

Lone Fjorback is a leading clinical consultant and senior scientist at the Research Clinic for Functional Disorders and Psychosomatics, Aarhus University Hospital, and director of Danish Center for Mindfulness, Aarhus University *http://mindfulness.au.dk/*. She is a certified MBSR teacher and has run a large RCT on mindfulness and bodily distress syndrome which includes various conditions such as fibromyalgia, chronic fatigue syndrome, and somatization disorder. The trial demonstrated that mindfulness had substantial socioeconomic benefits over the control condition.

W. Kim Halford is a Professor of Clinical Psychology at the University of Queensland in Brisbane, Australia, and a registered clinical psychologist. He earned his doctoral degree from Latrobe University in Melbourne, Australia, in 1979. Previously, he was a Professor of Clinical Psychology at Griffith University (1995–2008) and before that Chief Psychologist of the Royal Brisbane Hospital (1991–1994). Kim has published 6 books and over 170 articles, primarily focused on couple therapy and couple relationship education. He works with clinically distressed couples, couples adjusting to major life challenges, including developing committed relationships, couples struggling with severe physical and mental health problems in a partner; couples becoming parents, couples forming stepfamilies, couples transitioning to retirement, parents negotiating co-parenting after separation, and intercultural couple relationships.

Sean Dae Houlihan is a Ph.D. student at the Massachusetts Institute of Technology in the Department of Brain and Cognitive Sciences and a research associate at the UMass Medical School Center for Mindfulness. His research interests include how meditation interacts with core neural systems of emotion, attention, and decision making. He studies Mahāmudrā, Dzogchen, and Bön practices with Dr. Daniel P. Brown.

Itai Ivtzan is passionate about the combination of psychology and spirituality. He is a positive psychologist, a senior lecturer, and the program leader of MAPP (Masters in Applied Positive Psychology) at the University of East London (UEL). He has published many books, journal papers, and book chapters and his main interests are spirituality, mindfulness, meaning, and self-actualization. For the last 15 years, Dr. Ivtzan has run seminars, lectures, workshops, and retreats, in the UK and around the world, in various educational institutions and at private events while focusing on a variety of psychological and spiritual topics such as positive psychology, psychological and spiritual growth, consciousness, and meditation. If you wish to get additional information about his work or contact him, please visit www.AwarenessIsFreedom.com

Kelli Johnson is a doctoral student at SUNY-Stony Brook. Her research interests are in the field of decision making. She earned her Bachelor of Science degree in Biology from Carroll University. There, she conducted meditation research under the supervision of Dr. Christopher May.

Brendan D. Kelly is an associate clinical professor of psychiatry at University College Dublin and consultant psychiatrist at the Mater Misericordiae University Hospital. In addition to his medical degree (MB BCh BAO), Professor Kelly holds master's degrees in epidemiology (M.Sc.), healthcare management (M.A.), and Buddhist studies (M.A.) and doctorates in medicine (MD), history (Ph.D.), governance (DGov), and law (Ph.D.). Professor Kelly has authored and coauthored over 180 peer-reviewed papers and 300 non-peer-reviewed papers. Recent books include *Custody, Care and Criminality: Forensic Psychiatry and Law in nineteenth-Century Ireland* (History Press Ireland, 2014), *Ada English: Patriot and Psychiatrist* (Irish Academic Press, 2014), *"He Lost Himself Completely": Shell Shock and its Treatment at Dublin's Richmond War Hospital (1916–1919)* (Liffey Press, 2014), and *Dignity, Mental Health and Human Rights: Coercion and the Law* (Ashgate, 2015). He is editor-in-chief of the *Irish Journal of Psychological Medicine.*

Maryanna D. Klatt is an Associate Professor in the College of Medicine at Ohio State University, Department of Family Medicine. Dr. Klatt's research focus has been to develop and evaluate feasible, cost-effective ways to reduce the risk of stress-related chronic illness, for both adults and children. Trained in Mindfulness and a certified yoga instructor through Yoga Alliance, she combines these two approaches in a unique approach to stress prevention/reduction. The environments in which she offers her evidence-based interventions are located where people spend their days—either at the worksite or in the classroom. She serves on the Executive Committee of the Academic Consortium for Integrative Medicine and Health.

Álvaro I. Langer is a clinical psychologist and member of the Psychological Intervention Unit for the treatment of psychosis at RedGesam Clinical Center, in Santiago de Chile. He also holds an adjunct researcher position at the Millennium Institute for Research in Depression and Personality (MIDAP) at Pontifical Catholic University of Chile. He earned a doctoral degree in Functional Analysis in Clinical and Health Contexts from the University of Almeria in Spain and a postdoctoral fellowship funded by the Chilean National Commission for Scientific and Technological Research. Dr. Langer pioneered research on mindfulness in psychosis and in distressing hallucinatory experiences in Spain. His research interests include psychotherapy for psychosis and depression, phenomenology of psychotic symptoms, and the influence of cultural practices on diverse views about mental health.

Tim Lomas is a lecturer at the University of East London, where he is the deputy program leader for the M.Sc. in Applied Positive Psychology. After undertaking an M.A. and M.Sc. in psychology at the University of Edinburgh, Tim completed his Ph.D. at the University of Westminster in 2012. His thesis focused on the impact of meditation on men's mental health and was published in 2014 as a monograph by Palgrave Macmillan. Tim is the lead author on numerous books (published by Sage), including a positive psychology textbook (entitled "Applied Positive Psychology: Integrated Positive Practice"), a six-volume Major Works in Positive Psychology series, and an encyclopedia. Tim has also just received two grants to develop mindfulness-based interventions for specific populations (at-risk youth and older adults).

William R. Marchand is a board-certified psychiatrist, author, and mindfulness teacher. He is the Chief of Psychiatry and Associate Chief of Mental Health at the George E. Wahlen Veterans Affairs Medical Center in Salt Lake City, UT. He is also an Associate Professor of Psychiatry (Clinical) at the University of Utah School of Medicine. His research has focused on using functional neuroimaging to study the neurobiology of mood disorders as well as normal brain function. He is the author of multiple scientific publications as well as two books, *Depression and Bipolar Disorder: Your Guide to Recovery* and *Mindfulness for Bipolar Disorder: How Mindfulness and Neuroscience Can Help You Manage Your Bipolar Symptoms.*

Christopher J. May is an associate professor of Psychology at Carroll University. He also serves as the Interim Director of the Carroll University Honors Center. He earned a doctoral degree in Psychology with an emphasis in biological psychology from the University of California at Davis. His primary research interest concerns individual differences in the cognitive, emotional, and physiological responses of beginning meditators.

Lucia McBee is a Lecturer at the Columbia School of Social Work and mindfulness teacher at the Center for Health and Healing, Mount Sinai Beth Israel, in New York, NY. She received master's degrees in Public Health and Social Work from Columbia University and is a certified yoga instructor. She has worked with elders and their caregivers for over 30 years in community, research, and institutional settings. Since 1994, she has adapted mindfulness practices and programs for frail elders, staff, and family caregivers. She has also taught Mindfulness-Based Stress Reduction to college students, persons with HIV, persons who have been incarcerated, medical students, and the general public. She is currently a freelance author, teacher, and consultant. Her book, *Mindfulness-Based Elder Care: A CAM Model for Frail Elders and Their Caregivers*, was published in 2008.

Donald McCown is an assistant professor of health, director of the minor in contemplative studies, and codirector of the center for contemplative studies at West Chester University of Pennsylvania. He holds a Master of Applied Meditation Studies degree from the Won Institute of Graduate Studies, a Master of Social Service from Bryn Mawr College, and a Ph.D. in Social Science from Tilburg University. His primary research interests include the pedagogy of mindfulness in clinical applications and higher education, applications of complementary and integrative medicine in the community, and the contemplative dimensions of the health humanities. He is the author of *The Ethical Space of Mindfulness in Clinical Practice* and the primary author of *Teaching Mindfulness: A practical guide for clinicians and educators* and *New World Mindfulness: From the Founding Fathers, Emerson, and Thoreau to your personal practice.*

Barbara L. Niles is a Principal Investigator in the Behavioral Science Division of the National Center for PTSD, VA Boston Healthcare System, and an Assistant Professor in the Department of Psychiatry at the Boston University School of Medicine. Dr. Niles is also a licensed psychologist. She earned a doctoral degree in clinical psychology from Rutgers University. Her primary research interests are in the evaluation of complementary and alternative medicine approaches in the treatment of PTSD; examination of health and lifestyle behaviors in individuals with PTSD and stress-related problems; and assessment of telehealth delivery of behavioral treatments.

Analise O'Donovan is a professor and Head of School of Applied Psychology, Griffith University, Australia. Previously, she was Director of the Psychology Clinic and Director of Postgraduate Clinical Training. She earned a doctoral degree with an emphasis on the effectiveness of postgraduate clinical training. Her primary research interests include supervision, positive psychology, mindfulness, emotional regulation, eating disorders, and posttraumatic stress disorder.

Karen Johanne Pallesen is a senior researcher at The Research Clinic for Functional Disorders and Psychosomatics at Aarhus University Hospital, Denmark. She studied biology (M.Sc.) and psychology and received her Ph.D. degree in

Neuroscience from the Faculty of Medicine at Aarhus University in 2008, based on an fMRI study of the interaction between cognitive and emotional processes in the brain. She continued as a postdoctoral researcher at Copenhagen University, where she studied dynamics in neuronal networks related to sound perception. In 2013, she moved into the clinical domain and became involved in stress-related diseases and mindfulness-based stress treatment, a topic on which she gives regular guest lectures at universities and public events. Her current primary interest is designing an experimental protocol to investigate biological and neurophysiological biomarkers in patients suffering from functional disorders and the modulation of these biomarkers by MBSR treatment.

Christopher A. Pepping is a Lecturer in Clinical Psychology at La Trobe University in Melbourne, Australia. Prior to this, he was a lecturer in Clinical Psychology at Griffith University. Chris is a clinical psychologist working primarily with distressed couples, as well as individuals with mood and anxiety disorders. His primary research areas are mindfulness, close relationships and couple therapy, and attachment theory.

Jacob Piet is a researcher, educator, and clinical psychologist at the Danish Center for Mindfulness, Aarhus University Hospital. He is also an MBSR teacher certified by the Center for Mindfulness, University of Massachusetts Medical School. He earned a doctoral degree in Psychology investigating the effect of mindfulness-based stress reduction (MBSR) and mindfulness-based cognitive therapy (MBCT) on stress, anxiety, and depression. He has published several clinical trials and meta-analyses in the field of mindfulness-based interventions.

Jeffrey B. Rubin practices psychoanalysis and psychoanalytically oriented psychotherapy and teaches meditation in New York City and Bedford Hills, New York. He is considered one of the leading integrators of the Western psychotherapeutic and Eastern meditative traditions. A Sensei in the Nyogen Senzaki and Soen Nakagawa Rinzai Zen lineage and the creator of meditative psychotherapy, a practice that he developed through insights gained from decades of study, teaching, and trying to helping people flourish, Jeffrey is the author of two ebooks, Meditative Psychotherapy and Practicing Meditative Psychotherapy, and the critically acclaimed books "The Art of Flourishing," "Psychotherapy and Buddhism," "The Good Life," and "A Psychoanalysis for Our Time." Dr. Rubin has taught at various universities, psychoanalytic institutes, and Buddhist and yoga centers. He lectures around the country and has given workshops at the United Nations, the Esalen Institute, the Open Center, and the 92nd Street Y. A blogger for Huffington Post, Psychology Today, Rewireme, and Elephant Journal, his pioneering approach to psychotherapy and Buddhism has been featured in The New York Times Magazine. His website is drjeffreyrubin.com

Saki Santorelli is a Professor of Medicine, Director of the acclaimed Mindfulness-Based Stress Reduction Clinic (MBSR) and, since 2000, Executive Director of the Center for Mindfulness in Medicine, Health Care, and Society (CFM) at the University of Massachusetts Medical School. During his 32 years at the CFM, he has worked with thousands of medical patients and mentored generations of clinicians and researchers. He is the author of *Heal Thy Self: Lessons on Mindfulness in Medicine.* In 2001, he envisioned and founded *Oasis Institute*—the CFM's school of professional education and training, serving more than 14,000 healthcare professionals from 80 countries and six continents. Between 2003 and 2014, he founded and Chaired an annual scientific meeting on mindfulness and, more recently, established *INDRA-M,* the first international database registry for MBSR, and *CommonGood*—the CFM's affiliate network focused on sustaining the integrity and fidelity of MBSR. Saki teaches and presents internationally.

Jon Vøllestad is a clinical psychologist at Solli District Psychiatric Centre at Nesttun, Norway, and associate professor II at the Department of Clinical Psychology at the University of Bergen. He has a Ph.D. from the University of Bergen on the subject of mindfulness in the treatment of anxiety disorders. Dr. Vøllestad is trained in mindfulness-based stress reduction and mindfulness-based cognitive therapy and uses both these approaches in his clinical work. His primary research interests include the application of mindfulness to anxiety and depression, as well as mentalization-based therapy for personality disorders.

Anka A. Vujanovic is an Assistant Professor in the Department of Psychiatry and Behavioral Sciences at the University of Texas Health Science Center at Houston. Dr. Vujanovic is also a licensed psychologist and the Director of Psychology Services at the University of Texas—Harris County Psychiatric Center. She earned a doctoral degree in clinical psychology from the University of Vermont. Her primary research interest is focused on better understanding biopsychosocial mechanisms underlying the co-occurrence of posttraumatic stress and substance use disorders, with the ultimate goal of developing more effective, evidence-based treatment programs. Her secondary, interrelated interest is rooted in examining etiological and maintenance processes pertinent to psychopathology among trauma-exposed populations and advancing research-driven early intervention programs.

Emaline Wise is a student research assistant at the Ohio State University. Ms. Wise earned her Bachelor's Degree in Biomedical Science from Ohio State with a minor in Integrative Approaches to Health and Wellness. Her research with Dr. Maryanna Klatt, Ph.D., is focused on mindfulness meditation and its usefulness as part of an intervention for worksite wellness and increasing resilience in cancer survivors.

Koa Whittingham is an NHMRC postdoctoral research fellow at the Queensland Cerebral Play and Rehabilitation Research Centre, The University of Queensland, and a psychologist with specializations in clinical and developmental psychology. Koa is cofounder and codirector of Possums Education, a wing of the not-for-profit organization Possums for Mothers and Babies, focused on evidenced-based health professional training in postpartum care. She is also the author of *Becoming Mum* (www.becomingmum.com.au), a self-help book for the transition to motherhood grounded in Acceptance and Commitment Therapy. Koa's research spans three key interests: parenting, neurodevelopmental disabilities, and mindfulness-based psychological therapies, particularly Acceptance and Commitment Therapy. She writes for professionals and parents about parenting-related topics in her blog *Parenting from the Heart* (www.koawhittingham.com/blog/).

Jared R. Weyker received his Bachelor of Science degree in Psychology from Carroll University. He conducted research on the effects of meditation practice under Dr. Christopher May.

Chapter 1
Mindfulness and Buddhist-Derived Treatment Techniques in Mental Health and Addiction Settings

Edo Shonin, William Van Gordon, and Mark D. Griffiths

Introduction

Mindfulness is a 2500-year-old Buddhist practice and is a fundamental part of the Buddhist path to spiritual awakening. The most popular definition of mindfulness in the mental health literature is the practice of *paying attention in a particular way: on purpose, in the present moment, and non-judgmentally* (Kabat-Zinn, 1994: p. 4). Other definitions employed in the clinical literature describe mindfulness as *the process of engaging a full, direct, and active awareness of experienced phenomena that is: (i) spiritual in aspect, and (ii) maintained from one moment to the next* (Shonin & Van Gordon, 2015: p. 900).

Until a few decades ago, there was limited public and scientific interest in the West concerning the properties, correlates and applications of mindfulness. However, mindfulness is now arguably one of the fastest growing areas of mental health research. It is difficult to pinpoint precisely why mindfulness and related Buddhist practices are growing in popularity in Western clinical settings, but some possible explanations are the need to (1) find alternatives to pharmacological treatments, (2) augment the efficacy of psychopathology treatments, and (3) offer culturally syntonic treatments to service users from increasingly diverse cultural and

E. Shonin (✉) • W. Van Gordon
Awake to Wisdom, Centre for Meditation and Mindfulness Research, Nottingham, UK

Bodhayati School of Buddhism, Nottingham, UK

Division of Psychology, Chaucer Building, Nottingham Trent University, Burton Street, Nottingham, UK
e-mail: e.shonin@awaketowisdom.co.uk

M.D. Griffiths
Division of Psychology, Chaucer Building, Nottingham Trent University, Burton Street, Nottingham, UK

E. Shonin et al. (eds.), *Mindfulness and Buddhist-Derived Approaches in Mental Health and Addiction*, Advances in Mental Health and Addiction,
DOI 10.1007/978-3-319-22255-4_1

religious backgrounds. Other factors likely to have asserted an influential role are the steady influx to the West of Buddhist teachers from the East, and what could be considered the growing acceptance in Western culture that responsibility for psycho-spiritual wellbeing rests with the individual rather than an external entity or divine being. A slightly less eloquent (albeit plausible) explanation is that the current mindfulness trend has arisen for no reason other than the fact that popularity tends to foster popularity and that researching, practising or administering mindfulness approaches is—at least for the time being—a fashionable undertaking.

In terms of its psychotherapeutic applications, emerging evidence suggests that mindfulness-based interventions (MBIs) have applications for treating diverse psychopathologies and mental health disorders including mood disorders, anxiety disorders, substance use disorders, gambling disorder, post-traumatic stress disorder, eating disorders, attention-deficit hyperactivity disorder and schizophrenia (Arias, Steinberg, Banga, & Trestman, 2006; Edenfield & Saeed, 2012; Shonin, Van Gordon, & Griffiths, 2014). Mindfulness currently features—with differing degrees of emphasis—in the treatment guidelines of the *American Psychiatric Association* [APA], the UK's *National Institute for Health and Care Excellence* [NICE] and the *Royal Australian and New Zealand College of Psychiatrists* [RANZCP] for the treatment in adults of either recurrent depression [APA and NICE] or binge-eating disorder [RANZCP] (Van Gordon, Shonin, & Griffiths, 2015a).

Since mindfulness was first introduced into research and clinical settings approximately 30 years ago, a significant number of MBIs have been formulated and empirically evaluated. These range from MBIs intended to target a specific psychopathology (e.g. mindfulness-based relapse prevention for the treatment of substance addiction) to MBIs that appear to have broader applications (e.g. mindfulness-based stress reduction). A further development in mindfulness research and practice has been the introduction in recent years of a second wave of MBI (Singh, Lancioni, Winton, Karazsia, & Singh, 2014). First-generation MBIs refer to interventions such as mindfulness-based stress reduction and mindfulness-based cognitive therapy (Shonin & Van Gordon, 2015). First-generation and second-generation MBIs are both invariably tailored for utilisation in Western clinical settings (e.g. they are generally secular in nature). However, relative to the first generation of MBIs, second-generation MBIs (such as meditation awareness training) tend to be more overtly spiritual in nature, and often teach mindfulness in conjunction with other meditative practices and principles (e.g. ethical awareness, impermanence, emptiness/nonself, loving-kindness and compassion meditation, etc.) that are traditionally deemed to promote effective mindfulness practice (Van Gordon, Shonin, Griffiths, & Singh, 2015b).

The recent development and empirical evaluation of second-generation mindfulness approaches has arguably arisen due to the fact that there has not always been complete agreement amongst researchers and clinicians as to (1) exactly what defines mindfulness and (2) what constitutes effective mindfulness practice (e.g. Chiesa, 2013; Rosch, 2007). Indeed, it is not uncommon for academic papers concerning mindfulness to include a statement to the effect that *there is currently a lack of consensus amongst Western psychologists in terms of how to define mindfulness*. However, it is our personal view that too much emphasis is placed by academicians on attempting to devise and disseminate an "absolute" or "all-encompassing" definition of mindfulness. This is not to say that certain aspects of Western psychological definitions of mindfulness would not benefit from additional clarification, but this should not detract from the important contribution that mindfulness research has made not only in terms of introducing a novel and cost-effective approach to treating mental illness, but to advancing understanding of the human mind more generally.

In addition to mindfulness, other Buddhist-derived interventions (BDIs) have recently been introduced into research and clinical settings. Some of the most widely researched and publicised techniques include loving-kindness meditation, compassion meditation (including self-compassion meditation) and meditation on emptiness and nonself. Based upon emerging findings, it appears that such techniques have an important role to play in the treatment of mental illness (including addiction). However, in much the same way that there have been calls to replicate and consolidate outcomes from studies of MBIs, further research is required in order to evaluate the full clinical utility of these additional Buddhist techniques.

The present volume on *Mindfulness and Buddhist-Derived Approaches in Mental Health and Addiction* includes contributions from some of the world's leading experts in mindfulness research and practice. It provides a timely synthesis and discussion of recent developments in the research and clinical integration of mindfulness. The role of other Buddhist-derived interventions that are gaining momentum in mental health and addiction is also discussed.

Part One

Part One focusses on the effective use of mindfulness and derivative Buddhist techniques during both the diagnostic and treatment phases of clinician–patient engagement. In the opening chapter of Part One (Chap. 2), Brendan Kelly examines how core Buddhist teachings can inform more skilful engagement with psychiatric classification systems such as the *Diagnostic and Statistical Manual of Mental Disorders* and *ICD-10 Classification of Mental and Behavioural Disorders*. This is followed by an exploration in Chap. 3 by Don McCown of the relational dimensions that underlie the activities of teaching and learning mindfulness. The chapter describes four basic skill sets for teaching mindfulness: (1) stewardship of the group, (2) guidance of meditation, (3) sharing of didactic information (e.g. psycho-education) and (4) enquiry into participants' direct experience in the present moment.

In Chap. 4, Jacob Piet, Lone Fjorback and Saki Santorelli focus on mindfulness-based stress reduction and mindfulness-based cognitive therapy and present a framework for the effective teaching of mindfulness within these interventional approaches. In the final chapter of Part One (Chap. 5), Christopher May, Kelli Johnson and Jared Weyker demonstrate that mindfulness meditation and loving-kindness meditation have differential effects within and between individuals. They emphasise a greater need for single-subject experimental designs and discuss how the idiopathic approach of the clinician can help to advance the science of meditation.

Part Two

Following a discussion in Part One concerning the key considerations for using mindfulness and derivative Buddhist approaches in clinician–patient practice, Part Two draws upon key empirical findings and undertakes an in-depth discussion of the role of mindfulness both in the treatment of specific psychopathologies and for promoting psychological wellbeing more generally. In the opening chapter of Part Two (Chap. 6), Jon Vøllestad provides a comprehensive review of studies of mindfulness- and acceptance-based interventions for the treatment of anxiety disorders. He concludes that although cognitive behavioural therapy (CBT) is still the treatment of choice for most anxiety disorders, mindfulness approaches constitute a viable treatment option for CBT nonresponders and may also be preferred by some patients.

In Chap. 7, William Marchand reviews evidence supporting the use of mindfulness for the treatment of depressive spectrum disorders. Based on empirical studies, he suggests that mindfulness may impact depressive symptoms by facilitating disengagement from ruminative self-referential thinking. In Chap. 8, Karen Johanne Pallesen, Jesper Dahlgaard and Lone Fjorback give an account of the stress response (*allostasis*) and discuss findings from recent research examining the damaging effects of long-term stress (*allostatic load*). They then discuss how mindfulness can be used to mediate neuroplastic changes that have the potential to reverse some of the harmful effects of chronic stress.

In Chap. 9, Sean Dae Houlihan and Judson Brewer focus on mindfulness for the treatment of addictions. They describe the overlap and similarities between early Buddhist and contemporary scientific models of the addictive process, review studies of mindfulness training for addictions (including discussion of their mechanistic effects on the relationship between craving and behaviour), and then discuss findings from recent neuroimaging studies that help to inform understanding of the neural mechanisms underlying mindfulness.

In Chap. 10, following an appraisal of both the quantitative and qualitative literature, Álvaro Langer, José Carmona-Torres, William Van Gordon and Edo Shonin examine the role of mindfulness in the treatment of psychosis. They conclude that whilst findings point towards improvements in quality of life along with reduced intensity and frequency of psychotic episodes, further high-quality empirical enquiry is required.

In Chap. 11, Anka Vujanovic, Barbara Niles and Jocelyn Abrams discuss the relevance of mindfulness-based approaches to the aetiology, maintenance and treatment of post-traumatic stress disorder (PTSD). They conclude that mindfulness may serve as an effective stand-alone or adjunctive treatment for PTSD, or as an effective preventive or early-intervention approach. This chapter is complemented by Chap. 12, in which Joanne Cacciatore and Jeffrey Rubin present three case study examples and propose a model for mindfulness-based bereavement care.

In Chap. 13, Christopher Pepping, Penelope Davis and Analise O'Donovan veer away from the use of mindfulness for the treatment of mental health issues and focus on the role of mindfulness in cultivating self-esteem. This is complemented by

Chap. 14 in which Tim Lomas and Itai Ivtzan examine how in recent years, the field of positive psychology has been at the forefront of efforts to create mindfulness-based interventions that foster wellbeing and flourishing, and that capture more of the missing spirit of the original Buddhist meditational teachings.

Part Three

Part Three explores the emerging use of mindfulness in other remits of applied psychology. In the opening chapter of Part Three (Chap. 15), Andrew Day considers the role of mindfulness-based approaches in the delivery of forensic mental health services. He argues that whilst mindfulness is likely to have beneficial effects on mental health and wellbeing, it also has an important role to play in the management of risk—particularly in reducing the risk of violence.

Chapter 16 examines the utility of mindfulness for promoting work-related wellbeing. Here, Maryanna Klatt, Emaline Wise and Morgan Fish refer to the various physiological and psychological benefits elicited by mindfulness across a diverse range of professions (e.g. nurses, physicians, police, firefighters, teachers, lawyers, etc.). They discuss how mindfulness may be a cost-effective intervention for organisations wishing to promote mental health and wellbeing at work. In Chap. 17, Lucia McBee and Patricia Bloom explore the applications of mindfulness for elders and their caregivers. They conclude that mindfulness holds promise for preventing the major ailments facing elders and caregivers, and for improving quality of life amongst these two groups.

In Chap. 18, Koa Whittingham focusses on the applications of mindfulness to parenting. She reviews the relevant literature and concludes that mindfulness-based interventions may improve antenatal and postnatal outcomes, decrease parental stress, improve parental wellbeing and foster better parent–child interactions. Finally, in Chap. 19, Christopher Pepping and Kim Halford provide an assessment of the benefits of mindfulness in cultivating healthy couple relationships. The chapter also appraises the relevant literature and examines potential mechanisms in terms of how mindfulness can alleviate couple relationship distress.

Conclusions

The current volume provides what we believe to be a comprehensive overview of recent developments in the research and practice of both mindfulness and related Buddhist-derived approaches within mental health contexts. We hope that the book will serve as a valuable resource for researchers and mental health practitioners wishing to keep up to date with developments in mindfulness clinical research, as well as any professional wishing to equip themselves with the necessary theoretical and practical tools to effectively teach or utilise mindfulness in mental health and addiction settings.

References

Arias, A. J., Steinberg, K., Banga, A., & Trestman, R. L. (2006). Systematic review of the efficacy of meditation techniques as treatments for medical illness. *Journal of Alternative and Complementary Medicine, 12*, 817–832.

Chiesa, A. (2013). The difficulty of defining mindfulness: Current thought and critical issues. *Mindfulness, 4*, 255–268.

Edenfield, T. M., & Saeed, S. A. (2012). An update on mindfulness meditation as a self-help treatment for anxiety and depression. *Psychology Research and Behaviour Management, 5*, 131–141.

Kabat-Zinn, J. (1994). *Wherever you go, there you are: Mindfulness meditation in everyday life*. New York: Hyperion.

Rosch, E. (2007). More than mindfulness: When you have a tiger by the tail, let it eat you. *Psychological Inquiry, 18*, 258–264.

Shonin, E., & Van Gordon, W. (2015). Managers' experiences of Meditation Awareness Training. *Mindfulness, 4*, 899–909. doi:10.1007/s12671-014-0334-y.

Shonin, E., Van Gordon, W., & Griffiths, M. D. (2014). The emerging role of Buddhism in clinical psychology: Toward effective integration. *Psychology of Religion and Spirituality, 6*, 123–137.

Singh, N. N., Lancioni, G. E., Winton, A. S. W., Karazsia, B. T., & Singh, J. (2014). Mindfulness-based positive behavior support (MBPBS) for mothers of adolescents with autism spectrum disorders: Effects on adolescents' behavior and parental stress. *Mindfulness*. doi:10.1007/s12671-014-0321-3.

Van Gordon, W., Shonin, E., Griffiths, M. D., & Singh, N. N. (2015a). There is only one mindfulness: Why science and Buddhism need to work together. *Mindfulness, 6*, 49–56.

Van Gordon, W., Shonin, E., & Griffiths, M. D. (2015b). Towards a second-generation of mindfulness-based interventions. *Australia and New Zealand Journal of Psychiatry, 49*, 591–591. doi:10.1177/0004867415577437.

Part I
Mindfulness in Clinician–Patient Settings

Chapter 2
Compassion, Cognition and the Illusion of Self: Buddhist Notes Towards More Skilful Engagement with Diagnostic Classification Systems in Psychiatry

Brendan D. Kelly

Introduction

Diagnoses in psychiatry are primarily based on elucidation of symptoms rather than detection of biological parameters that differ from biological norms (Burns, 2013). As a result, formal diagnostic classification systems, based on identifying clusters of symptoms which commonly co-occur, assume greater importance in psychiatry than in other areas of medicine in which diagnostic suspicions can be confirmed through the use of laboratory tests or imaging techniques. This situation poses both challenges and opportunities for psychiatry, and this chapter focuses on specific ways in which to navigate this complex, important and often controversial area of practice.

At present, there are two dominant classification systems in psychiatry. The system most commonly used in the USA is the *Diagnostic and Statistical Manual of Mental Disorders* (DSM) of the American Psychiatric Association (APA), first published in 1952 (APA, 1952) and now in its fifth edition, DSM-5 (APA, 2013). In Europe, the classification system most commonly used is the *ICD-10 Classification of Mental and Behavioural Disorders: Clinical Descriptions and Diagnostic Guidelines* (World Health Organization [WHO], 1992), which is similar to the DSM in format, but differs in its definitions of various mental illnesses.

Media interest in these classification systems, especially the DSM, which has greater global reach, is phenomenal (Cloud, 2012). In addition to this public attention, DSM also generates controversy within medicine and psychiatry, as each new edition brings further changes to diagnostic practices, introduces apparently 'new' mental illnesses and unleashes a fresh wave of controversy and soul-searching

B.D. Kelly (✉)
Department of Adult Psychiatry, University College Dublin, 62/63 Eccles Street, Dublin 7, Ireland
e-mail: brendankelly35@gmail.com

E. Shonin et al. (eds.), *Mindfulness and Buddhist-Derived Approaches in Mental Health and Addiction*, Advances in Mental Health and Addiction,
DOI 10.1007/978-3-319-22255-4_2

(Angell, 2011; Bentall, 2003, 2009; Davies, 2013; Frances, 2013; Frances & Nardo, 2013; Greenberg, 2010; Horowitz, 2002; Leader, 2010, 2011; Menand, 2010).

The aim of the present chapter is to explore these classification systems and the controversies they generate from a Buddhist perspective and identify ways in which DSM and ICD can be used more skilfully if their use is informed by Buddhist teachings about 'dependent arising' and 'nonself', compassion and cognition.

This chapter is divided into four sections. 'Diagnostic Classification Systems in Psychiatry' examines the fundamental nature of psychiatric classification systems, their advantages and disadvantages, their interpretation and use. 'Buddhist Teachings About Nonself' examines Buddhist teachings about dependent arising and nonself and how these can inform more skilful and enlightened engagement with psychiatric classification systems. 'Other Buddhist Teachings: Cognition and Compassion' examines other relevant Buddhist teachings, chiefly relating to cognition and compassion, and how these can further assist with fruitful interpretation and use of DSM and ICD. Finally, 'Conclusions: You Cannot Diagnose the Same Mental Illness Twice' presents relevant conclusions.

Diagnostic Classification Systems in Psychiatry

Classification Systems: DSM and ICD

The presence of two dominant systems of psychiatric diagnosis, DSM in the USA and ICD in Europe, generates significant controversy within psychiatry and beyond (Bentall, 2009; Frances & Nardo, 2013). However, given psychiatry's reliance on symptoms rather than demonstrated biological anomalies for diagnosis, it is perhaps surprising that there are *only* two well-developed classification systems with significant global reach. Given the infinite variety of human experience and psychological states, one might expect a far greater number of well-developed diagnostic systems, reflecting myriad different cultures and belief systems around the globe. Nonetheless, it remains the case that, for better or worse, DSM and ICD dominate the field.

Both DSM and ICD rely on lists of symptoms which need to be present to a specified degree of severity for a specified period of time in order for a given diagnosis to be made. For example, a DSM-5 diagnosis of major depressive disorder requires the presence of five or more out of nine key symptoms, for more than 2 weeks, and this must represent a change from previous functioning (APA, 2013). The nine key symptoms are:

- Generally depressed mood
- Reduced pleasure or interest
- Significant weight change (loss or gain)
- Insomnia or hypersomnia almost every day
- Psychomotor agitation or retardation almost every day

- Loss of energy or fatigue almost every day
- Feelings of guilt or worthlessness
- Reduced concentration or decisiveness
- Recurring thoughts of death, self-harm or suicide or related acts

For a DSM-5 diagnosis of major depressive disorder, at least one of the five symptoms must be either generally depressed mood or reduced pleasure or interest; symptoms must cause significant distress or impairment in functioning; symptoms must not be attributable to a substance, medical condition or other mental illness; and there must have never been an episode of mania or hypomania, which would suggest a diagnosis of bipolar affective disorder rather than major depressive disorder.

Criticisms and Controversy

DSM and ICD go on to define a wide array of mental illnesses and psychological states in this list-based fashion with the result that, ever since this practice commenced, it has generated a steady stream of criticism and controversy. These criticisms and controversies fall into two main categories: criticism of the very idea of psychiatric classification as it is currently conceptualised and practiced, and detailed criticisms relating to the expansion and redefinition of specific diagnostic categories in various iterations of the DSM and ICD.

The first area of contention is the very idea that psychiatric classification as it is currently conceptualised and practiced represents a reasonable medical, psychiatric and psychological endeavour in the first instance (Leader, 2010; Lynch, 2001; Watters, 2010). Given the apparently reductive nature of this enterprise, it seems entirely reasonable to ask: What is the precise purpose of these psychiatric classification systems? Should they exist at all? Do they not reduce complex, changeable human states to lists of symptoms and diagnostic codes, removing the humanity, complexity and beauty of each individual and replacing them with cold, impersonal categorisation? Are they simply tools for the invention of new mental illnesses, marketing of new pharmaceutical products and generation of revenue for healthcare providers? What do these categories *mean?*

There are several reasons why psychiatric classification systems need to exist. First, every year, hundreds of thousands of people around the world develop mental states that are sufficiently unpleasant, disturbing or worrying that they appear to exceed the capacity of the individual and those immediately around them (Kessler & Üstün, 2008). When such individuals present to psychological or mental health services, it is necessary for mental health professionals to have some guide as to which kinds of psychological or psychiatric treatments will work best to address the problems represented by the constellation of symptoms with which each individual presents (Barr Taylor, 2010). Classification is necessary in order to perform studies and clinical trials to inform such an evidence based and provide responsible, effective care (Craddock & Mynors-Wallis, 2014).

For example, evidence from 41 studies involving a total of 1806 children and adolescents who fulfilled DSM or ICD criteria for anxiety disorders showed that cognitive behavioural therapy (CBT) is an effective treatment for children and adolescents with this particular collection of symptoms (James, James, Cowdrey, Soler, & Choke, 2013). In order to generate this evidence based, it was necessary to test CBT on children and adolescents with defined sets of symptoms, rather than children and adolescents arbitrarily selected from the general population. In other words, diagnosis is necessary in order to identify evidence-based treatments that are proven to help with specific problems and avoid well-meaning but unproven interventions that may do more harm than good.

It is, of course, imperative that the identification of recurring states of psychological distress (later codified as 'new' mental illnesses) drives the search for new treatments, rather than having the requirements of pharmaceutical companies (Angell, 2011; Healy, 2002; Horowitz, 2002) or healthcare funders (Carlat, 2010; Leader, 2011) drive the creation of new mental illnesses or, indeed, shape information about the effectiveness of, and indications for, specific treatments (Davies, 2013; Whitaker, 2002). The DSM and ICD processes present the best possibility for protections in this regard: robust revision processes for these classification systems have the potential to defend against cynical manipulation by vested interests and create opportunity for open, ethical engagement of all stakeholders, including patients, families, carers, mental health professionals, voluntary agencies, healthcare providers and governmental bodies, in this process.

Second, a similar argument applies to efforts to discover the aetiology or underpinnings of various psychological states or mental illnesses. There is, for example, strong evidence that individuals are more likely to develop the constellation of symptoms that ICD and DSM call 'schizophrenia' if they have a first degree relative with that same constellation of symptoms (Van Os & Kapur, 2009). Indeed, heritability estimates for schizophrenia are around 80 % (compared with 60 % for osteoarthritis of the hip and 30–50 % for hypertension) which reflects a substantial body of evidence for a relatively unified biological process contributing to 'schizophrenia'. While specific genes have yet to be identified for certain mental illnesses, diagnostic practices have greatly facilitated steps towards better understandings of biological elements of the aetiology of many such illnesses, including schizophrenia. The same applies to the non-biological determinants of mental illnesses and states of psychological distress (e.g. psychological stressors, social environments, upbringing, etc.).

Third, there are compelling human rights reasons for establishing clear criteria for psychiatric diagnoses, chiefly because involuntary admission and treatment have been long-standing features of the management of severe mental illness (Porter, 2002). Such mental health laws affect only a small minority of individuals: most individuals with mental illness are treated in primary care by family doctors (i.e. entirely voluntarily); among the minority referred to secondary (i.e. hospital-based) care, most are treated as outpatients rather than inpatients (again, voluntarily); and, finally, among those admitted to inpatient care, the vast majority are treated on a voluntary basis, and only a small minority ever require involuntary admission or treatment (Ng & Kelly, 2012). Nonetheless, for the tiny minority who become subject to involuntary treatment, there is a strong need for as much clarity as possible in diagnosis, in order to ensure appropriate treatment and accountability. In this context, clinically based classification systems are vital in protecting individuals from being labelled mentally ill for purposes of political or societal convenience (Clare, 1976).

Today, this argument is as relevant as ever: despite the clear limitations to classification systems such as the DSM and ICD, it is still apparent that transparent diagnostic systems are crucial in protecting human rights. If these systems had been introduced and implemented in an open, accountable fashion in the past, they held the potential to help protect against the alleged labelling of political dissidents as mentally ill in the former Soviet Union in the 1970s and 1980s (Bloch & Reddaway, 1984). Today, these classification systems, once used correctly and with an awareness of their limitations, hold similar potential in parts of the world where psychiatric diagnosis may still be used for political rather than therapeutic purposes (Munro, 2006). Other potential benefits include reducing stigma, alleviating blame or guilt that individuals or families may feel, guiding patients in choosing treatments and assisting with the construction of networks of individuals or families affected by similar symptoms (Craddock & Mynors-Wallis, 2014).

Expansion and Redefinition of Diagnostic Categories

The second area of common criticism of DSM and ICD relates to the expansion and redefinition of specific diagnostic categories in various iterations of the DSM or ICD. This is a vital and important area of debate (Batstra & Frances, 2012; Burns, 2013; Sommers & Satel, 2005). Over the past six decades, myriad critics and commentators have expressed concern and alarm at the expansion of diagnostic categories and, especially, the apparent medicalisation of parts of everyday life which were not hitherto considered to be disordered psychological states or mental illnesses, such as grief (Davies, 2013; Kramer, 1994).

Psychiatry is, of course, by no means unique in this regard, as thresholds for diagnosis and treatment are falling in all areas of medicine, not just mental health (Burns, 2013). Nonetheless, the issue appears especially acute in psychiatry (Frances, 2013). Most recently, DSM-5 generated significant and predictable controversy with some of its categorisations and reclassifications, including a compelling argument that the reconceptualised DSM-5 diagnosis of 'somatic symptom disorder' may now mislabel medical illness as mental disorder (Frances & Chapman, 2013). This kind of debate, far from striking at the heart of the DSM or ICD processes, is, in fact, a vital part of those processes. These kinds of arguments, once articulated clearly and presented with supporting evidence, can and should influence the next revisions of DSM and ICD and thus help generate a more reflexive, responsive and responsible classification process. Therefore, far from threatening the psychiatric classification process, these kinds of discussions are essential components of it.

These two areas of criticism and debate—relating to the idea of psychiatric classification as it is presently conceptualised and practiced, and questioning the validity of specific categories within DSM and ICD—reflect a high degree of public and professional engagement with psychiatric classification systems. These debates, however, also commonly reveal a great deal of misunderstanding about the precise role of diagnostic systems and how they might best be used in clinical practice. In other words, despite the apparent merits of DSM and ICD, some commentators argue that the ways in which they are sometimes used in clinical practice render them little more than inflexible lists (Carlat, 2010) that dehumanise the individual experience of mental illness and undermine valuable psychological, philosophical, cultural and political interpretations of suffering.

This is a central concern of the present chapter. Must the manner in which DSM and ICD are used really deny the individualised meanings that are often reflected, symbolised and distilled in complex states of psychological distress? How can we better understand and engage with these elaborate diagnostic systems so as to use the knowledge and experience embedded within them while retaining and deepening the unique interpersonal values that the therapeutic encounter demands, merits and (at its best) reflects? In the next section of this chapter, I argue that Buddhist teachings about 'dependent arising' and 'nonself' offer a deeply valuable perspective on these questions.

Buddhist Teachings About 'Nonself'

What Does 'Nonself' Mean?

The word 'Buddhism' refers to a collection of philosophical, psychological and cultural traditions, all of which find their roots in the original story of Buddha (Gethin, 1998). According to traditional accounts, Siddhartha Gautama was born in north-east India around 566 BC and, having become dissatisfied with his life of privilege, left home to become a wandering ascetic. After several years, he sat to meditate beneath a sacred Bodhi tree at Isipatana and achieved enlightenment, becoming a 'Buddha', or awakened one, who saw the nature of reality as it really is.

Buddha spent much of the rest of his life teaching about the 'four noble truths' which are *dukkha* (suffering, unsatisfactoriness or unease, which is everywhere), the causes of *dukkha* (craving, hatred and delusion, which are also everywhere), the cessation of suffering (by overcoming craving, hatred and delusion, one can achieve the cessation of suffering) and precisely how to overcome *dukkha*, by following the 'eightfold path', based on the principles of wisdom, moral virtue and meditation. The eightfold path involves right view (i.e. seeing things as they really are), right resolve, right speech, right action, right livelihood, right effort, right mindfulness and right concentration (e.g. meditation) (Das, 1997; Gethin, 1998, 2001).

According to this paradigm, the word 'right' means insightful or skilful (a term common in Buddhist teaching) and refers to well-motivated and clear-sighted thought and behaviour, free of craving, hatred and delusion. As a result of these teachings, Buddhism is at once a philosophy, a psychology and an ethics (Bodhi, 1999), i.e. it provides a specific system of beliefs about reality (philosophy), a theory of the human mind and behaviour (psychology) and recommendations for appropriate conduct (ethics) (Kelly, 2008a).

'Dependent arising' is another central concept in Buddhism and refers to the idea that phenomena arise, abide and pass away because of specific causes and conditions (Powers, 2000). Since phenomena are entirely dependent on these causes and conditions for their arising, endurance and cessation, such phenomena are without essence or underlying substance in and of themselves: they are empty. These phenomena include the self, which is also without substance, permanence or independent existence. In other words, for every phenomenon (including the self) there is a collection of causes and conditions which give rise to it, and all of these causes, conditions and phenomena (including the self) are in a state of continuous change (Bodhi, 1999). There is, therefore, no fixed or identifiable self, only the passing, changing impression of one.

Given that perceived and experienced phenomena are devoid of substantive or enduring reality, what, then, is going on around us? How is it that I feel like the same person from moment to moment, from day to day? To explain why transitory phenomena devoid of substance come to appear so concrete, Buddhism refers to the five 'aggregates' (Pāli, *khandhas*; Sanskrit, *skandhas*) which construct the apparent reality that surrounds us. These are (a) form (Pāli/Sanskrit: *rūpa*) which we perceive with our bodily senses; (b) feelings (Pāli/Sanskrit: *vedanā*) produced by these perceptions; (c) recognition and classification of experiences (Pāli, *saññā*; Sanskrit, *saĐjñā*); (d) volitional forces or formations (Pāli, *saĐkhāra*; Sanskrit, *saĐskāra*) provoked by experiences, such as wishes or desires; and (e) conscious self-awareness (Pāli, *viññāṇa*; Sanskrit, *vijñāna*) (Epstein, 2001; Gethin, 1998). This process is conceptualised as a circular one which results in the erroneous consolidation of self-image and conviction of self (Brazier, 2003).

Various combinations of these five aggregates are responsible for all aspects of apparent reality, including the self. In Buddhism, then, the self is merely a conceptual construct reflecting a constantly changing collection of aggregates and is otherwise without substance (Gethin, 2001; Powers, 2000). Each 'self' is simply a bundle of these aggregates, and while it remains operationally convenient to label a given bundle 'Helen' or 'John' or 'Peter', it is a mistake to ascribe permanence, substance or too much reality to such constructs (Williams & Tribe, 2000). This is the essence of the Buddhist teaching of 'nonself' (Pāli, *anattā*; Sanskrit, *anātman)*: not that individual human beings do not exist (Brazier, 2003; Midgley, 2014), but rather that the 'selves' we perceive are without permanence or substance and are so utterly dependent on surrounding causes and conditions that they are devoid of lasting substance or reality in themselves.

This teaching of nonself is the subject of constant discussion in various traditions and schools of Buddhism, with some conceptualising it as an absence of inherent existence rather than literal non-existence of a self (Thanissaro, 2014; Williams, 1989, 2009). Regardless of how it is conceptualised, however, the importance of the teaching is that, if brought to its logical conclusion, the idea of nonself assists with the cessation of suffering (*dukkha*) by fatally undermining the reasons for craving and delusion, which are root causes of *dukkha* (Williams & Tribe, 2000); i.e. if we shed the delusion that everyday phenomena possess significant or lasting substance, then why crave them? If we accept the impermanence and instability of all phenomena, shouldn't this end our futile, self-defeating search for acquisition and permanence? Moreover, if we accept the teaching of nonself, there isn't even a permanent self to do the craving or searching for permanence in the first instance.

These are profound and challenging perspectives on the world, rooted in ancient Buddhist tradition. What implications, if any, do these ideas hold for contemporary psychiatric classification systems?

Nonself and Psychiatric Classification Systems

The Buddhist teaching of nonself has attracted significant interest in the Western world (Gethin, 2001) not least in the fields of social justice (Cho, 2000; Ward, 2013) and psychotherapy (Epstein, 2001, 2007) and, to a lesser extent, science (Lopez, 2008). Can the teaching of nonself assist with the skilful use of DSM and ICD?

In the first instance, the teaching of nonself points to the fact that the apparent self is in a state of constant change, so any detailed descriptions of the apparent self or its associated phenomena (such as symptoms of mental illness) are likely to prove transitory at best. According to the Buddhist paradigm, the individual is in such a state of continual change that he or she exists solely as a collection of aggregates that form the *pattern* of a human being, and, while a certain connectedness maintains apparent identity over time, change is the only constant, not least because the human body is constantly replacing itself, cell by cell (Gethin, 1998). This is a salutary thought when seeking to characterise the precise features of mental illness in any given individual at any given point in time: if the person himself or herself is in a constant state of change, is it not likely that the mental illness will also constantly change in form and character, rendering it more or less impossible to characterise in detail at any given point in time, let alone over a period of time?

Notwithstanding this constant change—or, possibly, because of it—Buddhist psychology places enormous emphasis on describing and classifying cognitive and emotional phenomena. In the broader scheme, indeed, Buddhism displays a remarkable fondness for lists and systematisation in general: there are four noble truths, an eightfold path, five aggregates and many more such classifications and tabulations throughout Buddhist texts. The *Abhidhamma* (Pāli; Sanskrit: *Abhidharma*), or 'higher doctrine' of Buddhist psychology (Powers, 2000), in particular, presents what is possibly the most extraordinary array of lists and classifications in all Buddhism, centred on the myriad cognitive, emotional and experiential phenomena stemming from the apparent self and aiming to characterise and categorise all human mental experiences (Bodhi, 1999).

The ultimate focus of the *Abhidhamma* and other Buddhist teachings is the elimination of *dukkha* or suffering. The *Abhidhamma* is especially important because Buddhism teaches that, while *dukkha* is everywhere and is closely related to our cognitive and emotional habits, these phenomena change all the time, and clear-sighted description and understanding of the nature of, and our cognitive and emotional responses to, *dukkha* is a vital step in understanding and resolving it. This is consistent with the fundamental ideas underpinning DSM and ICD, at least in theory, i.e. the idea that clear-sighted description and classification of specific mental states can assist with the resolution of suffering through guiding research, facilitating discussion and pattern recognition, and increasing phenomenological understanding of complex states of psychological distress.

The teaching of nonself, however, warns against according too much reality both to the apparent self that is suffering and to other phenomena, such as the 'diagnosis' indicated by DSM or ICD. Both the self and the diagnosis are convenient labels that are useful for defined purposes (e.g. to guide treatment choices or facilitate research), but it would be a mistake to accord too much reality to them. Regrettably, it is common to see people accord far too much reality to the categories in DSM and ICD, with the result that diagnoses that were originally meant as research or treatment guidance tools come to be seen as concrete, immutable disease entities (Horowitz, 2002: 213). In other words, people confer too much reality on DSM and ICD diagnoses, eventually coming to regard them as real, stand-alone entities, rather than mere descriptions that are useful for certain purposes (e.g. testing treatments for specific sets of symptoms) but can be actively harmful if misused (e.g. disempowering people, ignoring the uniqueness of individualised distress, dominating the individual's self-image).

As the categories outlined in DSM and ICD are clearly based on symptoms rather than demonstrated biological aberrations, this kind of over-interpretation of their categorisations is a real risk. This risk is, however, well recognised in both DSM and ICD. In DSM-5, the APA (2013: 19) emphasises that the symptom lists are not comprehensive definitions of mental disorders, which are substantially more complex than such summaries suggest; that each case formulation must be broad and multifactorial; and that a tick-box system of diagnosis is insufficient and inappropriate. The APA (2013: 24) adds that the DSM-5 reflects current opinion in an evolving field: change is constant. The WHO makes precisely the same point in ICD-10 (WHO, 1992: 2).

In other words, both DSM and ICD clearly and openly acknowledge that their criteria are not to be used in an unthinking, tick-box fashion; mental disorders are significantly more complex than a simplistic reading of these criteria might suggest; and the categories presented are intrinsically impermanent and subject to change. An approach to DSM and ICD that is explicitly informed by the Buddhist teaching of dependent arising will not only underpin this point and lead to more flexible, skilful use of DSM and ICD, but will also go one step further, pointing to the impermanence of the 'self' that is experiencing these symptoms in the first instance. Consequently, significant difficulties arise if the transitory natures of the diagnostic categories and the self are ignored, and DSM or ICD are used as rigid, inflexible tools, rather than guides or simply structured ways of enquiring into psychological distress, which must always be combined with broad-based engagement with the unique position of each individual patient. An awareness of the Buddhist teachings of dependent arising and nonself can assist greatly with maintaining the flexibility, humility and humanity required for this task, as can a nuanced understanding of two other key areas of Buddhist teaching: cognition and compassion.

Other Buddhist Teachings: Cognition and Compassion

Cognition

Buddhist teaching and practice place strong emphasis on the workings of the mind as it relates to both cognition and emotion. The most detailed account of Buddhist theories of mind is presented in the *Abhidhamma* or 'higher doctrine' of Buddhist psychology. Vast and intricate, the seven books of *Abhidhamma* were, according to Thervāda tradition (but not all traditions), conceived by the Buddha 21 days after his awakening (Gethin, 1998) and present a highly disciplined, detailed classification of all mental phenomena (Bodhi, 1999).

Unlike the DSM and ICD, the *Abhidhamma* focuses not on mental illnesses or states of psychological distress, but on the broader scheme of human consciousness and workings of the mind. The *Abhidhamma* outlines levels of categorisation, subcategorisation and sub-subcategorisation of mental phenomena that are vastly more complex and systematised than those presented in either DSM or ICD.

By way of an overview of the *Abhidhamma*, it is instructive to consider the contents of the seven books of the Therāvada *Abhidhamma* (linked to the oldest Buddhist tradition, from India), which clearly demonstrate Buddhism's emphasis on the centrality of understanding specific psychological concepts, the significance of various cognitive practices, the definition and attainment of certain states of consciousness and the centrality of cognitive discipline (e.g. meditation) (Kelly, 2012):

(a) *Dhammasangani:* The first of the seven books of the Theravada *Abhidhamma* provides an outline of the *Abhidhamma*, presenting its categorisation of material phenomena and states of consciousness, as well as explanations of key terms.
(b) *Vibhanga*: This book analyses critical Buddhist concepts such as sense bases, mindfulness, dependent arising, the eightfold path, types of knowledge and *dhammahadaya* (the essence of the doctrine).
(c) *Dhātukathā*: This book analyses all phenomena in relation to Buddhist concepts of sense bases, elements and aggregates.
(d) *Puggalapannatti*: This book studies different levels of spiritual development and different types of individuals, using an approach similar to that of the *Suttas* (Pāli; Sanskrit: *Sūtras*) (or more general teachings) rather than the *Abhidhamma* itself.
(e) *Kathāvatthu*: This book comprises a collection of undecided or debatable points in *Abhidhamma* teachings.

(f) *Yamaka*: This book is centred in the use of *Abhidhamma* terminology and resolution of ambiguities in relation to sense bases, latent dispositions and consciousness, among other areas.
(g) *Patthāna*: This book is also known as the 'Great Treatise' and presents an analysis of the interrelations between different *Abhidhamma* teachings, according to 24 varieties of conditional relations. This constitutes an extremely detailed overview of much of Buddhist psychology and forms the centre of the *Abhidhamma* teachings (Bodhi, 1999).

This substantial emphasis on studying and categorising mental phenomena in the *Abhidhamma* is further reflected in the unique emphasis that Buddhism places on the practice of meditation as a key element of the path to enlightenment (Gethin, 1998). This includes meditation for the attainment of calm (Pāli, *samatha*; Sanskrit, *śamatha*) and meditation for the development of insight (Pāli, *vipassanā*; Sanskrit, *vipaśyanā*). In recent years, this emphasis that Buddhism places on meditation (especially for the attainment of calm) and cognitive training has been translated and modified in the Western world into the form of 'mindfulness' (Siegel, 2010).

Mindfulness essentially means paying attention to the present moment, simply and directly. It involves maintaining a careful awareness of thoughts, emotions and actions, but not judging them. It involves staying focussed on the present moment as much as possible and attaining calmness. There is now evidence to support the use of mindfulness-based techniques for a range of psychological states and mental illnesses (Kelly, 2008a, 2008b; Mace, 2008) including, most notably, preventing recurrence of depression (Segal, Williams, & Teasdale, 2013).

One of the key messages of the *Abhidhamma*, broader Buddhist teachings and, indeed, the practice of mindfulness (Michie, 2004) is that all of our mental phenomena are subject to dependent arising, i.e. occur due to surrounding causes and conditions, are subject to constant change and are devoid of substantive, permanent reality. These mental phenomena can be categorised at any given moment in time according to the *Abhidhamma* (and, in the case of states of psychological distress or mental illnesses, according to the DSM or ICD) but are also subject to constant change, at least some of which can be volitional or brought under conscious control. As a result, the practices of meditation and mindfulness can change our mental phenomena significantly, just as the practice of cognitive-behaviour therapy can help shift our cognitive habits in a more positive direction (Beck, 2011). Given this plasticity in our mental processes and phenomena, it is unsurprising that routine interaction with elaborate systems designed to guide cognitive decision-making in clinical situations (e.g. DSM, ICD) can affect patterns of thought.

Consistent with this, Carlat (2010: 61), a psychiatrist, in a uniquely thoughtful and constructive critique of contemporary psychiatry, describes a cognitive phenomenon that he terms 'DSM-think', which occurs when DSM starts to reshape thinking above and beyond what it merits and produces fundamental shifts in the way clinicians interpret and conceptualise human suffering, and their responses to it. This phenomenon can be exacerbated by the need for clinicians in certain countries (e.g. USA) to document DSM diagnoses in order to receive payment or by pharmaceutical companies seeking to develop and promote medications linked with specific DSM diagnoses.

Most of all, perhaps, 'DSM-think' may emerge from the feelings of confusion that clinicians sometimes feel when faced with complex psychological problems that threaten to overwhelm the clinician, just as they overwhelmed the patient. Faced with this situation, clinicians commonly feel a strong social pressure and real human need to act, and DSM and ICD provide apparent refuge from this confusion in the reassuring form of detailed lists of symptoms which appear to provide a ready-made 'diagnosis' and point to a path forward. The fact that the patient is likely to identify with at least some of the criteria listed in at least one of the categories in DSM and ICD reassures both patient and the clinician that, however confusing the present circumstances appear, this has happened before: they are not alone.

From a Buddhist perspective, the most skilful response to this situation involves, in the first instance, sitting mindfully with the feelings of confusion and being overwhelmed and recognising that these feelings fluctuate (and are thus less substantial than they appear), are dependent on specific causes and circumstances for their apparent existence (and should thus be accorded less reality than might be initially imagined) and eventually start to abate (and are thus impermanent). In addition, Buddhism's overall emphasis on cognitive discipline and mindfulness is intended to assist in seeing things 'as they really are', and this approach is especially useful when faced with apparently unbounded phenomena (e.g. panic attack) or an apparently overwhelming emotion (e.g. depression), which can be examined with greater equanimity, either during or after the phenomenon, if one has previously habituated oneself to mindful cognitive practice.

In this context, mindful and measured engagement with DSM or ICD can offer real guidance and genuine reassurance in relation to states of complex psychological distress or mental illness, in much the same way as the *Abhidhamma* offers guidance in relation to other apparent mental phenomena and levels of consciousness or awareness. This kind of measured engagement with DSM and ICD is more likely to be measured and appropriate if the cognitive habits of both patient and clinician are characterised by mindfulness and various other elements of the eightfold path including, most notably, right view (i.e. seeing things as they really are), right resolve, right speech, right effort, right mindfulness and right concentration.

In this way, Buddhism's emphasis on recognising the transient, dependent nature of cognitive and emotional experiences can assist with skilful engagement with DSM and ICD. More specifically, an awareness of, and engagement with, these basic Buddhist concepts can increase habitual cognitive flexibility when interpreting DSM and ICD criteria, promote mindful awareness of the transitory nature of such systems, deepen consciousness of the complexity of mental phenomena (as outlined in the *Abhidhamma* and elsewhere) and embed an awareness that the self and associated psychological phenomena lack permanent reality and are subject to constant change. These useful concepts, especially Buddhism's emphasis on mindful cognitive awareness and training, are usefully complemented by consideration of another key theme in Buddhist thought: the centrality of compassion.

Compassion

To complete this discussion of Buddhist perspectives on psychiatric classifications systems, it is useful to consider three other key concepts in Buddhist thought: *kamma* (Pāli; Sanskrit: *karma*), rebirth and compassion. These ideas come together in the concept of compassion, which is highly relevant to clinical encounters in psychiatry and more skilful engagement with DSM and ICD.

Kamma refers to the idea that every volitional act, which results from a deliberate choice, leads to a series of events which produces concordant results, i.e. results may be pleasant or unpleasant, depending on the nature and motivation of the original act (Keown, 2005; Powers, 2000; Ward, 2013). According to Buddhist thought, these results may be immediate or delayed and may even be delayed until a future life (Williams & Tribe, 2000). This is linked with the Buddhist idea of rebirth (Lopez, 2008), which refers to the idea that all sentient beings (including human beings) are caught in a repetitive cycle of birth, death and rebirth (Pāli/Sanskrit: *saĐsāra*) (Harvey, 2000). One of the key ways to break this cycle is through meditation on the true nature of reality, which leads to clear-sighted awareness of the mechanisms of the cycle and release from it through enlightenment (Brazier, 2003). The nature of future rebirths is determined by the *kammic* results of previous actions; rebirth as a human, with consequent opportunity for spiritual advancement, is the *kammic* result of previous good actions. Rebirth as an insect, which offers less opportunity for advancing towards enlightenment, is the *kammic* result of previous bad actions. The teachings of *kamma* and rebirth thus provide Buddhists with powerful incentives for good or skilful behaviour.

The ideas of *kamma* and rebirth are strongly consistent Buddhism's emphasis on compassion (Pāli/Sanskrit: *karuṇā*) (Williams, 1989). In the Western world, the word compassion refers to an emotion such as pity which inclines one to help others (Pearsall & Trumble, 1996). In Buddhism, compassion refers to a specific wish for the suffering of all beings to cease, and it constitutes the basis for the Buddhist concept of 'loving kindness', a feature of many meditation practices (Gethin, 1998). The idea of rebirth suggests that this compassion should extend not only to one's self and other humans but to all sentient beings, because any sentient being (e.g. an insect) may have been a human in a previous life, or may be one in a future life, and is thus to be treated with compassion and respect.

The teaching of rebirth, interpreted literally, is the subject of considerable debate within Buddhism (Powers, 2000). Nonetheless, it remains a central concept, possibly because it is amenable to many interpretations. For example, given Buddhism's teachings about the impermanence and emptiness of the concept of self, it is not unreasonable to imagine that one might experience multiple rebirths during the course of a single human life. Practicing compassion will lead to good *kammic* results and better rebirth, be it conceptualised as rebirth following a human death or rebirth within the span of a single human life (i.e. reinvention of the 'self' as one proceeds through life).

So, how is compassion linked to the more skilful use of DSM and ICD? First, compassion is immediately relevant to psychiatry anyway, owing to psychiatry's strong focus on relieving suffering though effective treatment of mental illness and provision of assistance to people in states of psychological distress. In this way, compassion is central to all aspects of medicine (Lown, 1999) and the psychiatric enterprise in particular (Spandler & Stickley, 2011), including the use of DSM and ICD, regardless of one's position on Buddhist teachings and ideas.

Second, Buddhist teachings about nonself, *kamma* and rebirth provide specific support for the idea that compassion can and should permeate all aspects of psychiatry, including the use of DSM and ICD in individual cases. The teaching of nonself, for example, does not deny that individuals exist or suggest that they are without meaning (Brazier, 2003), but rather that the concept of a self is dependent on a range of causes and conditions which change constantly and produce a range of outcomes that include the apparent self. In this way, the suffering (*dukkha*) that one 'self' experiences is continuous with the suffering of others, i.e. we are all a single, unified phenomenon, without distinction between artificially constructed 'selves' (Harvey, 2000), and this is a powerful argument in favour of compassion towards all.

Thus, Buddhist teachings about *kamma* and rebirth articulate the connections between volitional actions and their consequences; the teaching of nonself emphasises that our apparent 'selves' are not as substantive as we imagine, and we are essentially continuous with others; and all three teachings, taken together, point to the centrality of compassion in all areas of life, including psychiatry: if there is no self, there can be no self-interest, and if the suffering of others is continuous with one's own, then compassion for one's 'self' is compassion for all sentient beings (Cho, 2000; Ward, 2013). In this way, the Buddhist conception of compassion provides a powerful incentive to relieve the suffering attributable to mental illness for the benefit of *all* sentient beings, including the patient, the apparent 'self' and all other beings (there being no meaningful distinction between these groups). This further emphasises the logic supporting compassion as a key value in all aspects of psychiatric diagnosis and treatment, including use of DSM and ICD.

Third, the teaching of *kamma* suggests that the *kammic* results of compassionate actions, such as relieving the mental suffering of others, will produce good *kammic* results for the 'self' and for others. Such actions need to be motivated by genuine compassion for others and taken with mindful awareness of context. In psychiatry, this means diagnosing and practicing with a broad-based awareness of the suffering of the individual patient in all of his or her complexity. In the more specific context of DSM and ICD, this clearly points to a need to move away from a tick-box approach to diagnosis and towards an approach that is applied mindfully and compassionately and demonstrates the flexibility required to interact compassionately with all suffering beings. This is highly consistent with the emphasis the WHO places on having a flexible attitude towards diagnosis (WHO, 1992: 1–2), something which may be especially important towards the start of the diagnostic process (Callard, 2014): all diagnoses are provisional to begin with, and all remain subject to revision forever.

Fourth, mindful awareness of compassion can not only lead to more skilful diagnosis but also, in due course, help inform therapy. Compassion-focussed therapies are now being used and explored for a broad range of mental illnesses and psychological states (Gilbert, 2009) including anxiety (Tirch, 2012), post-traumatic stress disorder (Lee & James, 2011; Bowyer, Wallis, & Lee, 2014), disordered eating (Goss, 2011), personality disorder (Lucre & Corten, 2013) and even psychosis (Braehler et al., 2013; Laithwaite et al., 2009; Wright et al., 2014). These developments build on existing traditions of Buddhist-informed psychotherapies (Epstein, 2001, 2007; Kelly, 2008a, 2008b, 2012) and articulate further the importance of compassion at all stages of the therapeutic process, from the point of initial diagnosis (e.g. using DSM or ICD) through the provision of both general mental healthcare and specific psychological therapies and the ultimate resolution of psychological and psychiatric symptoms.

Conclusions: You Cannot Diagnose the Same Mental Illness Twice

The media commonly describe the DSM as the 'psychiatrists' bible', despite both DSM-5 and ICD-10 stating clearly that their descriptions are merely guidelines, to be interpreted flexibly and with a broad awareness of the multifactorial nature of psychological and psychiatric distress. Nonetheless, the description of DSM as the 'psychiatrists' bible' is not entirely without truth in one important respect: the majority of individuals in most religious traditions engage with their 'bible' or scripture in a nuanced fashion, taking certain sections literally, interpreting other sections metaphorically (Kelly, 2011) and completely ignoring other sections. It is useful and sensible and necessary for thinking clinicians to look at DSM and ICD in a similar fashion, depending on specific circumstances that present themselves.

In this context, and despite the controversies associated with psychiatric classification systems, there are compelling reasons why these systems should be retained and continuously revised. Not least of these are the facts that these systems facilitate research into treatment and aetiology of mental illnesses and states of psychological distress, help guide alleviation of suffering and help protect human rights, especially the right to liberty (i.e. protection against inappropriate or unlawful involuntary treatment). Until such time as the true aetiological underpinnings of mental illnesses and psychological distress are more clearly established, and the stigma associated with mental illness finally dispelled (Sartorius & Schulze, 2005), DSM and ICD will continue to generate controversy. This is to be expected and is not unwelcome.

It is, however, notable that many of the controversies surrounding DSM and ICD stem not from problems with the diagnostic systems themselves, but rather the inappropriate use of such systems, despite clear and emphatic warnings against inappropriate, over-literal or tick-box approaches in both DSM and ICD. The misuse of such systems is especially regrettable because nuanced, thoughtful use of these tools can help greatly with enhancing diagnostic transparency and understanding in individual cases, once their use is tempered by an awareness of their limitations and combined with genuine therapeutic engagement with individual patients and families.

In this context, more skilful engagement with DSM and ICD would be facilitated by an awareness of Buddhist teachings about dependent arising and nonself which, as already discussed, refer to the idea that perceived phenomena (including the self) are entirely dependent on specific causes and conditions for their apparent existence and are thus without substance, permanence or, in a sense, independent existence. This approach emphasises that specific clusters of co-occurring symptoms (such as the diagnoses outlined in DSM and ICD) are deeply impermanent and thus to be interpreted very flexibly and that the self experiencing such symptoms is similarly devoid of lasting substance and subject to change and constantly transforming forms of *dukkha* (suffering). Ultimately, it is the patient and his or her suffering, and not DSM or ICD, who guides diagnosis, treatment and resolution (Kelly, 2013).

Skilful engagement with DSM and ICD can be further advanced through an awareness of Buddhism's emphasis on the importance and *complexity* of mental phenomena (as outlined in the *Abhidhamma*), the need for cognitive flexibility (e.g. when interpreting DSM or ICD criteria) and mindful awareness of the transitory nature of such classification systems, complemented by a deep awareness that the self and associated psychological phenomena (e.g. symptoms) lack permanent reality and are also subject to constant change. This is highly consistent with Buddhism's emphasis on compassion, which, in the context of these other Buddhist concepts, is another construct necessary for skilful use of DSM or ICD: if there is no self, there can be no self-interest, and the suffering of others is continuous with one's own. Compassion should therefore underpin all aspects of psychiatric diagnosis and treatment, as well as informing specific, compassion-based psychological therapies.

Humility is another key value that complements compassion in mental healthcare and is highly consistent with the Buddhist world view (Harvey, 2000). In psychiatry, for example, it is important and appropriate to cultivate genuine humility about how much we really know about the biology of the brain, the biological correlates of mental illness (Kirsch, 2009), and, therefore, how medications work (Kramer, 1994). From a Buddhist point of view, new perspectives on knowledge about the brain has been a key (if controversial) feature of recent dialogues between Buddhism and neuroscience (Kelly, 2008a; Lopez, 2008; Shaheen, 2012) and will undoubtedly further shape concepts of both brain and mind in the coming decades.

In this context, what is important for clinicians, in the midst of the controversies surrounding DSM and ICD, is that the core tasks of mental healthcare do not become obscured: the core tasks remain the alleviation of suffering among individuals in states of psychiatric and psychological distress and the promotion of health and social care systems which promote wellness, enhance human rights, deepen social inclusion and optimise autonomy (Kelly, 2013). Accurate, sensible, flexible and compassionate diagnosis is central to this task.

Ultimately, an approach that combines DSM or ICD with flexible, individualised interpretation, an awareness of nonself, skilful cognition and deep compassion can recognise both that (a) identifiable patterns of suffering recur in different individuals, reflecting a commonality of experience and unity of suffering, and (b), at the same time, each individual is unique and constantly changing, so that all diagnosis is subject to revision—forever. The Greek philosopher Heraclitus stated that *you cannot step into the same river twice*; in psychiatry, you cannot diagnose the same person or the same illness twice: all the parts are moving parts, and change is the only constant.

Future research and development of classification systems can and should take account of changes in psychiatric and psychological knowledge, practice and thought, in order to make revised diagnostic categories reflect more accurately current experiences of mental illness and psychological distress (Frances & Nardo, 2013). Future editions of DSM and ICD could also usefully re-emphasise and elaborate ICD-10's guidance on careful, mindful use of diagnostic criteria (WHO, 1992) and DSM-5's stern warning against a tick-box approach to diagnosis (APA, 2013).

An approach to psychiatric classification and revision of diagnostic guidelines that was explicitly informed by compassion would also help ameliorate some of the suspiciousness and bitterness that occasionally surrounds ideological debates about DSM and ICD and help refocus attention on the common task: the alleviation of the suffering of all beings, including not only our patients but also ourselves and all sentient beings—regardless of their DSM or ICD diagnosis (if any) and regardless of their stage on the path to enlightenment. Further exploration of the relevance of Buddhist psychology to this process is likely to prove helpful, inclusive, insightful and even, perhaps, enlightening.

References

American Psychiatric Association. (1952). *Diagnostic and statistical manual of mental disorders* (1st ed.). Washington, DC: American Psychiatric Association.

American Psychiatric Association. (2013). *Diagnostic and statistical manual of mental disorders* (5th ed.). Washington, DC: American Psychiatric Association.

Angell, A. (2011). The illusions of psychiatry. *The New York Review of Books, 28*, 20–22.

Barr Taylor, C. (2010). *How to practice evidence-based psychiatry: Basic principles and case studies*. Arlington, VA: American Psychiatric.

Batstra, L., & Frances, A. (2012). Diagnostic inflation: causes and a suggested cure. *Journal of Nervous and Mental Diseases, 200*, 474–479.

Beck, J. S. (2011). *Cognitive behavior therapy: Basics and beyond* (2nd ed.). New York: The Guilford Press.

Bentall, R. P. (2003). *Madness explained: Psychosis and human nature*. London: Allen Lane/ Penguin Books.

Bentall, R. (2009). *Doctoring the mind: Why psychiatric treatments fail*. London: Allen Lane/ Penguin Books.

Bloch, S., & Reddaway, P. (1984). *Soviet psychiatric abuse: The shadow over world psychiatry*. London: Gollancz.

Bodhi, B. (Ed.). (1999). *A comprehensive manual of Abhidhamma: The philosophical psychology of Buddhism*. Seattle, WA: BPS Pariyatti Editions.

Bowyer, L., Wallis, J., & Lee, D. (2014). Developing a compassionate mind to enhance trauma-focused CBT with an adolescent female: a case study. *Behavioural and Cognitive Psychotherapy, 42*, 248–254.

Braehler, C., Gumley, A., Harper, J., Wallace, S., Norrie, J., & Gilbert, P. (2013). Exploring change processes in compassion focused therapy in psychosis: Results of a feasibility randomized controlled trial. *British Journal of Clinical Psychology, 52*, 199–214.

Brazier, C. (2003). *Buddhist psychology: Liberate your mind, embrace life*. London: Robinson/Constable & Robinson.
Burns, T. (2013). *Our necessary shadow: The nature and meaning of psychiatry*. London: Allen Lane/Penguin Books.
Callard, F. (2014). Psychiatric diagnosis: The indispensability of ambivalence. *Journal of Medical Ethics, 40*, 526–530.
Carlat, D. J. (2010). *Unhinged: The trouble with psychiatry – a doctor's revelations about a profession in crisis*. New York, NY: Free Press.
Cho, S. (2000). "Selflessness": Towards a Buddhist vision of social justice. *Journal of Buddhist Ethics, 7*, 76–85.
Clare, A. W. (1976). *Psychiatry in dissent: Controversial issues in thought and practice*. London: Tavistock.
Cloud, J. (2012, December 17). Redefining mental illness: New guidelines will change how we assess what ails the mind. *Time, 180*, 18.
Craddock, N., & Mynors-Wallis, L. (2014). Psychiatric diagnosis: Impersonal, imperfect and important. *British Journal of Psychiatry, 204*, 93–95.
Das, L. S. (1997). *Awakening to the Buddha within: Tibetan wisdom for the western world*. London: Bantam.
Davies, J. (2013). *Cracked: Why psychiatry is doing more harm than good*. London: Icon Books.
Epstein, M. (2001). *Going on being: Buddhism and the way of change – a positive psychology for the West*. London/New York: Continuum.
Epstein, M. (2007). *Psychotherapy without the self: A Buddhist perspective*. New Haven/London: Yale University Press.
Frances, A. (2013). *Saving normal: An insider's revolt against out-of-control psychiatric diagnosis, DSM-5, big pharma, and the medicalization of ordinary life*. New York: HarperCollins.
Frances, A., & Chapman, S. (2013). DSM-5 somatic symptom disorder mislabels medical illness as mental disorder. *Australian and New Zealand Journal of Psychiatry, 47*, 483–484.
Frances, A. J., & Nardo, J. M. (2013). ICD-11 should not repeat the mistakes made by DSM-5. *British Journal of Psychiatry, 203*, 1–2.
Gethin, R. (1998). *The foundations of Buddhism*. Oxford/New York: Oxford University Press.
Gethin, R. M. L. (2001). *The Buddhist path to awakening*. Oxford: Oneworld.
Gilbert, P. (2009). *The compassionate mind (Compassion focused therapy)*. London: Constable & Robinson.
Goss, K. (2011). *The compassionate mind-guide to ending overeating: Using compassion-focused therapy to overcome bingeing and disordered eating (Compassionate-mind guides)*. Oakland, CA: New Harbinger.
Greenberg, G. (2010). *Manufacturing depression: The secret history of a modern disease*. London: Bloomsbury.
Harvey, P. (2000). *An introduction to Buddhist ethics*. Cambridge: Cambridge University Press.
Healy, D. (2002). *The creation of psychopharmacology*. Cambridge, MA/London: Harvard University Press.
Horowitz, A. V. (2002). *Creating mental illness*. Chicago, IL/London: University of Chicago Press.
James, A. C., James, G., Cowdrey, F. A., Soler, A., & Choke, A. (2013). Cognitive behavioural therapy for anxiety disorders in children and adolescents. *Cochrane Database of Systematic Reviews, 6*, CD004690.
Kelly, B. D. (2008a). Buddhist psychology, psychotherapy and the brain: A critical introduction. *Transcultural Psychiatry, 45*, 5–30.
Kelly, B. D. (2008b). Meditation, mindfulness and mental health. *Irish Journal of Psychological Medicine, 25*, 3–4.
Kelly, B. D. (2011). Self-immolation, suicide and self-harm in Buddhist and western traditions. *Transcultural Psychiatry, 48*, 299–317.
Kelly, B. D. (2012). Contemplative traditions and meditation. In L. Miller (Ed.), *Oxford handbook of psychology and spirituality* (pp. 307–325). Oxford: Oxford University Press.

Kelly, B. D. (2013). DSM-5 – Plus ça change, plus c'est la même chose? *Irish Medial Times, 47*, 22.
Keown, D. (2005). *Buddhist ethics: A very short introduction*. Oxford: Oxford University Press.
Kessler, R. C., & Üstün, B. D. (Eds.). (2008). *The WHO world mental health survey: Global perspectives on the epidemiology of mental disorders*. Cambridge: Cambridge University Press/World Health Organization.
Kirsch, I. (2009). *The emperor's new drugs: Exploding the antidepressant myth*. London: Bodley Head.
Kramer, P. D. (1994). *Listening to Prozac*. London: Fourth Estate.
Laithwaite, H., O'Hanlon, M., Collins, P., Doyle, P., Abraham, L., Porter, S., et al. (2009). Recovery after psychosis (RAP): A compassion focused programme for individuals residing in high security settings. *Behavioural and Cognitive Psychotherapy, 37*, 511–526.
Leader, D. (2010, July 30). *Being mad is one thing, going mad quite another*. Guardian, p. 31.
Leader, D. (2011). *What is madness?* London: Hamish Hamilton/Penguin Books.
Lee, D. A., & James, S. (2011). *The compassionate-mind guide to recovering from trauma and PTSD: Using compassion-focused therapy to overcome flashbacks, shame, guilt, and fear (Compassionate-mind guides)*. Oakland, CA: New Harbinger.
Lopez, D. S., Jr. (2008). *Buddhism and science: A guide for the perplexed*. Chicago, IL/London: The University of Chicago Press.
Lown, B. (1999). *The lost art of healing: Practicing compassion in medicine*. New York: Ballantine Publishing Group/Random House.
Lucre, K. M., & Corten, N. (2013). An exploration of group compassion-focused therapy for personality disorder. *Psychology and Psychotherapy, 86*, 387–400.
Lynch, T. (2001). *Beyond Prozac: Healing mental suffering without drugs*. Dublin: Marino Books.
Mace, C. (2008). *Mindfulness and mental health: Therapy, theory and science*. East Sussex, UK: Routledge.
Menand, L. (2010, March 1). Head case: Can psychiatry be a science? *New Yorker, 86*, 68.
Michie, D. (2004). *Buddhism for busy people: Finding happiness in an uncertain world*. Crows Nest: Allen & Unwin.
Midgley, M. (2014). *Are you an illusion?* Durham: Acumen.
Munro, R. (2006). *China's psychiatric inquisition: Dissent, psychiatry and the law in post-1949 China (Law in East Asia Series)*. London: Wildy, Simmonds & Hill.
Ng, X. T., & Kelly, B. D. (2012). Voluntary and involuntary care: Three-year study of demographic and diagnostic admission statistics at an inner-city adult psychiatry unit. *International Journal of Law and Psychiatry, 35*, 317–326.
Pearsall, J., & Trumble, B. (1996). *The Oxford English reference dictionary* (2nd ed.). Oxford/New York: Oxford University Press.
Porter, R. (2002). *Madness*. Oxford: Oxford University Press.
Powers, J. (2000). *A concise encyclopedia of Buddhism*. Oxford: Oneworld.
Sartorius, N., & Schulze, H. (2005). *Reducing the stigma of mental illness: A report from a global programme of the world psychiatric association*. Cambridge: Cambridge University Press.
Segal, Z. V., Williams, J. M. G., & Teasdale, J. D. (2013). *Mindfulness-based cognitive therapy for depression* (2nd ed.). New York: The Guilford Press.
Shaheen, J. (2012). A gray matter. *Tricycle, 22*(2), 15.
Siegel, R. D. (2010). *The mindfulness solution: Everyday practices for everyday problems*. New York: The Guilford Press.
Sommers, C. H., & Satel, S. (2005). *One nation under therapy: How the helping culture is eroding self-reliance*. New York: St Martin's.
Spandler, H., & Stickley, T. (2011). No hope without compassion: The importance of compassion in recovery-focused mental health services. *Journal of Mental Health, 20*, 555–566.
Thanissaro, B. (2014). What the Buddha never said: "There is no self". *Tricycle, 23*, 88–89.
Tirch, D. D. (2012). *The compassionate-mind guide to overcoming anxiety: Using compassion-focused therapy to calm worry, panic, and fear (Compassionate-mind guides)*. Oakland, CA: New Harbinger.
Van Os, J., & Kapur, S. (2009). Schizophrenia. *Lancet, 374*, 635–645.

Ward, E. (2013). Human suffering and the quest for cosmopolitan solidarity: A Buddhist perspective. *Journal of International Political Theory, 9*, 136–154.
Watters, E. (2010). *Crazy like us: The globalization of the American psyche*. New York: Free Press.
Whitaker, R. (2002). *Mad in America: Bad science, bad medicine, and the enduring mistreatment of the mentally ill*. New York: Basic Books.
Williams, P. (1989). *Mahāyāna Buddhism: The doctrinal foundations*. London/New York: Routledge/Taylor & Francis Group.
Williams, P. (2009). *Mahāyāna Buddhism: The doctrinal foundations* (2nd ed.). London/New York: Routledge/Taylor & Francis Group.
Williams, P., & Tribe, A. (2000). *Buddhist thought: A complete introduction to the Indian tradition*. London/New York: Routledge/Taylor & Francis Group.
World Health Organization. (1992). *The ICD-10 classification of mental and behavioural disorders: Clinical descriptions and diagnostic guidelines*. Geneva: World Health Organization.
Wright, N. P., Turkington, D., Kelly, O. P., Davies, D. R. T., Jacobs, A. M., & Hopton, J. (2014). *Treating psychosis: A clinician's guide to integrating acceptance and commitment therapy, compassion-focused therapy, and mindfulness approaches within the cognitive behavioral therapy tradition*. Oakland, CA: New Harbinger.

Chapter 3
Being Is Relational: Considerations for Using Mindfulness in Clinician-Patient Settings

Donald McCown

Introduction

The most obscure fact in the use of mindfulness in clinical practice may actually be its most obvious feature—that we learn mindfulness 'together'. Because the chapters that follow begin to open into the range of applications, this relational basis of mindfulness becomes a central consideration. In any undertaking in the clinical use of mindfulness, there is a teacher and at least one participant. This may be a group, as in mindfulness-based stress reduction (MBSR) or one of the many mindfulness-based interventions (MBI) that are targeted to specific clinical populations, or it may be that a therapist and patient undertake to apply mindfulness in their work together. In any case, we need to develop an understanding of both the person of the teacher and the nature of the relational situation of the pedagogy. Yet, we encounter obscurity in both.

Much of this obscurity might be traced to more than three decades of scientific research that has been modelled on or has aspired to the 'gold standard' of the randomised controlled trial (RCT), endowing scientific legitimacy, while factoring out potential 'teacher effects', and insisting on a strong individualist view of the pedagogy. Assuredly, this effort has elaborated an evidence base that has been powerfully persuasive in encouraging adoption of mindfulness for a wide range of clinical applications. Yet, much has been and continues to be lost. That is, as colleagues and I have suggested (McCown, Reibel, & Micozzi, 2010; McCown, 2013; McCown & Wiley, 2008, 2009) and as others have concurred (Crane, Kuyken, Hastings, Rothwell, & Williams, 2010; Crane et al., 2014), the concerns in teacher training

D. McCown (✉)
Center for Contemplative Studies, West Chester University of Pennsylvania, 855 South New Street, West Chester, PA, 19383, USA
e-mail: dmccown@wcupa.edu

E. Shonin et al. (eds.), *Mindfulness and Buddhist-Derived Approaches in Mental Health and Addiction*, Advances in Mental Health and Addiction,
DOI 10.1007/978-3-319-22255-4_3

and pedagogical study are in a different discourse from the outcome studies. The RCT approach assumes the view of mindfulness as an analogue to a pharmaceutical compound. Mindfulness is reified, a thing to be placed 'inside' the patient to effect individual change. Moreover, this thing is placed there via a teacher who is simply a delivery vehicle, a 'vector', even, that must be pure and controlled.

The intention of this chapter is to attempt to counteract this individualist and positivist view, by exploring the relational dimensions of mindfulness that underlie the activities of teaching and learning it, and in the process to identify and define practical theories and skills for teachers that are valuable across the range of mindfulness-based approaches delivered in groups, as well as in more tailored applications for individuals. These theories and skills will offer answers to essential questions: Who is it that can engage in the use of mindfulness in clinical work with patients, that is, who are we as teachers? How do we understand the rich, non-verbal experience of being together with participants in the classroom or consulting room? How do we know that what we are doing is 'working'? And what do we do when it is not? As answers to these questions unfold, we will also consider the nature of teacher training, a context for pedagogical theory and practice, a non-foundational ethical stance for clinicians when using mindfulness and an aesthetics of the pedagogy.

All of these explorations will start from the relational dimensions of mindfulness, which is newer theoretical territory in the development of the use of mindfulness in clinician-patient settings. What follows, then, relies on language and descriptions that are mostly different from the more established discourses within the medical, scientific and Western Buddhist communities. It is hoped that this more neutral language will have the dual effect of allowing new descriptions of the space in which teachers and participants practice the pedagogy to come to the foreground while allowing the unresolved tensions between clinical and Western Buddhist framings of mindfulness (e.g. Lindahl, 2015; Monteiro, Musten, & Compton, 2015; Purser, 2015; Van Gordon et al., 2015; Williams & Kabat-Zinn, 2011, 2013) to recede into the background.

Perhaps, for the reader, the most pressing questions are about the person of the teacher—who am I and what do I do? Yet, to best answer those questions, it is necessary to consider another set of questions—how do we understand the experience of being mindful together? It is the context that defines the teacher, not the other way around, as the following section will describe.

Context First: It All Starts With Relationship

In considering the pedagogy of the mindfulness-based interventions, my colleagues and I (McCown & Reibel, 2009; McCown et al., 2010; McCown, 2013, 2014) have adopted a social constructionist view (e.g. Gergen, 2009, 2015), in which relationship defines who we are and what we do in any situation. This approach defines the activities of teaching and learning mindfulness as an ongoing co-creation, involving and affecting all participants. Each instance of co-creation is unique, arising in the moment, and therefore unrepeatable. These characteristics may begin to suggest the challenges to the teacher, as well as the broad margins for engagement and even pleasure.

Confluence

A clear evocation of co-creation comes in Gergen's (2009) description of confluence. In the dominant discourse of individualism, participants in a class or dyad are seen as autonomous individuals first, bound up in their chosen identities and only (perhaps even grudgingly) accountable to others. In opposition to that discourse, the concept of confluence sees participants as relational beings first, with identities shaped in each instant by the unfolding of the shared activities.[1] For example, in an MBI class, when the curriculum calls for learning sitting meditation, the participants mutually define meditators who sit quietly and a teacher who 'guides' with their voice. Participants know what to do (who they are) in that moment. Then, when the confluence that is formal meditation practice ends, the meditators are redefined as dyad partners that speak aloud to each other. A further change in action, as a plenary dialogue takes form, defines students who speak and listen and a teacher who listens and offers answers or inquires into the student's experience in the moment. These shifting ways of being are not seen as forced on participants from outside nor are they compelled by inner pressures to act as they do. What happens next in the class is moderated by the relationships throughout the confluence.

Confluence is a philosophical concept, but not as speculative as one might think. With this concept in mind, we can turn to a description, if not an explanation, that makes use of our emerging physiological and neurophysiological understanding of mindfulness.

[1] This discourse of bounded individuals dominates our culture and therefore our language. Gergen (2009) notes that it is nearly impossible to find terms in English that suggest the relationships of the confluence. Rather than creating a new set of terms, the reader could readjust their thinking, and when they see the term, say, 'participants' to consider the mutually defining and shifting identities of the confluence. In comparing the pedagogy of mindfulness-based interventions in the United States and Korea (McCown, under review), Korean terms are found to describe the confluence situation clearly. The term 'Ahwoolim' connotes a meeting of more than two different persons or things that become harmonious; however different they were, they come to resonate with each other and lose their ordinary self-boundaries. The term *Shinmyong* describes an ecstatic state of aliveness and mutual sense of becoming one another; it literally means a state when a divine force becomes brightened and connotes the fullness of vital life force when something bottled inside is completely released.

A Scientific Description

Nearly 30 years after the first study of mindfulness as defined within MBSR, Imel, Baldwin, Bonus and MacCoon (2008) pushed against the dominant discourse and looked at the effect of the relationships in the group on participants' outcomes. With data from 60 groups—about 600 participants—they applied multi-level statistical modelling to calculate the group effect on the differences in symptom change from pre- to post-intervention while factoring out any teacher effects and adjusting for pre-intervention symptom severity. The effect of the group, they reported, accounts for 7 % of variability in outcomes—a significantly large number. To give perspective, the most significant predictor of outcomes in psychotherapy, the client-therapist alliance, accounts for only about 5 % of variability in outcomes (Horvath & Bedi, 2002).

Such power in being together has always been obvious to MBI teachers, who often hear in last-class reflections how strongly the participants value the sense of support of the class, how much easier they find it to practice with others and how 'close' they feel to people with whom they've spent precious little time—and whose names they may not even know.

The scientific explanation for this closeness starts with the mirror neurons in our brains that allow us literally to feel in our bodies the movements and even the intentions of those who are with us (Gallese, Fadiga, Fogassi, & Rizzolatti, 1996; Gallese & Goldman, 1998). It may be that a 'resonance circuit' (Siegel, 2007) brings us together. It runs like this (Carr, Iacoboni, Dubeau, Mazziotta, & Lenzi, 2003): We become aware of an action or expression in another (it may not even be seen but might be heard or otherwise sensed), which is 'tried on' by the mirror neuron system. Next, the superior temporal cortex predicts how that will feel to us. Then, that information goes through the insula to the limbic system, which establishes the emotional tone and returns the information back through the insula to the prefrontal cortex for higher level interpretation—so now we know the situation.

Through this circuit, we feel what others are feeling. What's more, we know their intentions—their next move. We attune to one another through this circuit. It is active in the bonding of infant and caregiver, of lovers, of family and further outward in social circles. As an evolutionary fact, it is active in our cooperation, our competition and even our fighting (Cozolino, 2006).

This effect of the group helps to describe the quality of a typical pedagogical situation. Yet, we must also consider the effect of the mindfulness practice on the group or dyad in teaching and learning mindfulness. Here the resonance circuit may come into play 'intrapersonally' as well as 'interpersonally', with meditators attuning to their own intentions and resonating with themselves. The most important part of the resonance circuit in the description that we are developing is the final move of activation of the prefrontal cortex to name the feeling. Activity in the prefrontal cortex reduces negative reactivity by calming the limbic system, particularly the right amygdala—the seat of fear (Creswell, Way, Eisenberger, & Lieberman, 2007; Lieberman et al., 2007).

To most fully explain the pedagogical situation of a mindfulness group or dyad, there is one move left to make: during a formal group practice, some or many of the participants may come to intrapersonal resonance, resulting in a feeling that they might label as peaceful or relaxed. That feeling is evident in their expressions and postures, even in their breathing and speaking, all of which is information available to all in the room. As the formal practice closes and participants look around, whether they are 'peaceful' or not, their mirror neurons react to all those who are gathered—peaceful ones included. The whole group has a chance to 'try on' the feeling of resonance. That, indeed, creates a unique situation. And we can explain it, in some detail, through Stephen Porges' 'polyvagal theory' (2011).

Porges suggests that not only do we have subcortical reactions to awareness of threats in the environment—the fight or flight reaction to moderate threat or the freeze reaction to overwhelming threat—but we also have a subcortical reaction to awareness of safety. This reaction prepares us for social engagement. It is mediated by the myelinated vagus nerve, which enervates the heart, and the muscles of the head and neck as well. So, when our subcortical threat detection system perceives the environment as safe (as with a group of peaceful meditators), the hypothalamic-pituitary-adrenal (HPA) axis and sympathetic nervous system response of fight or flight is suppressed, the heart rate slows and the social response possibilities of the head and neck are enhanced. That is, for better communication, the eyes open further to exchange glances, the eardrums tune to the frequency of the human voice, the muscles of the face and neck gain tone for finely shaded expressions and gestures, while the larynx and pharynx get set for articulate speech. And, for bonding, there is a release of the 'love hormone' oxytocin, encouraging approach and embrace.

Now, perhaps, it is possible to consider the group effect described at the outset as so potent for bringing about positive participant outcomes. In the practice of mindfulness, in a class or dyad, we co-create, again and again, an environment that feels safe. The many potentially peaceful faces, postures, voices and gestures help even those who are struggling for emotional balance to move towards social engagement behaviours. In a sense, that response moves through the group as resonance moves through a circuit, bringing openness to approach—making it more possible for the group and each participant to meet the experience of the moment (whether wanted or unwanted) in a friendly way.

Three Descriptions of the Pedagogy

We are back, at last, to consider what the relational dimension adds to teaching and learning mindfulness. What happens when we are together—in a group or dyad—may be more powerful and of more lasting effect than a pedagogy pointed towards some ideal of the individual practicing alone. The space we create together is immensely valuable. Perhaps the neurophysiological story is persuasive for you. Or you may find that other descriptions make more sense, in your experience.

To better understand the qualities of this 'homeland' of the teacher and to better prepare for the unique, dynamic and unrepeatable events in class or dyad, let's walk through three different representations of the pedagogical space and process. First, we will investigate the nonconceptual, embodied ways that we respond to the ongoing flow of the moment in the group that is the background in which the pedagogy takes place. Second, we will examine the ways that we are shaped by the nonconceptual, embodied experiences of the moments of the pedagogy. Finally, we will consider how participants' capacities for action in the moment grow, change and become potentials for the future.

1. Joint Action

John Shotter, investigating the deep processes of social construction, insists that our living bodies are spontaneously responsive to the 'others or othernesses' (e.g. 2012, p. 84) around us, which make up the background in which we are embedded. This background shapes us far more than we contribute to its ever-shifting shape. There is not simply our action or the other's action, it is 'joint action' (1984). Shotter uses resources of the Russian literary theorist Mikhail Bakhtin to describe this as 'dialogical', that each in the dialogue is responsive to the other and any utterance is shaped by the prior and anticipated utterance of the other (2008). Shotter thickens this description further through the phenomenology of Maurice Merleau-Ponty, for whom dualisms such as body-mind or self-other are overlapping or 'chiasmically intertwined'. Thus, we make sense of a situation because the living body can integrate the range of our perceptions and impulses to orient us in the present moment, with others (Shotter, 2011). Joint action is not dependent upon intentions of particular participants (or the teacher). It is, rather, the actuality of the unpredictable exchanges among them and, in fact, can be seen as inviting further actions from any and all. The situation of joint action, then, is dialogically or socially constructed and is in flux from moment to moment. The world of the participants changes with each silence, each word, each motion and each feeling. Shotter (2011) describes it:

> But more than simply responding to each other in a sequential manner—that is, instead of one person first acting individually and independently of another, and then the second also by acting individually and independently of the first in his/her reply—the fact is that in such a sphere of spontaneously responsive dialogically structured activity as this, *we all act jointly as a collective-we*. (p. 58, emphasis added)

Of powerful significance, as we will see as each of the three representations of the pedagogical space and process unfold for us, is the part the collective-we plays in the development of new ontological possibilities. Through the shared activity of the group, Shotter (1984) notes, participants come away with new, different ways of being. Spend time sharing space and activities with musicians, and musician becomes a way of being. Spend time with brewers brewing beer, and brewing becomes a way of being. Share mindfulness practice—being within the experience of the moment in the group—and come away as one who can stay longer (perhaps!) in the present.

This is not the usual way of thinking about pedagogy. As teachers, scientists or clinicians, we are trained to take an intellectual, conceptual approach to our activities. From what is a continuous flow of events, we focus on and abstract particular parts, which become concepts that we can grasp—that we can hold on to in the flow. This allows us to both orient ourselves to general patterns and to create protocols, principles or rules to ensure repeatable responses. Further, through such a process, the conceptual becomes a world in which we live and act. This has undoubted value in certain areas of life: we can fix cars or perform heart surgery; there, we benefit from keeping the sense of continuous flow and change at bay.

In different undertakings, however, continuous flow and change may be the key. In the pedagogy of mindfulness, we are learning to be within the experience of the moment, regardless of its emotional valence for us. We learn to be with the experience of the moment by navigating it, again and again, together, as a group. As Shotter (2012) has it, 'we turn our intellectual powers in a rather unusual, ontological rather than epistemological direction' (p. 91). That is, we work on 'how to get ourselves ready, so to speak, to go out to meet the events confronting us, rather than ...working out how, instrumentally, to influence those events themselves' (Shotter, 2012, p. 91). The overall experience of being a participant in a mindfulness group produces a way of being in the continuously flowing and changing world, as opposed to a conceptual understanding of navigating a mapped and defined account of a world.

2. An Omelette in a Kitchen

The anthropologist Tim Ingold (2008) insists that we do not learn by bringing knowledge from 'outside' to 'inside' us. Rather, he suggests that we 'grow into' knowledge within a relationship located in a specific place with specific objects. As he describes, 'The minds of novices are not so much 'filled up' with the stuff of culture, as 'tuned up' to the particular circumstances of the environment' (2008, p. 117). He refers to this not as learning or education but as 'enskillment' and provides the example of a child learning to make an omelette. There is no one right way to crack a given egg, because each egg is different. The child learns the feel for it from hands that are skilled being placed on or over theirs. What is more, this process happens in a particular kitchen, with particular bowls and pans. The knowledge is in the system, not inside the child. Ingold notes that 'you only get an omelette from a cook-in-the-kitchen' (2008, p. 116).

Ingold's image of the knowledge in the system—cooking or being mindful—arises from a powerful critique of the dominant view of beings and their development. Ingold (2006) calls this dominant view the *logic of inversion*, in which the being's involvement in the continually changing outside world (consider the moment in the kitchen with egg, bowl and teacher) is seen as a cognitive schema or cultural model installed inside the being that is brought out when needed. Through the logic of inversion, 'beings originally open to the world are closed in upon themselves, sealed by an outer boundary or shell that protects their inner constitution from the traffic of interactions with their surroundings', notes Ingold (2006, p. 11). To invert this inversion, then, is to open the being to the world again, to come to experience continual flow and change and to be within each moment, which is, in fact, the central move of the pedagogy of mindfulness. An open being, then, is unbounded, moving in the world along a line (actually many lines) of development, interweaving relationships. Such an unbounded being is tangled, enmeshed with the texture (or textile!) of the world—in the kitchen, classroom or consulting room. Knowing is not inside but all around.

3. Potentials

Gergen's (2009) concept of confluence, as described at the outset of this section, may now have more resonance. Beings that are open may act jointly in the 'collective-we' that Shotter (2011, p. 58) mentions and may interweave to a thick texture in relationship with others, as Ingold (2006) suggests. A confluence and the mutually defining relationships that it comprises bestow on participants 'potentials' for being and acting in particular ways, according to Gergen (2009). A participant may attend to another's way of being as a model, will surely take on a particular way of being and will come to some level of prowess in the coaction of the confluence. Such potentials are not merely cognitive; they are embodied in action, movement, gesture, posture, facial expression, gaze, vocal tone and more. They are established by familiarity, by repetition within particular confluences, and are then available as seems sensible in particular situations. Through experiences, we develop a vast store of ways of being, or multi-being, as Gergen calls it (2009). This is not problematic, as questions of coherence and integration of the many potentials bestowed by relationships do not arise within the discourse of open, unbounded beings. In multi-being, coherence and integration may be valued within specific relationships, but are not essential to some overall self. As Gergen states, 'For the relational being there is no inside versus outside; there is only embodied action with others. Authenticity is a relational achievement of the moment' (2009, p. 138).

The pedagogy of mindfulness, then, is a question of potentials that are bestowed within the relationships of the class or therapeutic dyad. Everyone steeps in what is co-created in the confluence. This is not simply true of the participants, clients and patients—whatever word we use—but is also true of the teacher. All of those gathered are part of the confluence, all have potentials from past relationships and all help to bestow further potentials each to each, all to all, each to all and all to each. In this exhaustive situation, it begins to make sense to explore who it is that teaches.

The Teacher: Who (and How) Are You?

If the pedagogy of mindfulness is a relational undertaking, a process by which potentials are endowed among participants, the typical assumptions about the formation and identity of mindfulness teachers for clinical applications must come under rigorous scrutiny. Education and training need to be considered from the capacity to catalyse the central move of the pedagogy, that is, of helping participants to stay within their experience of the moment, however aversive or distracting it may be. This is a subtle and intimidating job that requires tacit as well as theoretical understanding of mindfulness as relational practice. It is not enough to know the practice of meditation for oneself (although this is certainly a requirement), for one must also be skilful with the other participants. It is not enough to be deeply experienced or knowledgeable in one or more meditative or contemplative tradition (although, again, this has significant value), for mindfulness in clinical work is most often presented with secular language and under time restraints that limit contextual explanations. Likewise, it is not enough to have clinical training (although, once more, this is an important background), since the confluence works without diagnoses, therapist/patient hierarchy or instrumental therapeutic moves.

Mindfulness Training

If all of this is the case, how is a teacher to be educated and trained for the subtle and intimidating job of catalysing and maintaining the move of turning towards and being within the experience of the moment? As suggested above, training must be multidimensional while maintaining the singular focus of the pedagogy of mindfulness as the key practice. Through spending time in MBI groups and dyads as a participant, participant/observer, co-teacher and teacher, the teacher in training is endowed with the potentials found within the pedagogy. This 'steeping' in the practice of the pedagogy is a definition of teacher training. Certainly, teachers are also endowed with different potentials from steeping in other forms of confluence, such as professional training in a clinical discipline or meditative training in a specific tradition, and these potentials may be more or less germane to MBI pedagogy from moment to moment in a class. Ultimately, however, steeping in the MBI confluence is the most simple, direct and effective mode of teacher training. After all, the practice of the confluence is the pedagogy of mindfulness, and those potentials are constantly being endowed, refined and endowed again to the teacher and all participants.

The priority of steeping in the confluence of mindfulness pedagogy for teacher training does not decrease the importance of the teacher's personal daily practice of mindfulness meditation and regular retreat attendance. The phrase in the MBI community appears to be 'having your own practice' and is a marker of existential commitment to an identity as a diligent and ethically aware MBI teacher. For example, the formal statement of 'principles and standards' for teaching MBSR teachers (Kabat-Zinn et al., 2012) states, 'MBSR instructors need to have their own personal meditation practice and attend retreats in the spirit of 'continuing education' and the ongoing deepening of their practice and understanding'. In mindfulness-based cognitive therapy (MBCT), developed on the armature of MBSR, the explicit requirement for therapists of 'having your own practice' (Segal, Williams, & Teasdale, 2002, p. 83) is rooted in the developers' failed attempts to teach without it, as well as with their positive experiences with the senior MBSR teachers at the UMASS Center for Mindfulness, whose existential commitments to mindfulness were embodied in their lives. With such a correlation of personal practice time and commitment as a teacher, it would be simple to move to 'a more is better' outlook. However, this has not been the case in clinical application of mindfulness, as demonstrated in an attitudinal statement from the MBSR community. 'We have had instructors with 5 or 6 years of meditation experience who do very well in the classroom. Conversely, we have met people seeking jobs who have 20 or more years of meditation practice in their background who we did not feel at the time were capable of teaching in the classroom' (Santorelli, 2001, p. 11–8:4).

We could begin to understand this more deeply by returning to a relational discourse, leaving behind the discourse of personal practice as individualistic and internal. Thus, the practice away from the group, so-called practice in solitude, may be reframed relationally as unfinished dialogue (McCown, 2013). The discourse of self-improvement and self-exploration shifts to ongoing practice of the turning towards and being within the emerging moment that is the central move of mindfulness pedagogy. Meditating alone is then the invocation of dialogue with one's current and past teachers (necessarily one sided, although with a background of profundity) to maintain that central move.

Likewise, then, requirements for retreat practice may be reframed as steeping in the practice of the pedagogy of mindfulness, so that the potentials endowed are relational in origin and intent. This, of course, problematises retreats that do not use MBI or other clinical mindfulness practice modes. Steeping in alternative confluences cannot endow the same potentials as MBI-style retreats and develops teachers in divergent ways. This is acknowledged to a certain extent, for example, in MBSR training recommendations for developing teachers to attend retreats in the 'Western Vipassana or other Buddhist mindfulness meditation traditions' (CFM/retreat), because the experience 'mirrors and expresses many aspects of MBSR' (CFM/retreat). When considered in the discourse in which mindfulness is a relational accomplishment, such retreats would endow very different relational potentials versus MBSR. The secular MBI language game and the form of life in which it is instantiated—to borrow useful terms from Wittgenstein (1953)—are significantly different from those encountered in a retreat in Western Buddhism. There, the life world is tinged with more or less Buddhist language, views and actions that would need to be carefully translated for application in the secular arena of the MBIs. This is difficult work and requires significant knowledge of both sides of the translation. Thus, neither retreat practice nor meditation training through resources outside the secular, clinical mindfulness community would be ideal for endowing new teachers with the potentials that are most valuable in secular, clinical uses of mindfulness. On reflection, this may answer the riddle of Santorelli's (2001) observation that teachers with relatively few years of meditation experience were found who notably outperformed meditators with 20 years or more of experience. The endowed potentials of the former may be traced to secular, clinical sources and, thus, more closely match the language game and form of life in which they come to be actuated.[2]

[2] This does not call into question the existential commitment to mindfulness of either a Western Buddhist or a secular practitioner. It is simply that the fit for the situation may be more or less close and thereby more or less successful. This suggests that staying within the practice "lineage" of secular and clinical mindfulness may have value in establishing oneself as a valuable therapist/teacher. This should not be seen in any way as a less spiritual path; the commitment is to the other

Clinical Training (and Unlearning)

Because this book is focussed on mindfulness uses in mental health and addictions contexts, it might be assumed that the reader has been trained as a clinician in one of a range of possible disciplines, including psychiatry, nursing, psychology, social work and professional counselling, among others. Such an education has significant value in endowing relational potentials that may be actuated by particular situations that arise, say, in screening interviews with potential MBI participants or with participants who find themselves in great distress during MBI class sessions. In a specific area, that of codes of ethics and rules of professional conduct, a clinical education offers an irreplaceable resource, as will be described in the section on ethics further below. The background knowledge, skills and confidence offered by professional education cannot be gainsaid, yet much of what is required in the application of mindfulness in clinician-patient settings is new and contradictory and often requires of clinicians a process of 'unlearning'. This section will consider the three areas where unlearning may be necessary, and the section to follow will present an overview of the new skills that may be endowed in the pedagogy of mindfulness.

There are three essential differences between clinical uses of mindfulness and the vast majority of other clinical interventions; they are located in three areas that are immediately problematised by both a relational approach and the application of mindfulness: (1) diagnostic practices, (2) the clinician-patient relationship and (3) the intention of practice.

1. Diagnostic Practices

Kabat-Zinn (2011) foreshadows the difference in the MBIs (and other uses of mindfulness) with the well-known statement made at the start of MBSR classes, 'We often say that from our perspective, as long as you are breathing, there is more "right" with you than "wrong" with you, no matter what is wrong. In this process, we make every effort to treat each participant as a whole human being rather than as a patient, or a diagnosis, or someone having a problem that needs fixing' (p. 292). When such expression of disinterest in an imposed and limiting identity is urged by the teacher, freedom and possibility are awakened in participants. Anything may happen. The next moment can be different. We need not rehearse old stories or look for patterns of continuity. Change is happening in each moment and is a resource available to all.

---

as the central concern, meaning the sense of self-sacrifice or selflessness is primary and noteworthy. As Shonin and Van Gordon (2015) note, "Belonging to a lineage theoretically ensures that a person has the necessary 'credentials' to be an effective meditation teacher, and as such, knowing an individual's lineage can help us make an informed decision about their suitability as a teacher. However, just because a given meditation or mindfulness teacher is from a scientific background and/or is not particularly interested in being part of a Buddhist lineage or tradition, this does not by default mean that they are not authentic. Likewise, just because a teacher belongs to an 'established' Buddhist or meditation lineage, this does not, by default, mean that they are able to impart an authentic transmission of the teachings" (p. 143).

The release from diagnostic identities, particularly those drawn from psychiatric manuals such as the DSM 5, is not limited to the classroom; when the teacher lets go of diagnostic thinking, participants may be endowed with a potential to let go of such constructs in other contexts of their lives as well. Foucault (1995) reminds us that participants tend to subject themselves to the same ongoing scrutiny that is operative in many clinicians' ways of relating. Once labelled 'depressive', for instance, a patient is under surveillance by self and others. The patient comes to feel well, but 'It may come back!' Those who subject themselves are never free. Foucault describes how participants take on the limits set by their diagnoses and treatments:

> He who is subjected to a field of visibility and who knows it, assumes responsibility for the constraints of power; he makes them play spontaneously upon himself; it inscribes in himself the power relation in which he simultaneously plays both roles; he becomes the principle of his own subjection. (1995, pp. 202–203)

Foucault encourages us to resist such subjectification, and the MBI class or mindfulness dyad may be seen as a site of collective resistance. The confluence, then, is a counter-culture in which it is possible for participants to explore new identities and different ways of being through the central pedagogical move of turning towards and staying within the experience of the present moment.

2. Clinician-Patient Relationship
The pedagogy of mindfulness is inherently democratic. Because the teacher is part of the confluence in practice, that role is more one of catalyst (getting the process started) and steward (maintaining the central move of the pedagogy) than of director. Further, as the class (or dyad) grows in its capacity to be within experience, the urgency of catalytic and stewardship interventions diminishes. In effect, teachers are subsumed more and more in the confluence.

In moving towards such a situation, there are pitfalls for those used to thinking in other clinical modes. The language of mindfulness pedagogy is specific and crucial; the stakes are high. Kabat-Zinn (2004) notes that verbal and non-verbal communication can misdirect the class. For example, there is a tone that he names 'idealising', which suggests 'I know how to do this and I'm going to teach you'. On the contrary, in competent mindfulness pedagogy, the teacher's language, expression, gesture and posture would convey an invitation to shared exploration, emphasising the not-knowing position of mindfulness—a 'Well, we can investigate this together and see what comes of it'. Such an approach makes the pedagogy's central move the focus for the confluence—turning towards and being within the moment's experience.

Another tension between typical clinical approaches and applications of mindfulness is in the teacher's use of 'self-disclosure'. In the confluence, the teacher's moment-to-moment experience is as formative as any other. Shotter (1995) reminds us that the joint action of the group or dyad proceeds on a moment-by-moment basis of embodied (or practical) responsive understandings:

> a structure of presumptions and expectations of a non-cognitive, gestural kind that unfolds in the 'temporal movement' of the speaker's voice…The very act of saying a word in a practical circumstance is a joint action: it is open to the influences of both past and present others at the very moment of its performance, and their influences may be present in it too. (p. 66)

The co-creation of mindfulness depends upon moments of self-disclosure for all participants. The proviso here is that self-disclosure is an expression of the shared pedagogy; it is in and of the moment. The MBI teacher is inevitably transparent and self-disclosing.

3. Intention of Practice

Mindfulness pedagogy diverges—sometimes dramatically—from many established clinical approaches. Kabat-Zinn (2010) suggests the obvious gap, noting that mindfulness is not 'just one more method or technique, akin to other familiar techniques and strategies we may find instrumental and effective in one field or another' (p. xi). Rather, he continues, mindfulness pedagogy has 'a way of being, of seeing, of tapping into the full dimensionality of our humanity, and this way has a critical non-instrumental essence inherent in it' (p. xi). These statements highlight the essential credo that derives from the moment-to-moment, not-knowing position of the pedagogy: no one needs to be fixed, because no one is broken.

Even in extremis, in deep sadness or intense pain, for example, the central move of the pedagogy may be maintained. This is both useful and potentially a misdirection, depending upon the intention. A 'staying with' pain or sadness that is instrumental in intention, seeking a change, a way out, may, in the words of Crane and Elias (2006):

> work to subvert a strong internal and external tendency to look for certain (sometimes quite fixed) kinds of improvement or resolution of difficulties. This is a tendency that can play out in therapeutic and mental health contexts in familiar and unhealthy ways for both practitioners and clients at times. (p. 32)

However, a 'staying with' that rests on not knowing and existential curiosity works in a different register, to provide the individual—and the group—with:

> the possibility to experience a sense of "OKness" in the midst of "not OKness," is a broader influence offered by the meditative traditions, which can inform not merely process but also potentially a different approach to content. (p. 32)

The pedagogical move of turning towards and being within experience often brings participants to a choice point. Does one allow the experience? Or does one change it if that is possible? The teacher does not decide in some calculated way what is best; rather, the participant assumes the responsibility. The quality of intention in this situation is of curiosity and fearlessness.

For clinicians who begin their MBI teaching with a history of meditation training and practice from specific spiritual traditions, adjusting to the differences inherent in the pedagogy of mindfulness may be challenging. For clinicians without such histories, the pedagogy of the MBIs may become home ground. In fact, becoming a teacher may even call into question their identity as a 'clinician'. There is a possibility that steeping in mindfulness pedagogy could potentiate a shift of paradigm away from conventional diagnostic theory and hierarchical practice in medicine (e.g. Sauer, Lynch, Walach, & Kohls, 2011) and mental health care (e.g. Grossman, 2010). As a start, we might point to the choice that UK training programmes for MBSR and MBCT (Crane et al., 2010) have made to use the term 'teacher' rather than 'therapist' for those trained. The mindfulness pedagogue may be seen as a clinician working at the extreme edges of the clinical paradigm—or, perhaps, beyond the edges. As such, pedagogues apply a unique set of skills, which are worth profiling.

The Teacher's Skills: Stewardship, Guidance and Inquiry

As my colleagues and I found in trying to identify and categorise the skills of the teacher (McCown et al., 2010), even with an almost elemental scheme of four, it is difficult to divide the skills, as each includes the other three to some extent. For example, stewardship of the group requires not simply concrete actions but also language choices that help to catalyse the co-creation of the pedagogy of mindfulness. The teacher may use figures of speech and rhetorical turns that they bring or extract from the conversation in the confluence. This connects stewardship closely to the language-centred skills of guidance and homiletics. Further, the skill dubbed inquiry generates language, gesture and other non-verbal expressions in the moment in the class, and these, in turn, shape guidance and homiletics and ultimately stewardship. The four skill sets belong ultimately to the confluence—yet they start with the teacher. Let us consider them in a logical order for their interrelationship.

Stewardship

The word itself comes from *sty-ward*, the Old English term for the one who guards the meeting hall. The word denotes the action of the person and connotes the humility of the service. This is evident to those who teach, as we are often left to take down tables and set up chairs in a repurposed clinical space, making a circle and ensuring what comfort we can. That circle is emblematic of the stewardship skill set. The circle creates an outside, upon which the world beyond the group may act; likewise the circle has an inside, which belongs to the group, the confluence, and eschews hierarchy in the way of King Arthur's Round Table.

Stewardship skills are applied on both sides of the circle. The outside skills are mainly concrete—recruiting, organising, finding a meeting space and tending the space before and after the session. The inside skills are those of maintaining the central move of the pedagogy of turning towards and being within the experience of the moment.

Outside Skills

These are skills of the working as well as possible with a world that may not understand or be concerned with mindfulness meditation. Worldliness, compromise, business acumen, may come into play. Depending on the teacher's situation, demands may include entrepreneurial skills of setting up a programme, finding a setting and space. Even marketing, public relations and advertising may need to be accessed. How might it be possible for the teacher to accomplish these tasks while maintaining a mindful balance? This part of stewardship may be more challenging than it at first appears.

Recruiting and screening are perhaps the most important stewardship skills. The question is not so much who is appropriate for the group as it is who may be inappropriate. Screening out those who have a potential to be disruptive is mostly unseen by participants, yet it is essential for their safety, comfort and possibilities for transformation. Well-honed clinical skills are an advantage here. Exclusion of potential participants should be considered carefully, and a teacher's honest appraisal of their own skill in maintaining the central move of the pedagogy in difficult situations is paramount.

Hayes and Feldman (2004) state the issue clearly; the judgment is of participants' abilities to face their own negative material while suspending use of their current coping strategies to try on new possibilities. This is a tall order for anyone. The teacher must feel confident that, with help as required, this is possible. As such, a teacher's exclusion parameters will no doubt change over time and with greater endowment of potentials will come to allow more and more inclusion.

For beginning teachers, some rules of thumb may be useful. The exclusion criteria used by the UMASS Center for Mindfulness (Santorelli, 2014) are clear and offer confidence for teachers with differing levels of clinical training. They specifically exclude folks in active addiction or in recovery less than a year and patients with suicidality, psychosis (refractory to medication), post-traumatic stress disorder, major depression, other psychiatric disorders if they interfere with group participation and social anxiety unworkable in a group environment. Exceptions are individual—if the participant is highly motivated and engaged in supportive professional treatment and agrees to the teacher communicating with the professionals and the professionals agree to act as primary care givers and first contacts in emergencies, enrolment may be considered. Other exclusion issues include language comprehension, logistical possibilities of attendance (not related to physical impairment) and scheduling issues that would result in missing three or more classes. It cannot be emphasised enough that the teacher's intuitive feel for the participant and confidence in their skills must always be the deciding factor.

The final outside skill is that of caring for the space, literally, meaning the room and its furnishings. The room may be made as comfortable and attractive as possible, yet 'fussiness' about décor and overcontrol of temperature fluctuations and outside noise may ultimately become distractions and undermine the central move of the pedagogy. It is often worth making statements about obvious 'drawbacks' to the physical set up, noting that we practice for real life, which is seldom perfect or the way we would prefer. The message that most supports the pedagogy is that 'we do what we can and accept what we must'. The setting of the circle of chairs or cushions marks the transition from outside to inside skills, so it will be taken up next.

Inside Skills

A circle of chairs or cushions is indeed the emblem of stewardship. The use of a circle (or some other sensitive arrangements of seating that allow participants to see and experience one another's expressions, gestures and postures) optimises the potential for social engagement responses, as described using theories from Porges

(2011) above, and thereby aids in establishing a space that supports the pedagogy of mindfulness. It is stewardship skills that begin the process and keep it going. The circle, particularly, undercuts the sense of anyone, even the teacher, having a preferred seat. All have equal potential, and all can see themselves as part of something larger. In fact, a stewardship skill is to turn participants towards each other, rather than towards the teacher, by establishing the value of the other members. This can be achieved through the use of dyads and small groups, to process experiences before dialogue in the larger group takes place. These conversations develop more fluidity in relationships around the circle—especially as participants are asked again and again to talk to someone they have not yet talked with—while also establishing that there are no experts, no right answers, yet there is wisdom to be found.

As the capacity of the group to stay with the central move of the pedagogy develops, it is often tested, by the environment, dramatic distractions or emotion or conflict within the gathering. The teacher's skill here is simply the pedagogy of mindfulness—aiding the group in turning towards difficult experiences as they arise or letting go of attractive experiences as they pass. Take a simple example of an outside distraction that cannot be avoided, say, a series of fire engines passing with sirens in the street, the teacher can (in good voice) ask the group to 'drop in' to meditation and to pay attention to what is in their awareness moment to moment. When the distraction has passed, the group can engage in small group and plenary dialogues around the experience. In this way, an extraordinary experience becomes an ordinary example of mindfulness practice, and participants come away with new potentials.

If the group is tested in its dialogues by conflict, crosstalk or dominating participants, the teacher may invoke stewardship skills of a formal approach to conversation that may equalise the situation. First is to remind all that the mindfulness skill in dialogue is located in listening. Then a formal practice for dialogue could be introduced. A simplified version of the subgrouping technique from Systems-Centred Therapy (Agazarian, 1997) may be valuable, as may a basic approach to Council Circle (Zimmerman & Coyle, 1996).

In subgrouping, as part of mindfulness pedagogy, the instructions to the group are three. First, participants are asked to come to awareness of the body and to maintain that awareness throughout the process of listening and speaking. This move brings them into the moment and helps ensure that whatever is spoken is present-focussed, not rushing off into past or future. Second, one person is speaking and all are listening. The listeners are asked to attempt to make a connection between what is being said and their own present-moment experience. If this is possible, they may choose to speak of that experience—to build on what has been said. Third, then is the instruction for when the participant does not connect to what is being said. They are asked to simply hold their own truth, in quiet, listening while those who have connected explore their topic. They are also told that when one exploration is complete, they may bring in a difference, which may then be explored with others. Using this technique, slowly and without conflict, all sides of a topic may be given voice.

Council Circle again makes listening a mindfulness practice and offers opportunities for participants to be aware of their inner reactivity and the unfinished dialogues we call thinking and to be with those in quiet while others speak. The process is simple. A talking piece moves around the circle. The participant with the talking piece may speak or offer silence, while the others in the group listen. There are four basic intentions involved in the practice. When translated into the language of mindfulness pedagogy, they might be stated: (1) speaking the truth of your present-moment experience; (2) listening by being present with your whole being for what is spoken by the other; (3) expressing what is true for you, without elaborating with story or analysis; and (4) do not rehearse as the talking piece nears you—keep returning your attention to the speaker and trust that what you need to say (or not say) will come to you. This is a mindfulness practice that endows the potentials to be found in keeping one's own counsel over time.

In both these practices, it may be noticed that participants are free to choose to be silent. This highlights what is perhaps the most important stewardship fact: participation is not easy to define. Folks may be quiet during spoken dialogues and yet be deeply engaged with their own unfinished dialogue. They may be transformed by what looks like simply sitting in the circle.

Homiletics

Another word study reveals that homiletics, at its Greek root, denotes friendly conversation and connotes dialogue in a group assembled to talk together—which is how it has come to its specific modern use referring to making sermons. Today, the word suggests much more of a sense of hierarchy than is intended in the usage here. The skill is definitely not one of sermonising, not of speaking from expertise, but rather of a curious collaborator in conversation. In the practice of the skill, the teacher, who does have information to impart, starts from the 'text' that the group creates in dialogue and explores and illuminates that text. As Santorelli (2014) describes it:

> rather than "lecturing" to program participants, the attention and skill of the teacher should be directed towards listening to the rich, information laden insights and examples provided by program participants and then, in turn, to use as much as possible these participant-generated experiences as a starting point for "weaving" the more didactic material into the structure and fabric of each class. (p. 9)

The experiences of the participants become living texts that are available for all to appreciate and interpret. A class, in fact, is a democracy of texts, because each participant has the opportunity to be an author. This increases the sense of deep sharing. Whether or not a participant speaks, he or she is nevertheless involved with this form of study. Thus, when the teacher is required by the curriculum to deliver specific information—say, describing the stress response—the teacher attempts to solicit contributions and conversation. For example, participants might be asked to imagine a scene, such as being stuck in traffic and late for a meeting, and to respond with the body sensations, thoughts and emotions that appear. The teacher then has references to heart rate, breathing, muscle tension, anxiety, catastrophic thoughts and many more contributions with which to work.

Another literal form of text is often used skilfully in the pedagogy of mindfulness within the MBIs: poems, stories and children's books (e.g. Baer & Krietemeyer, 2006; Segal et al., 2002). Read aloud, with mindful listening as a practice; such texts bring the group together. The wisdom of a poem or story is not the teacher's wisdom, so the democracy of texts asserts itself. Further, the content and the ideas shared around any text are a form of wisdom that is available to all.

Guidance

Guidance is simply using language to catalyse the pedagogy of mindfulness. The forms of that language are different from teacher to teacher, yet there are considerations that would seem to be inherent in the practice. Kabat-Zinn (2004) developed a style that is replicated in many of the MBIs. It is designed to support participant's understanding of mindfulness and is a feature of the pedagogy. He identifies four ways that language, expression, gesture and posture can undermine both understanding and practice. First, the teacher could convey 'striving' for things to change, as in 'if you did this long enough, you'd be better'. Second, the teacher may be 'idealising', as in 'I know how to do this and I'm going to teach you'. Third, the participant may hear an offer of 'fixing', implying that there is something wrong with the participant that mindfulness is meant to address. Fourth, the participant may detect 'dualism', assuming that there is an observed and an observer.

Guidance, then, must avoid placing these stumbling blocks in participants' paths. Further, and this is the most salient characteristic of the MBI style, teachers' language must reduce the resistance of participants. This is achieved by inviting the participants, rather than directing them. In a discursive analysis of a Kabat-Zinn audio recording of the body scan practice for MBSR, Mamberg, Dreeben and Salmon (2015) identified three features of language use that are of interest here. What they call 'inclusivity' involves the use of the first person plural in guidance, rather than second person, implying that all in the group are participating together. It sounds like 'Now, let's let the focus of our attention move on…'. What they call 'process over ownership' involves, among other tropes, the use of the definitive article, rather than first or second person possessive. That is, 'Raising the left leg', not 'your left leg', which suggests that the action is already underway and participants may join in, or not. Bringing us to the third feature, which Mamberg et al., call 'Action without agency'. This involves the inevitability of the present participle, together with constructions that diminish rather than intensify the call for doing. It sounds something like 'If you're ready, just raising the left leg and perhaps noticing…'. The impression on the participant is that, come what may, these actions are taking place in the present in the room. There is a sense of joining, a sense that reflects the concept of confluence.

A less specific and therefore potentially more flexible way of considering language use comes from the work of the sociologist Richard Sennett, who, across two books, *The Craftsman* (2009) and *Together* (2012), works towards an understanding of the very real practices that humans use to foster cooperation. When craftspersons are confronted with resistance from their material or when diplomats are working with difficult relationships, both have strategies that can be applied to the situation of an MBI teacher guiding meditation. Perhaps it is possible to read Sennett's description here as useful in encountering MBI participants:

> Applying minimum force is the most effective way to work with resistance. Just as in working with a wood knot, so in a surgical procedure: the less aggressive the effort, the more sensitivity. Vesalius urged the surgeon, feeling the liver more resistant to the scalpel than surrounding tissues, to 'stay his hand', to probe tentatively and delicately before cutting further. In practicing music, when confronted by a sour note or a hand-shift gone wrong, the performer gets nowhere by forcing. The mistake has to be treated as an interesting fact; then the problem will eventually be unlocked. (2012, p. 210)

The concept of minimum force may be used to shape the language of guidance, and specifics will follow. As an aside, however, the concept is wonderfully applicable to a teacher's own development: mistakes are simply interesting facts to be explored, not overcome. Sennett even notes that the use of minimum force links to mastering the tools one has—whether leaning to drive a nail, bow a cello or begin a meditation session. Reducing aggression towards oneself as teacher will shift the environment in the classroom.

In applying minimum force to dialogical or collaborative situations, such as the MBI classroom, there are three distinctive insights that Sennett (2012) offers from diplomatic practice, which deserve serious consideration as rules of thumb. First, one may refrain from insisting on one's own ideas and take on another's view of the situation. From whose position are we guiding? Second, one may deploy the 'subjunctive mood' in one's language: the 'what if…' and 'perhaps…' way of talking that opens possibilities for dialogue—that is, as an unfinished dialogue experienced by the participant. Third is that technique known as 'sprezzatura', recommended by Baldassare Castiglione, in that sixteenth-century diplomat's *Book of the Courtier*. Sprezzatura is a lightness of touch, a nonchalance that makes it difficult for others to find offence in what one says. In the MBI classroom, such lightness and such a sense humour are a powerful unguent. The reference is not to comedy—teachers don't need to do 'schtick'—but to the generation of a pleasant and informal atmosphere.

As this eschewing of comedy in favour of humour suggests, guidance is not performance. The language and expression of guidance arises within the experience of the teacher, who uses their own moment-to-moment experience of the practice they are leading to understand the environment in which the meditation is unfolding. That is, the teacher is a 'sensor', an instrument reading the quality of the confluence, using their embodied understanding of the practice and the group to shape their speaking in the moment. Yet it is not only the teacher's experience that is voiced. The language, expression, gesture and posture are considered, to allow an infinite range of possibilities for participants' subjective experiences, as well.

On a concrete level, the teacher senses and uses whatever arises in the environment, say, hallway sounds of whispered conversations or noisy groups or squeaky cart wheels—even the sounds and substance of HVAC systems can bring participants closer to their experience.

The most important of all manifestations of guidance is the specific meditations provided as audio recordings for participants to use in their 'homework' practice between classes. Language choices and expressive speaking must carry the entire experience. Because a practice will be listened to repeatedly, the recording needs to offer many layers of information, direction and permission to explore the new moment. In fact, permission to explore may be expanded, subtly, beyond the allowance offered in the classroom, since the home contexts from week to week, even year to year, will vary widely. A recording cannot become a document; as much as possible, it should allow the living moment to unfold, beyond any scripting or attempts to control experience.

Inquiry

As noted above, inquiry and dialogue are salient features of the MBIs: 'It is recommended that a significant amount of time in each class be dedicated to an exploration of the participants' experience of the formal and informal mindfulness practices and other weekly home assignments', suggests Santorelli (2001). The reference is not to plenary dialogue sessions but rather to teacher-participant engagement that inquires into a subjective experience. What is it like for this person, right now? Bringing tacit knowledge into language in this way may offer insights not only to the participant so engaged but to all of those listening as it happens.

Inquiry is a collaboration of two parties that incorporates the confluence. The interlocutors work from a 'not-knowing' position that is not directed towards any fixed outcome. The process is about recognising and knowing what is happening. It is, from the teacher's seat, an offering friendship. Stephen Batchelor (1997) describes this offering from a Western Buddhist context, parsing the participant's experience of a skilful inquiry:

> [F]riends are teachers in the sense that they are skilled in the art of learning from every situation. We do not seek perfection in these friends but rather heartfelt acceptance of human imperfection. Nor omniscience but an ironic admission of ignorance… For true friends seek not to coerce us, even gently and reasonably, into believing what we are unsure of. These friends are like midwives, who draw forth what is waiting to be born. Their task is not to make themselves indispensable but redundant. (pp. 50–51)

The friendship of inquiry is expressed not only through a willingness to accept whatever comes but also through a genuine curiosity—expressed in the open questions that characterise inquiry. 'How was it for you?' is a simple but ultimately unfathomable starting point. The participant may respond tentatively, and the teacher may prompt another, perhaps deeper, exploration—'Can you say more about that?' A process of reflection and speech may reveal new ways of encountering the world for the participant.

Inquiry is not a late-in-the course undertaking, but rather may be entered into from the start, as in this exchange during class one (McCown & Ahn, under review):

Participants around the circle introduce themselves with more or less detail about 'What brings you here?' And the moment comes for 'I'm Maria, and I don't think I can do this'.

'What's this', asks the teacher.

'This course... being quiet and meditating and stopping my thinking... I've never been able to manage that. My mind is racing all the time, like now. I'm always full of worries, so every time I try to stop and be quiet like I know you're supposed to, it just gets that much louder in my head. And so I can't sit still. At home, I'd already be up and doing something, washing dishes, doing laundry, something to distract me. That's the only thing that works...'.

'So Maria', the teacher reflects, 'That's not what I'm seeing in the present moment. I'm seeing someone who is focused and engaged and sitting in one place'.

'I guess', she says.

The teacher suggests, 'Can you put the story you're telling on hold for a moment, and simply check in with what it's like for you right now?' Then, looking around the group, the teacher connects others to the inquiry, saying, 'This is something you all can try, too. Maybe there's a way that you can explore this idea for yourself'.

Turning back to Maria, the teacher offers potential for exploration, 'Maybe checking in to how it is now—in this moment. Just knowing that you're sitting here, feeling your feet on the floor, and feeling the chair holding you.... Maybe closing your eyes, if that's comfortable...'. A long ten seconds of quiet, and then, 'Taking a little while with it... Noticing your body and where it's touching down'. Another longer pause, and then, 'So how is it with you right now, Maria? In this moment, without your story?'

'Right now, it's not too bad... It's OK. I know I'm still in the chair, and my mind feels less racy', she says.

'So, maybe the thought 'I can never be still' is just a thought, a part of a story that's not true in this moment?'

Maria says, 'I guess so'.

'It's a possibility', the teacher says and turns to the rest of the group. 'Do you see this difference Maria is noticing, between a story about what's happening in the moment and what you can find out is happening when you pay attention?' Hands go up around the circle. 'That's a way of thinking about mindfulness. It's always available, even when your mind is racing... Thanks, Maria, for being willing to do this'.

Maybe there was no shattering revelation, yet Maria worked towards some new experiences. What's more, the other participants engaged in their own 'unfinished' dialogues and noticed whatever they noticed—perhaps something important to them. Inquiry is subtle work, shared work and work that no one may own or control.

A Space to Hold Us: The Ethical Work of the Group

As my colleagues and I (McCown et al., 2010) analysed the pedagogy of the MBIs in order to write the first textbook about teaching mindfulness and as we went on to help develop curricula for training MBI teachers, we identified the key qualities of what I have come to call the 'ethical space' of mindfulness in clinical practice (McCown, 2013). These qualities are located in both the actions of teaching and the unspoken framing of the space by the teacher for the participants. The model I have suggested has seven key qualities, divided into two dimensions and one quality that pervades all others. It may sound like the ethical space is an abstraction, a construction of the confluence. This is not the case, however. The space of which I speak is an actual architectural volume—a place where people act together in site-specific ways. This will be evident in the description of each dimension, perhaps more in the 'doing dimension' than in the 'non-doing dimension', yet each is made concrete. A graphic depiction of the space may be helpful in orienting to the different dimensions.

The Doing Dimension

There are three qualities of action that define the work of the MBI confluence. These qualities are endowed by participation in the pedagogy of mindfulness, the ongoing attempt to turn towards and stay within the experience of the present moment.

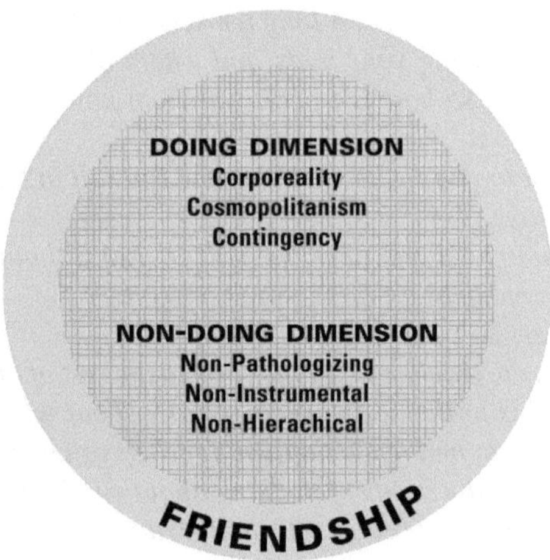

The interweaving of the doing and non-doing dimensions is ultimately infused with the quality of friendship, which can be compared to Aristotle's concept of perfect friendship, teleia philia

'Corporeality' foregrounZds the experience of the body, which participants quickly recognise as different from the typical modes of investigation in mental

health interventions. Mindfulness meditation at its foundation is a practice of the body. Participants recognise that it is founded on available sensations—particularly of the breath moving in the body. This sense of the body brings the participants into intimate contact with their ongoing experience—one cannot feel sensation in the future or the past—and helps make aesthetic and affective experiences available and tolerable for participants to explore directly and through dialogue.

'Contingency' deconstructs these experiences, particularly of aversive affect. In the formal and informal practices of the confluence and the homework, participants track the arising and subsiding of their emotions, the feelings in their bodies and the sometimes oppressive awareness of their thoughts. Participants see how sensations continually change and pass away. They encounter and are often able to turn towards and be within distressing moments of affect. When this can be investigated, particularly through observation of the affect as body sensation, the tendency towards change becomes evident. Things may be 'worse' or 'better' in the moment, but they are constantly moving. It is that kind of experience that helps to deconstruct an emotion—what is it really?—and that opens for participants different possibilities for self-regulation. Finally, they notice the instability of the stream of thought. In such a situation, insight and meaning may arise.

'Cosmopolitanism' holds any new insight or meaning. The term is chosen to describe the acceptance of the meaning that arises in the moment, without a drive to abstract it, reduce it or fit it into any system or set of values. Meaning, in other words, is revealed as contingent. This is a particularly consequential quality, because mindfulness practice often opens participants to the spiritual dimension of their lives. Although empirical evidence is thin in the literature of the MBIs, a meta-analysis of controlled trials (Chiesa & Serretti, 2009) found five studies that measured aspects of spirituality and results suggesting that MBSR significantly enhances spirituality compared to inactive but not active control groups. Two studies not in the meta-analysis (Carmody, Reed, Kristeller, & Merriam, 2008; Greeson et al., 2011) also suggest significant spiritual engagement. Teachers using mindfulness with participants are witness to a great deal more of this kind of meaning-making than researchers, and cosmopolitanism is one way of allowing such meanings to unfold in the classroom.

The Non-doing Dimension

In the dimension of 'non-doing', it would be easy to focus on the teacher as the actor establishing the qualities. Yet, as I hope you've seen in our explorations of the pedagogy, that is not usually the case. In the illustration of inquiry with Maria, above, the non-doing qualities are actually inherent in and activated through actions within the confluence.

'Non-pathologising' refers to that defining perspective that 'if you are breathing there is more right with you than there is wrong'. Ideally, no labels are invoked in the dialogues that are spoken aloud, and there is a possibility to allow the unfinished

dialogue called thinking to be deconstructed and any pathologising self-surveillance to be undermined as well.

'Non-hierarchical' certainly refers to the teacher's position of not-knowing when confronted with participants' experiences, and it also refers beyond the teacher, to describe the group relationship in dialogue—the rule that no one needs to be fixed because no one is broken is the key. One can impose meanings on one's own ever-changing experience, yet no one is the expert on the unfolding of the present moment. To phrase it in American vernacular speech, the teacher is as clueless as anyone else and is committed to exploring whatever experience is available 'within' the confluence.

'Non-instrumental' may be the most difficult to grasp of the qualities. The class does not practice the pedagogy of mindfulness in order to be changed or transformed in a particular way. Participants don't practice 'because' or 'in order to' but rather as exploration of the unknown of the present moment. This does not, however, rule out transformation. In fact, transformation may be seen as the nature of the confluence. Together, participants are observing that all contingent structures of sensation, affect and thought deconstruct themselves as they unfold within the ethical space and its associated qualities. Guided by the unfolding relationships in the moment and steeping in the experiences of silence, practice, spoken and unspoken dialogue, participants may come to be endowed with new potentials—that change life in and out of the confluence.

The Character of the Confluence

Friendship is neither a dimension nor a quality; rather it is the total character of the confluence of the pedagogy of mindfulness. It is not 'held' by the teacher in some way; it is not a choice to be friendly. Rather, friendship is a 'possibility of being' arising through the practice of the pedagogy, which participants steep in and may be endowed with and carry away from the confluence. Friendship, then, may be reflected in actions in relationships of other confluences and even in relationships of unfinished dialogue—the care and compassion for self that is a strong characteristic of the MBIs (Kuyken et al., 2010) and, by extension the secular, the clinical pedagogy of mindfulness.

Ethics in the Ethical Space

The ethical space arises from the group or dyad's practice of the pedagogy.

Gergen (2009, 2011) would say that participants are fully immersed within a first-order morality, which means the confluence has defined and may create its own goods, which become new ways of being, which Gergen has dubbed 'potentials', for participants. Those in a first-order morality cannot act otherwise than in accordance with those goods: the confluence, the ethical space and a first-order morality are identical. However, participants and teacher all have potentials from other first-order moralities as well—allegiances to other communities. Gergen (2009) suggests that such instability of allegiance can be problematic. However, teachers of mindfulness may also find this fact congenial; their allegiances (potentials) as psychologist, social worker, nurse or physician are available if required.

When the confluence is steeping in the pedagogy of the MBIs, the qualities of the ethical space are evident, and the teacher is a seamless part of that. However, should a participant find themselves incapable of maintaining the key move of the pedagogy, even with assistance from the teacher, that participant may enact other potentials from other first-order moralities, disturbing the confluence. In such a case, the teacher may 'step out' of the ethical space and align instead with the ethical code of their particular profession—potentials from another first-order morality.

It is also possible that it is the teacher that lacks the capacity to maintain the key move of the pedagogy in a particular situation or encounter. In this case, the teacher may 'step out' of the ethical space and actuate ethical potentials of a clinical professional identity. The character of this stepping out is different than the first, in that the impulse is to protect the teacher rather. Such reflexive self-protection does also protect the participants—offering codified control in an ambiguous situation.

Within the co-created ethical space, the participants steep in the potentials of the confluence. They grow more and more in capacity to turn towards and be within what is arising in the moment. Therefore, the less the participants or teacher 'step out' and interrupt that steeping, the more 'trust' in the practice develops within the relationships of the gathering—endowing valuable potential in all. Yet, stepping out is a live option for all, as well. There is safety in both the ethical space and within the alternative first-order moralities of the health-care professions, with well-accepted professional and legal commitments. We might say that the ethical space as first-order morality is transparent to participants and is a useful pragmatic situation for teachers.

Sublime Moments: The Aesthetic Work of the Group

Clinical work with mindfulness is different from mindfulness in education and organisational development and, particularly, from personal development and spiritual practice. There is an aesthetic experience available in clinical applications that is not easily found in the others. It can be described as a form of the sublime. Imagine a confluence that is well steeped in the central move of the pedagogy, so that the participants find it possible to approach aversive moments of experience. Imagine, as well, that one particular participant is willing to enter into dialogue—inquiry with the teacher—about an emerging experience. It might sound something like this, arising from the continuation of the introductions from a first class that appear above:

'What brings me here is my panic disorder… Oh, my name is Jessica… sorry', says a young woman. 'My therapist thinks that this course can help me not react so big and fast. I start to get anxious, and I don't like the feelings I get… they scare me… and so I need to take something, or call my Mom or my boyfriend, before I end up in a panic'.

'That doesn't sound like the easiest way to be', the teacher ventures.

'It's tiring… for everyone', she says.

'How is it with you right now?' the teacher asks. 'Is there anxiety here?'

'Yeah, a bit'.

'Would you be willing to explore it, just a little, in a mindful way? Maybe there's a way to be with it that's different than what you've been doing. You're in charge, so you can stop any time, OK?' (The teacher has been very much reading the person and the opportunity in the group in the moment, before making this attempt to engage.)

'OK', says Jessica.

To the group, the teacher says, 'While Jessica and I explore her experience, maybe you can find a way— not to watch, exactly, yet to be connected to your own experience. I suspect that quite a few of you may be interested in ways to be with anxiety. Yes?' Hands sprout around the circle. Jessica looks around, maybe settling a little more in her chair.

'So, Jessica, are you still noticing some anxiety?' the teacher asks.

'Some, yeah', she says quietly.

The teacher asks, also quietly, 'If you bring attention to your body right now, can you feel where that anxiety is showing up? Just take your time and feel into it…'.

Quickly she answers, 'In my back. That's where it's been a lot recently. It sort of moves around…'.

From the teacher, 'Can you bring your attention there? And see what you find out about that feeling?'

'That's scary, but I'll try'. A longish pause. 'OK, I am… I'm paying attention'.

'And what is the feeling like?'

'It's like, constricted… tight'.

'Do you know anything more? Like how big the area is, or, maybe, what shape it is…'. And the teacher waits quietly, with a curious and patient expression and attitude.

With her thumbs and forefingers Jessica makes a long, horizontal oval. 'It's a rectangle, about this big, in the centre of my back. It's really tight'.

'OK', says the teacher. 'You're right there with it… I wonder if you can find a way to give it a little room, to open some space around it? Maybe you can use your breath to soften around it…'. She looks puzzled, and the teacher elaborates. 'Can your breath go to that part of your back when you breathe in? Do you know what I mean?'

'I think so… Yeah'

'So when you breathe in, letting some space open up around that rectangle…and when you breathe out, letting it stay soft…'. Jessica, the teacher and the participants

in the space breathe in the quiet for thirty seconds—a long time. The teacher asks, 'What more do you know about that spot now? Anything?'

'It's gotten smaller', Jessica replies. 'Much smaller… It's like the size of my finger, now'.

'So it changed… You gave it space and it stopped taking up so much space in you. OK. Maybe you want to keep in touch with it, keep breathing and softening', the teacher says to Jessica. Then to the whole group, 'That's sometimes what happens. It's not a guarantee of a particular outcome not a technique to get rid of something. Jessica was just paying attention to what was there, opening space for it to be, and for herself to see what it was. The willingness to be with… and to pay attention to her experience is the important thing here. Her courage in showing up for it… that's what matters'.

This was not an easy dialogue for Jessica. Nor was it easy for the other members of the class to have their own incomplete dialogues as they watched and listened. This was not so much an encounter of teacher and participant as it was an encounter of the class with an affective charge—the question of turning towards and being within one's own anxiety. This was an initial steeping in the deeply human, seriously committed, way of being that it is possible to experience in a mindfulness-based group or therapeutic dyad. One potential description of such experiences is of the sublime.

The term is borrowed from aesthetics and rendered with particular connotations for mindfulness pedagogy. A detailed discussion of the history of the many uses and interpretations of the sublime is far beyond the scope of this chapter (e.g. Shaw, 2006). However, Burke's (1759/1999) view of the sublime and its activities on the person offers a historically influential and useful discussion. His attempt at definition makes 'terror' a central idea. It might be found in overwhelming natural phenomena, such as storms at sea or ascents of mountains. The inexpressibility of such views and experiences takes them beyond the rational and carries one, as observer, beyond oneself. The ego is diminished, the 'I', is reduced, and one is more open to the experience. In mindfulness pedagogy, the term sublime may be used to point to those moments when participants confront more of the fullness and contingency of human existence—the possibilities of death and madness, to name the extremes—than is typical for in a classroom. In the scene above, the affect for many may have been strong and may have opened them to Jessica's and their own experience of anxiety. Along with this opening may arise, as well, a contradictory or paradoxical sense of pleasure, which, Burke suggests, is possible when there is space for observation. The ability to observe that which imbues a sense of terror is not merely a requirement for experience of the sublime; it is also the central move of the pedagogy of mindfulness—the turning towards and being within the experience. Mindfulness, then, makes the experience of the sublime possible for the participants of a class or dyad.

The sublime has particular value for the teacher in the MBIs or other modes of mindfulness application; when it is part of the experience of a session, it may be assumed that the pedagogy is 'working' and that participants are steeping—being endowed with potentials for living in more profound and authentic ways.

The experience of the sublime is in contrast to the beautiful, as Burke (1759/1999) notes. Shaw (2006) quotes Burke pithily that:

> Where the sublime 'dwells on large objects, and terrible' and is linked to the intense sensations of terror, pain, and awe, the focus of the beautiful, by contrast, is on 'small ones, and pleasing' and appeals mainly to the domestic affections, to love, tenderness, and pity. Crucially, with the sublime 'we submit to what we admire', whereas with the beautiful 'we love what submits to us. (p. 57)

The beautiful is what brings us closer together through our agreement on the pleasure of an experience; the sublime does bring us together but through terror—as if the participants all faced a fearful prospect together. Continual experience of the beautiful, not interspersed with the sublime, therefore, may be considered as a measure of the weakness of a mindfulness group or dyad. When the currency, so to speak, of the experiences of the participants is restricted to the beautiful, the steeping, the development of potentials is likewise restricted. We might use the sublime-beautiful distinction to distinguish the effective use of mindfulness in clinical practice from other applications. The clinical uses are different because they are sublime. In other uses, such as in business, organisations or education, where, for many reasons, the default is to the pleasure of togetherness and shared taste, the beautiful dominates, and the capacity for endowing new potentials is in consequence reduced.

Conclusion: Continuous Development

When mindfulness is seen as a relational achievement, the considerations for using mindfulness in clinician-patient settings become clear: the pedagogy is the practice, and the practice has no end. Together, whether in a group or a therapeutic dyad, patients and clinicians (or, better, participants and teachers) co-create a space in which it is possible for all to turn towards and be within their experience of the moment. The space is living and responsive, with a neurophysiological background that may create a safety that resonates throughout the group and allows deep social engagement (Porges, 2011). Participants and teachers are able to steep in that atmosphere, that space, and as a result are endowed with potential ways of being that comprise mindfulness, ways that they may bring to old, new and different situations in their lives.

There is a balance and reciprocity in the pedagogy and the formation of teachers in clinical mindfulness applications, particularly the MBIs. Just as participants are changed and shaped through the availability of new potentials, so too are teachers developed by being in the classroom, and that development has no end. The skills of caring for the group and its space, of speaking in ways that reinforce the practice of the pedagogy, of guiding formal meditation practice and of inquiring into participants' moment-to-moment experience become, once a teacher has been introduced to them, self-reinforcing. That is, the skills assist the co-creation of the space in which participants and teacher simply 'are' together: 'being is relational'.

When all are engaged in the pedagogy, learning to turn towards and be within each moment of experience, it is likely that the qualities of the ethical space arise. Participants connect more closely to bodily experiences, which helps to deconstruct emotions as feelings. They are continually expecting and tracking change, as they learn to live in contingency. Further, they are making their own meaning from their experiences, rather than having meanings imposed on them. And it is the non-doing in the pedagogy that helps the environment as well. There is little interest in people's diagnoses from the teacher or other participants, which allows participants to distance the diagnoses as well and to come with beginner's mind to the possibility of each moment. No one can be one-up on another—not even the teacher—since all are experts on their own experience. And, within the pedagogy, mindfulness practice does not aim to cause or create anything; rather, it is an expression of curiosity and courage, an openness, a willingness to turn towards and be within how it is in the moment, whether pleasurable or aversive. A space with such qualities is inherently a space where participants and teacher can be friendly towards their experience and towards others. It may be that a clear definition of the pedagogy of mindfulness is perfect friendship, *teleia philia*, in which the friends are together turned towards the good, rather than towards each other. The good certainly is the central move of the pedagogy—turning towards and being within each moment of experience.

The pedagogy reinforces itself: friendship deepens friendship. It also allows participants, individually and as a reflective group, to encounter that which might terrify them in any other context. Thus, the sublime becomes a measure of the transformative power of the pedagogy in a group or dyad. Touching the extremes offers that paradox of being broken open and becoming more whole, together.

References

Agazarian, Y. M. (1997). *Systems centered therapy for groups*. New York: Guilford.

Baer, R. A., & Krietemeyer, J. (2006). Overview of mindfulness- and acceptance-based treatment approaches. In R. A. Baer (Ed.), *Mindfulness-based treatment approaches: Clinician's guide to evidence base and applications*. Academic: Burlington, MA.

Batchelor, S. (1997). *Buddhism without beliefs: A contemporary guide to awakening*. New York: Riverhead Books.

Burke, E. (1999). *A Philosophical enquiry into the origins of the sublime and beautiful: And other pre-revolutionary writings*. London: Penguin.

Carmody, J., Reed, G., Kristeller, J., & Merriam, P. (2008). Mindfulness, spirituality, and health-related symptoms. *Journal of Psychosomatic Research, 64*, 393–403.

Carr, L., Iacoboni, M., Dubeau, M.-C., Mazziotta, J., & Lenzi, G. (2003). Neural mechanisms of empathy in humans: A relay from neural systems for imitation to limbic areas. *Proceedings of the National Academy of Sciences, 100*, 5497–5502.

CFM. (n.d.). *Mindfulness meditation retreats*. http://www.umassmed.edu/cfm/training/detailed-training-information/meditation-retreats/. Accessed April 27, 2015.

CFM/TDI. (n.d.). *Teacher development intensive*. http://www.umassmed.edu/cfm/training/detailed-training-information/teacher-development-intensive---tdi/. Accessed April 27, 2015.

Chiesa, A., & Serretti, A. (2009). Mindfulness-based stress reduction for stress management in healthy people: A review and meta-analysis. *Journal of Alternative and Complementary Medicine, 15*(5), 593–600.

Cozolino, L. (2006). *The neuroscience of human relationships*. New York: Norton.
Crane, R., & Elias, D. (2006). Being with what is. *Therapy Today, 17*(10), 31–33.
Crane, R., Kuyken, W., Hastings, R. P., Rothwell, M., & Williams, J. M. (2010). Training teachers to deliver mindfulness-based interventions: Learning from the UK experience. *Mindfulness, 1*, 74–86.
Crane, R. S., Stanley, S., Rooney, M., Bartley, T., Cooper, L., & Mardula, J. (2014). Disciplined improvisation: Characteristics of inquiry in mindfulness-based teaching. *Mindfulness*. doi:10.1007/s12671-014-0361-8 [published online 29 November].
Creswell, J. D., Way, B. M., Eisenberger, N. I., & Lieberman, M. D. (2007). Neural correlates of dispositional mindfulness during affect labeling. *Psychosomatic Medicine, 69*, 560–565.
Foucault, M. (1995). Discipline & Punish. New York: Vintage.
Gallese, V., Fadiga, L., Fogassi, L., & Rizzolatti, G. (1996). Action recognition in the premotor cortex. *Brain, 119*, 593–609.
Gallese, V., & Goldman, A. (1998). Mirror neurons and the simulation theory of mindreading. *Trends in Cognitive Sciences, 2*(12), 493–501.
Gergen, K. (2009). *Relational being: Beyond self and community*. Oxford, UK: Oxford University Press.
Gergen, K. (2011). From moral autonomy to relational responsibility. *Zygon, 46*(1), 204–223.
Gergen, K. (2015). An invitation to social construction, third edition. London: SAGE.
Greeson, J. M., Webber, D. M., Smoski, M. J., Brantley, J. G., Ekblad, A. G., Suarez, E. C., et al. (2011). Changes in spirituality partly explain health-related quality of life outcomes after mindfulness-based stress reduction. *Journal of Behavioral Medicine, 34*(6), 508–518 [published online March 1].
Grossman, P. (2010). Mindfulness for psychologists: Paying kind attention to the perceptible. *Mindfulness, 1*, 87–97.
Hayes, A., & Feldman, G. (2004). Clarifying the construct of mindfulness in the context of emotion regulation and the process of change in therapy. *Clinical Psychology: Science and Practice, 11*(3), 255–262.
Horrigan, B. J. (2007). Saki Santorelli, EdD, MA: Mindfulness and medicine. *Explore, 3*(2), 137–144.
Horvath, A., & Bedi, R. (2002). The alliance. In J. Norcross (Ed.), *Psychotherapy relationships that work: Therapist contributions and responsiveness to patients* (pp. 37–70). New York: Oxford University Press.
Imel, Z., Baldwin, S., Bonus, K., & MacCoon, D. (2008). Beyond the individual: Group effects in mindfulness-based stress reduction. *Psychotherapy Research, 18*(6), 735–742.
Ingold, T. (2006). Rethinking the animate, reanimating thought. *Ethnos, 71*(1), 9–20.
Ingold, T. (2008). The social child. In A. Fogel, B. J. King, & S. G. Shanker (Eds.), *Human development in the twenty-first century: Visionary ideas from systems scientists* (pp. 112–118). Cambridge: Cambridge University Press.
Kabat-Zinn, J. (2004). The uses of language and images in guiding meditation practices in MBSR. Audio Recording from 2nd Annual Conference sponsored by the Center for Mindfulness in Medicine, Health Care and Society at the University of Massachusetts Medical School. March 26.
Kabat-Zinn, J. (2010). Foreword. In D. McCown, D. Reibel, & M. Micozzi (Eds.), *Teaching mindfulness: A practical guide for clinicians and educators* (pp. ix–xxii). New York: Springer.
Kabat-Zinn, J. (2011). Some reflections on the origins of MBSR, skillful means, and the trouble with maps. *Contemporary Buddhism, 12*(1), 281–306.
Kabat-Zinn, J., Santorelli, S., Blacker, M., Brantley, J., Meyer, F. M., Grossman, P., et al. (2012). *Training teachers to deliver mindfulness-based stress reduction: Principles and standards*. Downloaded from http://www.umassmed.edu/cfm/trainingteachers/index.aspx. Accessed January 15, 2012.
Kuyken, W., Watkins, E., Holden, E., White, K., Taylor, R. S., Byford, S., et al. (2010). How does mindfulness-based cognitive therapy work? *Behaviour Research and Therapy, 48*(11), 1105–1112.

Lieberman, M. D., Eisenberger, N. I., Crockett, M. J., Tom, S. M., Pfeifer, J. H., & Way, B. M. (2007). Putting feelings into words: Affect labeling disrupts amygdala activity in response to affective stimuli. *Psychological Science, 18*(5), 421–427.

Lindahl, J. R. (2015). Why right mindfulness might not be right for mindfulness. *Mindfulness, 6*, 57–62.

Mamberg, M. H., Dreeben, S. J., & Salmon, P. (2015). *MBSR Languaging: Discursive analysis of the body scan* (in preparation).

McCown, D. (2013). *The ethical space of mindfulness in clinical practice*. London: Jessica Kingsley.

McCown, D. (2014). East meets West in the pedagogy of the mindfulness-based interventions. In A. Ie, C. Ngnoumen, & E. Langer (Eds.), *Wiley-Blackwell handbook of mindfulness*. Oxford: Wiley-Blackwell.

McCown, D., & Ahn, H. *Dialogical and Eastern perspectives on the self in practice: Teaching mindfulness-based stress reduction in Philadelphia and Seoul* (unpublished manuscript).

McCown, D., & Reibel, D. (2009). Mindfulness and mindfulness-based stress reduction. In A. Weil (Ed.), *Integrative psychiatry*. New York: Oxford.

McCown, D., Reibel, D., & Micozzi, M. (2010). *Teaching mindfulness: A practical guide for clinicians and educators*. New York: Springer.

McCown, D., & Wiley, S. (2008). Emergent issues in MBSR research and pedagogy: Integrity, fidelity, and how do we decide? *6th annual conference: Integrating mindfulness-based interventions into medicine, health care, and society,* Worcester, MA, April 10–12.

McCown, D., & Wiley, S. (2009). Thinking the world together: Seeking accord and interdependence in the discourses of mindfulness teaching and research. *7th annual conference: Integrating mindfulness-based interventions into medicine, health care, and society,* Worcester, MA, March 18–22.

Monteiro, L. M., Musten, R. F., & Compton, J. (2015). Traditional and contemporary mindfulness: Finding the middle path in the tangle of concerns. *Mindfulness, 6*, 1–13.

Porges, S. W. (2011). *The polyvagal theory: Neurophysiological foundations of emotions, attachment, communication, and self-regulation*. New York: Norton.

Purser, R. E. (2015). Clearing the muddled path of traditional and contemporary mindfulness: a response to Monteiro, Musten, and Compson. *Mindfulness, 6*, 23–45.

Santorelli, S. (2001). Interview with Saki Santorelli, Stress Reduction Clinic, Massachusetts Memorial Medical Center. In L. Freedman (Ed.), *Best practices in alternative and complementary medicine* (pp. 11-8–1–4). Frederick, MD: Aspen.

Santorelli, S. (Ed.). (2014). *Mindfulness-based stress reduction (MBSR) standards of practice*. Worcester, MA: UMASS Medical School, Center for Mindfulness in Medicine, Health Care & Society.

Sauer, S., Lynch, S., Walach, H., & Kohls, N. (2011). Dialectics of mindfulness: Implications for western medicine. *Philosophy, Ethics, and Humanities in Medicine, 6*, 10.

Segal, Z. V., Williams, J. M. G., & Teasdale, J. D. (2002). *Mindfulness-based cognitive therapy for depression: A new approach to preventing relapse*. New York: Guilford Press.

Sennett, R. (2009). *The Craftsman*. New Haven: Yale.

Sennett, R. (2012). *Together: The rituals, pleasures and politics of cooperation*. New Haven: Yale.

Shaw, P. (2006). *The sublime*. New York: Routledge.

Shonin, E., & Van Gordon, W. (2015). The lineage of mindfulness. *Mindfulness, 6*, 141–145.

Shotter, J. (1984). *Social accountability and selfhood*. Oxford, UK: Blackwell.

Shotter, J. (1995). In conversation: Joint action, shared intentionality, and ethics. *Psychology and Theory, 5*, 49–73.

Shotter, J. (2008). *Conversational realities revisited: Life, language, body and world*. Chagrin Falls, OH: Taos Institute Publications.

Shotter, J. (2011). *Getting it: Witness-thinking and the dialogical…in practice*. New York: Hampton Press.

Shotter, J. (2012). Ontological social constructionism in the context of a social ecology: The importance of our living bodies. In A. Lock & T. Strong (Eds.), *Discursive perspectives in therapeutic practice* (pp. 83–105). Oxford: Oxford University Press.
Siegel, D. (2007). *The mindful brain*. New York: Norton.
Van Gordon, W., Shonin, E., Griffiths, M. D., & Singh, N. N. (2015). There is only one mindfulness: Why science and Buddhism need to work together. *Mindfulness, 6*, 49–56.
Williams, M., & Kabat-Zinn, J. (2011). Mindfulness: Diverse perspectives on its meaning, origins, and multiple applications at the intersection of science and dharma. *Contemporary Buddhism, 12*(1), 1–18.
Williams, M., & Kabat-Zinn, J. (Eds.) (2013). *Mindfulness: Diverse perspectives on its meaning, origins, and applications*. New York: Routledge.
Wittgenstein, L. (1953). *Philosophical investigations*. Oxford, UK: Blackwell.
Zimmerman, J., & Coyle, V. (1996). *The way of council*. Las Vegas: Bramble Books.

Chapter 4
What Is Required to Teach Mindfulness Effectively in MBSR and MBCT?

Jacob Piet, Lone Fjorback, and Saki Santorelli

Introduction

In a book on *Mindfulness and Buddhist-derived Approaches in Mental Health and Addictions*, why devote an entire chapter to the subject matter of skills, capacities and competencies required to teach mindfulness effectively? Might it not be sufficient simply to read the treatment manuals to familiarise oneself with the structure and content of specific mindfulness-based intervention programmes? Let us consider the background for even addressing such a question in the first place.

The majority of mindfulness-based intervention programmes, which are now increasingly being integrated into fields of medicine, health care, education, business, social care and leadership, are either based on or derived from mindfulness-based stress reduction (MBSR), which was developed by Jon Kabat-Zinn in the late 1970s and subsequently refined in close collaboration with his colleagues at the Center for Mindfulness in Medicine, Health Care, and Society, University of Massachusetts Medical School (Kabat-Zinn, 2013; Santorelli, 1999).

MBSR is the coming together of two distinct epistemological traditions or ways of knowing: contemporary empirical science and traditional contemplative practice. Since the development of MBSR, scientific research has been carried out to investigate its health-related benefits. During the last few decades, there has been a dramatic and exponential rise in the number of peer-reviewed published articles on

J. Piet (✉) • L. Fjorback
Danish Center for Mindfulness, Aarhus University Hospital, Noerrebrogade 44, 8000 Aarhus C, Denmark
e-mail: jacobpiet@cfm.dk

S. Santorelli
Center for Mindfulness in Medicine, Health Care, and Society, University of Massachusetts Medical School, Worcester, MA, 01655, USA

E. Shonin et al. (eds.), *Mindfulness and Buddhist-Derived Approaches in Mental Health and Addiction*, Advances in Mental Health and Addiction,
DOI 10.1007/978-3-319-22255-4_4

mindfulness, including numerous clinical trials documenting the beneficial effects of mindfulness-based interventions (Williams & Kabat-Zinn, 2011).

In this chapter, mindfulness-based interventions (MBIs) refer to MBSR and programmes modelled on MBSR that have been adapted to specific clinical and non-clinical populations. The two main MBIs we will focus on are MBSR (Kabat-Zinn, 2013) and mindfulness-based cognitive therapy (MBCT) (Segal, Williams, & Teasdale, 2013). These programmes are well structured, based on systematic training in mindfulness meditation, and have an extensive base of scientific evidence. Indeed, as the empirical evidence has grown strong, MBSR and MBCT are now supported by results from several recently published meta-analyses (e.g. Hoffmann, Sawyer, Witt, & Oh, 2010; Khoury et al., 2013; Piet & Hougaard, 2011; Piet, Würtzen, & Zachariae, 2012).

While the results derived from empirical investigation are highly promising, it is worth noting that in the majority of published studies of MBSR and MBCT, the intervention was carried out by highly skilled and well-trained MBI teachers, many of whom are dedicated long-term students of contemplative practice with deeply integrated and embodied knowledge of mindfulness acquired through decades of ongoing daily practice of mindfulness meditation, coupled with a detailed grasp of the MBSR/MBCT curriculum and solid interpersonal and didactic teaching skills.

However, it cannot be taken for granted that the inherent integrity and quality of the first generation of MBI teachers have been or will be successfully passed on to future generations. Indeed, as mindfulness is becoming increasingly popular and integrated into the mainstream of society, the proposition becomes more tenuous. Many health-care professionals, who are oriented towards evidence-based clinical interventions, now seek professional education and training in MBSR and MBCT without prior experience of training in mindfulness meditation. While this is encouraging, it also presents a huge challenge to the people responsible for training future MBI teachers. Given the statement below by Jon Kabat-Zinn, the professional training of MBI teachers may be of uttermost importance to ensure the quality and integrity of interventions based on training in mindfulness:

> … the quality of MBSR as an intervention is only as good as the MBSR instructor and his or her understanding of what is required to deliver a truly mindfulness-based programme. (Kabat-Zinn, 2011, pp. 281–282)

Indeed, if the teacher is a significant moderator of the intervention outcome, in particular, the extent to which he or she embodies genuine knowledge and understanding of mindfulness and the specific mindfulness-based programme, then inadequate training of novice teachers, with no prior experience of mindfulness meditation, will have serious implications for future research. The worst-case scenario is that future studies with inadequately trained MBI teachers may no longer find and report any beneficial effects of MBSR and MBCT, nor be able to replicate positive findings found in previous studies. As such, we strongly suggest that the professional trajectory for educating and training teachers to competently deliver a mindfulness-based programme is a critical necessity for maintaining the quality and integrity of MBSR and MBCT as well as their adaptations.

Effective Teachers

The attempt to write and decide on the main content of a chapter on effectively teaching mindfulness within MBSR and MBCT is immediately humbling. Why is that? One might ask. Experiencing highly effective MBSR teachers over long periods of time, aspiring professionals often report observing the following: these teachers are apparently not using any specific technique; they rarely respond in a stereotypical manner; they do not give lectures to the programme participants; they do not put on a professional attitude or persona; they often make no attempt to position themselves as teachers, and they do not appear to be so caught up in the tendency of wanting to be liked. They are deeply and personally engaged in teaching. They are not afraid to turn towards people in the midst of suffering, as suffering takes the form of pain, loss, anger, aggression, sadness, sorrow, despair, doubt, agitation, jealousy, etc. They appear to really listen to what is being said, sometimes you may even get the impression that they manage to comprehend the fuller meaning of what is being expressed beneath the spoken words, as they are not exclusively focussed on the verbal forms of communication. They appear to be in tune with what is unfolding in the present moment. Importantly, independent assessors, using the mindfulness-based interventions–teaching assessment criteria (MBI:TAC), have observed the embodiment of these teacher qualities and competencies (Crane et al., 2013). However, as we shall see below, these 'advanced' teachers are not 'special'. In fact, they exhibit a lot of the same qualities of any well-seasoned teacher across a wide array of fields.

In the educational literature, the question of 'what makes an expert teacher?' has been thoroughly investigated. Similar to the description of highly effective MBSR teachers, expert teachers across disciplines are characterised by traits such as autonomy and flexibility. Moreover, their teaching reflects a rich and integrated knowledge base, they demonstrate a high degree of awareness of important contextual variables, they have accurate pattern recognition, and they show creative problem-solving together with highly developed improvisational skills for relating to the immediacy and unpredictability of classroom events (Tsui, 2003; Berliner 2004a, 2004b).

Apparently, innate talent is not the most critical factor for the development of a high degree of expertise. Rather, people identified as experts have all studied with devoted teachers and practised intensively while being deeply engaged in the demanding process of continuously learning from feedback (see Ericsson, Charness, Feltovich, & Hoffman, 2006). According to Ericsson, Prietula, & Cokely (2007), the development of genuine expertise involves struggle, sacrifice and honest and often painful self-assessment.

While seasoned and highly effective mindfulness teachers, like most expert teachers in general, often function as a source of great inspiration, as living evidence of what might be possible in terms of learning and growing as a human being on the path of becoming a teacher, their level of integrity and competency should not represent 'the' benchmark for prospective teachers in terms of what is required to begin teaching. This is simply because the traits and qualities that such expert teachers manifest and embody are the consequence of many years of deliberate practice and teaching in a process of being highly committed to lifelong learning.

To help guide prospective and novice MBSR and MBCT teachers, it is therefore much more appropriate to explore professional training and teaching skills and competencies that may be considered competent or 'good enough' to begin teaching. In fact, models have been proposed that may serve to provide systematic and sustained guidance as one enters into the territory of becoming an MBI teacher.

In the following parts of this chapter, we identify key elements of professional teacher education and training, standards for teaching and proposed competencies considered 'good enough' to effectively deliver mindfulness-based interventions.

An Integrative Model of Quality and Integrity

In the Japanese Zen tradition, the term *koan* is sometimes used to refer to a story, question or statement to be meditated upon in order to reach a deeper understanding of aspects of reality, not merely based on logic and intellectual reasoning. The *koan* of this chapter, so to speak, is to try to uncover the very fabric that good teachers are made of. What makes a teacher effective? Is it their academic background? Is it their professional training as a mindfulness instructor? Is it because they are in alignment with established good practice standards of teaching mindfulness-based interventions? Is it a matter of acquired competencies or skills? Is it the ethical foundation of their behaviour? Might it concern the teacher's ability to be fully human, knowing intimately the human condition? If so, can this be taught? Or might it have everything to do with the first-person experience of being committed to a life fully lived? Is it possible that highly effective MBI teachers may at times hold an awareness that sees things as they are, with great compassion and the urge to relieve suffering? Might they in their interaction with others be guided by a form of perception that is not clouded by personal preferences, opinions, strategies and agendas and therefore able to relate much more directly in order to actually be of service? How many of us teachers can live up to such standards? Perhaps at our inherent 'best', we all can, as the potential for awareness and compassion is already ours, already intact and 'simply' needs to be discovered or uncovered, nurtured and applied through practice and teaching.

To begin with, let's have a look at one available map of the territory of becoming a competent teacher. Figure 4.1 is an extension of a working model presented by Crane et al. (2012) of three interconnected aspects of quality and integrity in teaching mindfulness-based courses, namely, (a) *professional training*, (b) *good practice standards* and (c) *teaching competencies*. To highlight that the process of becoming an effective teacher is by far a professional undertaking alone, we have added an outer circle to the model called 'life practice' based on an 'inner ethical foundation' and 'awareness as the essential ground' for living and teaching mindfulness, together with an orientation towards 'contemplative traditions and lineages' that have been deeply engaged in cultivating and refining mindfulness over millennia.

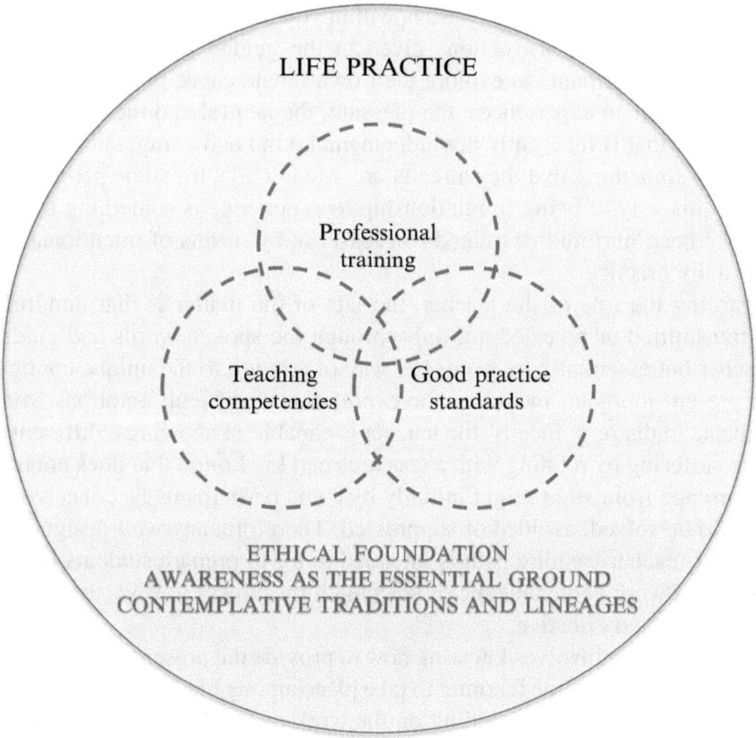

Fig. 4.1 The life practice of integrity and quality in teaching mindfulness

As such, the model serves to illustrate how an all-integrating view of teaching mindfulness may support the field in the long-term perspective of maintaining integrity and quality among mindfulness-based teachers. We find it especially important that teaching mindfulness is not viewed as some professional endeavours separate from the foundational intention and practice of bringing awareness to all aspects of one's life nor separate from the vast wisdom of contemplative traditions and practicing lineages. The different interconnected components of the model will be explained in detail in the following parts of this chapter.

Professional Training and Education

Because mindfulness is a capacity of mind that cannot be discovered and refined through intellectual understanding alone, the act of teaching mindfulness takes on a certain complexity different from that of other forms of academic knowledge acquired and assimilated primarily through reading and study. Teaching mindfulness can be likened to the well-known metaphor of a finger pointing at the moon. If you look too much at the finger, you are likely to miss the full beauty of the moon and, more so, the 'moon-like' qualities within you that allow you to 'recognise' the moon. In parallel, the instructions given in the guided practices of MBSR and MBCT invite participants to explore their own innate capacity for attending to the full range of human experiences, the pleasant, the neutral and the unpleasant, with an awareness that is inherently nonjudgemental, kind and compassionate. They are discovering something that they already are. Meanwhile, for some people, it is possible that this way of being in relationship to experience is something that has not previously been nurtured or trained—at least not by means of intentional and systematic daily practice.

Regarding the role of the teacher, the fact of the matter is that mindfulness is being transmitted or revealed not only through the spoken words and guidance of the teacher but essentially by his or her way of relating to the unique configuration of the present moment, including the expression of difficult emotions from class participants in distress. Ideally, the teacher is capable of showing a different way of meeting suffering by relating with a spacious and kind mind that does not try to fix, alter or escape from what might initially by some participants be conceived of as a problem to be solved, avoided or suppressed. Therefore, any well-designed professional MBI teacher-training path is intended to try to prepare students for entering into the great work and challenge of teaching mindfulness in ways that are actually transformative and effective.

Importantly, this involves knowing how to provide the present moment space and ground needed for genuine learning to take place among class participants. It resembles what Robert Kegan, expanding on the work of D. H. Winnicott, has termed a healthy holding environment characterised by (1) 'confirming' people where they are while validating their absolute rightness; (2) skilfully introducing 'contradiction', often using questions to spur curiosity and further investigation; and (3) offering 'continuity' to support learning over time (for a detailed description of these three core processes within the context of teaching MBSR, see Santorelli, 2015).

As mindfulness continues to be integrated within the mainstream of society, professional training institutes have been established within university settings around the world. These include Center for Mindfulness in Medicine, Health Care, and Society, University of Massachusetts Medical School (http://www.umassmed.edu/cfm/); Oxford Mindfulness Centre, University of Oxford (http://oxfordmindfulness.org); Centre for Mindfulness Research and Practice, Bangor University (http://www.bangor.ac.uk/mindfulness/); Danish Center for Mindfulness, Aarhus University Hospital (http://mindfulness.au.dk).

Any professional training path that remains true to the integrity of mindfulness-based interventions such as MBSR and MBCT will often include the following successive phases:

1. Prerequisites

   To begin with, prospective teachers must complete the relevant MBI as a class participant. This initial phase provides an opportunity for learning from the inside what it actually means to be engaged in bringing mindfulness into everyday life by participating in a structured mindfulness-based programme.

Throughout the teacher training and beyond, this first-person perspective of direct experience of mindfulness is further cultivated, strengthened, refined and stabilised through ongoing daily meditation practice as well as regularly attending mindfulness meditation retreats. Indeed, attending 5–10 days silent teacher-led retreat is usually another prerequisite for embarking on a path of professional teacher training in MBSR or MBCT. Furthermore, a professional degree in mental or physical health care, education or social care and prior knowledge and experience of the particular clinical or nonclinical population, for whom the intervention is adapted for, are often required.

2. Foundational teacher training

This phase involves attending several professional training courses intended to prepare the students to begin teaching. One such training course might include attending the 8-week MBSR or MBCT programme as a so-called participant-observer. This involves full participation in the programme with fellow class participants, followed by weekly reflection, and study together with other prospective teachers, led by a senior teacher. This format is highly praised as it allows future teachers to enter into dialogue and inquiry with an experienced teacher about the actual unfolding of each in vivo session of the 8-week programme. Likewise, it mirrors an aspect of mindfulness practice itself: the capacity to both observe (observer) and feel (participant) the full range of body sensations, thoughts and emotions arising in the continually changing field of awareness. Bhante Gunaratana says it like this:

> Mindfulness is participatory observation. The meditator is both participant and observer at one and the same time. If one watches one's emotions or physical sensations, one is feeling them at that very same moment. Mindfulness is not an intellectual awareness. It is just awareness. The mirror-thought metaphor breaks down here. Mindfulness is objective, but it is not cold or unfeeling. It is the wakeful experience of life, an alert participation in the ongoing process of living. (Gunaratana, 2011, p. 135)

Usually, completion of one or more 5–10 days silent, teacher-led mindfulness meditation retreat is required before attending the next level of professional training. Retreats are considered an absolute necessity for developing one's own meditation practice, for refining and stabilizing attention and awareness, for cultivating greater kindness towards oneself and others, and for developing one's understanding and effectiveness as a teacher (Santorelli, 1999, 2015; Kabat-Zinn, 2011). Additional training courses are often weeklong intensive trainings in which the cultivation of mindfulness is closely interwoven with learning and observing specific core teaching skills. Furthermore, at this stage, led by experienced teacher trainers, students may start to guide one another in a series of different mindfulness practices while learning how to give and receive nuanced and constructive feedback.

In this second phase, essential study courses are also offered, including subjects on, for example, the science of mindfulness, stress physiology, psychoeducation on depression, interpersonal mindfulness, group dynamics, the use of story and metaphor in teaching, introduction to relevant aspects of Buddhist psychology, etc.

3. Advanced teacher training

   In addition to further teacher training, aimed at refining essential teaching skills, this phase encourages teachers to enter into a period of teaching under supervision by an experienced senior MBI teacher. This allows for a deepening of their understanding of the 8-week programme as well as of themselves as an MBSR or MBCT teacher, including shedding light on any barriers that may prevent effective teaching. As for all other phases in the formation of teachers, attending silent meditation retreats is a mandatory discipline.
4. Ongoing professional and personal development

   This phase involves a deep commitment to sustain and refine mindfulness through daily formal and informal practice, as well as attending silent retreats on a regular basis. Also, the teacher needs to keep up with the relevant literature and evidence base of mindfulness. Supervision when needed is strongly recommended as well as familiarisation with the current good practice standards for teaching MBSR and MBCT. In addition, ongoing participant evaluation of intervention outcome is regarded as good practice. Finally, this phase may include a teacher certification review.

Good Practice Principles and Standards

For people wishing to teach mindfulness as a mind-body intervention, in ways that ideally correspond with the quality and integrity of the original MBSR approach, good practice guidelines, principles and standards are now available.

The following six points to be considered and embodied over time by any teacher of MBSR and related MBIs have been emphasised by Kabat-Zinn (1996). They include the guiding principles of:

(a) Making experience and the act of observing one's life mindfully an adventure to be lived and a challenge to be met
(b) Prioritising individual effort, motivation and discipline in the daily formal practicing of mindfulness, regardless of whether one 'feels' like it or not
(c) Understanding the immediate change of lifestyle required to fully participate in MBSR, given extensive daily homework
(d) Deliberately prioritising the full experience of each unfolding moment during formal and informal practice
(e) A group format and time-limited structure with an educational orientation as the foundation for forming a community of learning and practicing to cultivate ongoing support and motivation together with feelings of acceptance and belonging
(f) A generic approach focussing on common humanity, and what is right with people rather than what is wrong, on deep inner resources rather than limitations and on active involvement in one's own healing process rather than adopting a passive attitude

Although substantial research has found therapeutic effects of MBSR (e.g. reduced symptoms of stress, anxiety and depression), it has been underscored that MBSR is 'not' therapy; it is a way of being (Kabat-Zinn, 2006).

More recently, a number of standards and guidelines have been proposed to promote good practice in teaching mindfulness to people in the mainstream of society and to help maintain and protect the quality and integrity of research-supported mindfulness-based intervention programmes. The key principles and aspects of these standards and guidelines are summarised below:

1. MBI teachers need to have a strong commitment to the practice of mindfulness meditation sustained through (a) daily practice and (b) ongoing participation in retreats, in order to deepen their own practice and understanding which provide the very ground of teaching mindfulness.
2. Adherence to the principle of never asking more of participants in terms of daily practice requirements than you as a teacher ask of yourself. On a similar account 'Do not teach what you do not know'. For example, by not guiding participants in mindfulness practices that you do not know intimately through your own direct experience or so-called first-person perspective. This form of knowledge, while rooted in the present moment, is gained from the teachers' own long-term practice of mindfulness meditation practice.
3. Understanding the noninstrumental nature of teaching mindfulness. That mindfulness, rather than being a set of techniques to be acquired or a particular mental state to be attained, essentially is a way of being in wise relationship to experience.
4. Commitment to ongoing learning and development as a teacher through (a) further training and regular supervision by senior MBI teachers, (b) continuing collaboration with MBI colleagues, (c) keeping updated with the relevant scientific literature on mindfulness and (d) gaining an understanding of the historical roots of mindfulness by studying some of the essential texts from relevant contemplative traditions, in particular Buddhism, that are grounded in mindfulness practice and remain informative for bringing mindfulness into the lives of people in modern society. To begin an exploration of mindfulness at the intersection of science and dharma, *Contemporary Buddhism, volume 12, issue 1*, is a helpful place to start.
5. Adherence to ethical guidelines, including a fair pricing structure for mindfulness-based courses as well as for professional training of mindfulness-based teachers.

In addition, in a paper on practical recommendations for teaching mindfulness effectively, Shonin and Van Gordon (2014a, 2014b) have emphasised the importance of remembering to practice mindfulness while teaching and guiding others. To support this intention, they strongly recommend taking time to restabilise attention and re-establish oneself in the present moment immediately before teaching a class or group of people. Such an effort, to actually pause before teaching MBSR or MBCT, can provide a powerful shift from (a) the usual doing mode of mind to (b) being present and available to others in ways that embody the practice of mindfulness.

Furthermore, these authors caution teachers against trying to appear 'too mindful'. They also point out some of the characteristics that may define a teacher who does not have much presence of mind. These include (1) an overly pious demeanour, (2) constant and/or inappropriate smiling, (3) not being able to introduce genuine joy and light-heartedness into their teachings and (4) doing things excessively slowly when others are watching while rushing around mindlessly at other times. These characteristics may be worth looking for, at least in ourselves as teachers, as they are all based on a 'mental idea' of how a teacher who is mindful should behave, rather than actually teaching from within present moment awareness in ways that are embodied, authentic, relaxed and transparent to reality. In addition to a regular practice of mindfulness, it may be very beneficial continuously to remind oneself that the work of teaching mindfulness is all about being at the service of other people. To actually be at service may require that we learn to get out of our own way. Being caught up by our personal preferences, needs and agendas, e.g. the need to be seen, heard and respected, can easily create a barrier for helping others towards growth and well-being. In Buddhism, too much attachment to one's ego or self-image is a root cause of suffering, and it may indeed be the greatest hindrance for maturing as a person and teacher to effectively teach mindfulness. While many people may begin teaching with pure intentions, there is a real risk for all of us to become inflated and corrupted by even the slightest bit of fame or success (ibid.). This is one reason why it is important for mindfulness teachers to have (1) a mentor (teacher), (2) access to teachings and practical guidelines for travelling the path of awakening (dharma) and (3) a community (sangha) of fellow meditation practitioners. Such fortunate circumstances, in Buddhism referred to as the three jewels, can provide immediate feedback and regulation to protect against crucial pitfalls on the journey of becoming an authentic and effective teacher.

For further details on standards of good practice of teaching MBSR and MBCT, please see the following documents, as well as practical recommendations for teaching mindfulness by Shonin and Van Gordon (2014a, 2014b):

http://www.umassmed.edu/cfm/stress-reduction/mbsr-standards-of-practice/
http://www.umassmed.edu/cfm/training/principles--standards/http://mindfulnessteachersuk.org.uk

In addition, at the Center for Mindfulness in Medicine, Health Care, and Society (CFM), University of Massachusetts Medical School, standards of practice for trainers of MBSR instructors have been outlined. Apart from having (1) completed the MBSR professional training path, (2) taught a minimum of 15 8-week MBSR courses and (3) received MBSR teachers certification granted by the CFM, MBSR teacher trainers are required to (4) engage in ongoing MBSR teacher training consultation, (5) regularly attend teacher-led silent meditation retreats, (6) maintain a sustained personal practice of mindfulness meditation and mindful Hatha yoga and (7) embody learner-centred teaching skills, a capacity for deep listening, regard and compassion for all participants, highly developed sensitivity to the use of language, knowledge of the art of dialogue and inquiry with class participants and an ability to create and maintain a safe container for exploration and learning in the face of stress, pain, illness and suffering (for details, see http://www.umassmed.edu/cfm/training/principles--standards/). Similarly, the UK Network for Mindfulness-Based Teacher Trainer Organizations has proposed good practice guidelines for trainers of mindfulness-based teachers (see http://mindfulnessteachersuk.org.uk).

Teaching Skills and Competencies

Given the effort of novice teachers to adhere to the professional standards of practice, committing oneself to the path of meditation, and being called by the imperative to begin to turn towards suffering with skilful means, what essential teaching competencies might hopefully be discovered, developed and refined over time?

First of all, the foundation or basic ground of teaching mindfulness within MBSR and MBCT is awareness itself. For mindfulness to be truly effective, the capacity for nonjudgemental awareness, clear seeing and genuine compassion needs to be directly known and embodied by teachers, in their life and in their teachings. By genuine compassion, we mean compassion that is felt and experienced from the inside to the extent that it naturally and effortlessly flows out in the form of deeply caring about the well-being of others. When such qualities of being are embodied by the teacher, and inform the teaching process moment by moment, it allows for being in direct relationship to other people with an open mind and heart that is capable of listening deeply by offering a form of attention that is not caught up in discursive thinking based on theory and analysis, or personal ideas, beliefs, preferences and opinions, all of which may characterise our 'default' state of mind. Therefore, as emphasised in a paper on dialogue and inquiry in the MBSR classroom:

> The MBSR teacher's capacity for appreciating and cultivating mutually-ennobling relationships with participants, for sympathetic resonance, gratitude, warmth, clarity and flexibility in making moment-by-moment choices in response to class participants' experiences requires them to be firmly committed to a keen and persistent observation of their own experience. (Santorelli, 2015)

This of course is asking a lot of people, perhaps especially of those who may enter into a professional training pathway to learn MBSR or MBCT based on the assumption that mindfulness is simply a set of skills or competencies that can easily be observed, learned, imitated and then applied in order to successfully carry out the intervention. While some people, these days, may come to a professional training pathway with a limited understanding of what it takes, many may, over time, come to see that a lot more is at stake. In fact, this recognition may give rise to an even deeper motivation and reorganisation of their initial intention for learning and studying MBSR or MBCT.

In a book on teaching mindfulness, McCown, Reibel and Micozzi (2010) identify four sets of interrelated skills that appear to be shared among MBI teachers. These are:

1. 'Stewardship' of the group, which emphasises a nonhierarchical, participatory-oriented form of teaching in which the teacher holds the space in a certain way that creates a sense of freedom and belonging to allow participants to explore and share their direct experience of the joys and sorrows of the human condition.
2. 'Homiletics', used by the authors to refer to a certain way of delivering didactic material to convey principles of the pedagogy of MBSR. Rather than presenting information from an 'expert lecturing' stance, information is co-created by engaging participants using skilful questioning, reflections, stories and poetry. This approach can provide a starting point for delivering didactic material in ways that make central themes of MBSR (e.g. perception, stress and communication) personally relevant. For example, people in an MBSR class already know a lot about stress in terms of their direct personal experience, and probing this knowledge may be very helpful in order to cocreate and unfold knowledge about stress physiology.
3. 'Guidance' of formal and informal practices and exercises using language that is non-commanding and invitational in ways that allow people to feel and experience what they are actually feeling and experiencing beyond judgements or expectations. Most importantly, the teacher needs to be anchored in the present moment in order to effectively guide others towards paying attention nonjudgementally to the unfolding of different aspects of their moment-by-moment experience.
4. 'Inquiry' into participants' direct experience of practicing mindfulness. Inquiry is a form of conversation or dialogue based on the presence, openness and curiosity on behalf of the teacher in ways that support participants in exploring, acknowledging and discovering the full territory of their own direct experience of themselves and their lives.

Interestingly, the authors emphasise that these four skill sets completely depend upon the teacher's authenticity, authority and friendship, in particular, the teacher's capacity for remaining present and responding thoughtfully and compassionately to whatever arises in the present moment (ibid.). The topic of dialogue and inquiry between teacher and class participants in MBSR and MBCT is further addressed later in this chapter.

In parallel, in a series of papers, Crane et al. (Crane et al., 2010, 2012, 2013) have proposed a number of core competencies for teaching mindfulness-based interventions that provide the foundation for assessing MBSR/MBCT intervention integrity. These competencies are reflected in the following six domains:

1. Coverage, pacing and organisation of each session
2. Relational skills
3. Embodiment of mindfulness
4. Guiding mindfulness practices

5. Conveying course themes through interactive inquiry and didactic teaching
6. Holding the group learning environment

Based on the above six domains (or teaching assessment criteria), the scale developed by Crane and colleagues, the mindfulness-based interventions–teaching assessment criteria (MBI:TAC), has been reported to be a reliable and valid tool for evaluating the integrity of MBSR/MBCT by means of assessing teacher competencies (Crane et al., 2013). The MBI:TAC may prove useful for assessing teacher competencies in order to:

(a) Support the development and formation of future MBI teachers in professional training programmes by monitoring their level of competency. Such routine may help to both evaluate the effectiveness of the professional training process and to identify specific skills that need further refinement before prospective teachers are ready to deliver MBSR/MBCT in real-world settings in alignment with the integrity of the approach.
(b) Optimise the quality and integrity of MBSR/MBCT in future research studies. In particular, the MBI:TAC may help to select highly competent teachers to ensure a high degree of teacher fidelity in future clinical trials. Indeed, several reviews and meta-analyses (e.g. Baer, 2003; Grossman et al., 2004) have pointed to the lack of assessment of teacher fidelity in trials investigating the effects of mindfulness-based interventions. As discussed earlier in this chapter, the quality and integrity of the MBSR/MBCT teacher may actually be a significant moderator of the intervention effect. Although plausible, this hypothesis remains to be tested, confirmed or rejected, by empirical research.

Life Practice

As emphasised previously in this chapter, the foundation for teaching mindfulness rests on the capacity of the teacher to stay present and open with a nonjudgemental attitude. This way of being in relationship to whatever arises in the field of awareness, even in the midst of difficult situations and painful experiences, is very different from the usual habit of relating to experience through the filter of judgement and personal opinions of right and wrong. Indeed, it may be, in and of itself, a radical form of loving-kindness.

Initially, we have the rich texture of our personal life as a training arena to explore and implement new ways of being in wise relationship to our own suffering. This work of individual liberation over a lifetime is informed by our meditation practice. In Buddhism, it is sometimes referred to as the journey of the foundational vehicle, which is considered necessary for learning how to stay present to other people who are suffering (Trungpa, 2013a, 2013b).

From this perspective, teaching mindfulness is not separate from the intention to be present to what Jon Kabat-Zinn has called the full catastrophe, namely, life itself. The term *life practice* or *integral life practice* is sometimes used to refer to specific complementary and mutually supportive practices for developing one's body, mind, emotional capacities and interpersonal skills (see Leonard & Murphy, 1995; Wilber, Patten, Leonard, & Morelli, 2008; Risom, 2010). However, we use the term *life practice* in a broader sense to refer to the intention of bringing the same quality of awareness and attention that is cultivated through the formal practice of mindfulness meditation into every imaginable aspect of life, sometimes called informal practice, including the interpersonal domains, the act of cooking and eating, working, exercising, making love, taking out the garbage, caring for the children, etc. It also involves periodically going into therapy to help resolve or coming to terms with personal trauma as well as other aspects of one's personality and relational patterns that may at times in very real ways prevent one from relating to others with clarity and compassion.

This ongoing commitment to personal growth and self-development together with several other factors—including a sustained practice of mindfulness meditation, consistent silent retreats, regular mentoring and supervision by senior teachers, as well as self-inquiry into the questions of who and what I am—is what Saki Santorelli has called 'the real work of an MBSR teacher' (Santorelli, 2015).

A lack of this kind of knowledge of oneself may cause a great barrier to being effective as an MBSR or MBCT teacher. For example, unresolved anger or sadness may arise in a teaching situation, and to the extent that the teacher is taken over by such strong emotions, it may completely prevent him or her from seeing the situation clearly. Rather than responding with clarity and kindness, it may lead to automatic and fearful reactions based on old habitual patterns. This therapeutic work, which is considered part of an integrative life practice leading to greater self-knowledge, may be required in order to start navigating more freely in one's life and teaching—perhaps in ways that may at times to some degree dissolve the perceived barrier between oneself and others. The Japanese Zen meditation master Dogen beautifully expresses the way of transcending the experience of being an isolated self that is separate from others:

> To study the Way is to study the self. To study the self is to forget the self. To forget the self is to be enlightened by all things. To be enlightened by all things is to remove the barriers between one's self and others. (Dogen, 2002)

Thus, we view teaching mindfulness as something that is by no means separate from one's life. Awareness is the essential ground of all of life, including teaching others to discover their own full potential for attention and awareness as necessary means for learning, and growing, and for coming to terms with things as they are. For a clear and simple presentation of mindfulness meditation as a practice of life awareness, please see Risom (2010).

Ethical foundation

> MBSR is at its healthiest and best when the responsibility to ensure its integrity, quality, and standards of practice is being carried by each MBSR instructor him or herself. (Kabat-Zinn, 2011, p. 295)

Integrity of the approach is fundamentally carried by each individual teacher and therefore involves carefully attending to how we as teachers live our personal and professional lives. This endeavour is supported by the intention to bring full awareness to the present moment, including one's own state of body and mind, in order to skilfully relate in ways that prioritise right conduct and the well-being of others. For many of us, to actually be in touch with awareness of our interior experience in a moment-by-moment manner, while relating to others, may not be all that easy. However, it can be cultivated, stabilised and refined through the practice of mindfulness. Indeed, this present moment capacity, to know one's emotional state with the configuration of thoughts that usually comes along with it, can make a real difference by virtue of awareness itself that allows for freedom to choose to respond (or not to respond) in alignment with the intention to benefit others. This contrasts the usual process in which we are normally hooked and triggered by potentially harming emotional states such as anger, rage, jealousy, envy, pride, etc. With no awareness of our own interior landscape, we run the risk of being driven by automatic habitual reactions that manifest through words and behaviour that can cause unforeseen harm to our relationships and to ourselves.

As such, ethics are not primarily guided by a set of external values, rules or guidelines. Rather ethical behaviour arises from having, to some extent, developed genuine empathy and compassion for others and also from having gained insight into the causes of suffering. In teaching mindfulness, this involves present moment skilful means in order to differentiate between (a) behavioural responses, including any form of communication, that may support others to discover their own innate capacity for awareness, wisdom, kindness and compassion and (b) behavioural responses that are likely not to be helpful to the learning, growing and healing of other people.

This perspective on ethics, the imperative of the teacher to live with care and attention, invites there to be no separation between one's practice and one's life. At the same time, MBSR and MBCT rest on an ethical foundation that lies at the very root of medicine and health care, namely, the Hippocratic oath or principle of *primum non nocere*, meaning above all 'to first do no harm'. It is remarkable how this guiding principle at least to some extent resembles the Bodhisattva vow which in classical and contemporary Buddhism reflects the intention to devote one's life to work for the well-being of others (Kabat-Zinn, 2011; Harvey, 2013; Santorelli, 1999, 2015). For a more detailed description of the ethos of MBSR, please see Santorelli (2015).

Tradition, Lineage and Modern Society

> MBSR is simply a contemporary expression of a twenty six hundred year old meditation tradition that has at its heart, the cultivation of a human being's familiarity with the one awareness that already is. (Santorelli, 2015)

Given that the practice of mindfulness meditation within many ancient contemplative traditions, in particularly Buddhism, has been passed on from one generation to the next for at least 2500 years, let us consider some of the traditional requirements for teaching mindfulness.

In general, within these traditions, you would receive authorisation to teach the dharma (the teachings of the Buddha), including guiding practitioners in the life-long process of working with mindfulness meditation, through what is commonly known as 'lineage transmission'. Traditionally, this responsibility was, and still is, granted by lineage holders within each particular contemplative tradition, only to highly devoted, gifted and dedicated long-term students, who, in their way of conducting themselves with integrity of thought, speech and action, to a large extent, embody what the dharma is all about. This embodied knowledge and insight are presumably acquired through intensive and prolonged study and practice of the dharma, including formal and informal practice of mindfulness meditation. However, lineage can be transmitted in several different ways, e.g. oral transmission, written transmission or mind-to-mind transmission. Ultimately, and beyond any formal means of transmission and approval, a lineage holder is someone who embodies genuine presence with the mark of wisdom, unconditional compassion and steadfast awareness. Therefore, inner realisation of the dharma, recognition of the essence of consciousness, may be the only true credential that counts (for details on lineage transmission, please see Shonin & Van Gordon, 2014a, 2014b). For readers interested in a nuanced description of the functions of ordinary consciousness that covers the essence of mind, please see Bertelsen (2013).

Thus, traditionally, only relatively few people had achieved a level of personal maturation considered adequate for effectively teaching others the practice of meditation.

A basic view in many traditions of contemplative practice is that the innate human capacity for clarity of awareness, kindness and compassion and essentially the wisdom needed to respond in a manner that does not cause harm to people, is something that can be nurtured and developed through sustained practice and right livelihood. In many of these traditions, and explicitly addressed in Mahayana Buddhism, a fundamental motivation is the cultivation of *bodhichitta,* which means 'mind of awakening', and *metta* which means 'loving-kindness', namely, human qualities needed to effectively guide and help suffering beings. To take on this lifelong work and responsibility—to nurture and cultivate these important aspects of the human mind and heart to relieve suffering in oneself and others—may be exactly what is needed, not only for the future generation of mindfulness-based teachers but for humanity all together. We are as a species, and as part of the larger order of sentience, in a very precarious place in human history. Potentially, we could do enormous damage to the planet and all life forms that inhabit this small sphere. It is well known that we, due to ever-greater consumption, have depleted the Earth of many of its resources. According to Rifkin (2009), we now have a world in crisis that more than ever needs a global shift towards greater empathy to save the Earth and improve on our species' ability to survive and flourish in the future. The practice of mindfulness meditation is one means of bringing about such a shift towards greater empathy and compassion.

Now, as mindfulness is increasingly integrated within the mainstream of society, including health care, education, business and leadership—mainly due to scientific research documenting the effect and applicability of MBSR and MBCT in a broad range of clinical and nonclinical populations—there is a need to increase the capacity of people who can effectively deliver interventions based on mindfulness.

The downside to the popularisation of mindfulness, what we might call worst-case scenarios, is the training courses offered for becoming a certified mindfulness instructor by attending a single weekend course or two. Such initiatives run the risk of seriously compromising the quality and integrity of mindfulness-based interventions. These interventions, carried out by less competent teachers, are in fact likely not to be based on mindfulness. If mindfulness, as a core trait and way of being in relationship to oneself, others and the world, could be taught and acquired in just a few days or weeks, without previous experience of practicing mindfulness, this would be no problem. But it turns out—as with training of any genuine human capacity, including the acquisition of different languages, mathematics, athletics and musical skills—that it takes time and effort to develop, nurture and refine the inherent capacity for being present to whatever is unfolding in the mind-body-heart moment by moment.

The rigorous traditional requirements for teaching mindfulness, embodied by some living teachers within contemplative traditions, may provide an inspiring perspective in terms of the potential possibilities for human growth and development. However, as described in the beginning of this chapter, it is not helpful to view the marks of an expert as standards of what is required to begin teaching—simply because the characteristics of an expert teacher are the result of decades of practice and learning. Rather, to sum up, we suggest that the proposed MBI teacher competencies and standards of good practice, outlined in this chapter, reflect what might be considered adequate or 'good enough' to begin teaching mindfulness in MBSR and MBCT.

To assist novice teachers in the process of further growth and development, a competent mentor or senior teacher is highly recommended. In the poem below, the Sufi master Rumi beautifully describes the process of transformation from being raw to being cooked by one's teacher and undone by the heat of life. All in service of one day becoming effective as a teacher—capable of teaching others to discover their own innate capacity for living life fully with awareness and the courage of an open heart that is responsive and responsible to oneself, others and the world—perhaps with an increasing sense that the perceived separation between self and others may be somewhat artificial.

Chickpea to Cook

A chickpea leaps almost over the rim of the pot where it's being boiled.
'Why are you doing this to me?'
The cook knocks him down with the ladle.
'Don't you try to jump out. You think I'm torturing you. I'm giving you flavour, so you can mix with spices and rice and be the lovely vitality of a human being. Remember when you drank rain in the garden. That was for this'.

Grace first. Sexual pleasure, then a boiling new life begins, and the friend has something good to eat.

Eventually, the chickpea will say to the cook, 'Boil me some more. Hit me with the skimming spoon. I can't do this by myself. I'm like an elephant that dreams of gardens back in Hindustan and doesn't pay attention to his driver. You're my cook, my driver, my way into existence. I love your cooking'.

The cook says, 'I was once like you, fresh from the ground. Then I boiled in time, and boiled in the body, two fierce boilings. My animal soul grew powerful. I controlled it with practices, and boiled some more, and boiled once beyond that, and became your teacher'.

Rumi, translated by Coleman Barks (Coleman & Moyne, 1995). Reprinted with permission by Coleman Barks

Relevance of the Four Noble Truths

In addition to principles and standards of teaching mindfulness, agreed upon by experts in the field, a number of complementing facets of what is actually required to teach mindfulness effectively need to be highlighted with reference to the four noble truths, as described in various Buddhist traditions.

The first noble truth of the Buddhadharma, which in essence is no different from a universal dharma operating independently of Buddhism or any other religion for that matter, is the recognition that suffering (stress) is part of the human condition.

A helpful distinction is often made between (a) a first order or natural form of suffering caused by sickness, old age and death, including the inevitable loss of people we love, and (b) a second order or extra form of suffering, sometimes referred to as adventitious suffering, which causes the majority of suffering in a human being's life (Kabat-Zinn, 2012). Mark Twain is known for having expressed this heart breaking observation in the following sentence: 'I am an old man and have known a great many troubles, but most of them never happened'. This extra form of suffering is self-imposed on top of the unavoidable natural suffering, and according to Buddhism, it is largely caused by (a) the tendency to try to secure our own happiness by grasping on to pleasant experiences while trying to avoid the unpleasant and (b) ignorance of the impermanent and interconnected nature of ourselves and reality. Indeed, the second noble truth of the Buddha is the recognition that there is a cause to all suffering, including this form of self-created suffering. The third noble truth recognises that the cessation of this suffering is possible, while the fourth noble truth concerns the actual path of the dharma that may eventually lead to the liberation of self-imposed suffering. By practicing meditation, we gradually come to see many ways in which we actually cause and maintain our own suffering.

The path of becoming a teacher of mindfulness and the dharma in its universal manifestation essentially involve the courage to meet the suffering of this world. Initially this involves turning towards one's own suffering in order to begin learning to relate to suffering in new ways, rather than trying to avoid or deny its existence.

Through meditation practice, by relating directly to the experience of one's own suffering, the wish and urge to be at service to alleviate the suffering of others may arise naturally over time. Indeed, the teacher may then gradually come to view and prioritise the well-being of other people as equally or more important than their own well-being. This radical orientation may arise from the recognition or insight that others are not fundamentally separate from oneself.

Dialogue and Inquiry

To navigate as a teacher by means of intimately knowing the present moment is central to the process of dialogue and inquiry. In the context of MBSR and MBCT, the terms inquiry and dialogue refer to the open intimate conversation between teacher and participants in ways that allow for further exploration and investigation of the experience of being alive and awake to the present moment. This includes bringing close attention to the full range of experiences' characteristic of the human condition—the full catastrophe of life with all of its joys and sorrows.

Interestingly, 'dialogue' in MBSR has been described as the outward counterpart to the inward cultivation of present-moment-centred, nonjudgemental awareness (Santorelli, 1999; Kabat-Zinn, 2012). It is radically different from the process of 'discussion', which tends to be the norm or stereotype of verbal communication in the interpersonal domain. Discussions are often characterised by strong personal opinions and strategies and often driven by hidden agendas and power differentials between people. Dialogue on the other hand provides a relational space of openness and safety based on the faculty of nonjudgemental deep listening and seeing that can allow each and every voice to be heard and known as a valid contribution to the collective process of inquiry and investigation (Kabat-Zinn, 2012). Such a sensitive approach to communication may lead to important insight and discovery that cannot be uncovered if the process is primarily fuelled by personal and fixed agendas. With fundamental attitudes, such as nonjudgemental deep listening and no attachment to outcome, the process of dialogue and inquiry may provide enough relational space for new knowledge to emerge. This in turn may guide action in more creative, innovative and compassionate ways.

In the MBCT treatment manual (Segal, Williams, & Teasdale, 2013), the practice of inquiry has been described in terms of three concentric circles or layers. The first layer is concerned with the direct experience of the practice of mindfulness by inviting participants to describe any thoughts, feelings and bodily sensations that they were aware of during the practice. The second layer involves skilful questioning and reflection to place experience in a personal context of understanding. In the third layer, however, learning is generalised and situated to a larger context, making it relevant for the whole group of participants.

A note of caution: If this step-by-step model to dialogue and inquiry is rigidly applied with too much interruption and intervening, driven by a perceived directionality and goal-oriented behaviour on behalf of the teacher, the risk may be that participants are not allowed enough space to investigate and express their actual experience, whatever it may be. The authors seem to be well aware of this. In fact, they underscore what may be one of the most important aspects of inquiry and dialogue, namely, the quality of the relationship to experience that is lived and embodied by the teacher. If this relationship is one of awareness infused with kindness, gentleness, compassion and understanding, especially towards difficult and painful experiences, it may help participants themselves to integrate this way of being in relationship to their own experience. Indeed, it may serve as a powerful antidote to self-criticism and self-judgement, which is not an uncommon habitual response to difficult experiences. To witness the conduct of a human being or expert teacher with such capacity of mind and heart can make a long lasting impression and is a powerful inspiration for practicing mindfulness meditation, at least in our experience.

According to Santorelli (2015), while detailed frameworks and maps of the process of inquiry and dialogue may have limited value, there is no doubt that as a teacher, with the intention to 'first do no harm', the capacity to mindfully investigate one's own experience of being human essentially provides the context required to actually meet other people in ways that are helpful for human growth and transformation. A fundamental view of human nature, embedded in the teachings of MBSR, is expressed in the following line: 'As long as you are breathing, there is more right than wrong with you' (Kabat-Zinn, 2013). In other words, the capacity to live this human life with awareness is available within each of us as a deep resource for healing and for coming to terms with things as they are and as such not restricted by adversity, loss, illness and pain.

Based on the ethos of MBSR, Santorelli (2015) has outlined 21 guiding principles that express the essence of the dialogue and inquiry process within MBSR. Some of these guiding principles are the following: Dialogue and inquiry are an expression and reflection of mindfulness meditation practice. They are grounded in the body and grounded in present centred awareness. Dialogue and inquiry are respectful and directed towards inner growth and the implications of this learning in everyday life. Dialogue and inquiry are non-goal oriented, and they are not directed towards changing or fixing anyone or anything. Even when painful, they are always directed towards the sovereignty of every human being and the principle of ennobling. Through direct experience, they are a learning to 'turn towards' the difficult and/or unwanted. Importantly, dialogue and inquiry occur in a community that learns to bear witness to the self-revealing of another without giving advice (ibid.).

While inquiry is an art form that essentially is creative and responsive to the unique configuration of the present moment, Santorelli (2015) has described a typology of Socratic questions that can be integrated into the MBSR learning environment. These types of questions include (1) 'conceptual clarification' which invites participants to expand on and clarify what they report from their own experience; (2) 'wondering about assumptions' that participants may have about themselves, others and the world; (3) 'probing rationale and evidence' for a certain point of view; (4) 'challenging viewpoints and perspectives' that may no longer serve; (5) 'probing implications and consequences'; and (6) asking questions about questions (ibid.). How do you know this? Are you sure? Do you benefit from this view? What might happen if…? What do you make of that? These are a few examples of such open questions. Now, the teacher's willingness to live with and inside such open questions, to inquire into their own experience of life, is exactly what provides them with the licence to ask such questions to their students (ibid.). Again, this is not a technique or manual-based approach but rather a response in the form of a question arising from deep listening and attending to participants as they communicate and express their experience of being aware in the present moment. The intention is to be at service to others with great sensitivity to the present moment and to be in touch with the range of present-moment information that can provide the foundation for responding with wisdom and skilful means in ways that may allow each individual as well as the group to further their understanding and growth towards wholeness and greater well-being.

Closing Comments

If the principles of 'first do no harm' and 'teach only what you know'—along with a direct recognition that MBSR and MBCT 'rest in the view that the essential nature of human beings is luminous and unimpeded' (Santorelli, 2015)—become an embodied ethos within an MBI teacher and they continue their deep commitment to practice and study and silent retreats and a working relationship with a teacher and with life itself, they may be able to do some genuine good in this world.

Acknowledgement The authors thank Edo Shonin and Jens-Erik Risom for helpful comments to the first draft of the chapter manuscript.

References

Baer, R. A. (2003). Mindfulness training as a clinical intervention: A conceptual and empirical review. *Clinical Psychology: Science and Practice, 10*, 125–143.

Berliner, D. C. (2004a). Describing the behavior and documenting the accomplishments of expert teachers. *Bulletin of Science Technology Society, 24*, 200–212.

Berliner, D. C. (2004b). Expert teachers: Their characteristics, development and accomplishments. In R. Batllori i Obiols, A. E Gomez Martinez, M. Oller i Freixa & J. Pages i Blanch (eds.), *De la teoria....a l'aula: Formacio del professorat ensenyament de las ciències socials* (pp. 13–28). Barcelona, Spain: Departament de Didàctica de la Llengua de la Literatura I de les Ciències Socials, Universitat Autònoma de Barcelona

Bertelsen, J. (2013). *Essence of mind: An approach to Dzogchen*. Berkeley, CA: North Atlantic Books.

Coleman, B., & Moyne, J. (1995). *The essential Rumi*. New York: Harper Collins.

Crane, R. S., Eames, C., Kuyken, W., Hastings, R. P., Williams, J. M., Bartley, T., et al. (2013). Development and validation of the mindfulness-based interventions – Teaching assessment criteria (MBI:TAC). *Assessment, 2*, 681–688.

Crane, R. S., Kuyken, W., Hastings, R. P., Rothwell, N., & Williams, J. M. G. (2010). Training teachers to deliver mindfulness-based interventions: Learning from the UK experience. *Mindfulness, 1*, 74–86.

Crane, R. S., Kuyken, W., Williams, J. M. G., Hastings, R. P., Cooper, L., & Fennell, J. V. (2012). Competence in teaching mindfulness-based courses: Concepts, Development and assessment. *Mindfulness, 3*, 76–84.

Dogen (Ed.). (2002). *The heart of Dogen's Shobogenzo*. Albany, NY: SUNY.

Ericsson, K. A., Charness, N., Feltovich, P. J., & Hoffman, R. R. (2006). *The Cambridge handbook of expertise and expert performance*. New York: Cambridge University Press.

Ericsson, K. A., Prietula, M. J., & Cokely, E. T. (2007). The making of an expert. *Harvard Business Review, 85*, 114–121.

Grossman, P., Niemann, L., Schmidt, S., & Walach, H. (2004). Mindfulness-based stress reduction and health benefits: A meta-analysis. *Journal of Psychosomatic Research, 57*, 35–43.

Gunaratana, B. H. (2011). *Mindfulness in plain English*. Boston: Wisdom.

Harvey, P. (2013). *An introduction to Buddhism: Teachings, history and practices*. New York: Cambridge University Press.

Hofmann, S. G., Sawyer, A. T., Witt, A. A., & Oh, D. (2010). The effect of mindfulness-based therapy on anxiety and depression: A meta-analytic review. *Journal of Consulting and Clinical Psychology, 78*, 169–183.

Kabat-Zinn, J. (1996). Mindfulness meditation: What it is, what it isn't, and it's role in health care medicine. In Y. Haruki, Y. Ishii, & M. Suzuki (Eds.), *Comparative and psychological study on meditation* (pp. 161–169). Netherlands: Eburon.

Kabat-Zinn, J. (2006). *Coming to our senses: Healing ourselves and the world through mindfulness*. New York: Hyperion.

Kabat-Zinn, J. (2011). Some reflections on the origins of MBSR, skillfull means, and the trouble with maps. *Contemporary Buddhism, 12*, 281–306.

Kabat-Zinn, J. (2012). *Mindfulness for beginners: Reclaiming the present moment and your life*. Boulder, CO: Sounds True.

Kabat-Zinn, J. (2013). *Full catastrophe living: Using the wisdom of your body and mind to face stress, pain, and illness*. New York: Bantam Books.

Khoury, B., Lecomte, T., Fortin, G., Masse, M., Therien, P., Bouchard, V., et al. (2013). Mindfulness-based therapy: A comprehensive meta-analysis. *Clinical Psychology Review, 33*, 763–771.

Lonard, G., & Murphy, M. (1995). *The life we are given: A long-term program for realizing the potential of body, mind, heart, and soul*. New York: Penguin Putnam.

McCown, D., Reibel, D., & Micozzi, M. S. (2010). *Teaching mindfulness: A practical guide for clinicians and educators*. New York: Springer.

Piet, J., & Hougaard, E. (2011). The effect of mindfulness-based cognitive therapy for prevention of relapse in recurrent major depressive disorder: A systematic review and meta-analysis. *Clinical Psychology Review, 31*, 1032–1040.

Piet, J., Würtzen, H., & Zachariae, B. (2012). The effect of mindfulness-based therapy on symptoms on anxiety and depression in adult cancer patients and survivors: A systematic review and meta-analysis. *Journal of Consulting and Clinical Psychology, 80*, 1007–1020.

Rifkin, J. (2009). *The empathic civilization: The race to global consciousness in a world in crisis*. London: Penguin Books.

Risom, J.-E. (2010). *Presence meditation. The practice of life awareness*. Berkeley, CA: North Atlantic Books.

Santorelli, S. (1999). *Heal thy self: Lessons on mindfulness in medicine*. New York: Bell Tower.

Santorelli, S. (2015). Remembrance: Dialogue and inquiry in the MBSR classroom. In D. McCown, D. Reibel, & M. Micozzi (Eds.), *Resources for teaching mindfulness: A cross-cultural and international handbook*. New York: Springer.

Segal, Z. V., Williams, J. M. G., & Teasdale, J. D. (2013). *Mindfulness-based cognitive therapy for depression: A new approach to preventing relapse*. New York: The Guildford Press.

Shonin, E., & Van Gordon, W. (2014a). Practical recommendations for teaching mindfulness effectively. *Mindfulness*. doi:10.1007/s12671-014-0342-y. Published online: September 16, 2014.

Shonin, E., & Van Gordon, W. (2014b). The lineage of mindfulness. *Mindfulness*. doi:10.1007/s12671-014-0327-x. Published online: August 05, 2014.

Trungpa, C. (2013a). *The profound treasury of the ocean of Dharma. Volume one: The path of individual liberation*. Boston/London: Shambhala.

Trungpa, C. (2013b). *The profound treasury of the ocean of Dharma. Volume two: The bodhisattva path of wisdom and compassion*. Boston/London: Shambhala.

Tsui, A. B. M. (2003). *Understanding expertise in teaching: Case studies of second language teachers*. New York: Cambridge University Press.

Wilber, K., Patten, T., Leonard, A., & Morelli, M. (2008). *Integral life practice: A 21st-century blueprint for physical health, emotional balance, mental clarity, and spiritual awakening*. Boston/London: Integral Books.

Williams, J. M. G., & Kabat-Zinn, J. (2011). Mindfulness: Diverse perspectives on its meaning, origins, and multiple applications at the intersection of science and dharma. *Contemporary Buddhism, 12*, 1–18.

Chapter 5
Experimental Approaches to Loving-Kindness Meditation and Mindfulness That Bridge the Gap Between Clinicians and Researchers

Christopher J. May, Kelli Johnson, and Jared R. Weyker

Introduction

Mindfulness meditation (MM) and loving-kindness meditation (LKM) are two broad types of meditation stemming from the Buddhist tradition. MM has numerous salutary effects in both clinical and non-clinical populations (Brown, Ryan, & Creswell, 2007; Chiesa & Serretti, 2011; Cullen, 2011; Eberth & Sedlmeier, 2012; Goyal et al., 2014; Grossman, Niemann, Schmidt, & Walach, 2004; Kabat-Zinn, 2003; Ludwig & Kabat-Zinn, 2008). Increasingly, researchers are also investigating kindness-based meditations (for reviews, see Galante, Galante, Bekkers, & Gallacher, 2014; Shonin, Van Gordon, Compare, Zangeneh, & Griffiths, 2014a). MM and LKM emphasize different psychological domains (Wallace & Shapiro, 2006). Mindfulness practice cultivates attention, typically to the breath, with an awareness of phenomena arising in the body, mind, and environment (Shonin, Van Gordon, Griffiths, 2014b). Loving-kindness meditation cultivates the affective domain as the practitioner directs heartfelt intentions to others (Salzberg, 1995). Because psychiatric conditions, such as depressive and anxiety disorders, involve both attention and affect, mindfulness and loving-kindness meditations may provide complimentary therapeutic interventions.

A small number of studies have begun to directly examine the relative effects of these two types of meditation (Barnhofer, Chittka, Nightingale, Visser, & Crane, 2010; Crane, Jandric, Barnhofer, & Williams, 2010; Feldman, Greeson, & Senville, 2010; Lee et al., 2012; May, Weyker, Spengel, Finkler, & Hendrix, 2014). Barnhofer et al. (2010)

C.J. May (✉) • J.R. Weyker
Carroll University, Waukesha, WI, 53186, USA
e-mail: cmay@carrollu.edu

K. Johnson
SUNY Stony Brook, Stony Brook, NY, 11794, USA

E. Shonin et al. (eds.), *Mindfulness and Buddhist-Derived Approaches in Mental Health and Addiction*, Advances in Mental Health and Addiction,
DOI 10.1007/978-3-319-22255-4_5

demonstrated that both MM and LKM increased left-hemisphere anterior EEG asymmetry, a pattern associated with positive affect. Interestingly, participants scoring higher on a measure of brooding tended to respond more strongly to MM while low brooders exhibited a greater leftward shift following LKM. May et al. (2014) found that MM and LKM both increase mindfulness and positive affect, with LKM having a greater effect on positive affect. May et al. (2014) also identified a dissociation where MM had a greater impact on self-acceptance, while LKM had a greater effect on participants' sense of presence. Feldman, Greeson, and Senville (2010) found that MM increased decentering (viewing thoughts and emotions from a more objective point of view) relative to LKM and progressive relaxation. In Lee et al. (2012), MM was associated with enhanced sustained attention and changes in attention-related brain areas not seen in LKM. MM and LKM also led to the recruitment of distinct brain networks in processing affective images. Collectively, these studies suggest that particular types of meditation practice may be more helpful for a given personality/disposition, disorder, or symptom. A natural follow-up research program would be to match meditation types with individual psychological profiles.

Research on contemplative practices, such as MM and LKM, is complicated, however, by the substantial individual differences in response to beginning meditation. May et al. (2014) found that 48–71 % of the study variance was attributable to individual differences, rather than assignment to MM or LKM groups. A number of studies have also shown either no or minimal associations between meditation time and significant effects (Carmody & Baer, 2008, 2009; Davidson et al., 2003; Leppma, 2011). This should not be taken to mean that there is no effect of practice time—indeed, long-practicing monks exhibited striking differences compared to novice meditators (e.g., Lutz, Greischar, Rawlings, Ricard, & Davidson, 2004)—but rather that there is substantial variability in the relationship between meditation time and observed effects. Some individuals may respond rapidly, while others more slowly. There are also likely to be nonlinear effects of practice time, with periods of relative gain or stagnancy.

High between-subject variability means that studies must have higher sample sizes in order to isolate experimental effects. This need for higher sample sizes is further compounded when comparing two or more types of meditation. The different effects of MM and LKM reported by Barnhofer et al. (2010), Feldman, Greeson, and Senville (2010), Lee et al. (2012), and May et al. (2014) were derived from sample sizes much too small to be considered robust. Their results should therefore be regarded as suggestive. Obtaining large sample sizes can be problematic for contemplative research, however. Experimental studies assessing changes over time in response to a treatment generally require more resources, in terms of time, labor, and money, than do cross-sectional or correlational studies. Moreover, for meditation research, experienced meditators should be used to providing initial instruction to meditation-naïve participants (Crane, Kuyken, Hastings, Rothwell, & Williams, 2010; Kabat-Zinn, 2003; Shonin & Van Gordon, 2014). Participants should also have opportunities to discuss difficulties arising in their practice and receive informed feedback from a teacher. These best practices put constraints on the number of participants that can be ably taught meditation at a time.

One remedy to the difficulty of obtaining adequate sample sizes for comparing the effects of different types of meditation is to more extensively employ single-subject experimental designs. Single-subject designs focus on an individual, such as a patient, exemplifying the idiopathic approach (Molenaar, 2004). In these designs, the subject serves as their own control. For example, patient or client symptoms can be compared during periods when they have been instructed to meditate with periods when they have been instructed not to meditate. Single-subject designs differ from case studies in that there is an explicit manipulation (e.g., whether and when a patient is practicing a certain type of meditation) and thus are considered experiments (for an accessible review, see Kratochwill et al., 2010). Because clinical work is also typically idiopathic, there may be a natural synergy between clinicians and single-subject experimental designs. Importantly, multiple single-subject experiments can be collated for collective analysis (see Shadish, 2014a). This presents an opportunity to "crowdsource" the experimental study of meditation, effectively distributing the relatively high cost of conducting such work. In other words, the clinician can, and we believe should, play a vital role in advancing the science of meditation.

In the next section, we present an example of a single-subject experiment looking at the relative effects of MM and LKM. We conducted this experiment with multiple subjects, simulating a clinician that is working with multiple patients. As we will discuss at the end, the results from this experiment further reinforce the value, if not the need, for an idiopathic approach to studying meditation.

Experiment

We conducted an exploratory alternating-treatment experiment to examine the relative effects of mindfulness and loving-kindness meditation. Though an alternating-treatment experiment is a type of single-subject design, we simultaneously conducted the experiment with 16 participants. Participants with no previous regular meditation practice were recruited through campus advertisements. Participants alternated weekly over the course of 8 weeks between MM and LKM.

Guided meditations created by the first author (a practitioner of 10 years) were provided to participants. They were asked to practice at least 4 days per week for 15 min at a time. In MM, participants were instructed to attend to their breathing, returning their attention to their breath whenever they noticed their mind had wandered. In the loving-kindness meditation, participants directed intentions ("may you be well; may you be happy; may you be free from suffering") first to a loved one and then to themselves.

Each week, participants completed the Five Facet Mindfulness Questionnaire (FFMQ; Baer, Smith, Hopkins, Krietemeyer, & Toney, 2006; Baer et al., 2008) and the Profile of Mood States-Short Form (POMS; Curran, Andrykowski, & Studts, 1995; Shacham, 1983). The FFMQ contains subscales for "observing," "describing," "acting with awareness," "non-reacting," and "nonjudging." Participants were asked how frequently they had had certain experiences (e.g., "I perceive my feelings and emotions without having to react to them," "I find it difficult to stay focused on what's happening in the present") in the past week on a 5-point scale. In the POMS, participants were asked to rate to what extent each of 37 adjectives (such as tense, cheerful, bitter, and lively) described how they had been feeling in the past week on a 5-point scale. We also employed additional measures, such as the Navon task and heart rate variability; however we are able to demonstrate all pertinent points using results from just the FFMQ and POMS. For the sake of brevity and clarity, we omit those other measures (results were consistent with those to be presented). The FFMQ and POMS took participants 5–10 min to complete.

During our alternating-treatment experiment, there were a total of seven alternations between meditation conditions (A-1-B-2-A-3-B-4-A-5-B-6-A-7-B). Half of the participants began with MM, while the other half started with LKM. We predicted that the data would follow one of two patterns: a sawtooth pattern where scores increased in the first transition, decreased in the second, and alternated for the remaining transitions or the reverse sawtooth pattern where scores decreased in the first transition, increased in the second, and alternated for the remaining transitions. Given seven transitions in which scores either increased or decreased, there are $2^7 = 128$ permutations of these transitions.[1] The probability of obtaining one of the two predicted patterns is 2/128 or 0.015. The probability of obtaining 6 transitions following the predicted patterns within the range of 7 transitions is $6/128 = 0.047$.[2] We therefore considered six or more consecutive pattern-following transitions as statistically significant evidence for a causal effect of meditation type on a particular dependent variable.

Results

For the FFMQ, three participants exhibited a significant effect of meditation type on the "observing" facet (see Fig. 5.1). For all three, "observing" scores decreased following a week of mindfulness meditation and increased after a week of loving-kindness meditation. One individual had systematically higher "acting with awareness" scores following MM compared to LKM. Another participant scored higher on the "nonjudging" scale of the FFMQ following LKM compared to MM. Three participants scored differentially from week to week on the "non-reacting" subscale of the FFMQ. One participant scored lower following MM, while two participants scored lower following LKM. One participant with lower "non-reacting" scores following MM also had lower "observing" scores following MM. Indeed, their total FFMQ score was lower following MM compared to LKM.

[1] Some scores did not change in successive weeks. We believe, however, that adding the possibility of unchanged scores to that of increased and decreased scores would produce an excessively conservative probability: $2/(3^7) = 0.0009$.

[2] The six possible hypothesized combinations of increasing (I) and decreasing (D) scores were IDIDIDI, IDIDIDD, IIDIDID, DIDIDID, DIDIDII, and DDIDIDI.

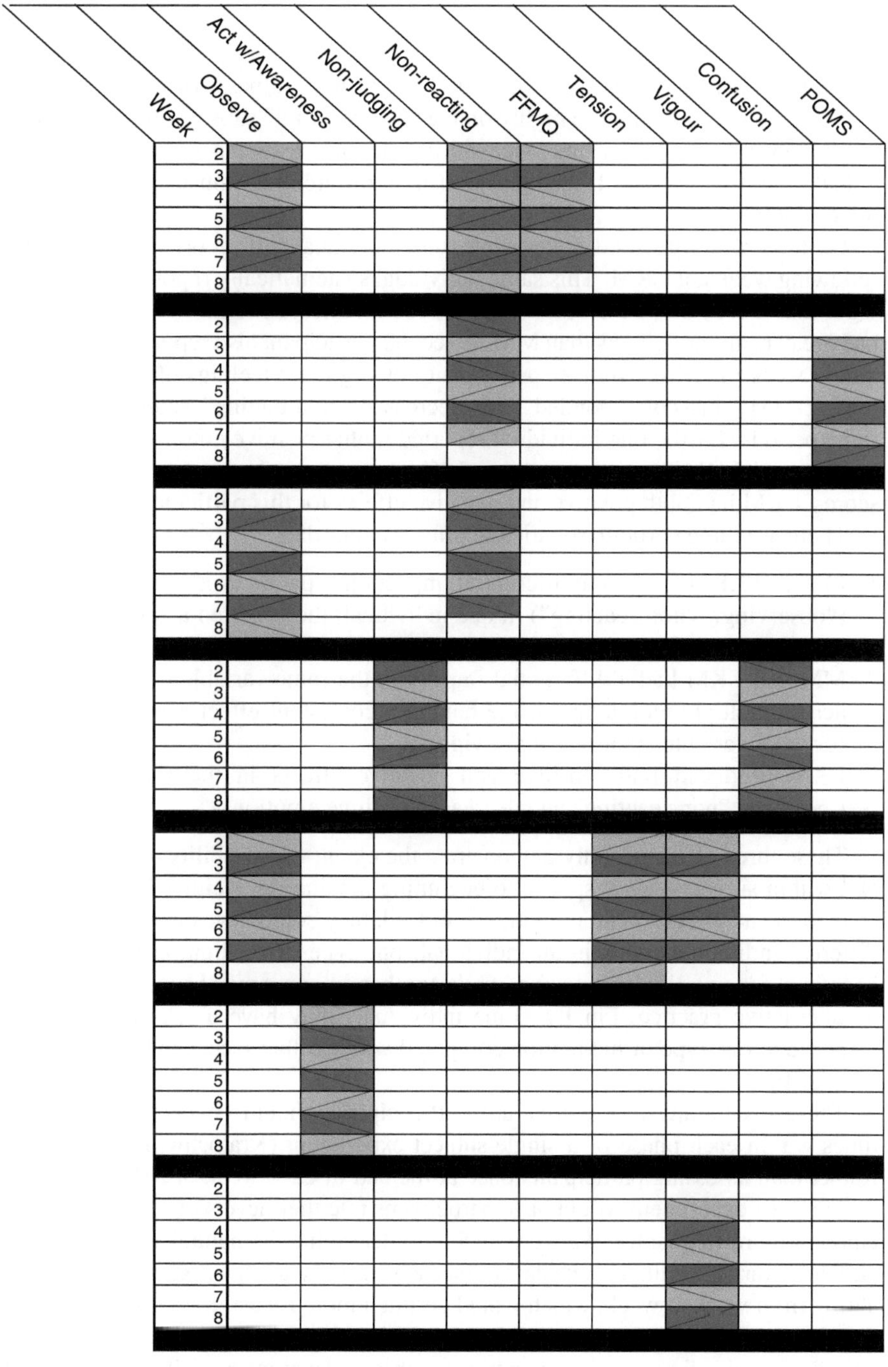

Fig. 5.1 Weekly changes in FFMQ and POMS scores following a week of mindfulness meditation (MM) or loving-kindness meditation (LKM). Only participants and variables with significant effects are included in the graph. *Light gray shading* indicates participants had practiced MM in the previous week; *dark gray shading* corresponds to LKM in the previous week. *Diagonal lines* extending from the *upper left* to the *lower right* indicate decreases in scores from the previous week. *Diagonal lines* extending from the *lower left* to the *upper right* denote increases in scores from the previous week. A *single block of rows* starting from week 2 and ending at week 8 corresponds to a single individual

For this participant, LKM led to higher levels of mindfulness. However, a second participant, who scored more highly on the "non-reacting" subscale following MM, scored lower on the "observing" facet during the same testing periods. For this individual, the two types of meditation had a differential impact on aspects of mindfulness.

On the Profile of Mood States scale, one individual self-reported lower tension following weeks of LKM. This same individual systematically reported heightened vigor and increased "observing" after practicing LKM. For this individual, LKM had greater salutary effects than MM. A second participant also reported more vigor after a week of LKM. Another participant noted greater feelings of confusion following MM; this corresponded with decreased "nonjudging" scores during the same periods. Lastly, one individual reported higher positive emotions (as indexed by the total POMS score) following LKM as well as decreased "non-reacting" scores. LKM had both positive and negative effects for this particular individual.

There are three particularly notable effects in our data:

1. MM and LKM exerted a differential impact on separate aspects of mindfulness ("observing," "non-reacting") in one individual; they exerted a consistent effect in another.
2. MM and LKM had a differential impact on the same variable ("non-reacting") across multiple individuals while having a consistent effect across individuals for other variables ("observing," "vigor").
3. LKM produced both positive and negative effects in the same individual (increased "non-reacting" and decreased positive emotion).

These three effects vividly demonstrate the extent of variability—both between and within subjects—in response to beginning meditation. Neither MM nor LKM have the same effects on all individuals. Indeed, they could have opposing effects in different individuals. Within an individual, one type of meditation may be more beneficial for a particular outcome, while another outcome may be more sensitive to an alternative practice. Finally, some individuals may have a relatively negative response to one type of meditation compared with another (see also Crane, Jandric et al. 2010).

These results are very conservative. Participants should be measured multiple times within each phase of a single-subject experiment (Kratochwill et al., 2010). Rather than assessing participants once at the end of each week of MM or LKM, a more robust experiment would have participants rate their levels of mindfulness and emotion more frequently. We were unable to determine the natural variability for a particular variable with just one data point each week. Without an estimate of the variability from week to week, which would permit a more robust inference of the mean for each week, results were more likely to deviate from the predicted sawtooth pattern. Despite this limitation, we nonetheless observed a number of illustrative effects.

These results highlight the importance of an idiopathic approach to the study of mindfulness and meditation. Group analyses of this data would not reveal effects of meditation type on any variable (Johnson, Weyker, & May, 2013). However, with a single-subject design, we were able to determine that certain types of meditation had demonstrable effects for particular individuals. In group analyses, individual differences can obscure individual effects. This complicates using evidence-based practice (see Spring, 2007) with patients. In general, the higher the individual variability in a particular domain, such as meditation, the less the average effect reported in the literature will be reflective of a particular individual. For this reason, clinicians may find single-subject designs both more appealing and more useful.

The academic study of meditation would also benefit from the wide-scale use by clinicians of single-subject experiments. Limitations imposed by the resource-intensiveness of longitudinal meditation research can be mitigated by distributing the load over hundreds of clinicians. To maximally profit from this work, the field should develop an international database for clinicians and researchers to publish their data and methods. Even in the absence of such a database, however, experiments can be collated by individual researchers and analyzed using increasingly sophisticated methods (see Moeyaert, Ferron, Beretvas, and Van den Noortgate, 2013; Shadish, Kyse, and Rindskopf, 2013; Shadish, 2014a, 2014b). With sufficient adoption, researchers will be better positioned to determine the effects of different meditation types (or combinations of practices) for particular personality profiles, disorders, or symptoms. This, in turn, would provide clinicians with more skillful means for improving the mental health of their patients.

References

Baer, R. A., Smith, G. T., Hopkins, J., Krietemeyer, J., & Toney, L. (2006). Using self-report assessment methods to explore facets of mindfulness. *Assessment, 13*, 27–45.

Baer, R., Smith, G. T., Lykins, E., Button, D., Krietemeyer, J., Sauer, S., et al. (2008). Construct validity of the five facet mindfulness questionnaire in meditating and non-meditating samples. *Assessment, 15*, 329–342.

Barnhofer, T., Chittka, T., Nightingale, H., Visser, C., & Crane, C. (2010). State effects of two forms of meditation on prefrontal EEG asymmetry in previously depressed individuals. *Mindfulness, 1*, 21–27.

Brown, K. W., Ryan, R. M., & Creswell, J. D. (2007). Mindfulness: Theoretical foundations and evidence for its salutary effects. *Psychological Inquiry, 18*, 211–237.

Carmody, J., & Baer, R. A. (2008). Relationships between mindfulness practice and levels of mindfulness medical and psychological symptoms and well-being in a mindfulness-based stress reduction program. *Journal of Behavioral Medicine, 31*, 23–33. doi:10.1007/s10865-007-9130-7.

Carmody, J., & Baer, R. A. (2009). How long does a mindfulness-based stress reduction program need to be? A review of class contact hours and effect sizes for psychological distress. *Journal of Clinical Psychology, 65*, 627–638. doi:10.1002/jclp.20555.

Chiesa, A., & Serretti, A. (2011). Mindfulness based cognitive therapy for psychiatric disorders: A systematic review and meta-analysis. *Psychiatry Research, 187*, 441–453.

Crane, C., Jandric, D., Barnhofer, T., & Williams, J. M. (2010). Dispositional mindfulness meditation and conditional goal setting. *Mindfulness, 1*, 204–214.

Crane, R. S., Kuyken, W., Hastings, R. P., Rothwell, N., & Williams, J. M. G. (2010). Training teachers to deliver mindfulness-based interventions: Learning from the UK experience. *Mindfulness, 1*, 74–86. doi:10.1007/s12671-010-0010-9.

Cullen, M. (2011). Mindfulness-Based interventions: An emerging phenomenon. *Mindfulness, 2*, 186–193.

Curran, S. L., Andrykowski, M. A., & Studts, J. L. (1995). Short Form of the Profile of Mood States (POMS-SF): Psychometric information. *Psychological Assessment, 7*, 80–83.

Davidson, R. J., Kabat-Zinn, J., Schumacher, J., Rosenkranz, M., Muller, D., Santorelli, S. F., et al. (2003). Alterations in brain and immune function produced by mindfulness meditation. *Psychosomatic Medicine, 65*, 564–570.

Eberth, J., & Sedlmeier, P. (2012). The effects of mindfulness meditation: A meta-analysis. *Mindfulness, 3*, 174–189.

Feldman, G., Greeson, J., & Senville, J. (2010). Differential effects of mindful breathing progressive muscle relaxation and loving-kindness meditation on decentering and negative reactions to repetitive thoughts. *Behaviour Research and Therapy, 48*, 1002–1011.

Galante, J., Galante, I., Bekkers, M. J., & Gallacher, J. (2014). Effect of kindness-based meditation on health and well-being: A systematic review and meta-analysis. *Journal of Consulting and Clinical Psychology, 82*, 1101–1114.

Goyal, M., Singh, S., Sibinga, E. M. S., Gould, N. F., Rowland-Seymour, A., Sharma, R., et al. (2014). Meditation programs for psychological stress and well-being. *JAMA Internal Medicine, 174*, 357–368.

Grossman, P., Niemann, L., Schmidt, S., & Walach, H. (2004). Mindfulness-based stress reduction and health benefits: A meta-analysis. *Journal of Psychosomatic Research, 57*, 35–43.

Johnson, K., Weyker, J. R., & May, C. J. (2013). *Examining the effects of alternating treatments of concentration and loving-kindness meditation*. Poster presented at the 25th annual convention of the association for psychological science, Washington, DC, May 23–26, 2013.

Kabat-Zinn, J. (2003). Mindfulness-based interventions in context: Past present and future. *Clinical Psychology: Science & Practice, 10*, 144–156.

Kratochwill, T. R., Hitchcock, J., Horner, R. H., Levin, J. R., Odom, S. L., Rindskopf, D. M., et al. (2010). *Single-case designs technical documentation*. Available at: What Works Clearinghouse website http://ies.ed.gov/ncee/wwc/pdf/wwc_scd.pdf

Lee, T. M., Leung, M. K., Hou, W. K., Tang, J. C., Yin, J., So, K. F., et al. (2012). Distinct neural activity associated with focused-attention meditation and loving-kindness meditation. *PLoS ONE, 7*, e40054.

Leppma, M. (2011). *The effect of loving-kindness meditation on empathy perceived social support and problem-solving appraisal in counseling students* (Doctoral dissertation). Retrieved from: http://etd.fcla.edu/CF/CFE0003656/Leppma_Monica_201105_PhD.pdf

Ludwig, D. S., & Kabat-Zinn, J. (2008). Mindfulness in medicine. *JAMA, 300*, 1350–1352.

Lutz, A., Greischar, L. L., Rawlings, N. B., Ricard, M., & Davidson, R. J. (2004). Long-term meditators self-induce high-amplitude gamma synchrony during mental practice. *Proceedings of the National Academy of Sciences of the United States of America, 101*, 16369–16373.

May, C. J., Weyker, J. R., Spengel, S. K., Finkler, L. J., & Hendrix, S. E. (2014). Tracking longitudinal changes in affect and mindfulness caused by concentration and loving-kindness meditation with hierarchical linear modeling. *Mindfulness, 5*, 249–258.

Moeyaert, M., Ferron, J. M., Beretvas, S. N., & Van den Noortgate, W. (2013). From a single-level analysis to a multilevel analysis of single-case experimental designs. *Journal of School Psychology, 52*(2), 191–211.

Molenaar, P. C. (2004). A manifesto on psychology as idiographic science: Bringing the person back into scientific psychology: This time forever. *Measurement, 2*, 201–218.

Salzberg, S. (1995). *Loving-kindness: The revolutionary art of happiness*. Boston: Shambhala.

Shacham, S. (1983). A shortened version of the profile of mood states. *Journal of Personality Assessment, 47*, 305–306.

Shadish, W. R. (2014a). Statistical analyses of single-subject designs: The shape of things to come. *Current Directions in Psychological Science, 23*, 139–146.

Shadish, W. R. (2014b). Analysis and meta-analysis of single-case designs: An introduction. *Journal of School Psychology, 52*, 109–122.

Shadish, W. R., Kyse, E. N., & Rindskopf, D. M. (2013). Analyzing data from single-case designs using multilevel models: New applications and some agenda items for future research. *Psychological Methods, 18*, 385–405.

Shonin, E., & Van Gordon, W. (2014). Practical recommendations for teaching mindfulness effectively. *Mindfulness*. doi:10.1007/s12671-014-0342-y.
Shonin, E., Van Gordon, W., Compare, A., Zangeneh, M., & Griffiths, M. D. (2014). Buddhist-derived loving-kindness and compassion meditation for the treatment of psychopathology: A systematic review. *Mindfulness*. doi:10.1007/s12671-014-0368-1.
Shonin, E., Van Gordon, W., & Griffiths, M. D. (2014). The emerging role of Buddhism in clinical psychology: Toward effective integration. *Psychology of Religion and Spirituality, 6*, 123–137.
Spring, B. (2007). Evidence-based practice in clinical psychology: What it is, why it matters; what you need to know. *Journal of Clinical Psychology, 63*, 611–631.
Wallace, B. A., & Shapiro, S. L. (2006). Mental balance and well-being: Building bridges between Buddhism and western psychology. *The American Psychologist, 61*, 690–701.

Part II
Mindfulness for the Treatment of Psychopathology

Chapter 6
Mindfulness- and Acceptance-Based Interventions in the Treatment of Anxiety Disorders

Jon Vøllestad

Introduction

Anxiety Disorders

Humans have a hard-wired ability to respond with fear to threatening situations and to solve problems by anticipating potential aversive outcomes. Unfortunately, these adaptive capacities can sometimes go awry, inhibiting the person in a number of ways. When this impairment becomes significant, we speak of anxiety disorders—a set of clinical conditions characterised by excessive fear, worry, or anxious apprehension (Barlow, 2002). Epidemiological data show anxiety disorders to be the second most common group of mental disorders after substance use, with an overall lifetime prevalence of 25 % (Kessler, Chiu, Demler, & Walters, 2005). Anxiety disorders incur large costs in terms of reduced quality of life and everyday functioning, poorer academic achievements, relationship instability, and low occupational and financial status (Lépine, 2002; Marciniak, Lage, Landbloom, Dunayevich, & Bowman, 2004; Olatunji, Cisler, & Tolin, 2007). For individuals with an early onset, these disorders lead to increased risk of comorbid mental and substance use disorders (Kessler, Ruscio, Shear, & Wittchen, 2010). Anxiety disorders are also independently linked to increased mortality due to heightened risk for coronary heart disease (Kubzansky, Davidson, & Rozanski, 2005) and suicide (Bolton et al., 2008).

Studies of the clinical course of anxiety disorders show that they are unlikely to remit without treatment and are highly likely to recur after observed recovery (Bruce et al., 2005; Ramsawh, Raffa, Edelen, Rende, & Keller, 2009; Wittchen, Lieb,

J. Vøllestad (✉)
Solli District Psychiatric Centre (DPS), Nesttun, Norway

Department of Clinical Psychology, University of Bergen, Bergen, Norway
e-mail: jon.vollestad@uib.no

E. Shonin et al. (eds.), *Mindfulness and Buddhist-Derived Approaches in Mental Health and Addiction*, Advances in Mental Health and Addiction,
DOI 10.1007/978-3-319-22255-4_6

Pfister, & Schuster, 2000). A substantial proportion of sufferers never seek treatment (Roness, Mykletun, & Dahl, 2005). For those who do, there is a considerable delay from onset of the disorder to referral for treatment (Wang et al., 2005). Concurrent with underutilisation of mental health services, anxiety disorders are associated with overutilisation of other health services, including emergency care (Deacon, Lickel, & Abramowitz, 2008; Greenberg et al., 1999). There is a need for interventions that are cost-efficient, easily disseminated, and attractive to individuals less likely to seek help for their problems.

Of the psychological treatments, cognitive behavioural therapy (CBT) has proven particularly effective in the treatment of anxiety disorders (Hofmann & Smits, 2008; Hollon & Beck, 2004; Norton & Price, 2007). However, current CBT interventions have not reached optimal levels of efficiency for anxiety disorders. Meta-analyses report dropout rates in the range of 9–21 %, and approximately a third of patients are classified as nonresponders (Taylor, Abramowitz, & McKay, 2012). For specific disorders, 40–50 % of patients suffering from social anxiety disorder treated with CBT show minimal improvement (Hofmann & Bögels, 2006; Rodebaugh, Holaway, & Heimberg, 2004) and continue to report considerable dissatisfaction with their lives following treatment (Heimberg, 2002). Research on generalised anxiety disorder (GAD) indicates that partial remission is a twice as likely outcome of CBT as full remission, and a number of responders continue to be troubled by residual symptoms (Ninan, 2001). A number of authors have argued that current interventions should be expanded upon or supplemented in order to meet the public health challenge of anxiety disorders in the twenty-first century (e.g. Antony, 2002; McManus, Grey, & Shafran, 2008). Mindfulness- and acceptance-based interventions constitute one potential avenue of expansion.

Mindfulness- and Acceptance-Based Interventions

'Mindfulness' is a mental state characterised by a present-centred and non-judging mode of awareness. Originally a Buddhist practice, mindfulness training aims to facilitate an adaptive way of relating to experience that can alleviate distress and suffering. A mindful state allows the person to be aware of what happens perceptually, psychologically, or physiologically, without being absorbed in it and without reacting to it in a habitual or non-reflective manner. Instead, the person cultivates an attitude of friendly acknowledgement of whatever arises in the present moment. The related notion of 'acceptance' captures the same allowing stance toward experience. Taken together, present-centred awareness and openness to experience constitutes a form of psychological flexibility (Hayes, 2004) that can enable the person to relate more adaptively to the bodily distress, strong emotions, and negative thinking characterising a number of clinical disorders.

A seminal contribution in the clinical use of mindfulness is *mindfulness-based stress reduction* (MBSR) created by Jon Kabat-Zinn (1990). This programme implements a secularised version of various mindfulness practices in the structured format of an 8-week course. MBSR was originally aimed at chronically ill patients in a behavioural medicine setting but has subsequently been applied to a wide variety of presenting problems. Reviews of the research on MBSR show significant reductions in psychological symptoms secondary to medical illness, as well as the mitigation of stress and enhanced emotional well-being in nonclinical samples (Chiesa & Serretti, 2009; de Vibe, Bjørndal, Tipton, Hammerstrøm, & Kowalski, 2012).

Building on the MBSR programme, Segal, Williams and Teasdale (2012) developed mindfulness-based cognitive therapy (MBCT) for patients with recurring depressive problems. MBCT aims to prevent depressive relapse by familiarising patients with their own experience through mindfulness practice and by enabling them to view their thoughts and feelings as events in the mind rather than the truth about themselves and the world. The cultivation of a 'decentred' perspective on thoughts, feelings, and bodily sensations is presumed to inhibit the pattern of depressive rumination that could otherwise trigger new episodes of depression. Several randomised controlled trials have shown that MBCT significantly reduced the rate of relapse in recurrent major depression compared to treatment as usual (Bondolfi et al., 2010; Godfrin & van Heeringen, 2010; Ma & Teasdale, 2004; Teasdale et al., 2000). MBCT has also proven to be as effective as long-term maintenance treatment with antidepressants in preventing relapse (Kuyken et al., 2008; Segal et al., 2010).

MBSR and MBCT employ mindfulness training as the main intervention. As a second—although partially overlapping—developmental trajectory, several multicomponent treatment packages have integrated interventions from CBT into a conceptual framework of mindfulness and acceptance. This synthesis of models is argued by some to be a novel psychotherapeutic paradigm, constituting a 'third wave' in the historical development of CBT (see Hayes, 2004). The overall goal is to enable clients to relate in a non-identificatory and flexible way to experience, but the range of interventions employed in the service of this goal is typically broader than in stand-alone mindfulness-based therapies.

Acceptance and commitment therapy (ACT) combines principles of mindfulness and acceptance with treatment components from behavioural therapy and experiential psychotherapy (Hayes, Strosahl, & Wilson, 1999). The ACT model holds that psychopathology is due to relating to thoughts as literal truths (cognitive fusion), as well as maladaptive attempts to escape from or control unwanted experience (experiential avoidance) (Hayes, 2004). The strategies in ACT include metaphors, experiential work, exposure in the service of valued goals, as well as traditional mindfulness exercises to promote non-judgmental and nonreactive awareness of internal experiences. In ACT terms, these are all known as 'defusion techniques', aimed at undermining contexts of literality that constrict psychological flexibility (Hayes, Luoma, Bond, Masuda, & Lillis, 2006). Meta-analytic reviews have found ACT to outperform control conditions on primary and secondary outcomes after treatment and follow-up for a variety of conditions (Powers, Zum Vörde Sive Vörding, & Emmelkamp, 2009). There were no significant differences in effect sizes when comparing ACT to active control conditions, suggesting equal effectiveness relative to established treatments (Powers et al., 2009).

Acceptance-based behaviour therapy (ABBT) is a multicomponent intervention augmenting CBT with components from ACT, dialectical behaviour therapy (DBT), and MBCT (Roemer & Orsillo, 2007; Roemer, Orsillo, & Salters-Pedneault, 2008). ABBT has been developed specifically for the treatment of generalised anxiety disorder (GAD) and aims to decrease experiential avoidance through increased awareness and willingness to carry out valued action in important life domains.

One issue that needs to be considered is that of mindfulness-based interventions in a narrow sense versus treatment packages comprising a greater range of components. As noted, MBSR and MBCT aim most exclusively at the cultivation of mindfulness skills, while ACT, DBT, and ABBT include a broader array of therapeutic interventions from the cognitive behavioural tradition. However, these interventions share an overarching conceptualisation of the nature of mental processes, the causes of suffering, and the development of well-being. I argue that they have more shared than unique features, both conceptually and in terms of practical implementation. Their common denominator is an emphasis on changing the individual's relationship to experience, enabling a present-centred and nonevaluative stance that facilitates valued action in the face of distress. There is also a shared understanding of the tendency of discursive thoughts and linguistic processes to reify experience in ways that contribute to psychological suffering. Rather than changing the content of thoughts or verbal rules, these interventions aim for insight into the transient and non-veridical nature of mental phenomena. As such, mindfulness- and acceptance-based interventions (MABIs) can be seen as a family of interventions, with different treatment packages offering different routes to a common goal.

However, it must be noted that some authors disagree. For instance, Hofmann, Sawyer, Witt, and Oh (2010) and Strauss, Cavanagh, Oliver, and Pettman (2014) chose to exclude acceptance-based approaches from their recent reviews and meta-analyses on the grounds that the behaviour analytic framework constitutes a different therapeutic model. Also, Chiesa and Malinowski (2011) raise the question whether mindfulness is an adequate umbrella term for the diversity of backgrounds, aims, and practices found in different MABIs.

For the present purpose, I will use the term MABIs to refer to mindfulness- and acceptance-based interventions in the broad sense. When referring to the group-based modalities of MBSR and MBCT that offer mindfulness training in the pure form, the term mindfulness-based interventions (MBIs) will be used. Although a conceptual equivalence is assumed here, it is important to note that the comparative efficacy of pure or mixed approaches can only be assessed empirically. It is possible that as the field progresses, points of conceptual or empirical distinction between these approaches might emerge more clearly than is the case today.

Outline of the Chapter

In this chapter, I will present a more detailed rationale for why MABIs may be of relevance to the treatment of anxiety disorders. My point of departure will be the variety of transdiagnostic processes characterising these clinical conditions, before

I go on to consider more specifically how strategies of mindfulness and acceptance can modify these processes within the domains of cognition, emotion, behaviour, and self-experience. I then review the empirical status of MABIs for both transdiagnostic samples and samples with homogeneous anxiety disorders, before discussing their clinical implementation and recommendations for future research.

The Relevance of Mindfulness and Acceptance for the Treatment of Anxiety Disorders

Anxiety as such is, strictly speaking, not the problem in anxiety disorders. Rather, it is the way the person relates to his or her experience that creates distress and problems in functioning. Flexible adaptation is characterised by an ability to view thoughts, feelings, and bodily sensations as transient events. When this is the case, irrational thoughts, worry, and anxious arousal can arise and pass in awareness without being given too much credence or focus. By contrast, anxiety as a disorder manifests itself in cases where there is a reactive relationship to experience—that is, a state of being overly absorbed in thinking or arousal—and concurrent attempts to control, suppress, or avoid experience (Baer, 2007; Roemer, Erisman, & Orsillo, 2008). This inflexible relationship to the contents of awareness serves to maintain loops of avoidance and safety behaviours and related distress. As a somewhat paradoxical antidote, mindfulness- and acceptance-based interventions aim to facilitate willingness to stay in contact with whatever is present in a non-judgmental way and may thus be helpful for patients' suffering from anxiety disorders. Instead of fighting symptoms or trying to achieve control over them, the person practises attending to his or her experience as a temporary mental state. Thereby, reactive behavioural tendencies are expected to diminish, and the detrimental cognitive-affective processes characteristic of anxiety can be prevented from unfolding (Roemer, Erisman, & Orsillo, 2008). Additionally, therapeutic work is consistently embedded in a framework de-emphasising the removal of unpleasant thoughts and feelings. Instead, the focus is on valued action and the possibility of living a meaningful life regardless of anxiety-related discomfort (Eifert & Forsyth, 2005).

It is fair to assume that individuals vary in terms of how they habitually relate to their experience, including anxious arousal and distress. A number of self-report instruments have been developed to assess mindfulness, acceptance, and psychological flexibility. Research shows that measures of mindfulness as a dispositional variety or trait are inversely related to anxiety symptoms in nonclinical samples (Baer, Smith, Hopkins, Krietemeyer, & Toney, 2006; Bränström, Duncan, & Moskowitz, 2011; Brown & Ryan, 2003; Cash & Whittingham, 2010). Research on dispositional mindfulness in samples with clinical levels of anxiety is more limited, but a recent study of patients seeking treatment for anxiety and depression found that the mindfulness facets of 'nonreactivity' and 'describing' were particularly indicative of lower levels of anxious distress (Desrosiers, Klemanski, & Nolen-Hoeksema, 2013). Also, a recent meta-analysis of studies incorporating a much-used measure of acceptance and psychological flexibility, the Acceptance and Action Questionnaire (AAQ), found consistent negative correlations between the AAQ and both general measures of anxiety as well as measures of severity of specific anxiety disorders (Bluett, Homan, Morrison, Levin, & Twohig, 2014). This indicates that present-centred, non-judging awareness and value-oriented action constitute a potential counterpart to the psychophysiological state of anxiety. How might we understand this obverse relationship in greater detail?

The current diagnostic taxonomy for anxiety disorders contains a number of distinct phenotypes, characterised by specific cognitions, behaviours, symptoms, and maintaining factors. For instance, an individual with panic disorder (PD) will typically be cognitively preoccupied with signals of bodily harm (Austin & Richards, 2001), while an individual with social anxiety disorder (SAD) will rather be hypervigilant with regard to potential interpersonal embarrassment (Voncken, Bögels, & de Vries, 2003). The various diagnostic categories will be presented in more detail later, as clinical research on anxiety usually targets discrete disorders. However, in addition to diagnostically distinct symptom profiles, a number of processes are involved in the instigation and maintenance of the various anxiety disorders (Mansell, Harvey, Watkins, & Shafran, 2009; Norton & Philipp, 2008). When considering the potential for mindfulness and acceptance in the treatment of anxiety disorders, there is reason to consider both approaches. Emphasis on disorder-specific expressions could allow more effective targeting of unique symptoms and maintaining factors but requires that clinicians train in a variety of models and may be less suited to address cases where several diagnoses are present. Transdiagnostic approaches, on the other hand, can be applied to patient groups with different presenting problems. Theoretically and conceptually, MABIs emphasise mental and emotional processes that generate distress irrespective of diagnostic categories. Instead, these are seen as inherent tendencies in human psychology as such, but in clinical disorders are present in more extreme forms. I now go on to consider these shared features as they relate to anxiety disorders, and how the psychological processes associated with mindfulness may be beneficial with regard to the anxiety spectrum in general. Specifically, the following transdiagnostic features of anxiety disorders are addressed: dysfunctional cognitive processes (including attentional biases), avoidance behaviours, emotional dysregulation, and maladaptive self-relatedness. Table 6.1 presents an overview of these transdiagnostic features, their corresponding counterpoints in MABIS, as well as examples of relevant practices and interventions.

The Cognitive Domain

In the cognitive domain, anxiety disorders are characterised by attentional biases to threat (Craske et al., 2009), aversive self-focussed attention (Ingram, 1990; Mor & Winquist, 2002), as well as a tendency to catastrophic interpretations and repetitive negative thinking in the form of worry or rumination (Ehring & Watkins, 2009;

Table 6.1 MABIs and transdiagnostic features of anxiety disorders

Domain	Transdiagnostic psychopathological processes	Beneficial psychological processes from MABIs	Examples of practices from MABIs
Cognition	Attentional bias to threat, self-focussed attention	Self-regulation of attention/contact with the present moment	Awareness of breathing (MBSR/MBCT)
	Cognitive fusion and reactivity (worry, rumination, and catastrophising)	Metacognitive insight/decentring/defusion	Awareness of thinking (MBSR/MBCT) Defusion exercises (ACT/ABBT)
Emotion	Hyperarousal Emotional reactivity Experiential Avoidance	Body awareness: attending to internal sensations and feelings with non-judging attitude	Body scan, yoga (MBSR/MBCT)
		Acceptance-facilitated interoceptive exposure and emotion regulation	Working with difficulty (MBCT)
Behaviour	Avoidance Passivity Social isolation	Value clarification	Value work, establishing chosen life directions (ACT/ABBT)
		Committed action	Determining effective action guided by values (ACT)
	Reactivity/impulsivity Automatic pilot	Behavioural self-regulation/acting with awareness	Breathing space (MBCT)
Self	Attachment to narrative/conceptualised self and rigid self-standards	Self as process/context	Choiceless awareness (MBSR/MBCT) Observer exercises (ACT)
	Self-criticism	Self-compassion	Loving kindness/Metta meditation (MBSR)

MABIs mindfulness- and acceptance-based interventions, *MBSR* mindfulness-based stress reduction, *MBCT* mindfulness-based cognitive therapy, *ACT* acceptance and commitment therapy, *ABBT* acceptance-based behaviour therapy

Mathews & MacLeod, 2005). Experientially, this leads to an erratic or rigid attentional focus and a narrowing down of the bandwidth of information that is available from both the environment and about oneself. This frenzied hypervigilance exists alongside a state of 'cognitive fusion' that causes thoughts to be experienced as dominant in awareness and as factual and convincing despite their often dramatic one-sidedness. I now go on to consider separately the attentional and thought-related transdiagnostic processes implicated in anxiety disorders, as well as the potential of MABIs to counteract these processes.

Well-regulated attention is a central aspect of well-being and optimal performance in any kind of activity. To deal with challenges and arousal, the person needs to be able to voluntarily and flexibly direct, sustain, and disengage attention (Baumeister, Heatherton, & Tice, 1994; Wadlinger & Isaacowitz, 2010). It is also of value to be able to broaden the field of awareness in a manner that enables integration of information from the surroundings with ongoing mental events. One of the clinical features of anxiety disorders is the tendency for scarce attentional resources to be bound up in a hypervigilant scanning for cues of threat or danger. Reviews of the research conclude that threat-related biases in information processing have been found in all anxiety disorders (Bar-Haim, Lamy, Pergamin, Bakermans-Kranenburg, & van Ijzendorn, 2007; Mathews & MacLeod, 2005). Conversely, a central facet of approaches based on mindfulness and acceptance is the 'self-regulation of attention' (Bishop et al., 2004; Carmody, 2009).

In order to cultivate contact with the here and now, the individual must practise engaging with present-moment stimuli, sustain attention, and redirect it whenever it wanders onto past- or future-focussed cognitive processing. The practice of sustaining and redirecting attention is assumed to lead to greater stability in attention and a corresponding greater deliberate control of what one is attending to. Furthermore, mindfulness practice also aims to strengthen a capacity to broaden the attentional focus, enabling the individual to accommodate more aspects of experience in the field of awareness, as well as learning to monitor his or her state of mind (Carmody, 2009). Most commonly, early phases of training involve a focussing of attention through concentrating on specific objects of awareness, while later phases gradually reduces the focus on an explicit object and instead emphasises an open monitoring of any element of awareness (Lutz, Slagter, Dunne, & Davidson, 2008). It is therefore conceivable that MABIs could exert positive effects on anxiety disorders by increasing the effective and flexible allocation of attentional resources.

A common mindfulness practice that can illustrate how MABIs facilitate self-regulation of attention is awareness of breathing as it is practised in MBSR and MBCT. The person here gathers attention and awareness around the felt physical sensation of breathing either in the abdomen or wherever else in the body that the breath can be sensed most clearly. The instruction is to follow the breath, and whenever one becomes aware that the mind has wandered, merely to notice what has caught one's attention and to return to breathing. This seemingly simple exercise most likely recruits a number of neural subsystems required for focussing, sustaining, and redirecting attention as needed. A related practice from MBSR/MBCT is awareness of sounds. This entails a greater degree of expansive awareness or open monitoring, as the person focusses on the sense modality of hearing—adopting an allowing and investigative stance toward sounds from the environment as they come and go.

One of the most consistent findings across brain imaging studies of meditation is the functional upregulation of brain regions involved in the mediation of attention control (Hölzel et al., 2011; Marchand, 2014). This is evidence of neural plasticity: experience and practice shape neural sculpture, leading to increased connectivity in brain areas underlying the capacity being exercised. Meditation techniques, including mindfulness training, have been shown to be associated with outcomes such as enhanced ability to concentrate and inhibit distracting stimuli, reduced expectancy response when presented with unexpected stimuli, and improved sustained attention and attention switching (Ivanovski & Malhi, 2007; Rubia, 2009). Research on basic attentional processes also shows that mindfulness training modifies subsystems of attention, as indicated by performance on the attention network test (Jha, Krompinger, & Baime, 2007; van den Hurk, Giommi, Gielen, Speckens, & Barendregt, 2010) and the Stroop test (Chan & Woollacott, 2007; Kozasa et al., 2012). Taken together, these findings indicate that attentional performance and cognitive flexibility are positively related to mindfulness. Consequently, mindfulness training and its incorporation in acceptance-based behaviour therapies could serve to counteract the maladaptive attention deployment often seen in anxiety disorders.

Turning to the form and content of cognitive processes involved in anxiety, negative repetitive thinking is a central feature of these disorders (Ehring & Watkins, 2009; Mathews & MacLeod, 2005). Rumination is the repetitive focussing on negative feelings and thoughts in response to low mood, presumably in an effort to understand and cope with distress. Ironically, however, elaborating on negative emotional states and their corresponding mental content maintains the mood it seeks to reduce (Nolen-Hoeksema, 2000; Watkins, Moberly, & Moulds, 2008). Rumination is often focussed on the present or past, while worry is a process of future-focussed thinking characterised by overestimating negative outcomes and related tension and anxious apprehension (Barlow, 2002). Interwoven with the lack of flexible attention described above, rumination and worry constitute forms of negative self-absorption (Mor & Winquist, 2002; Ingram, 1990) that prevents the individual from relating in an adaptive manner to current situations and challenges.

Furthermore, negative or catastrophic interpretations or expectations are a prominent feature of anxiety disorders. For instance, individuals with PD/AG typically interpret descriptions of bodily sensations as indicative of impending physical collapse, and those with social phobia predict that social situations will have disastrous outcomes (e.g. Austin & Richards, 2001; Stopa & Clark, 2000; Voncken et al., 2003). Rumination, worry, and catastrophising are all characterised by cognitive fusion, that is, a quality of mental experience as being predominant in awareness, factually accurate, and requiring urgent action (Hayes, 2004). Phenomenologically, this feels as being 'zoned out', lost in a stream of thoughts that have an adhesive, sticky quality, with little freedom in choosing how to respond.

Mindfulness can be seen as an alternative behaviour to ruminating about the past and worrying about the future, where the person is clinging less to his or her thoughts or interpretations (Hayes, 2004). Although mindfulness practice is sometimes misconstrued as a form of emptying the mind of thoughts, it is better understood as a more flexible and less identified relationships to thinking. Both mindfulness training and acceptance-based interventions cultivate a mental mode that lets the person disengage somewhat from maladaptive cognitive processes while at the same time being aware of the patterns of thinking as they are unfolding in the mind. In that way, it gradually becomes clear that thoughts and mental images are temporary phenomena that do not always give actual representations of the self or reality. As a consequence, mental processes need not be identified with too strongly and don't necessarily have to be acted upon. This form of spacious awareness of mental content is variously called 'metacognitive insight' (Teasdale et al., 2002), 'defusion' (Hayes, 2004), or 'decentring' (Shapiro, Carlson, Astin, & Freedman, 2006).

An illustrative exercise for the purpose of strengthening metacognitive skills is the practice of observing thinking. Here, the person practises mindful awareness of the content of the mind from a witnessing perspective, allowing thoughts to come and go without being absorbed in them and without trying to control them. Rather than avoiding mind wandering, the task is to observe such wandering as it is happening with a gently detached attitude. Similarly, in ACT, there are various interventions designed to facilitate defusion from thoughts, such as visualisations inviting one to relate to thoughts as one would to cars passing by outside one's house or leaves sailing by on a stream. Also, the 'milk exercise' is a way of facilitating defusion by repeating a word until it is experienced as meaningless, thereby garnering insight into the arbitrary and non-veridical nature of linguistic signifiers (and, by extension, thinking as such).

By developing the capacity for mindful awareness of thoughts, the mental proliferation or cognitive reactivity often seen in anxiety disorders may be diminished. This capacity for broadening the field of awareness can serve to facilitate a decoupling from negative cognitive loops or merely allowing processes of rumination and worry to play themselves out without being absorbed in them (Carmody, 2009). In line with this, evidence indicates that mindfulness training is associated with decreases in negative repetitive thinking (Deyo, Wilson, Ong, & Koopman, 2009; Frewen, Evans, Maraj, Dozois, & Partridge, 2008; Jain et al., 2007; Kumar, Feldman, & Hayes, 2008). There is also evidence from patients with depressive disorders indicating that MBCT leads to a more decentred perspective on mood and mental processes that may serve to counteract depressive relapse (Hargus, Crane, Barnhofer, & Williams, 2010; Kuyken et al., 2010).

The Domain of Behaviour

Behaviourally, anxiety disorders are characterised by avoidance of situations and activities seen as fear-provoking (Shear, Bjelland, Beesdo, Gloster, & Wittchen, 2007). This restricts the behavioural repertoire of patients and contributes to the functional impairment and reduced quality of life associated with these diagnoses (Mendlowicz & Stein, 2000). The lack of positive reinforcement and sense of disconnection caused by pervasive avoidance can also serve as a partial explanation for the high rates of comorbidity between anxiety and depressive disorders. That is, avoiding situations, or enduring them despite strong discomfort, contributes to a lack of mastery and a sense of helplessness that increase the risk of a secondary depressive disorder developing.

Mindfulness and acceptance might serve to counteract avoidance behaviours through the encouragement to seek out meaningful activities and situations despite the discomfort they engender. This theme is most fully developed in the interventions in ACT, which to a large extent frames therapeutic work in terms of how it might help the client reconnect with important life goals. In this sense, mindfulness and acceptance can serve an important self-regulatory function—in accordance with self-determination theory which posits open awareness as a prerequisite for facilitating choices consistent with the individual's needs, values, and interests (Brown & Ryan, 2003). However, MBSR and MBCT also emphasise the cultivation of awareness as something different from and beyond a mere strategy for reducing distress. Instead, mindfulness training is seen as a reconfiguration of one's way of being in the world, also opening up to the aspects of life that give the individual enjoyment, occasion for relational connections, and a sense of purpose (Kabat-Zinn, 2003; Santorelli, 1999).

Interventions facilitating behavioural self-regulation include value work in ACT, where the person is assisted in exploring valued life directions and making them more explicit. In turn, this 'moral compass' serves to determine avenues of action to bring oneself more in line with overarching life goals. These exercises are similar to exposure interventions and behavioural activation strategies in traditional CBT but are consistently framed in terms of willingness to accept distress in the service of living an engaged life, as opposed to reducing anxiety as such (see Hayes et al., 1999).

There is evidence that willingness to engage in valued action despite distress is associated with outcome in studies on various disorders. Early changes in acceptance and valued action have been shown to predict later changes in social anxiety (Dalrymple & Herbert, 2007; Kocovski, Fleming, & Rector, 2009). Changes in acceptance and valued action have been found to mediate effects on depression at follow-up (Bohlmeijer, Fledderus, Rokx, & Pieterse, 2011), as well as predicting posttreatment responder status for patients with GAD (Hayes, Orsillo, & Roemer, 2010).

Behaviour in anxiety disorders is furthermore characterised by a lack of deliberate choice, as ingrained proclivities for avoidance cause people to act in an automatic or habitual manner. Mindfulness training aims to increase the ability to flexibly respond rather than mindlessly react to stressors and emotionally challenging situations (Kabat-Zinn, 1990). An example of an exercise supporting such flexibility is the 'three-minute breathing space' found in MBCT. In this brief practice, the person starts by bringing a spacious, non-judging awareness to his or her current experience (thoughts, feelings, and bodily sensations). As a next step, attention is narrowed for a brief period of time to focus on the breath, as a means of stabilising attention. The third step is to expand awareness again to include the totality of one's experience, allowing for the presence of worries, emotional distress, and physical discomfort/tension. This alternation between open monitoring and focussed attention may help the person step out of behavioural automaticity and gain a more decentred perspective on his or her situation. This can help him or her to see potential behavioural options that were previously unavailable. It also entails a form of emotion regulation, a process to which I now turn.

The Domain of Emotion Regulation

Emotional distress is considerable in all anxiety disorders, as they are characterised by physiological tension and hyperarousal (Craske et al., 2009). In addition to overt avoidance of anxiety-provoking activities and situations, individuals suffering from anxiety disorders usually display deficiencies in emotion regulation in the form of overreliance on covert strategies aimed at removing, diminishing, or controlling their distress (Amstadter, 2008; Campbell-Sills & Barlow, 2007). These strategies are usually counterproductive and serve to maintain or exacerbate the disorder in question (Clark, 1999; Salkovskis, 1991). By contrast, 'acceptance' is the active and aware embrace of current private events without attempting to change their form or frequency (Hayes et al., 2006). It involves a 'turning toward' experience regardless of its emotional valence and an emphasis on processing the concrete details of physical sensations in the body as opposed to judging, ruminating about, or trying to eliminate internal experiences (Williams, 2010). In this sense, regular mindfulness and acceptance can be seen as facilitating a form of interoceptive exposure (Barlow, 2002) that offers opportunities for desensitisation to internal events that would habitually be avoided or suppressed. This may lead to corrective learning experiences whereby fear and anxious apprehension can be attenuated or extinguished and a corresponding expansion in the range of behaviours engaged in (Treanor, 2011).

Mindfulness and acceptance can be seen as modes of emotion regulation that are not based on the deliberate manipulation of the affective experience itself. Instead, it entails a shift from representational experience (an evaluative, instrumental mode of processing) to a more direct mode of experiencing. In a mindful state, the individual is able to see more clearly the difference between direct perceptions or sensations and the reactions he or she has to these experiences (Williams, 2010). The ability to stand back and observe with an open-hearted curiosity enables the individual to relate to aversive experience as shifting patterns of thoughts and sensations, rather as something to be elaborated on or changed. Mindfulness is thus conceptualised as being in opposition to both avoidance and over-engagement by being *an emotional balance that involves acceptance of internal experiences, affective clarity, and ability to regulate one's emotions and moods* (Hayes & Feldman, 2004, p. 257). This does not imply passivity or resignation in the face of distress, but rather an acknowledgement that unpleasant experience is a part of life that can be coped with more adaptively if one does not try to fight or control it.

Notable practices that illustrate the process of emotion regulation in MBIs include those aimed at facilitating bodily awareness, such as body scan or yoga. By attending to shifting patterns of sensation in a non-judging manner, people can familiarise themselves with their bodies and can use its signals as information that can be acted upon intentionally instead of automatically. There are also exercises more explicitly targeting subjective distress, such as 'working with difficulty' from MBCT. Here, the person is asked to contemplate a distressing situation and, rather than thinking about it, is encouraged to stay experientially present with the way distress is sensed in the body. Instructions invite the person to allow the experience, to open up to it, and to observe it from moment to moment with a caring attitude (see Segal, Williams, & Teasdale, 2012 for more detailed instructions).

Research in nonclinical samples show that attempts to suppress mental content or emotional arousal tends to backfire, leading to greater accessibility of unwanted thoughts and increased arousal (Gross, 2002; Wegner & Erber, 1992; Wegner, Broome, & Blumberg, 1997). Such ironic effects of experiential avoidance have also been demonstrated in subclinical and clinical samples. Laboratory studies show that when subjects with anxiety disorders or high anxiety sensitivity are instructed to accept their experience as opposed to suppressing it during biological challenge paradigms (CO_2 trials), they either report less anxiety symptoms (Eifert & Heffner, 2003) or evaluate their symptoms less negatively (Levitt, Brown, Orsillo, & Barlow, 2004). These findings on the benefits of acceptance with regard to panicogenic stimuli might be particularly relevant to panic disorder (PD), but studies indicate that patients with different anxiety disorders display lower degrees of present-centred awareness and an overreliance of suppression and avoidance strategies (Campbell-Sills, Barlow, Brown, & Hofmann, 2006a; Roemer et al., 2009). There is also evidence to suggest that distress may be related to more adaptively by applying present-centred acceptance as an intentional emotion regulation strategy (Campbell-Sills, Barlow, Brown, & Hofmann, 2006b).

Brain imaging studies support the notion that mindfulness training beneficially impacts brain areas associated with emotion regulation. Longitudinal studies indicate that participation in an MBSR course is associated with reduced grey matter density in the amygdala, a part of the limbic system involved in stress- and anxiety-related reactivity (Hölzel et al., 2009, 2010). Also, mindfulness has been shown to be associated with increased functional connectivity in brain networks associated with emotion regulation and present-moment awareness and reduced activity in limbic areas associated with fear and distress, including the amygdala. This pattern of findings have been reported for individuals scoring higher on dispositional mindfulness (Creswell, Way, Eisenberger, & Lieberman, 2007), for individuals having undergone a brief mindfulness induction (Lutz et al., 2014), and for individuals with generalised anxiety disorder having participated in MBSR (Hölzel et al., 2013). Hölzel et al. (2011) note that there appears to be striking similarities in brain regions influenced by mindfulness meditation and those involved in mediating fear extinction, suggesting that mindfulness meditation could facilitate the extinguishing of learned fear by enhancing brain networks involved in safety signalling.

Mindful emotion regulation involves an ability to accurately perceive and appraise ongoing emotional and physiological processes. Hölzel et al. (2008) found that meditators as opposed to non-meditators had increased grey matter concentration in the right anterior insula, an area involved in detecting interoceptive stimuli. Similarly, Farb, Segal, and Anderson (2012) found that MBSR participants showed plasticity in the middle and anterior insula relative to controls, indicating that mindfulness practice alters the way in which interoceptive attention is represented in the brain. Specifically, this is suggested to entail a shift in which experience is processed less by evaluative and elaborative cognitive activity involving cortical midline structures and more by way of attention to the shifting landscape of sensory input as it is represented in interoceptive networks of the brain (Farb, Segal, & Anderson, 2012). Although there are many unanswered questions with regard to mindfulness and the brain, these investigations provide preliminary support that mindfulness training affects discrete neural networks in a way that might facilitate more adaptive emotion regulation.

The Domain of Self-experience

Anxiety disorders involve a sense of the self as precarious and vulnerable. At the same time, certain facets of the self become more salient, such as self-critical and demanding standards for one's own behaviour, performance, and control and the acceptability of bodily and mental experience. All of the facets of anxiety disorders detailed above (attentional and cognitive distortions, avoidance behaviours, and deficits in emotion regulation) contribute to a particular constellation of self-relatedness, characterised by heightened self-focus and a reactive relationship to experience. Interweaving this heightened self-salience and vulnerability, Barlow (2002) points to low expectations of mastery and self-efficacy with regard to perceived distress, akin to a state of learned helplessness. Interventions based on mindfulness and acceptance might facilitate different self-perceptions that could serve to counteract maladaptive self-relatedness.

Anxiety entails a perception of one's self as a distinct and static entity opposed to one's surroundings, whose experiences are identified with and whose current state is being monitored with regard to threats from within or without. By contrast, the mindful stance allows for experience to ebb and flow more freely, without putting rigid demands on sensations, thoughts, or emotions. In the process, a change in the sense of self may occur that entails a movement from a fixed sense of self (vulnerable, subject to self-critical performance standards, a high need for control, and low tolerance for fluctuation in affect) to what is termed 'self as process' or 'self as context' (Hayes, 2004)—a more relaxed and open way of being in the world, regardless of the ongoing emotional valence of experience. Instead of the pervasive self-criticism often seen in anxiety disorders, this mode of being is characterised by 'self-compassion'—that is, a sense of care, warmth, and kindness toward the experiencing self (Neff, 2003).

The practice of 'choiceless awareness' from MBSR captures well how mindfulness training may support the development of an observing self-experience rather than one based on narrative and self-evaluation. This is a form of open-monitoring meditation wherein the person practises mindfulness and acceptance of whatever enters the field of awareness, be it body sensations, feelings, sounds, or thoughts. Similarly, ACT features 'observer exercises' that invite a similar stance toward the various streams of experience while at the same time discerning between the objects of attention and the neutral core of the observing self watching the arising and passing of mental and physical phenomena. Finally, a number of mindfulness exercises emphasise friendliness and compassion for self and others in a way that supports a less atomistic self-experience, such as 'loving-kindness' or 'Metta' meditation.

Theoretically, there is a compelling convergence between traditional Buddhist notions of 'non-self' and contemporary investigations of neurally based self-experience as it relates to well-being and distress. There is also some evidence from brain imaging studies indicating that mindfulness practice is associated with downregulation of conceptual-linguistic representations of the self (Farb et al., 2007; Goldin, Ramel, & Gross, 2009). These studies indicate that there is a network of cortical midline structures involved in maintaining a sense of the self as a permanent, cognitively elaborated, and narratively based entity that may also be implicated in processes of anxiety, rumination, and worry. Conversely, by engaging networks associated with moment-to-moment somatosensory experiencing, the person may be able to redeploy attention away from the reactive, maladaptive egocentric loops characterising anxiety and mood disorders (Farb, Anderson, & Segal, 2012).

Clinical Trials

Heterogeneous Anxiety Disorders

As detailed above, there is a sound theoretical and empirical rationale for expecting MABIs to impact transdiagnostic processes involved in all anxiety disorder. The first ever study of mindfulness-based interventions for anxiety disorders was carried out on a sample with different anxiety disorders (Kabat-Zinn et al., 1992). These authors studied the effects of MBSR in an open trial of 22 patients with generalised anxiety disorder or panic disorder with or without agoraphobia. Twenty of the twenty-two participants showed significant decreases over the course of treatment on both clinician-rated and self-report measures. Treatment gains on anxiety, agoraphobia, and panic frequency were maintained after 3 months and at a 3-year follow-up investigation (Miller, Fletcher, & Kabat-Zinn, 1995). The results from this pioneering study indicate that mindfulness training constitutes a potentially effective treatment for anxiety disorder that is responded to with compliance and lasting satisfaction from participants.

Despite these promising results, it took more than a decade for the next clinical trial for patients with anxiety disorders to appear (Ramel, Goldin, Carmona, & McQuaid, 2004). Subsequently, a number of open trials have yielded promising results in samples with heterogeneous anxiety disorders or mixed anxiety and depression (Finucane & Mercer, 2006; Ree & Craigie, 2007; Yook et al., 2008). These studies show MBSR and MBCT to be consistently associated with significant reductions in symptoms of anxiety, depression, worry, and rumination.

Several randomised controlled trials have investigated MABIs for samples with heterogeneous anxiety disorders. Vøllestad et al. (2011) compared MBSR to a wait-list control for 76 patients diagnosed with panic disorder with or without agoraphobia, social anxiety disorder, or GAD. Treatment completers showed medium to large effect sizes on measures of anxiety, depression, and sleep problems, and gains were maintained at follow-up after 6 months. Analysis of clinical significance showed that two thirds of MBSR participants reached either recovery status or reliable improvement on measures of anxiety, worry, and depression. The percentages of patients in the clinical range reaching recovery status at posttreatment were highest for anxiety (44 %) and depression (53 %) and lower for trait anxiety (36 %) and worry (26 %).

At a treatment site in South Korea, Lee et al. (2007) and Kim et al. (2009) examined the effectiveness of a meditation-based stress management programme and MBCT, respectively, for two different samples of 46 patients with PD/AG or GAD receiving concurrent pharmacotherapy. Participants were randomly assigned to an 8-week trial of either mindfulness training or an anxiety disorder education programme. Compared to the education group, patients in the mindfulness condition group showed significant improvement in anxiety severity. Kim et al. (2009) report that 16 patients in the MBCT group and none in the anxiety education group were categorised as remitters, and this difference was statistically significant.

How do MABIs perform when compared to established treatment for patients with mixed anxiety disorders? One study compared ACT to CBT for a sample of 128 participants with heterogeneous anxiety disorders (Arch et al., 2012). Both treatments were given in individual format. Results for ACT ($n=57$) and CBT ($n=71$) were equal on self-reported measures of worry, fear, and behavioural avoidance. Within-group effect sizes were very large for principal disorder severity and in the moderate to large range for other anxiety measures, indicating that both treatments were highly efficacious. After the end of treatment, a steeper curve of improvement was observed for treatment completers in the ACT condition, yielding a greater reduction in anxiety severity than CBT at 1-year follow-up. As hypothesised, at follow-up, patients in the ACT condition reported greater psychological flexibility. However, patients in the CBT condition had higher quality of life scores—contrary to expectations, as the emphasis of broader goals and living a valued life is prominent in ACT and less explicit in CBT. This study is among the few to assess adherence to treatment manual and therapist competence, which were found to be good for both conditions. It thus indicates that ACT performs as well as a bona fide treatment of choice for anxiety disorders in the short term and even showing a potential edge over CBT in reducing anxiety severity in the long term.

Arch et al. (2013) compared adapted MBSR and Group CBT for a sample of 105 US combat veterans with one or more anxiety disorders. Care was taken to maximise external validity by carrying out the trial in a real-life veteran hospital setting with economically disadvantaged patients and by limiting exclusion criteria. The initial prediction that CBT ($n=60$) would outperform MBSR ($n=45$) on anxiety-specific outcomes was not supported, as both showed very large improvement in clinician-rated anxiety severity. A pattern of differential effects emerged at follow-up, where CBT was more effective at reducing perceived anxious arousal, whereas MBSR was more effective at reducing worry and comorbid disorders. There were no significant differences in clinically significant improvement, with 54 % in the CBT sample and 68 % in the MBSR sample showing reliable and clinically significant change based on one or more primary outcomes. The authors note that overall, MBSR performs better in this study than in the other study comparing MBSR to CBT (Koszycki, Benger, Shlik, & Bradwejn, 2007), suggesting that MBSR may be a more favourable treatment choice than CBT for more severe and complex patients with anxiety disorders. However, attrition was high, with only half of patients completing the recommended number of sessions. Also, despite large effects on clinician-rated disorder severity, effects on self-report measures were considerably lower than those found in other trials for CBT for mixed anxiety disorders (Arch et al., 2013).

Finally, a Swedish study compared Internet-based mindfulness training to a discussion forum control group in a sample of 91 patients with PD, SAD, GAD, or anxiety not otherwise specified (Boettcher et al., 2014). Participants in the mindfulness condition ($n=45$) showed a large decrease of symptoms of anxiety, depression, and sleep problems relative to the control group ($n=46$). The between-group effect size posttreatment indicated a large group difference for both anxiety and depression, with no significant difference in effects for the different anxiety disorders and maintenance of gains for anxiety (but not depression) at follow-up. Forty percent of the participants in the mindfulness condition met criteria for clinically significant change, as opposed to only four participants in the control group. These results indicate that an Internet-delivered mindfulness intervention is associated with effects of the same magnitude as found for face-to-face MBSR as reported by Vøllestad et al. (2011). Boettcher et al. (2014) note that the between- and within-group effect sizes found in their trial are comparable to results from other trials on computerised CBT for anxiety disorders. Interestingly, the results of Boettcher et al. (2014) were obtained despite low amount of home practice (only 7 min a day) and low adherence (participants completed on average only half of the treatment protocol).

Generalised Anxiety Disorder

Generalised anxiety disorder (GAD) is primarily characterised by pervasive chronic worry about a number of different everyday events or problems, where worry is difficult to control and accompanied by muscle tension or other physical symptoms (American Psychiatric Association, 1994; Tyrer & Baldwin, 2006). Cognitive conceptualisations of the disorder also emphasise maladaptive psychological processes such as intolerance of uncertainty (Dugas, Buhr, & Ladouceur, 2004), as well as worry over everyday matters serving as a defensive strategy distracting from both larger life concerns and from current emotional experience (Borkovec, Alcaine, & Behar, 2004). From the mechanisms and evidence reviewed above, it is clear that MABIs have the potential to reduce rumination and worry and related distress by way of present-centred attention, increased metacognitive awareness, and more adaptive emotion regulation. Through increased acceptance and commitment to valued action, the anxious person might also be able to live with greater ease with the unknown and unexpected in life. How does research on MABIs for GAD bear out these hypotheses?

Several pilot studies have explored MABIs in the treatment of GAD. Evans et al. (2008) found MBCT to be associated with decreases in anxiety, worry, and depression in a small sample of 11 patients, with about half of the participants who exhibited clinical levels of anxiety or worry dropping below the nonclinical range at posttreatment. Craigie, Rees, Marsh, and Nathan (2008) examined effects of MBCT in a larger GAD sample of 23 patients. They found significant improvements in pathological worry, stress, depression, and one of two anxiety scales, with moderate to large effect sizes for each. However, the authors note that effects in this study were smaller than those observed for the most effective trials of CBT for GAD and the rate of clinically significant improvement in pathological worry scores was very small (Craigie et al., 2008). Roemer and Orsillo (2007) carried out a small open trial of acceptance-based behaviour therapy (ABBT) for 16 patients with GAD, finding significant reductions in clinician-rated severity of GAD as well as self-reported improvement in anxiety, depressive symptoms, fear/avoidance of internal experience, and quality of life.

Turning to randomised controlled trials, a wait-list-controlled study by Roemer, Orsillo, and Salters-Pedneault (2008) found large effects of ABBT on GAD-specific outcomes as well as depressive symptoms. At posttreatment, 77 % of the treated sample met criteria for high end-state functioning, and 78 % no longer fulfilled diagnostic criteria for GAD. These effects were stable at follow-up after 9 months. The intervention group also showed significant change in the expected direction on measures of mindfulness and experiential avoidance and a subsequent study of process variables found changes in acceptance and valued action to predict responder status (Hayes et al., 2010).

Hoge et al. (2013) compared a slightly modified MBSR ($n = 48$) programme to an attention control group (Stress Management Education—SME) ($n = 45$). Both interventions led to significant reductions in clinician-rated anxiety on the Hamilton Anxiety Rating Scale (HAMA), with a large effect size. However, MBSR was associated with significantly greater reduction in anxiety on the three other clinical outcome measures. Furthermore, clinician-rated 'responder' status (being rated as 'very much' or 'much' improved) was higher for MBSR (66 %) than CME (40 %). MBSR participants also showed reduced ratings of distress and anxiety following a laboratory stress paradigm, suggesting that mindfulness training may have improved coping in challenging situations (Hoge et al., 2013).

Two studies have featured active and credible control groups. A recent RCT compared ABBT to applied relaxation (AR), an evidence-based treatment for GAD (Hayes-Skelton, Roemer, & Orsillo, 2013). Both ABBT ($n = 40$) and AR ($n = 41$) led to large effects on clinician-rated GAD severity, anxiety symptom severity, as well as on self-reported worry, anxiety, depressive symptoms, and quality of life. Results were comparable to, or better than, what has been reported in trials of conventional CBT for GAD, with between 60 and 80 % of participants in both conditions manifesting clinically significant change both at posttreatment and follow-up. The authors had expected ABBT to outperform AR; however, they note that their version of AR was designed to be maximally effective—and may also be operative through some of the same mechanisms such as mindfulness, acceptance, and decentring (Hayes-Skelton et al., 2013).

Finally, ACT in a group format has been compared to cognitive behavioural group therapy (CBGT) for a sample of 51 patients (Avdagic, Morrissey, & Boschen, 2014). Both treatments led to significant improvement on all measures from pre- to post-assessment, with large within-group effect sizes for all symptom scales. The ACT group ($n=25$) showed more rapid gains in reduction of worry, distress, and symptom interference than the CBT group ($n=26$). However, at follow-up after 3 months, the treatments were equivalent. Also, a greater number of ACT participants achieved reliable and clinically significant change on worry symptoms at posttreatment (72 % vs. 42 %). Similarly to what was found for symptom scores, there were no differences between the treatments at follow-up, with both groups demonstrating rates of reliable and clinically significant change of 60 % (Avdagic et al., 2014).

Panic Disorder

Panic disorder (PD) is characterised by unexpected panic attacks, which are sudden surges of fear accompanied by physical sensations interpreted by the individual in a catastrophic manner. In PD, panic attacks lead to worry about the consequences of the attacks for one's physical health, safety, and well-being. PD is sometimes accompanied by agoraphobia, a pattern of phobic avoidance of situations or settings where it is difficult to escape or get help if a panic attack should occur (American Psychiatric Association, 1994; Roy-Byrne, Craske, & Stein, 2006).

How might the quality of awareness found in MABIs be brought to bear on PD? Fear of bodily sensations in PD often leads to watchful scanning for signs of an oncoming attack, as well as avoidance of both internal experience and of activities and external situations. In a sense, PD is clearly associated with heightened awareness—but this awareness is of the vigilant and fearful kind. Mindfulness, by contrast, entails a form of concrete and specific somatic awareness that is unlike the focus found in PD in that it is (a) inquiring in a gentle manner rather than fearful and (b) allowing for the natural ebb and flow of bodily sensations, rather than attempting to control or remove them. Individuals with PD are also often preoccupied with catastrophic thoughts, be it the possibility of a heart attack, fainting, or going mad/losing control. This thinking has a quality of absoluteness to it, where thoughts are seen as unquestionable facts rather than temporary mental phenomena that may or may not be true. By contrast, the processes of metacognitive awareness and defusion associated with the practice of mindfulness and acceptance could enable the individual to observe his or her thoughts from a witnessing perspective rather than being identified with them. The question is thus whether the cultivation of mindfulness and acceptance can counteract the psychological mechanisms triggering and exacerbating panic disorder.

The hypothesis would be that MABIs could provide what Barlow (2002) terms 'interoceptive exposure' by enabling the person to stay in touch with sensations of fear and panic without acting on them. It might facilitate a more relaxed and discerning attitude to bodily sensations, reducing the vigilant attention to them. Also, when panic occurs, allowing the physiological rush of it to arise and pass lends to an experiential realisation that the feared outcomes did not appear, thus constituting a form of extinction learning. A more spacious awareness of thoughts might make catastrophic interpretations either less salient or more liable to just fade away from awareness. Alternately, there is the possibility that the individual might also be able to challenge the veracity of these interpretations by way of merely becoming aware of them—or to counter them with more supportive and self-compassionate statements.

There is evidence from correlational studies that mindfulness and acceptance are inversely related to anxiety sensitivity, a heightened vulnerability to bodily symptoms that is seen as a precursor to developing a full-blown diagnosis of panic disorder (Vujanovic, Zvolensky, Bernstein, Feldner, & McLeish, 2007; McKee, Zvolensky, Solomon, Bernstein, & Leen-Feldner, 2007). Furthermore, analogue studies have shown that in laboratory paradigms designed to elicit panic symptomatology in both healthy subjects and subjects with anxiety disorders, behavioural strategies based on mindfulness and acceptance lead to better regulation of distress than what is the case for control groups (Eifert & Heffner, 2003; Levitt et al., 2004).

In sum, there exists a cogent theoretical rationale as to why mindfulness and acceptance may be beneficial for people suffering from PD/AG. According to both cross-sectional and analogue research designs, there are empirical indications that individuals high on measures of mindfulness and acceptance have less panic-related symptomatology. However, to this day, very few studies have examined the effect of MABIs on pure samples of patients with panic disorder.

An open trial of ACT for 11 patients with PD/AG found the intervention to be feasible and most likely effective. Large reductions in panic symptom severity were observed, comparing well to traditional CBT for panic disorder (Meuret, Twohig, Rosenfield, Hayes, & Craske, 2012). Another open trial investigated the effects of MBCT in combination with pharmacotherapy for a sample of 23 patients (Kim et al., 2010). Participants showed significant improvement on measures of panic severity, anxiety sensitivity, and specific catastrophic cognitions relating to bodily sensations. Effect sizes were large for clinician-rated scales but small for self-report outcome measures. Improvement was maintained at 1-year follow-up.

The first randomised controlled trial to examine a MABI for PD was recently published (Gloster et al., 2015). These authors examined the effects of ACT relative to a waiting list with delayed treatment for a sample of 43 patients with PD/AG who had failed to respond to previous evidence-based treatment. The ACT group ($n=33$) demonstrated improvement on panic symptoms, general symptom load, and functioning relative to the control group ($n=10$), with medium to large effect sizes that were maintained at follow-up after 6 months. Despite this being a small trial, the results indicate that ACT may be a viable treatment option for patients who do not respond to conventional CBT.

Social Anxiety Disorder

Social anxiety disorder (SAD)involves excessive anxiety and self-consciousness in social situations, with the primary concern in such situations being that the individual will say or do something that will result in embarrassment or humiliation (American Psychiatric Association, 1994; Stein & Stein, 2008). Like other anxiety disorders, social phobia constitutes the inverse of mindfulness as far as it involves negative self-focussed attention and a highly self-critical and judgmental stance toward oneself. The more adaptive form of attention toward thoughts and bodily sensations described above in relation to GAD and PD should thus be relevant also for SAD. In addition, mindfulness and acceptance as it is linked to the domain of self-experience might be particularly beneficial for individuals with SAD. The person could gently detach from reactive loops related to the narrative and evaluative self, instead allowing for thoughts and feelings as transient events and behaviour to be carried out in the service of broader life goals.

Bögels, Sijbers, & Voncken (2006) combined MBCT with task concentration training for nine patients with social phobia. They found significant decreases in self-reported symptoms of social phobia, and 7 out of 9 no longer met diagnostic criteria posttreatment. Patients kept improving from end of treatment to follow-up at 2 months. Effect sizes and the percentage of patients meeting criteria for high end-state functioning were within the range found for conventional CBT for social phobia (Bögels et al., 2006).

Ossman, Wilson, Storaasli, and McNeill (2006) investigated a group treatment protocol based on ACT for 22 patients with social phobia and reported significant decreases on measures of social phobia and experiential avoidance. In a pilot study of a 12-week programme integrating exposure therapy and ACT for patients with SAD, Dalrymple and Herbert (2007) found significant improvement and large effect sizes for social anxiety symptoms and quality of life.)Finally, Kocovski et al. (2009) assessed the feasibility and clinical effectiveness of mindfulness- and acceptance-based group therapy (MAGT) for 42 patients with social anxiety disorder in an open trial. MAGT resulted in significant reductions in social anxiety, depression, and rumination, as well as significant increases in mindfulness and acceptance. Gains were maintained at follow-up after 3 months. Most of the treatment completers met criteria for reliable change, and 43 % demonstrated clinically significant change on the Social Phobia Scale.

The most recent open trial examined the effects of ABBT for 38 patients with SAD and comorbid depression on concurrent pharmacotherapy (Dalrymple et al., 2014). Effect sizes for both clinician-rated and self-reported measures of social anxiety and depression were large for treatment completers. The authors note that while effects are lower than what is found in the most impressive efficacy trials of CBT for SAD, they compare well both to average effect sizes in meta-analyses of CBT for SAD, as well as to what is found in studies on real-world samples. Effects for broader measures of quality of life and everyday functioning were in the moderate range but also compare well to what has been found in trials of CBT for

SAD. However, the dropout rate was 32 %—fairly high, although not atypical for highly comorbid samples (Dalrymple et al., 2014).

Moving now to randomised controlled trials, Jazaieri, Goldin, Werner, Ziv, and Gross (2012) examined the effects of MBSR versus aerobic exercise for 56 patients with SAD ($n=31$ vs. 25). Both conditions showed equal reductions in social anxiety and depressive symptoms, as well as increases in well-being at posttreatment and 3-month follow-up. Within-group effect sizes were in the moderate range. About ¼ of participants in both groups evidenced clinically significant change in social anxiety symptoms as measured by LSAS-SR and SIAS-S, indicating that both interventions were less effective than what has been found in previous trials of CBT for SAD.

In a well-designed randomised trial, Koszycki et al. (2007) compared MBSR and cognitive behavioural group therapy (CBGT) for 53 patients with generalised SAD. Results revealed better response and remission rate on both clinician-rated and self-report outcome measures for CBGT, although the effects found for MBSR were also in the large range. The treatments were equally efficacious in improving functioning, self-rated depression, and quality of life. The authors conclude that despite MBSR being less effective than CBGT in reducing core symptoms of SAD, MBSR might still be a potentially useful alternative intervention for some patients with SAD. It should be noted that treatment dosage was unequal in the study, with the duration of CBGT being 12 weeks versus 8 weeks for MBSR.

Piet, Hougaard, Hecksher, and Rosenberg (2010) compared MBCT and group cognitive behavioural therapy (GCBT) in a small randomised pilot trial for 26 young adults with SAD. They report results similar to those of Koszycki et al. (2007), with both groups achieving moderate to large within-group effects on composite measures of social phobia. Unlike Koszycki and colleagues, Piet et al. (2010) did not find a significant difference between mindfulness training and GCBT. The authors conclude that MBCT is a useful low-cost treatment for patients with social phobia. However, they note that it is probably less efficacious than CBT, on the basis that the trial in question did not have large enough sample size for numerical trends favouring CBT to reach statistical significance.

Finally, Kocovski, Fleming, Hawley, Huta, and Antony (2013) compared mindfulness- and acceptance-based group therapy (MAGT) to cognitive behavioural group therapy (CBGT) and a wait-list control condition for 137 patients with SAD. Both interventions were more effective than the control group, and gains were maintained at 3-month follow-up. There were no significant differences for MAGT ($n=53$) and CBGT ($n=53$) on most outcome measures. For both groups, two thirds of participants were categorised as 'much' or 'very much' improved on clinician-rated clinical severity. Forty percent of treatment completers met criteria for clinically significant change on self-report measures of social anxiety, with no difference between the active treatment groups. Contrary to expectations, there was no difference between conditions on measures of valued living, mindfulness, acceptance, or reappraisal—the three former being outcome dimensions more directly addressed in MAGT, while the latter is seen as a core mechanism in CBT.

Post-traumatic Stress Disorder

Post-traumatic stress disorder (PTSD) is an anxiety disorder in which an individual's ability to function is impaired by cognitive and emotional responses to memories of one or more traumatic events. The diagnosis of PTSD requires exposure to an extreme stressor or traumatic event to which the individual responded with fear, helplessness, or horror. Symptoms include re-experiencing the event in the form of distressing images, nightmares, or flashbacks; avoidance of reminders of the event; and hyperarousal (American Psychiatric Association, 1994; Yehuda, 2002).

Whereas MABIs encourage present-centred awareness, PTSD powerfully illustrates how the past can intrude into the present to create suffering. Trauma-related cues trigger both cognitive and emotional reactivity, usually accompanied by physiological arousal that is difficult to regulate. The potential for mindfulness and acceptance to be directed toward intrusive mental images seems particularly promising with regard to PTSD, and so do the various strategies helping the individual to anchor himself or herself in the actuality of the present rather than in overwhelming memories of the past.

A few open trials have examined the effects of MBSR for patients with PTSD. Kimbrough and colleagues (2010) found large effect sizes for depression, anxiety, and PTSD symptoms for 27 adult survivors of childhood sexual abuse. A follow-up study after 2 ½ years with 19 of 27 original participants showed that these gains were largely maintained, indicating that MBSR may be effective in reducing emotional distress in the long term for individuals with childhood sexual trauma (Earley et al., 2014). Another open trial of MBSR for 92 US combat veterans found significant improvements in measures of PTSD, depression, experiential avoidance, and quality of life (Kearney, McDermott, Malte, Martinez, & Simpson, 2012). Effect sizes for mental health were medium to large, and nearly half of participants had clinically significant reductions in PTSD symptomatology at follow-up after 6 months. Mindfulness skills increased significantly during participation and were found to statistically mediate improvement in PTSD, depression, and quality of life (Kearney et al., 2012). Similarly, Serpa, Taylor, and Tillisch (2014) observed significant improvement in anxiety, depression, and general mental health for 79 US combat veterans, with increased mindfulness skills found to mediate these outcomes. This study also found MBSR to decrease suicidal ideation by almost half, an important metric in a patient population at far higher risk for suicide or self-injury than the general population (Kang et al., 2015).

Following up their 2012 open trial, Kearney, McDermott, Malte, Martinez, and Simpson (2013) carried out a randomised controlled pilot study comparing MBSR to treatment as usual for 47 veterans with PTSD. MBSR completers showed medium to large between-group effect sizes for depression, quality of life, and mindfulness from pre- to posttreatment. However, these results were attenuated when taking the entire intention-to-treat sample into consideration. Also, neither completer nor intention-to-treat analyses found reliable effects of MBSR on PTSD. In sum, this study found no evidence that MBSR was more effective than treatment as usual for trauma symptomatology in combat veterans, but there was some indication that mindfulness beneficially affects health-related quality of life for this population. The authors argue in favour of further trials to evaluate MBSR for veterans with PTSD and possibly augmenting the intervention to explicitly address the core symptoms of this disorder.

Another pilot study for combat veterans with long-term trauma symptoms compared MBCT modified for PTSD to treatment as usual (group-based psychoeducation or imagery rehearsal therapy) in a nonrandomised design (King et al., 2013). A reduction in clinician-rated PTSD symptoms was observed for MBCT participants, but not for the control condition. The effect size was moderate (0.67), and improvement was largely due to reduction in the avoidance subscale. Eleven of 15 treatment completers (73 %) in the MBCT condition showed 'clinically meaningful' improvement, as opposed to only 4 of 13 in the treatment as usual (33 %). As in the studies by Kearney et al. (2012) and Serpa et al. (2014), King et al. (2013) found indications that mindfulness was associated with better outcome, as decrease in intrusive symptoms was correlated with self-reported time spent on formal mindfulness exercises. The authors note that the findings are particularly noteworthy considering the brevity of the intervention and the long-standing trauma-related problems of the participants (all more than 10 years of PTSD, with the majority more than 30 years) (King et al., 2013).

Finally, one study has investigated MBSR as a telehealth intervention compared to psychoeducation for a)sample of 33 male combat veterans (Niles et al., 2012). MBSR participants showed an initial significant decrease in PTSD symptoms relative to the psychoeducation intervention, but returned to baseline levels of distress at follow-up after 6 weeks.

Other Anxiety Disorders

Obsessive-Compulsive Disorder

Obsessive-compulsive disorder (OCD) is characterised by intrusive thoughts or images (obsessions) and by repetitive or ritualistic actions or mental rituals (compulsions) which reduce anxiety (Stein, 2002). The most frequent symptoms in OCD are concerns about contamination and cleanliness with consequent washing or fear of harming oneself or others with consequent checking. However, there are a broad array of other obsessions and compulsions, including symmetry concerns and arranging, hoarding, as well as sexual, religious, and somatic concerns and corresponding rituals (American Psychiatric Association, 1994; Stein, 2002).

Two case series studies of patients with OCD found ACT protocols to be associated with reductions in compulsions in the magnitude of 80–90 %, as well as decreases in OCD severity (Dehlin, Morrison, & Twohig, 2013; Twohig, Hayes, & Masuda, 2006). In a more rigorous study design, Twohig et al. (2010) compared a short ACT protocol to relaxation training for 79 patients with OCD, finding greater improvement in OCD symptoms and depression symptoms at posttreatment and follow-up for the ACT condition. Half of the ACT participants (19 of 41) showed clinically significant change on the Yale-Brown Obsessive Compulsive Scale (Y-BOCS), as opposed to only 5 of 38 of those having received relaxation training. ACT participants also showed larger initial decreases in thought control and increased psychological flexibility relative to relaxation training.

Hypochondriasis

A pilot study found significant improvement in health anxiety, disease-related thoughts, and somatic symptoms for 10 patients with hypochondriasis (Lovas & Barsky, 2010). Building on these results, McManus, Surawy, Muse, Vazquez-Montes, and Williams (2012) compared MBCT to unrestricted health service utilisation for 74 patients with hypochondriasis. They found no difference in levels of general anxiety and depression or in comorbid states, but on a composite measure of health anxiety, the MBCT had significantly more improvement than the control condition both immediately after treatment and at follow-up after 1 year. Half of MBCT treatment completers (53 %) no longer met diagnostic criteria for hypochondriasis at the end of treatment, with this rate increasing to 72 % at 1-year follow-up. The authors also found support for increased mindfulness as being a mechanism of change, as changes in self-reported mindfulness served as a statistical mediator for changes in health anxiety (McManus et al., 2012).

Meta-Analyses

A benefit of the accumulating empirical investigation in any field is the possibility of quantitatively integrating the available evidence. Several recent large-scale meta-analyses have examined the impact of MABIs for anxiety disorders. Firstly, anxiety has been considered as an outcome across patient groups and diagnostic categories. Khoury et al. (2013) summed up the results of 209 clinical trials ($n = 12\ 154$) and found large effect sizes for anxiety both within groups (0.89) and when comparing active treatment and wait-list control groups (0.96). These effects were maintained at follow-up. When MBIs were compared to active control groups, an advantage was found for MBIs over some interventions (e.g. psychoeducation, supportive therapy, relaxation) but not over traditional CBT (Khoury et al., 2013).

A more stringent recent meta-analysis included only randomised controlled trials where comparison groups were either active treatment or nonspecific placebo (i.e. matched for time and attention) (Goyal et al., 2014). When comparing mindfulness meditation to nonspecific placebo, these authors found moderate effect sizes on measures of anxiety at posttreatment (0.38) relative to controls. This effect was attenuated somewhat at follow-up (0.22), but was still significant. The meta-analysis found no evidence that any meditation intervention was more effective than active comparisons including, among others, CBT, physical exercise, and progressive muscle relaxation. Nevertheless, they conclude that mindfulness meditation may serve to reduce anxiety and depression over and above the effects of time and attention—with effects akin to those of antidepressant medication, but without the potential side effects (Goyal et al., 2014).

Turning now to meta-analyses limited to clinical trials for patients diagnosed with anxiety disorders, the present author and colleagues (Vøllestad et al. 2011) found 19 studies examining the effects of MABIs for anxiety disorders (PD/AG, SAD, GAD, or mixed anxiety), with pre- to posttreatment effects yielding overall Hedge's g effect sizes of 1.08 for anxiety measures and 0.85 for depression symptoms, with treatment gains maintained over time. Effect sizes for measures of quality of life were in the medium range, indicating that MABIs do contribute to broader positive outcomes than reduced symptom distress. As the majority of the trials were uncontrolled, it is not possible to draw any definite conclusions about the contribution of the mechanisms assumed to be specific to MABIs to outcomes. The four trials employing proper randomisation procedures indicate that MABIs outperform no-treatment and placebo controls and either perform as well as or slightly poorer than established treatments (Vøllestad et al. 2012).

Strauss et al. (2014) focussed their meta-analysis on RCTs where participants met diagnostic criteria for a current episode of an anxiety or depressive disorder. The authors initially found reason to question the feasibility and effectiveness of MBIs for this purpose, as individuals in the midst of acute depression or anxiety might have difficulties bringing awareness to their present-moment experience, as well as difficulties in motivation and concentration inhibiting engagement in the therapeutic work of MBIs. The authors draw different conclusions for depression and anxiety. They report significant benefits of MBIs relative to control conditions for patients with primary diagnosis of depression, with a moderate to large between-group effect size (0.73). So contrary to the authors' expectations, a current depressive episode does not constitute a barrier to benefitting from MBIs. However, the authors did not find a similar significant effect for anxiety disorders—neither when examining participants with a confirmed diagnosis of anxiety nor when taking into account anxiety as an outcome irrespective of primary diagnosis. On this basis, they caution against offering MBIs to patients with anxiety disorders or when addressing anxiety severity as such in patients with other primary diagnoses. This more pessimistic conclusion is in opposition to what was found by Vøllestad et al. (2012) but Strauss et al. (2014) argue that their meta-analysis features more stringent inclusion criteria (restricted to MBIs and thus excluding acceptance-based interventions) and include more trials in the between-group analysis—and thus provides a more accurate picture of the (lacking) impact of MBIs on anxiety symptoms.

A recent review of ACT for anxiety disorders found modest support for the use of ACT with GAD, OCD, SAD, and mixed anxiety disorders (Bluett et al., 2014). These authors also conducted a preliminary meta-analysis of RCTs of ACT for anxiety disorders, including nine studies with a total sample size of 404 participants.

There were no significant differences between ACT and active comparison conditions on anxiety outcome measures or measures of change process (e.g. the Acceptance and Action Questionnaire). The authors conclude that although CBT should continue to be seen as the treatment of choice for anxiety disorder, there is sufficient evidence to recommend ACT to patients who choose to opt out of CBT or do not benefit from it.

Finally, Norton, Abbott, Norberg, and Hunt (2014) provide a systematic review of nine trials of MABIs (termed MABTs) for SAD (all of which have been presented in this chapter). They conclude that MABTs are associated with clinically significant reductions in social anxiety symptoms, with effect sizes in the moderate to large range at posttreatment and at follow-up after 3 or 6 months. However, they note that the observed effects are consistently smaller than those found in RCTs of CBT [1.24–2.63], as well as there being considerable methodological limitations in the current research on MABTs for SAD (small sample sizes, high attrition rates, lack of active control groups, or equivalent or slightly less favourable results when active comparisons are used).

Discussion

A Summary of the Evidence

We have seen in this chapter that there is a cogent theoretical rationale for employing mindfulness- and acceptance-based approaches to the treatment of anxiety disorders, detailing how the cultivation of non-judgmental, present-centred attention may alleviate the suffering associated with these clinical syndromes. Specifically, mindfulness and acceptance may serve to counteract the maladaptive psychological processes involved in anxiety disorders, such as attentional deficits, repetitive negative thinking, avoidance behaviours, emotional dysregulation, and maladaptive self-experience. Furthermore, correlational studies have shown mindfulness and acceptance to be inversely related to anxiety and related constructs; also basic laboratory research has demonstrated that strategies of present-centred awareness and acceptance constitute a viable response to distress. However, clinical trials have not as of yet unequivocally borne out the potential of these approaches.

In keeping with the transdiagnostic nature of MABIs, there is emerging evidence that they are consistently associated with significant reductions of anxiety and related problems for patients with heterogeneous anxiety disorders. They have outperformed wait-list (Vøllestad et al. 2011) and attentional control groups (Lee et al., 2007; Kim et al., 2009), and ACT and MBSR have proven equivalent to CBT in well-designed RCTs with adequate sample sizes (Arch et al., 2012; Arch et al., 2013). This would indicate that for samples of patients with heterogeneous anxiety disorders, MABIs may be regarded as empirically validated and even well-established treatments. It is also of interest that an Internet-delivered mindfulness intervention performs as well as face-to-face MBSR (Boettcher et al., 2014), giving grounds for optimism regarding alternative modes of delivery for MABIs.

When considering specific anxiety disorders, the picture is more mixed. The best evidence exists for the treatment of GAD, where clinical trials of MABIs have consistently found significant improvements in anxiety, worry, and comorbid depression. ABBT has outperformed wait-list control, demonstrating impressive effects with regard to end-state functioning and diagnostic remission (Roemer, Orsillo, & Salters-Pedneault, 2008). MBSR has outperformed an attentional control (Hoge et al., 2013), while a comparison of ACT and CBGT found both treatments to be equivalent (Avdagic et al., 2014). Finally, ABBT has also performed as well as an already established treatment for GAD, applied relaxation, with outcomes comparable to the strongest findings from trials of CBT for GAD (Hayes-Skelton et al., 2013). Similar to what was found for mixed anxiety disorders, the case could be made that MABIs are an empirically validated treatment option for GAD. However, comparisons between MABIs and CBT in trials with a greater number of participants are needed in order to clarify how well these interventions perform relative to the current treatment of choice for GAD.

For SAD, open trials of MABIs have demonstrated consistent reductions in social anxiety and related symptoms. One RCT found equivalent outcomes for MBSR and aerobic exercise, but the authors emphasise that the rate of clinically significant change is lower than what has been found for CBT in other trials (Jazaieri et al., 2012). In RCTs comparing MABIs to CBT, two studies have found equal outcomes, while one found CBT to be superior. However, the authors in both studies reporting equal effects conclude that CBT is most likely a more efficacious treatment for SAD. Piet et al. (2010) note that CBT would probably have proved more efficacious given a larger sample size, while Kocovski et al. (2013) point to the fact that larger effects are routinely found in individual CBT for SAD. It must also be noted that the UK guidelines for SAD caution against routinely offering MBIs to this patient group, on the basis of insufficient evidence (National Institute for Health and Care Excellence, 2013).

The current evidence suggests caution in offering MABIs as a first-line treatment for patients with SAD. However, there is a cogent theoretical rationale for employing MABIs for this disorder, as well as some evidence from laboratory and analogue studies showing strategies from these treatments to be effective in managing or counteracting psychopathological processes involved in SAD (Vassilopoulos, 2008; Vassilopoulos & Watkins, 2009) . It is possible that the strong negative self-focus and entrenched proneness to self-criticism and shame found in SAD require further tailoring of interventions for MABIs to fully benefit socially anxious individuals.

There is a gap between the strong theoretical rationale for MABIs and the promising analogue studies of mindfulness and acceptance for panic disorder and the paucity of research on this diagnostic category. This could be due to existing highly effective treatment in the form of CBT, with higher response rates than treatments for SAD and GAD. However, a recent open trial which shows effects for CBT nonresponders (Gloster et al., 2015) indicates that MABIs merit further consideration also for this diagnostic category.

A reactive relationship to experience and lack of present-centred awareness are prominent features of PTSD. There is also correlational research showing acceptance and mindfulness to be negatively associated with trauma symptomatology (Smith et al., 2011; Thompson & Waltz, 2010; Vujanovic, Youngwirth, Johnson, & Zvolensky, 2009). Despite this, clinical research on MABIs for PTSD has been lagging behind compared to the most-studied anxiety disorders. However, in recent years, both open and controlled trials comparing MBSR and MBCT to treatment as usual have produced promising results. Interestingly, pure-form mindfulness training seems to predominate in the trauma field. An exception here is dialectical behaviour therapy (DBT), which has been studied extensively for patients with borderline personality disorder, a clinical syndrome often featuring prominent trauma symptomatology (for a review, see Panos, Jackson, Hasan, & Panos, 2013). It will be interesting to see how ACT performs for patients with PTSD, as well as the relative efficacy of MBSR/MBCT compared to treatments already established as effective for PTSD (see Watts et al., 2013).

Clinical Implications

A considerable subset of patients with anxiety disorders does not respond to current treatment or suffers from residual symptoms or impairment after treatment (Hofmann & Bögels, 2006; Ninan, 2001). It is possible that MABIs could offer a novel way of relating to symptoms that might alleviate distress unsuccessfully targeted by CBT. The reasons for nonresponse or premature treatment termination are diverse, but one possibility is that the treatment format of CBT might not appeal equally to all patients. Matching treatments to patient preferences have been shown to beneficially affect outcome and reduce likelihood of premature termination. A recent meta-analysis found that matched clients have a 58 % chance of showing greater improvement, and further analyses indicate that they are about half as likely to drop out of treatment when compared with clients not receiving a preferred treatment (Swift & Callahan, 2009).

MABIs have features that might cause patients to prefer them over other treatment modalities, given the opportunity of patient choice. These include the downplaying of disorder-specific processes and symptom removal and an explicit focus on valued action and quality of life over and above that related to illness and mental health. MABIs typically engage more comprehensively with issues pertinent to the totality of the individual's life, advocating mindful awareness as a way of life rather than merely a more efficient way of managing symptoms.

MABIs come in different treatment modalities. The group format of MBSR, MBCT, and MAGT may confer potential advantages in terms of cost-effectiveness, although this has not hitherto been assessed in relation to patients with anxiety disorders. It could be argued that MABIs might be particularly suited for group administration: understanding of the somewhat counter-intuitive nature of mindfulness and acceptance strategies could be facilitated by vicarious learning, and the possibility for communal exercises could benefit motivation and commitment to therapeutic tasks. Also, many treatment centres are unable to recruit homogeneous groups within manageable time frames, and allowing for diagnostically heterogeneous groups enables treatment providers to easily recruit from a broader spectrum of patients. On the other hand, the individual format that ACT and ABBT is usually delivered in has the advantage of tailoring treatment by way of personalised case formulations and interventions targeting the most pressing problem areas.

Some authors and guidelines caution against applying MABIs to anxiety disorders given the current status of evidence (National Institute for Health and Care Excellence, 2013; Strauss et al., 2014). However, there are no reports of adverse effects of mindfulness for these disorders. MABIs are likely to be effective for some patients, but more research is needed to determine who might benefit from MABIs as compared to other treatments. It is also important to keep in mind that research on these modalities is ongoing and progressing, so conclusions from current meta-analytic reviews should not be seen as final assessments of their efficacy. But until further notice, as a general rule CBT should be treatment of choice, while MABIs could be an option for patients not benefiting fully from CBT or who decline CBT treatment.

There is also the issue of how similar or different MABIs are from CBT. Should they be seen as a separate family of treatments, or should they rather be subsumed as a potential set of interventions within the framework of CBT? It can sometimes be difficult to distinguish MABIs from traditional CBT, as many include elements that are similar to CBT interventions. Consequently, some authors have argued that they should be seen as part of the CBT family (Hofmann & Asmundson, 2008; Mennin, Ellard, Fresco, & Gross, 2013). However, as argued initially in this chapter, MABIs can be seen as operating according to common principles and mechanisms of change that serve to unite them conceptually while at the same time distinguishing them from conventional CBT. There is still a need to further clarify how well the varieties of MABIs perform relative to established treatments. Given the tendency to differential effects for different MABIs in anxiety disorders, it might also be relevant to compare different treatment modalities within this tradition head to head. However, an equally relevant issue is the investigation of how different approaches may be suited to different types of patients or presenting problems, as some findings are beginning to suggest (Wolitzky-Taylor, Arch, Rosenfield, & Craske, 2012).

On the other hand, there is potential for selective integration between MABIs and CBT, informed by theory and research evidence. There is no reason that current treatment options for anxiety should be seen as final in this regard. It does seem that therapeutic packages combining mindfulness and cognitive behavioural principles (i.e. ACT, ABBT, and MBCT) fare somewhat better than the pure-form mindfulness of MBSR. This would seem to go counter to the transdiagnostic approach that is integral to MABIs and that has been emphasised in this chapter. However, one cannot disregard the possibility that specific anxiety disorders do constitute particular forms of suffering, characterised by certain deeply engrained reactive patterns that need to be more explicitly addressed. Indeed, some authors have cautioned against applying mindfulness training with disregard for the specific characteristics of particular disorders (Teasdale, Segal, & Williams, 2003; Williams, 2010). The addition of certain cognitive behavioural techniques to an MBI could further help participants in disengaging from maladaptive patterns or biases in information processing. The behaviour-analytical approaches of ACT and ABBT are already practising this form of eclecticism. Such integration is also the foundation of MBCT, which in addition to the formal mindfulness exercises in MBSR features psychoeducational material and experiential exercises to address the particular modes of cognitive reactivity involved in depressive relapse. It is possible that the MBCT format could thus be tailored to address the specific pathogenic forms of information processing, behavioural avoidance, emotional dysregulation, and self-experience in different anxiety disorders. It would be relevant to further explore along these lines in future treatment development.

Recommendations for Research

There is a need for further studies that compare MABIs to CBTs, in order to clarify the relative benefit of these approaches to patients with anxiety disorders. It is advisable that such studies are sufficiently powered to test for statistical non-inferiority, i.e. equal efficacy. Also, few studies have provided adequate checks for fidelity and competence with regard to treatment manuals, and this is recommended to ensure that therapists are actually offering the treatment in question. It would also be of interest to compare different MABIs to each other, to test which mode of delivery is most useful with regard to anxiety disorders. However, it is possible that such head-to-head comparisons will demonstrate less of a difference between treatment groups, as is generally the rule rather than the exception in psychotherapy research when bona fide treatments are tested against each other. It will therefore be important to consider moderating variables that may tell us more about who benefits from what type of treatment.

A further avenue of investigation concerns mechanisms of action. There are indications that observed outcomes in clinical trials of MABIs can be ascribed to changes in the putative mechanisms of change, such as increased mindfulness and acceptance. However, future studies will benefit from designs that allow for stringent statistical tests of mediation, as this is rare in the extant research. Also, for MBIs it needs to be further investigated which role formal and informal mindfulness practice plays in bringing about outcomes. At present, neither changes in mindfulness/acceptance nor amount of practice have been established as prerequisites for observed benefits. As such, it cannot be ruled out that the effects of interventions are due to 'nonspecific' factors of treatment such as social support, group cohesion, therapeutic alliance, relaxation, increased self-efficacy, expectancy effects, and a host of other factors. It is also the case that particularly MBIs require therapists or mindfulness instructors to be sufficiently trained and grounded in meditative practice, in order to be able to embody the qualities of mindful awareness and non-judging inquiry in their clinical work. The relationship between such competencies and outcomes has of yet been largely neglected in the study of MABIs and may be a worthwhile path to follow in future investigations.

Conclusion

There is growing evidence that therapeutic strategies aimed at fostering a stance of mindfulness and acceptance are effective in reducing distress and improving functioning in individuals with anxiety disorders. The current evidence is strongest for mixed anxiety disorders and GAD, with equivocal findings for SAD and limited research on other anxiety disorders. At present, few trials of MABIs have demonstrated the same level of efficacy as found in both individual trials and meta-analytic reviews of CBT. These more modest findings suggest that despite a cogent theoretical rationale and evidence that mindfulness and acceptance is inversely correlated with anxiety, we still don't know how to optimally strengthen these important qualities in patients with anxiety disorders. However, given the level of nonresponding to CBT and varying patient preferences, there is reason to include MABIs as part of a differentiated set of treatment options. There may be reason to expect the further integration of strategies of mindfulness with conventional cognitive behavioural interventions to be a way forward. This might undercut the transdiagnostic foundation of MABIs somewhat, but could be necessary in order to effectively address the entrenched nature of psychological dysfunction in some of these disorders. MABIs may be of particular appeal as an empowering, non-pathologising approach emphasising the active participation of the individual in self-care and emotion regulation. They offer a broad range of coping mechanisms relevant not only to disorder-specific symptoms but also to everyday life more broadly conceived. Continued investigation of their implementation for patients with anxiety disorders is warranted.

References

American Psychiatric Association. (1994). *Diagnostic and statistical manual of mental disorders: DSM-IV* (4th ed.). Washington, DC: APA.

Amstadter, A. (2008). Emotion regulation and anxiety disorders. *Journal of Anxiety Disorders, 22*, 211–221.

Antony, M. M. (2002). Enhancing current treatments for anxiety disorders. *Clinical Psychology: Science and Practice, 9*, 91–94.

Arch, J. J., Ayers, C. R., Baker, A., Almklov, E., Dean, D. J., & Craske, M. G. (2013). Randomized clinical trial of adapted mindfulness-based stress reduction versus group cognitive behavioral therapy for heterogeneous anxiety disorders. *Behaviour Research and Therapy, 51*, 185–196.

Arch, J. J., Eifert, G. H., Davies, C., Vilardaga, J. C. P., Rose, R. D., & Craske, M. G. (2012). Randomized clinical trial of cognitive behavioral therapy (CBT) versus acceptance and commitment therapy (ACT) for mixed anxiety disorders. *Journal of Consulting and Clinical Psychology, 80*, 750–765.

Austin, D. W., & Richards, J. C. (2001). The catastrophic misinterpretation model of panic disorder. *Behaviour Research and Therapy, 39*, 1277–1291.

Avdagic, E., Morrissey, S. A., & Boschen, M. J. (2014). A randomised controlled trial of acceptance and commitment therapy and cognitive-behaviour therapy for generalised anxiety disorder. *Behaviour Change, 31*, 110–130.

Baer, R. A. (2007). Mindfulness, assessment, and transdiagnostic processes. *Psychological Inquiry, 18*, 238–271.

Baer, R. A., Smith, G. T., Hopkins, J., Krietemeyer, J., & Toney, L. (2006). Using self-report assessment methods to explore facets of mindfulness. *Assessment, 13*, 27–45.

Bar-Haim, Y., Lamy, D., Pergamin, L., Bakermans-Kranenburg, M. J., & van Ijzendorn, M. H. (2007). Threat-related attentional bias in anxious and nonanxious individuals: A meta-analytic study. *Psychological Bulletin, 133*, 1–24.

Barlow, D. H. (2002). *Anxiety and its disorders* (2nd ed.). New York: The Guilford Press.

Baumeister, R. F., Heatherton, T. F., & Tice, D. M. (1994). *Losing control: How and why people fail at self-regulation*. San Diego: Academic.

Bishop, S. R., Lau, M., Shapiro, S., Carlson, L., Anderson, N. D., Carmody, J., et al. (2004). Mindfulness: A proposed operational definition. *Clinical Psychology: Science and Practice, 11*, 230–241.

Bluett, E. J., Homan, K. J., Morrison, K. L., Levin, M. E., & Twohig, M. P. (2014). Acceptance and commitment therapy for anxiety and OCD spectrum disorders: An empirical review. *Journal of Anxiety Disorders, 28*, 612–624.

Boettcher, J., Åström, V., Påhlsson, D., Schenström, O., Andersson, G., & Carlbring, P. (2014). Internet-based mindfulness treatment for anxiety disorders: A randomized controlled trial. *Behavior Therapy, 45*, 241–253.

Bögels, S. M., Sijbers, G. F. V., & Voncken, M. (2006). Mindfulness and task concentration training for social phobia: A pilot study. *Journal of Cognitive Psychotherapy, 20*, 33–44.

Bohlmeijer, E. T., Fledderus, M., Rokx, T. A. J. J., & Pieterse, M. E. (2011). Efficacy of an early intervention based on acceptance and commitment therapy for adults with depressive symptomatology: Evaluation in a randomized controlled trial. *Behaviour Research and Therapy, 49*, 62–67.

Bolton J. M., Cox, B. J., Afifi, T. O., Enns, M. W., Bienvenu, O. J., & Sareen, J. (2008). Anxiety disorders and risk for suicide attempts: Findings from the Baltimore Epidemiologic Catchment area follow-up study. *Depression and Anxiety, 25*, 477–481.

Bondolfi, G., Jermann, F., der Linden, M. V., Gex-Fabry, M., Bizzini, L., Rouget, B. W., et al. (2010). Depression relapse prophylaxis with Mindfulness-Based Cognitive Therapy: Replication and extension in the Swiss health care system. *Journal of Affective Disorders, 122*, 224–231.

Borkovec, T. D., Alcaine, O., & Behar, E. (2004). Avoidance theory of worry and generalized anxiety disorder. In R. G. Heimberg, C. L. Turk, & D. Mennin (Eds.), *Generalized anxiety disorder: Advances in research and practice* (pp. 77–108). New York: Guilford Press.

Bränström, R., Duncan, L. G., & Moskowitz, J. T. (2011). The association between dispositional mindfulness, psychological well-being, and perceived health in a Swedish population-based sample. *British Journal of Health Psychology, 16*, 300–316.

Brown, K. W., & Ryan, R. M. (2003). The benefits of being present: Mindfulness and its role in psychological well-being. *Journal of Personality and Social Psychology, 84*, 822–848.

Bruce, S. E., Yonkers, K. A., Otto, M. W., Eisen, J. L., Weisberg, R. B., Pagano, M., et al. (2005). Influence of psychiatric comorbidity on recovery and recurrence in generalized anxiety disorder, social phobia, and panic disorder: A 12-year prospective study. *American Journal of Psychiatry, 162*, 1179–1187.

Campbell-Sills, L., & Barlow, D. H. (2007). Incorporating emotion regulation into conceptualizations and treatments of anxiety and mood disorders. In J. J. Gross (Ed.), *Handbook of emotion regulation* (pp. 542–559). New York: Guilford.

Campbell-Sills, L., Barlow, D. H., Brown, T. A., & Hofmann, S. G. (2006a). Acceptability and suppression of negative emotion in anxiety and mood disorders. *Emotion, 6*, 587–595.

Campbell-Sills, L., Barlow, D. H., Brown, T. A., & Hofmann, S. G. (2006b). Effects of suppression and acceptance of emotional responses of individuals with anxiety and mood disorders. *Behavior Research and Therapy, 44*, 1251–1263.

Carmody, J. (2009). Evolving concepts of mindfulness in clinical settings. *Journal of Cognitive Psychotherapy, 23*, 270–280.

Cash, M., & Whittingham, K. (2010). What facets of mindfulness contribute to psychological well-being and depressive, anxious, and stress-related symptomatology? *Mindfulness, 1*, 177–182.

Chan, D., & Woollacott, M. (2007). Effects of level of meditation experience on attentional focus: Is the efficiency of executive or orientation networks improved? *The Journal of Alternative and Complementary Medicine, 13*, 651–658.

Chiesa, A., & Malinowski, P. (2011). Mindfulness-based approaches: Are they all the same? *Journal of Clinical Psychology, 67*, 1–21.

Chiesa, A., & Serretti, A. (2009). Mindfulness-based stress reduction for stress management in healthy people: A review and meta-analysis. *Journal of Alternative and Complementary Medicine, 15*, 593–600.

Clark, D. M. (1999). Anxiety disorders. Why they persist and how to treat them. *Behaviour Research and Therapy, 37*, 5–27.

Craigie, M. A., Rees, C. S., Marsh, A., & Nathan, P. (2008). Mindfulness-based cognitive therapy for generalized anxiety disorder: A preliminary evaluation. *Behavioral and Cognitive Psychotherapy, 36*, 553–568.

Craske, M. G., Rauch, S. L., Ursano, R., Prenoveau, J., Pine, D. S., & Zinbarg, R. E. (2009). What is an anxiety disorder? *Depression and Anxiety, 26*, 1066–1085.

Creswell, J. D., Way, B. M., Eisenberger, N. I., & Lieberman, M. D. (2007). Neural correlates of dispositional mindfulness during affect labeling. *Psychosomatic Medicine, 69*, 560–565.

Dalrymple, K. L., & Herbert, J. D. (2007). Acceptance and commitment therapy for generalized social anxiety disorder – a pilot study. *Behavior Modification, 31*, 543–568.

Dalrymple, K. L., Morgan, T. A., Lipschitz, J. M., Martinez, J. H., Tepe, E., & Zimmerman, M. (2014). An integrated, acceptance-based behavioral approach for depression with social anxiety - Preliminary results. *Behavior Modification, 38*, 516–548.

de Vibe, M., Bjørndal, A., Tipton, E., Hammerstrøm, K. T., & Kowalski, K. (2012). Mindfulness based stress reduction (MBSR) for improving health, quality of life, and social functioning in adults. *Campbell Systematic Reviews, 8*.

Deacon, B., Lickel, J., & Abramowitz, J. S. (2008). Medical utilization across the anxiety disorders. *Journal of Anxiety Disorders, 22*, 344–350.

Dehlin, J. P., Morrison, K. L., & Twohig, M. P. (2013). Acceptance and commitment therapy as a treatment for scrupulosity in obsessive compulsive disorder. *Behavior Modification, 37*, 409–430.

Desrosiers, A., Klemanski, D. H., & Nolen-Hoeksema, S. (2013). Mapping mindfulness facets onto dimensions of anxiety and depression. *Behavior Therapy, 44*, 373–384.

Deyo, M., Wilson, K. A., Ong, J., & Koopman, C. (2009). Mindfulness and rumination: Does mindfulness training lead to reductions in the ruminative thinking associated with depression? *Patient Education and Counseling, 5*, 265–271.

Dugas, M. J., Buhr, K., & Ladouceur, R. (2004). The role of intolerance of uncertainty in etiology and maintenance. In R. G. Heimberg, C. L. Turk, & D. S. Mennin (Eds.), *Generalized anxiety disorder: Advances in research and practice* (pp. 77–108). New York: Guilford Press.

Earley, M. D., Chesney, M. A., Frye, J., Greene, P. A., Berman, B., & Kimbrough, E. (2014). Mindfulness intervention for child abuse survivors: A 2.5-year follow-up. *Journal of Clinical Psychology, 70*, 933–941.

Ehring, T., & Watkins, E. R. (2009). Repetitive negative thinking as a transdiagnostic process. *International Journal of Cognitive Therapy, 1*, 192–205.

Eifert, G. H., & Forsyth, J. P. (2005). *Acceptance and commitment therapy for anxiety disorders: A practitioner's treatment guide to using mindfulness, acceptance, and value-based behavior change strategies*. Oakland, CA: New Harbinger Publications.

Eifert, G. H., & Heffner, M. (2003). The effects of acceptance versus control contexts on avoidance of panic-related symptoms. *Journal of Behavior Therapy and Experimental Psychiatry, 34*, 293–312.

Evans, S., Ferrando, S., Findler, M., Stowell, C., Smart, C., & Haglin, D. (2008). Mindfulness-based cognitive therapy for generalized anxiety disorder. *Journal of Anxiety Disorders, 22*, 716–721.

Farb, N. A., Anderson, A. K., & Segal, Z. V. (2012). The mindful brain and emotion regulation in mood disorders. *Canadian Journal of Psychiatry, 57*, 70–77.

Farb, N. A. S., Segal, Z. V., Mayberg, H., Bean, J., McKeon, D., Fatima, Z., et al. (2007). Attending to the present: Mindfulness meditation reveals distinct neural modes of self-reference. *Social Cognitive and Affective Neuroscience, 2*, 259–263.

Farb, N. A., Segal, Z. V., & Anderson, A. K. (2012). Mindfulness meditation training alters cortical representations of interoceptive attention. *Social Cognitive and Affective Neuroscience, 8*, 15–26.

Finucane, A., & Mercer, S. W. (2006). An exploratory mixed methods study of the acceptability and effectiveness of mindfulness-based cognitive therapy for patients with active depression and anxiety in primary care. *BMC Psychiatry, 6*, 14.

Frewen, P. A., Evans, E. M., Maraj, N., Dozois, D. J., & Partridge, K. (2008). Letting go: Mindfulness and negative automatic thinking. *Cognitive Therapy and Research, 32*, 758–774.

Gloster, A. T., Sonntag, R., Hoyer, J., Meyer, A. H., Heinze, S., Ströhle, A., et al. (2015). Treating treatment-resistant patients with panic disorder and agoraphobia using psychotherapy: A randomized controlled switching trial. *Psychotherapy and Psychosomatics, 84*, 100–109.

Godfrin, K. A., & van Heeringen, C. (2010). The effects of mindfulness-based cognitive therapy on recurrence of depressive episodes, mental health and quality of life: A randomized controlled study. *Behaviour Research and Therapy, 48*, 738–746.

Goldin, P. R., Ramel, W., & Gross, J. J. (2009). Mindfulness meditation training and self-referential processing in social anxiety disorders: Behavioral and neural effects. *Journal of Cognitive Psychotherapy, 23*, 242–257.

Goyal, M., Singh, S., Sibinga, E. M., Gould, N. F., Rowland-Seymour, A., Sharma, R., et al. (2014). Meditation programs for psychological stress and well-being: A systematic review and meta-analysis. *JAMA Internal Medicine, 174*, 357–368.

Greenberg, P. E., Sisitsky, T., Kessler, R. C., Finkelstein, S. N., Berndt, E. R., Davidson, J. R. T., et al. (1999). The economic burden of anxiety disorders in the 1990s. *Journal of Clinical Psychiatry, 60*, 427–435.

Gross, J. J. (2002). Emotion regulation: Affective, cognitive, and social consequences. *Psychophysiology, 39*, 281–291.

Hargus, E., Crane, C., Barnhofer, T., & Williams, J. M. G. (2010). Effects of mindfulness on meta-awareness and specificity of describing prodromal symptoms in suicidal depression. *Emotion, 10*, 34–42.

Hayes, S. C. (2004). Acceptance and commitment therapy, relational frame theory, and the third wave of behavioral and cognitive therapies. *Behavior Therapy, 35*, 639–665.

Hayes, A. M., & Feldman, G. (2004). Clarifying the construct of mindfulness in the context of emotion regulation and the process of change in therapy. *Clinical Psychology: Research and Practice, 11*, 255–262.

Hayes, S. C., Luoma, J. B., Bond, F. W., Masuda, A., & Lillis, J. (2006). Acceptance and Commitment Therapy: Model, processes, and outcomes. *Behaviour Research and Therapy, 44*, 1–25.

Hayes, S. A., Orsillo, S. M., & Roemer, L. (2010). Changes in proposed mechanisms of action during an acceptance-based behavior therapy for generalized anxiety disorder. *Behaviour Research and Therapy, 48*, 238–245.

Hayes, S. C., Strosahl, K. D., & Wilson, K. G. (1999). *Acceptance and commitment therapy. An experiential approach to behavior change*. New York: The Guilford Press.

Hayes-Skelton, S. A., Roemer, L., & Orsillo, S. M. (2013). A randomized clinical trial comparing an acceptance-based behavior therapy to applied relaxation for generalized anxiety disorder. *Journal of Consulting and Clinical Psychology, 81*, 761–773.

Heimberg, R. G. (2002). Cognitive-behavioral therapy for social anxiety disorder: Current status and future directions. *Biological Psychiatry, 51*, 101–108.

Hofmann, S. G., & Asmundson, G. J. G. (2008). Acceptance- and mindfulness-based therapy: New wave or old hat? *Clinical Psychology Review, 28*, 1–16.

Hofmann, S. G., & Bögels, S. M. (2006). Recent advances in the treatment of social phobia: Introduction to the special issue. *Journal of Cognitive Psychotherapy, 20*, 3–5.

Hofmann, S. G., Sawyer, A. T., Witt, A. A., & Oh, D. (2010). The effect of mindfulness-based therapy on anxiety and depression: A meta-analytic review. *Journal of Consulting and Clinical Psychology, 78*, 169–183.
Hofmann, S. G., & Smits, J. A. (2008). Cognitive-behavioral therapy for adult anxiety disorders: A meta-analysis of randomized placebo-controlled trials. *Journal of Clinical Psychiatry, 69*, 621–632.
Hoge, E. A., Bui, E., Marques, L., Metcalf, C. A., Morris, L. K., Robinaugh, D. J., et al. (2013). Randomized controlled trial of mindfulness meditation for generalized anxiety disorder: Effects on anxiety and stress reactivity. *The Journal of Clinical Psychiatry, 74*, 786–792.
Hollon, S. D., & Beck, A. T. (2004). Cognitive and cognitive-behavioral therapies. In A. E. Bergin & S. L. Garfield (Eds.), *Handbook of psychotherapy and behavior change* (4th ed., pp. 428–466). Oxford: John Wiley & Sons.
Hölzel, B. K., Carmody, J., Evans, K. C., Hoge, E. A., Dusek, J. A., Morgan, L., et al. (2009). Stress reduction correlates with structural changes in the amygdala. *Social Cognitive and Affective Neuroscience, 5*, 11–17.
Hölzel, B. K., Carmody, J., Vangel, M., Congleton, C., Yerramsetti, S. M., Gard, K., et al. (2010). Mindfulness practice leads to increases in regional gray matter density. *Psychiatry Research: Neuroimaging, 1*, 36–43.
Hölzel, B. K., Hoge, E. A., Greve, D. N., Gard, T., Creswell, J. D., Brown, K. W., et al. (2013). Neural mechanisms of symptom improvements in generalized anxiety disorder following mindfulness training. *NeuroImage: Clinical, 2*, 448–458.
Hölzel, B. K., Lazar, S. W., Gard, T., Schuman-Olivier, Z., Vago, D. R., & Ott, U. (2011). How does mindfulness meditation work? Proposing mechanisms of action from a conceptual and neural perspective. *Perspectives on Psychological Science, 6*, 537–559.
Hölzel, B. K., Ott, U., Gard, T., Hempel, H., Weygandt, M., Morgen, K., et al. (2008). Investigation of mindfulness meditation practitioners with voxel-based morphometry. *Social Cognitive and Affective Neuroscience, 3*, 55–61.
Ingram, R. E. (1990). Self-focused attention in clinical disorders: Review and a conceptual model. *Psychological Bulletin, 107*, 156–176.
Ivanovski, B., & Malhi, G. S. (2007). The psychological and neuropsychological concomitants of mindfulness forms of meditation. *Acta Neuropsychiatrica, 19*, 76–91.
Jain, S., Shapiro, S. L., Swanwick, S., Roesch, P. J., Mills, P. J., Bell, I., et al. (2007). A randomized controlled trial of mindfulness meditation versus relaxation training: Effects on distress, positive states of mind, and distraction. *Annals of Behavioral Medicine, 33*, 11–21.
Jazaieri, H., Goldin, P. R., Werner, K., Ziv, M., & Gross, J. J. (2012). A randomized trial of MBSR versus aerobic exercise for social anxiety disorder. *Journal of Clinical Psychology, 68*, 715–731.
Jha, A. P., Krompinger, J., & Baime, M. J. (2007). Mindfulness training modifies subsystems of attention. *Cognitive Affective and Behavioral Neuroscience, 7*, 109–119.
Kabat-Zinn, J. (1990). *Full catastrophe living. Using the wisdom of your body and mind to face stress, pain, and illness*. New York: Bantam.
Kabat-Zinn, J. (2003). Mindfulness-based interventions in context: Past, present, and future. *Clinical Psychology: Research and Practice, 10*, 144–156.
Kabat-Zinn, J., Massion, A. O., Kristeller, J., Peterson, L., Fletcher, K. E., Pbert, L., et al. (1992). Effectiveness of a meditation-based stress reduction program in the treatment of anxiety disorders. *American Journal of Psychiatry, 149*, 936–943.
Kang, H. K., Bullman, T. A., Smolenski, D. J., Skopp, N. A., Gahm, G. A., & Reger, M. A. (2015). Suicide risk among 1.3 million veterans who were on active duty during the Iraq and Afghanistan wars. *Annals of Epidemiology, 25*, 96–100.
Kearney, D. J., McDermott, K., Malte, C., Martinez, M., & Simpson, T. L. (2012). Association of participation in a mindfulness program with measures of PTSD, depression and quality of life in a veteran sample. *Journal of Clinical Psychology, 68*, 101–116.
Kearney, D. J., McDermott, K., Malte, C., Martinez, M., & Simpson, T. L. (2013). Effects of participation in a mindfulness program for veterans with posttraumatic stress disorder: A randomized controlled pilot study. *Journal of Clinical Psychology, 69*, 14–27.

Kessler, R. C., Chiu, W. T., Demler, O., & Walters, E. E. (2005). Prevalence, severity, and comorbidity of 12-month DSM-IV disorders in the National Comorbidity Survey replication. *Archives of General Psychiatry, 62*, 617–627.

Kessler, R. C., Ruscio, A. M., Shear, K., & Wittchen, H.-U. (2010). Epidemiology of anxiety disorders. *Current Topics in Behavioral Neurosciences, 2*, 21–35.

Khoury, B., Lecomte, T., Fortin, G., Masse, M., Therien, P., Bouchard, V., et al. (2013). Mindfulness-based therapy: A comprehensive meta-analysis. *Clinical Psychology Review, 33*, 763–771.

Kim, Y. W., Lee, S., Choi, T. K., Young, S. Y., Kim, B., Kim, C. M., et al. (2009). Effectiveness of mindfulness-based cognitive therapy as an adjuvant to pharmacotherapy in patients with panic disorder or generalized anxiety disorder. *Depression and Anxiety, 26*, 601–606.

Kim, B., Lee, S., Kim, Y. W., Choi, T. K., Yook, K., Suh, S. Y., et al. (2010). Effectiveness of a mindfulness-based cognitive therapy program as an adjunct to pharmacotherapy in patients with panic disorder. *Journal of Anxiety Disorders, 24*, 590–595.

Kimbrough, E., Magyari, T., Langenberg, P., Chesney, M., & Berman, B. (2010). Mindfulness intervention for child abuse survivors. *Journal of Clinical Psychology, 66*, 17–33.

King, A. P., Erickson, T. M., Giardino, N. D., Favorite, T., Rauch, S. A., Robinson, E., et al. (2013). A pilot study of group Mindfulness-Based Cognitive Therapy (MBCT) for combat veterans with posttraumatic stress disorder (PTSD). *Depression and Anxiety, 30*, 638–645.

Kocovski, N. L., Fleming, J. E., Hawley, L. L., Huta, V., & Antony, M. M. (2013). Mindfulness and acceptance-based group therapy versus traditional cognitive behavioral group therapy for social anxiety disorder: A randomized controlled trial. *Behaviour Research and Therapy, 51*, 889–898.

Kocovski, N. L., Fleming, J. E., & Rector, N. A. (2009). Mindfulness and acceptance-based group therapy for social anxiety disorder: An open trial. *Cognitive and Behavioral Practice, 16*, 276–289.

Koszycki, D., Benger, M., Shlik, J., & Bradwejn, J. (2007). Randomized trial of a meditation-based stress reduction program and cognitive behavior therapy in generalized social anxiety disorder. *Behavior Research and Therapy, 45*, 2518–2526.

Kozasa, E. H., Sato, J. R., Lacerda, S. S., Barreiros, M. A., Radvany, J., Russell, T. A., et al. (2012). Meditation training increases brain efficiency in an attention task. *NeuroImage, 59*, 745–749.

Kubzansky, L. D., Davidson, K. W., & Rozanski, A. (2005). The clinical impact of negative psychological states: Expanding the spectrum of risk for coronary heart disease. *Psychosomatic Medicine, 67*, 10–14.

Kumar, S., Feldman, G., & Hayes, A. (2008). Changes in mindfulness and emotion regulation in an exposure-based cognitive therapy for depression. *Cognitive Therapy and Research, 32*, 734–744.

Kuyken, W., Byford, S., Taylor, R. S., Watkins, E., Holden, E., White, K., et al. (2008). Mindfulness-based cognitive therapy to prevent relapse in recurrent depression. *Journal of Consulting and Clinical Psychology, 76*, 966–978.

Kuyken, W., Watkins, E., Holden, E., White, K., Taylor, R. S., Byford, S., et al. (2010). How does mindfulness-based cognitive therapy work? *Behaviour Research and Therapy, 48*, 1105–1112.

Lee, S. H., Ahn, S. C., Lee, Y. J., Choi, T. K., Yook, K. H., & Suh, S. Y. (2007). Effectiveness of a meditation-based stress management program as an adjunct to pharmacotherapy in patients with anxiety disorder. *Journal of Psychosomatic Research, 62*, 189–195.

Lépine, J. P. (2002). The epidemiology of anxiety disorders: Prevalence and social costs. *Journal of Clinical Psychiatry, 63*, 4–8.

Levitt, J. T., Brown, T. A., Orsillo, S. M., & Barlow, D. H. (2004). The effects of acceptance versus suppression of emotion on subjective and psychophysiological response to carbon dioxide challenge in patients with panic disorder. *Behavior Therapy, 35*, 747–766.

Lovas, D. A., & Barsky, A. J. (2010). Mindfulness-based cognitive therapy for hypochondriasis, or severe health anxiety: A pilot study. *Journal of Anxiety Disorders, 24*, 931–935.

Lutz, J., Herwig, U., Opialla, S., Hittmeyer, A., Jäncke, L., Rufer, M., et al. (2014). Mindfulness and emotion regulation—An fMRI study. *Social Cognitive and Affective Neuroscience, 9*, 776–785.

Lutz, A., Slagter, H. A., Dunne, J. D., & Davidson, R. J. (2008). Attention regulation and monitoring in meditation. *Trends in Cognitive Science, 12*, 163–169.

Ma, S., & Teasdale, J. (2004). Mindfulness-based cognitive therapy for depression: Replication and exploration of differential relapse prevention effects. *Journal of Consulting and Clinical Psychology, 72*, 31–40.

Mansell, W., Harvey, A., Watkins, E., & Shafran, R. (2009). Conceptual foundations of the transdiagnostic approach to CBT. *Journal of Cognitive Psychotherapy, 23*, 6–19.

Marchand, W. R. (2014). Neural mechanisms of mindfulness and meditation: Evidence from neuroimaging studies. *World Journal of Radiology, 6*, 471.

Marciniak, M., Lage, M. J., Landbloom, R. P., Dunayevich, E., & Bowman, L. (2004). Medical and productivity costs of anxiety disorders: Case control study. *Depression and Anxiety, 19*, 112–120.

Mathews, A., & MacLeod, C. (2005). Cognitive vulnerability to emotional disorders. *Annual Review of Clinical Psychology, 1*, 167–195.

McKee, L., Zvolensky, M. J., Solomon, S. E., Bernstein, A., & Leen-Feldner, E. (2007). Emotional vulnerability and mindfulness: A preliminary test of associations among negative affectivity, anxiety sensitivity, and mindfulness skills. *Cognitive Behaviour Therapy, 36*, 91–101.

McManus, F., Grey, N., & Shafran, R. (2008). Cognitive therapy for anxiety disorders: Current status and future challenges. *Behavioural and Cognitive Psychotherapy, 36*, 695–704.

McManus, F., Surawy, C., Muse, K., Vazquez-Montes, M., & Williams, J. M. G. (2012). A randomized clinical trial of mindfulness-based cognitive therapy versus unrestricted services for health anxiety (hypochondriasis). *Journal of Consulting and Clinical Psychology, 80*, 817–828.

Mendlowicz, M. V., & Stein, M. B. (2000). Quality of life in individuals with anxiety disorders. *American Journal of Psychiatry, 157*, 669–682.

Mennin, D. S., Ellard, K. K., Fresco, D. M., & Gross, J. J. (2013). United we stand: Emphasizing commonalities across cognitive-behavioral therapies. *Behavior Therapy, 44*, 234–248.

Meuret, A. E., Twohig, M. P., Rosenfield, D., Hayes, S. C., & Craske, M. G. (2012). Brief acceptance and commitment therapy and exposure for panic disorder: A pilot study. *Cognitive and Behavioral Practice, 19*, 606–618.

Miller, J. J., Fletcher, K., & Kabat-Zinn, J. (1995). Three-year follow-up and clinical implications of a mindfulness-based stress reduction intervention in the treatment of anxiety disorders. *General Hospital Psychiatry, 17*, 192–200.

Mor, N., & Winquist, J. (2002). Self-focused attention and negative affect: A meta-analysis. *Psychological Bulletin, 128*, 638–662.

National Institute for Health and Care Excellence. (2013). *Social anxiety disorder: Recognition, assessment and treatment of social anxiety disorder* (Clinical guideline 159.) http://guidance.nice.org.uk/CG159

Neff, K. D. (2003). Self-compassion: An alternative conceptualization of a healthy attitude toward oneself. *Self and Identity, 2*, 85–102.

Niles, B. L., Klunk-Gillis, J., Ryngala, D. J., Silberbogen, A. K., Paysnick, A., & Wolf, E. J. (2012). Comparing mindfulness and psychoeducation treatments for combat-related PTSD using a telehealth approach. *Psychological Trauma: Theory, Research, Practice, and Policy, 4*, 538–547.

Ninan, P. T. (2001). Dissolving the burden of generalized anxiety disorder. *Journal of Clinical Psychiatry, 62*, 5–10.

Nolen-Hoeksema, S. (2000). The role of rumination in depressive disorder and mixed anxiety/depressive symptoms. *Journal of Abnormal Psychology, 109*, 504–511.

Norton, A. R., Abbott, M. J., Norberg, M. M., & Hunt, C. (2014). A systematic review of mindfulness and acceptance-based treatments for social anxiety disorder. *Journal of Clinical Psychology*. doi:10.1002/jclp.22144.

Norton, P. J., & Philipp, L. M. (2008). Transdiagnostic approaches to the treatment of anxiety disorders: A quantitative review. *Psychotherapy: Theory, Research, Practice, Training, 45*, 214–226.

Norton, P. J., & Price, E. M. (2007). A meta-analytic review of adult cognitive-behavioral treatment outcome across the anxiety disorders. *The Journal of Nervous and Mental Disease, 195*, 521–531.

Olatunji, B. O., Cisler, J. M., & Tolin, D. F. (2007). Quality of life in the anxiety disorders: A meta-analytic review. *Clinical Psychology Review, 27*, 572–581.

Ossman, W. A., Wilson, K. G., Storaasli, R. D., & McNeill, J. W. (2006). A preliminary investigation of the use of Acceptance and Commitment Therapy in group treatment for social phobia. *International Journal of Psychology and Psychological Therapy, 6*, 397–416.

Panos, P. T., Jackson, J. W., Hasan, O., & Panos, A. (2013). Meta-analysis and systematic review assessing the efficacy of dialectical behavior therapy (DBT). *Research on Social Work Practice*, Retrieved from: http://rsw.sagepub.com/content/early/2013/09/16/1049731513503047

Piet, J., Hougaard, E., Hecksher, M. S., & Rosenberg, N. K. (2010). A randomized pilot study of mindfulness-based cognitive therapy and group cognitive-behavioral therapy for young adults with social phobia. *Scandinavian Journal of Psychology, 51*. doi:10.1111/j.1467-9450.2009.00801.x/pdf

Powers, M. B., Zum Vörde Sive Vörding, M. B., & Emmelkamp, P. M. G. (2009). Acceptance and commitment therapy: A meta-analytic review. *Psychotherapy and Psychosomatics, 78*, 73–80.

Ramel, W., Goldin, P. R., Carmona, P. E., & McQuaid, J. R. (2004). The effects of mindfulness meditation on cognitive processes and affect in patients with past depression. *Cognitive Therapy and Research, 28*, 433–455.

Ramsawh, H. J., Raffa, S. D., Edelen, M. O., Rende, R., & Keller, M. B. (2009). Anxiety in middle adulthood: Effects of age and time on the 14-year course of panic disorder, social phobia and generalized anxiety disorder. *Psychological Medicine, 39*, 615–624.

Ree, M. J., & Craigie, M. A. (2007). Outcomes following mindfulness-based cognitive therapy in a heterogeneous sample of adult outpatients. *Behavior Change, 24*, 70–86.

Rodebaugh, T. L., Holaway, R. M., & Heimberg, R. G. (2004). The treatment of social anxiety disorder. *Clinical Psychology Review, 24*, 883–908.

Roemer, L., Erisman, S. M., & Orsillo, S. M. (2008). Mindfulness and acceptance-based treatments for anxiety disorders. In M. M. Antony & M. B. Stein (Eds.), *Oxford handbook of anxiety and related disorders* (pp. 476–487). Oxford: Oxford University Press.

Roemer, L., Lee, J. K., Salters-Pedneault, K., Erisman, S. M., Orsillo, S. M., & Mennin, D. S. (2009). Mindfulness and emotion regulation difficulties in generalized anxiety disorder: Preliminary evidence for independent and overlapping contributions. *Behavior Therapy, 40*, 142–154.

Roemer, L., & Orsillo, S. M. (2007). An open trial of an acceptance-based behavior therapy for generalized anxiety disorder. *Behavior Therapy, 38*, 72–85.

Roemer, L., Orsillo, S. M., & Salters-Pedneault, K. (2008). Efficacy of an acceptance-based behavior therapy for generalized anxiety disorder: Evaluation in a randomized controlled trial. *Journal of Consulting and Clinical Psychology, 76*, 1083–1089.

Roness, A., Mykletun, A., & Dahl, A. A. (2005). Help-seeking behaviour in patients with anxiety disorder and depression. *Acta Psychiatrica Scandinavia, 111*, 51–58.

Roy-Byrne, P. P., Craske, M. G., & Stein, M. B. (2006). Panic disorder. *Lancet, 368*, 1023–1032.

Rubia, K. (2009). The neurobiology of meditation and its clinical effectiveness in psychiatric disorders. *Biological Psychology, 82*, 1–11.

Salkovskis, P. M. (1991). The importance of behaviour in the maintenance of anxiety and panic. *Behavioural and Cognitive Psychotherapy, 19*, 6–19.

Santorelli, S. (1999). *Heal thy self: Lessons on mindfulness in medicine*. New York: Bell Tower.

Segal, Z. V., Bieling, P., Young, T., MacQueen, G., Cooke, R., Martin, L., et al. (2010). Antidepressant monotherapy vs sequential pharmacotherapy and Mindfulness-Based Cognitive Therapy, or placebo, for relapse prophylaxis in recurrent depression. *Archives of General Psychiatry, 67*, 1256–1264.

Segal, Z. V., Williams, J. M. G., & Teasdale, J. D. (2012). *Mindfulness-based cognitive therapy for depression*. New York: Guilford Press.

Serpa, J. G., Taylor, S. L., & Tillisch, K. (2014). Mindfulness-based stress reduction (MBSR) reduces anxiety, depression, and suicidal ideation in veterans. *Medical Care, 52*, 19–24.

Shapiro, S. L., Carlson, L. E., Astin, J. A., & Freedman, B. (2006). Mechanisms of mindfulness. *Journal of Clinical Psychology, 62*, 373–386.

Shear, M. K., Bjelland, I., Beesdo, K., Gloster, A. T., & Wittchen, H. (2007). Supplementary dimensional assessment in anxiety disorders. *International Journal of Methods in Psychiatric Research, 16*, 52–64.

Smith, B. W., Ortiz, J. A., Steffen, L. E., Tooley, E. M., Wiggins, K. T., Yeater, E. A., et al. (2011). Mindfulness is associated with fewer PTSD symptoms, depressive symptoms, physical symptoms, and alcohol problems in urban firefighters. *Journal of Consulting and Clinical Psychology, 79*, 613–617.

Stein, D. J. (2002). Obsessive-compulsive disorder. *Lancet, 360*, 397–405.

Stein, M. B., & Stein, D. J. (2008). Social anxiety disorder. *Lancet, 371*, 1115–1125.

Stopa, L., & Clark, D. M. (2000). Social phobia and interpretation of social events. *Behaviour Research and Therapy, 38*, 273–283.

Strauss, C., Cavanagh, K., Oliver, A., & Pettman, D. (2014). Mindfulness-based interventions for people diagnosed with a current episode of an anxiety or depressive disorder: A meta-analysis of randomised controlled trials. *PLoS ONE, 9*, e96110.

Swift, J. K., & Callahan, J. L. (2009). The impact of client treatment preferences on outcome: A meta-analysis. *Journal of Clinical Psychology, 65*, 368–381.

Taylor, S., Abramowitz, J. S., & McKay, D. (2012). Non-adherence and non-response in the treatment of anxiety disorders. *Journal of Anxiety Disorders, 26*, 583–589.

Teasdale, J. D., Moore, R. G., Hayhurst, H., Pope, M., Williams, S., & Segal, Z. V. (2002). Metacognitive awareness and prevention of relapse in depression: Empirical evidence. *Journal of Consulting and Clinical Psychology, 70*, 275–287.

Teasdale, J. D., Segal, Z. V., Williams, J. M. G., Ridgeway, V. A., Soulsby, J. M., & Lau, M. A. (2000). Prevention of relapse/recurrence in major depression by mindfulness-based cognitive therapy. *Journal of Consulting and Clinical Psychology, 68*, 615–623.

Teasdale, J. D., Segal, Z. V., & Williams, J. M. G. (2003). Mindfulness training and problem formulation. *Clinical Psychology: Science and Practice, 10*, 157–160.

Thompson, B. L., & Waltz, J. (2010). Mindfulness and experiential avoidance as predictors of posttraumatic stress disorder avoidance symptom severity. *Journal of Anxiety Disorders, 24*, 409–415.

Treanor, M. (2011). The potential impact of mindfulness on exposure and extinction learning in anxiety disorders. *Clinical Psychology Review, 31*, 617–625.

Twohig, M. P., Hayes, S. C., & Masuda, A. (2006). Increasing willingness to experience obsessions: Acceptance and commitment therapy as a treatment for obsessive-compulsive disorder. *Behavior Therapy, 37*, 3–13.

Twohig, M. P., Hayes, S. C., Plumb, J. C., Pruitt, L. D., Collins, A. B., Hazlett-Stevens, H., & Woidneck, M. R. (2010). A randomized clinical trial of acceptance and commitment therapy versus progressive relaxation training for obsessive-compulsive disorder. *Journal of Consulting and Clinical Psychology, 78*, 705–716.

Tyrer, P., & Baldwin, D. (2006). Generalised anxiety disorder. *Lancet, 368*, 2156–2166.

van den Hurk, P. A., Giommi, F., Gielen, S. C., Speckens, A. E., & Barendregt, H. P. (2010). Greater efficiency in attentional processing related to mindfulness meditation. *The Quarterly Journal of Experimental Psychology, 63*, 1168–1180.

Vassilopoulos, S. P. (2008). Social anxiety and ruminative self-focus. *Journal of Anxiety Disorders, 22*, 860–867.

Vassilopoulos, S. P., & Watkins, E. R. (2009). Adaptive and maladaptive self-focus: A pilot extension study with individuals high and low in fear of negative evaluation. *Behavior Therapy, 40*(2), 181–189.

Vøllestad, J., Nielsen, M. B., & Nielsen, G. H. (2012). Mindfulness- and acceptance-based interventions for anxiety disorders: A systematic review and meta-analysis. *British Journal of Clinical Psychology, 51*, 239–260.

Vøllestad, J., Sivertsen, B., & Nielsen, G. H. (2011). Mindfulness-based stress reduction for patients with anxiety disorders: Evaluation in a randomized controlled trial. *Behaviour Research and Therapy, 49*, 281–288.

Voncken, M. J., Bögels, S. M., & de Vries, K. (2003). Interpretation and judgmental biases in social phobia. *Behaviour Research and Therapy, 41*, 1481–1488.

Vujanovic, A. A., Youngwirth, N. E., Johnson, K. A., & Zvolensky, M. J. (2009). Mindfulness-based acceptance and posttraumatic stress symptoms among trauma-exposed adults without axis I psychopathology. *Journal of Anxiety Disorders, 23*, 297–303.

Vujanovic, A. A., Zvolensky, M. J., Bernstein, A., Feldner, M. T., & McLeish, A. C. (2007). A test of the interactive effects of anxiety sensitivity and mindfulness in the prediction of anxious arousal, agoraphobic cognitions, and body vigilance. *Behaviour Research and Therapy, 45*, 1393–1400.

Wadlinger, D. A., & Isaacowitz, D. M. (2010). Fixing our focus: Training attention to regulate emotion. *Personality and Social Psychology Review, 20*, 1–28.

Wang, P. S., Berglund, P., Olfson, M., Pincus, H. A., Wells, K. B., & Kessler, R. C. (2005). Failure and delay in initial treatment contact after first onset of mental disorders in the National Comorbidity Survey replication. *Archives of General Psychiatry, 62*, 603–613.

Watkins, E., Moberly, N. J., & Moulds, M. L. (2008). Processing mode causally influences emotional reactivity. Distinct effects of abstract versus concrete construal on emotional response. *Emotion, 8*, 364–378.

Watts, B. V., Schnurr, P. P., Mayo, L., Young-Xu, Y., Weeks, W. B., & Friedman, M. J. (2013). Meta-analysis of the efficacy of treatments for posttraumatic stress disorder. *The Journal of Clinical Psychiatry, 74*, 541–550.

Wegner, D. M., Broome, A., & Blumberg, S. J. (1997). Ironic effects of trying to relax under stress. *Behaviour Research and Therapy, 35*, 11–21.

Wegner, D. M., & Erber, R. (1992). The hyperaccessibility of suppressed thought. *Journal of Personality and Social Psychology, 63*, 903–912.

Williams, J. M. G. (2010). Mindfulness and psychological process. *Emotion, 10*, 1–7.

Wittchen, H.-U., Lieb, R., Pfister, H., & Schuster, P. (2000). The waxing and waning of mental disorders: Evaluating the stability of syndromes of mental disorders in the population. *Comprehensive Psychiatry, 41*, 122–132.

Wolitzky-Taylor, K. B., Arch, J. J., Rosenfield, D., & Craske, M. G. (2012). Moderators and non-specific predictors of treatment outcome for anxiety disorders: A comparison of cognitive behavioral therapy to acceptance and commitment therapy. *Journal of Consulting and Clinical Psychology, 80*, 786–799.

Yehuda, R. (2002). Post-traumatic stress disorder. *New England Journal of Medicine, 346*, 108–114.

Yook, K., Lee, S., Ryu, M., Kim, K., Choi, K. C., Suh, S. Y., et al. (2008). Usefulness of mindfulness-based cognitive therapy for treating insomnia in patients with anxiety disorders. *The Journal of Nervous and Mental Disease, 196*, 501–503.

Chapter 7
Mindfulness for the Treatment of Depression

William R. Marchand

Introduction

In recent years, mindfulness-based interventions have become increasingly popular as complementary treatment strategies for a number of medical and psychiatric conditions. In particular, there has been a focus on using mindfulness as an alternative treatment for depressive disorders. One of the most studied clinical mindfulness interventions, Mindfulness-Based Cognitive Therapy (MBCT) was developed specifically for the prevention for relapses in recurrent depression by Zindel Segal, Mark Williams, and John Teasdale (2002). Another evidence-based intervention, Mindfulness-Based Stress Reduction (MBSR) developed by Jon Kabat-Zinn (2005), has been shown to have benefit for depressive symptoms. This chapter will review what is known about the underlying mechanisms of action and discuss evidence for supporting the use of these interventions for depression. It will start with an explanation of mindfulness and meditation, including the development of mindfulness from classic Buddhist practices.

Basics of Mindfulness and Meditation

The language of mindfulness and meditation practices can be unclear. Mindfulness refers to a mental state that can occur while practicing meditation or at any time or place during one's daily life. Meditation refers to specific practices that can include mindfulness meditation. One practices mindfulness meditation to develop the ability to spend more of life in a state of mindful awareness.

W.R. Marchand (✉)
George E. Wahlen VAMC, 116, 500 Foothill Drive, Salt Lake City, UT, 84148, USA
e-mail: wmarchand@me.com

E. Shonin et al. (eds.), *Mindfulness and Buddhist-Derived Approaches in Mental Health and Addiction*, Advances in Mental Health and Addiction,
DOI 10.1007/978-3-319-22255-4_7

Mindfulness

The concept of mindfulness can be puzzling, but in fact, it is a very simple idea. Mindfulness is simply keeping one's attention focused on the present moment (Bishop et al., 2004; Kabat-Zinn, 2005). Mindfulness can be best understood by contrasting the mindful to the non-mindful state of mind.

Cognitive neuroscience considers mental processes to come in two varieties—controlled and automatic. Automatic processes may be innately automatic or become automatic through practice, such as when one learns a new skill. Automated processes are initiated unintentionally and cannot be easily interrupted or prevented (Raz & Buhle, 2006). In the non-mindful state, the mind automatically focuses attention. In the language of mindfulness, this is known as autopilot. When on autopilot, attention may be focused on whatever is occurring at the time, but often there is also stimulus-independent thought (Mason et al., 2007) or what we commonly think of as mind wandering. In fact, unless the current situation or task requires full attention, the mind will often be primarily engaged in stimulus-independent thought (SIT). SIT is a component of mind wandering (Smallwood & Schooler, 2006), is automatic, and occurs in the absence of a strong requirement to respond to external stimuli (McKiernan, D'Angelo, Kaufman, & Binder, 2006). A simple example is thinking about what happened at work while driving home in the evening. It is important to note the difference between making a conscious decision to spend time thinking about the work event versus the situation where these thoughts arise spontaneously. The latter mental state is autopilot/SIT.

In contrast, when practicing mindfulness, attention is directed on the incoming stimuli, mental activity, and actions that are occurring at the moment. When the practitioner notices the mind has wandered, attention is directed back to the present moment. The general practice of mindfulness then is simply keeping attention focused on whatever is occurring at the moment. This includes internal stimuli (thoughts, emotions, proprioception, pain, and interoception), external stimuli (auditory, olfactory, and visual stimuli as well as general awareness of the environment), and cognizance of any current motor behaviors. The overarching aim of a mindfulness practice is to spend more of one's time in mindful awareness and less on autopilot/SIT. As will be discussed in this chapter, autopilot/SIT thinking patterns contribute to depressive symptoms.

Meditation

Mindfulness meditation is the foundation of a mindfulness practice. The word "meditation" stems from the Latin *meditari*, meaning to participate in contemplation or reflection. Meditation in general includes a large number of practices. Though there are many variations, meditation practices are united by a general aim to bring mental processes under voluntary control by way of intentionally focusing attention and awareness (Walsh & Shapiro, 2006). Perhaps the most straightforward explanation of meditation is that it is a practice aimed at training one's attention to remain under voluntary control rather than being directed by autopilot/SIT. Two general forms of meditation have been described, focused attention (FA) and open monitoring (Lutz, Slagter, Dunne, & Davidson, 2008).

In the broadest sense, mindfulness meditation is simply a specific practice during which one attempts to keep attention under voluntary control and focused on the present moment and thus avoiding autopilot/SIT. An advanced mindfulness practice is a sitting meditation in which attention is on open awareness and one observes thoughts, emotions, and physical sensations arise and pass. This is the open monitoring (OM) meditation style. OM is difficult because of the strong tendency of the mind to engage in SIT. Thus, FA meditations are initially used to develop mindfulness skills. In FA, attention is typically focused on an anchor for the attention.

One of the most common FA practices is meditation with a focus on the physical sensations of breathing. The breath is a useful anchor because it is always available, lacks emotional valence, and occurs in the present moment. Keeping attention focused on the sensations of the breath automatically keeps awareness in the present moment and helps prevent the mind from being carried away with autopilot/SIT. Beginning mindfulness practitioners are instructed to sit for a specified period of time and do their best to keep awareness focused on the breath. When the mind wanders, the instruction is to gently redirect attention to the breath.

It is important for students of mindfulness to expect the mind to wander. The goal of meditation is not to completely avoid SIT, rather it is to recognize autopilot when it occurs and then return attention to the sensations of breathing. One useful technique is to count the breaths to ten and then start over. Whenever one notices they have lost count because the mind has wandered, then the instruction is to start over with one. By consistently practicing FA meditation, mindfulness students gradually develop their meditation skills and are able to practice mindfulness at other times when not engaged in formal meditation. Other practices used to develop mindfulness skills include doing simple activities, such as brushing one's teeth mindfully, with attention fully focused on the physical sensations of the activity.

The relevance for depression is that mindfulness practitioners develop the ability to recognize autopilot-/SIT-driven thinking patterns that worsen depressive symptoms as well as the automatic emotional responses associated with this illness. By shifting into mindful awareness, one is able to gain distance from mental and emotional processes such that these lose power and become less compelling.

Buddhist Roots and Advanced Mindfulness Concepts

Though the core of a mindfulness practice is maintaining the focus of awareness on the present moment, an understanding of more advanced concepts is necessary to comprehend the hypothetical mechanisms underlying the effectiveness of mindfulness-based interventions for depression. A brief review of the origins of mindfulness is a useful starting point.

Buddhist Traditions

Mindfulness-based interventions originated in Buddhist spiritual practices (Salmon et al., 2004). Though Buddhism is a complex religion and philosophy encompassing many schools, the fundamental concept of Buddhism is the relief of suffering. This is articulated in The Four Noble Truths, which are thought to represent the first instructions of the Buddha and the core teachings of Buddhism. The Four Noble Truths are expressed in a variety of translations. However, they can be understood as follows (Fischer-Schreiber, Ehrhard, & Diener, 1991).

The first truth says that all existence is characterized by suffering and does not bring satisfaction. The second truth declares that the cause of suffering is craving and desire. The third truth indicates that elimination of craving and desire can result in the end of suffering. Finally, the fourth truth indicates that Buddhist practice can bring the end of suffering. This practice is further described in the Eightfold Path.

Though generally considered a religion, Buddhism is essentially a method for the relief of suffering. The liberation from suffering does not require a deity, and the Buddha is not thought of as a divine being. In contrast, escape from suffering is entirely predicated on the actions that an individual can choose to take based upon the teaching of the Buddha. Buddhism postulates that engaging in a specific set of practices will result in the decrease or elimination of personal suffering. Sometimes this is interpreted as release from samsara, which is an endless cycle of death and rebirth (Fischer-Schreiber et al., 1991). However, many Buddhist traditions, such as Zen, interpret Buddhism as a way to move out of a cycle of suffering in one's current life and do not emphasize the concept of reincarnation.

Understanding Mindfulness from a Buddhist Perspective

There are several essential points from the above that inform an understanding of mindfulness and specifically how mindfulness practices may be beneficial for depression. The first point is that the First Nobel Truth indicates that life always results in suffering.

In this context, the definition of suffering is broad and ranges from severe physical or emotional pain to unhappiness or just a vague sense of unease or dissatisfaction. Another way to think about it is that suffering can be equated to a lack of joy and pleasure in life. This truth is very self-evident. We all experience dissatisfaction and unhappiness as a normal component of our lives. However, depression could be conceptualized as an extreme manifestation of the Buddhist concept of suffering, as it is a condition of sadness and loss of joy and pleasure in life. This is not to say that Buddhist philosophy explains the etiology of depression, but rather to suggest there are similarities between suffering as understood in Buddhism and the clinical manifestations of the illness of depression.

Importantly, the Second Noble Truth indicates that suffering is the result of the workings of the mind. This implies that changing one's own thinking patterns can lead to less suffering. It also suggests that increased happiness and satisfaction with life can be achieved by changing thought processes. In other words, Buddhist philosophy suggests that interventions, such as psychotherapy and mindfulness practices, may be beneficial. This is the point of the Third Noble Truth, which indicates that elimination of craving and desire is the method to decrease suffering.

The Third Noble Truth is often translated as above, that the process for the relief of suffering is through the elimination of craving and desire. However, what this really means is that through meditation practice, one learns to decrease the desire for life to be different than the reality of the moment. The core point of a mindfulness practice is to recognize that autopilot/SIT frequently is focused on wanting things to be different than reality. In other words, the mind tends to be dissatisfied.

Resistance to Physical and Emotional Pain

One way that wanting things to be different manifests is the natural human resistance to the pain of life. Mindfulness hypothesizes that this resistance often causes increased pain and suffering rather than resulting in a symptom decrease. Physical pain is a good example of this. If one is experiencing physical pain, the natural tendency of the mind is to wish that the pain would go away and think about ways to eliminate the pain. This can be a beneficial process if it leads to adaptive behaviors that may work, such as seeking medical treatment. However, often the mind's desire to be free of pain increases suffering.

This is particularly the case in chronic pain for which there is unlikely to be an easy solution. In this case, the tendency to think about the pain typically leads to increased suffering. Mindfulness is particularly effective for pain because practitioners learn to recognize that wishing the pain would go away actually makes it worse. In contrast, they discover that by simply being present with the pain in mindful awareness, there is a tendency for the discomfort to decrease (Segal et al., 2002).

One mechanism is that by focusing on the sensations of the moment, one may discover that subconscious tensing of the muscles in the painful area is causing increased pain [Is there a citation to support this statement?]. Sometimes by really paying close attention to pain, one may realize that it is not that uncomfortable and that it can be accepted without resistance.

By paying very close attention to the workings of the mind, practitioners may realize that autopilot/SIT is almost always focused on the past or future, rather than the present moment. In the situation of chronic pain, thinking about the distress associated with past pain is obviously not helpful. Perhaps more importantly, worrying about future pain clearly increases suffering. To put it another way, the pain of the present moment is likely to be tolerable. In contrast, if one thinks about the pain for the next moment, next day, etc., this may feel overwhelming.

In mindfulness language, the expression, "pain is mandatory, but suffering is optional" is used to assert this concept. A similar process occurs for emotional pain, which will be discussed later in the chapter.

The Human Tendency to Be Dissatisfied

Another manifestation of suffering because of the natural human tendency to be dissatisfied involves our inability to achieve lasting joy from success. The propensity to be dissatisfied drives human success by compelling us to always strive for new accomplishments and successes. However, by practicing mindfulness and paying attention to one's thinking patterns, it becomes apparent that the mind is very frequently dissatisfied. Practitioners also notice that accomplishments typically do not result in a long-term sense of satisfaction. The mind typically becomes dissatisfied quickly and thinking patterns focus on another goal. Mindfulness does not label this inclination as good or bad, but rather advocates for awareness of it.

By practicing mindfulness, one can develop the understanding that thoughts are just thoughts and not facts. Thoughts of dissatisfaction can exist, but practitioners can allow them to run in the background without believing them. Mindfulness, through watching one's thoughts, leads to the realization that many autopilot/SIT thoughts are irrational and some are absurd. Buddhist language calls autopilot/SIT "monkey mind," suggesting that thoughts are like the mindless chattering of a monkey. Practitioners become skeptical of their own thoughts and thus are less likely to be influenced by those that don't make sense or lead to a sense of dissatisfaction.

Finally, as stated above, the Fourth Noble Truth indicates that Buddhist practices can decrease or end suffering. This chapter describes how the secularized Buddhist practice of mindfulness meditation can decrease the suffering associated with depression.

Spiritual Awakening

Perhaps the most important Buddhist concept is that of enlightenment or awakening. This is traditionally understood as a profound insight into a transcendental truth (Shambhala, 1991). A more straightforward interpretation in the awakening is simply developing the ability to see life, as it really is, not obscured by one's ego-based irrational thinking patterns. In other words, awakening is the process through which one comes to the understanding that unhappiness and dissatisfaction with life come from the workings of the mind and not the external circumstances of the moment.

The aim of Buddhist practice is enlightenment and thus liberation from suffering. However, it is important to note that in many Buddhist traditions, the goal is awakening for oneself and for all other sentient beings.

Psychological Mechanisms of Mindfulness for Depression

This section of the chapter will discuss general psychological mechanisms of mindfulness and then review how mindfulness may impact depression from a psychological standpoint. The next section will integrate psychological and neural mechanisms.

Psychological Components of Mindfulness

One psychological model of mindfulness is that developed by Shapiro and colleagues (Shapiro, Carlson, Astin, & Freedman, 2006). They propose three constituents of mindfulness: (1) intention, (2) attention, and (3) attitude. These are not thought to be separate stages, but rather interwoven aspects of a single process.

The component of intention is the 'why' behind developing a mindfulness practice (Shapiro et al., 2006). In Buddhism, the intent is the attainment of enlightenment and thus liberation from suffering for oneself and for others. For those with depression, the initial intention will likely be to decrease their symptoms. Nevertheless, there is evidence (Shapiro, 1992) that over time, the intentions of mindfulness practitioners may shift from simply symptom control to self-exploration and finally to self-liberation. One potential advantage of using mindfulness as an intervention for depression is that it offers the possibility of self-exploration and spiritual development as well as symptom reduction.

Attention is the element of mindfulness that facilitates awareness of moment-to-moment experience (Shapiro et al., 2006). Attitude describes the 'how' one pays attention to moment-by-moment experience when practicing mindfulness. Practitioners focus attention on the here and now with an attitude of curiosity, openness, and acceptance. This attitude facilitates the capacity to accept things as they are and avoid the autopilot/SIT striving for pleasant and avoidance of aversive experiences (Shapiro et al., 2006).

An important point is that while mindfulness encourages accepting things as they are in the moment, the intent is not for individuals to become passive. Rather, the aim is to be able to take appropriate and beneficial actions based upon the awakened state of seeing reality clearly. In the context of depression, one would accept the feelings of sadness in the moment but then take suitable action to find symptom relief, such as going for a walk or engaging in physical exercise. This is in contrast to autopilot-/SIT-driven behaviors which might be maladaptive, such as self-medicating with substances or sitting and ruminating.

Mindfulness Changes Perspective Through Reperceiving

Shapiro and colleagues have also suggested that a fundament psychological mechanism of mindfulness is "reperceiving" or shifting perspective (Shapiro et al., 2006). Reperceiving is postulated to occur as a result of the mindfulness components of intention, attention, and attitude described above. Reperceiving is an alteration in perspective resulting in the ability to step back from, and be less identified with, one's own thoughts and emotions (Shapiro et al., 2006).

Reperceiving may be thought of as analogous to one component of the Buddhist concept of awakening. By being less identified with one's habitual thinking patterns and beliefs, it is possible to see reality more clearly. Mindfulness practitioners gain awareness that they are greater than their thoughts and emotions (Shapiro et al., 2006). In Buddhism, this is an important element in the process of becoming aware of one's own Buddha-nature. Buddha-nature is the concept that all humans are capable of becoming awake and achieving enlightenment, just as the Buddha is said to have done. One's own Buddha-nature is difficult, or impossible, to see when caught up in autopilot/SIT thinking patterns.

As Shapiro and colleagues state, reperceiving may manifest as awareness that "this pain is not me" or "this depression is not me." Becoming less identified with one's emotions and cognitions results in these mental processes losing power. Thus, negative thoughts may be less likely to lead to depression, and negative affect may be less likely to persist.

Decreased Identification with the Concept of Self

Reperceiving and watching one's monkey mind may also lead to the discovery that self is only a psychological concept made up of ever-changing memories, beliefs, and ideas (Shapiro et al., 2006). This is perhaps the most profound idea expressed by Buddhism and mindfulness. The memories of our experiences and beliefs about ourselves define how we see ourselves and who we see ourselves to be. Mindfulness leads to the realization that these are just ephemeral thoughts too, without any deep meaning. What is left after letting go of ideas and beliefs about the self is Buddha-nature.

Becoming less identified with the concept of self facilitates seeing reality more clearly; in Buddhist language this is considered to be part of the process of awakening (Shambhala, 1991). Decreased attachment to an egocentric worldview allows one to more readily see the perspectives of others. This perception shift can facilitate increased compassion and concern for both self and others. One becomes less likely to feel separate from others and to have an "us against them" mentality. There is greater awareness that all humans are very similar and want the same things. We are all more alike than different. Awakening leads to a profound sense of being connected to the entire universe rather than feeling separate and alone.

From the Buddhist perspective (Shambhala, 1991), the decreased identification with the idea of self that is associated with awakening leads to less distress when the concept of self is threatened, whether the threat is actual (e.g., old age and death) or perceived (e.g., negative thinking about the self). The impact of a mindfulness practice on self-referential thinking is thought to be a key component underlying the benefits of mindfulness for depression.

Self-referential Thinking and Depression

Dysfunctional self-referential thinking plays a key role in the etiology of depressive disorders. For example, aberrant self-schemas (beliefs and ideas about self) form the basis for Beck's classic approach to depression (Beck, 1967). Many studies indicate an association between low self-concept and/or negative self-schemas and depression, for example (Brown, Andrews, Harris, Adler, & Bridge, 1986; Evans, Heron, Lewis, Araya, & Wolke, 2005; King, Naylor, Segal, Evans, & Shain, 1993; Miller, Warner, Wickramaratne, & Weissman, 1999; Schafer & Keith, 1981). There is persuasive evidence that processing of self-referent information in general is abnormal in affective illness, for example (Blairy et al., 2004; Gara et al., 1993; Nilsson, Jorgensen, Craig, Straarup, & Licht, 2010; Shestyuk & Deldin, 2010). Lastly, the effectiveness of cognitive therapy interventions targeting negative schemas is well established (Gibbons et al., 2010; Jones, 2004; Lauder, Berk, Castle, Dodd, & Berk, 2010; Work Group On Major Depressive Disorder, 2010; Wright, Beck, & Thase, 2003). These studies suggest that mindfulness, which changes the way one thinks about the self, might be an effective intervention for depressive spectrum disorders.

Research indicates that in addition to the content of thoughts about self (i.e., schemas and self-esteem), the extent and type of self-referential thinking are also important in depression. Individuals with unipolar illness demonstrate a tendency toward generalized increase of self-focus (Ingram, 1990; Northoff, 2007). Furthermore, excessive self-focus in general is associated with negative affect (Mor & Winquist, 2002). Finally, self-focused rumination is specifically associated with depression (Burwell & Shirk, 2007; Sakamoto, 1999; Spasojevic & Alloy, 2001) including relapse of illness (Michalak, Holz, & Teismann, 2010). Therefore, interventions that might decrease the amount of time spent thinking about the self also have the potential to benefit depression.

The content of self-referential thinking is particularly relevant for depression. Narrative thoughts about the self include memories of the past and intentions for the future (Gallagher, 2000). Narrative thinking includes generalized autobiographical memory (Watkins & Teasdale, 2004) and is the basis for the sense of self, described above, that is composed of memories of subjective experiences across time. Narrative self-reference is composed of autopilot-/SIT-driven thinking patterns. SIT may take the form of self-referential rumination (Burwell & Shirk, 2007; Michalak et al., 2010; Sakamoto, 1999; Spasojevic & Alloy, 2001) and is analytical, for example, thinking analytically about self and depressive symptoms. This type of self-referential thinking is often maladaptive (Teasdale, 1999), frequently associated with negative self-judgments (Rimes & Watkins, 2005) and dysphoria (Lo, Ho, & Hollon, 2010; Williams & Moulds, 2010).

Psychological Changes of Mindfulness that Impact Depression

In contrast to the analytical/narrative style of self-referential thinking described above, experiential self-reference is the experience of self in the immediate moment without a story or theme. The aim of mindfulness practices is to facilitate the ability to experience experiential self-reference, which is adaptive (Watkins, 2004; Watkins & Teasdale, 2004).

Studies show that mindfulness is associated with enhanced emotional self-regulation and decreased emotional reactivity (Brown, Goodman, & Inzlicht, 2012; Delgado et al., 2010; Goldin & Gross, 2010; Hill & Updegraff, 2011; Kemeny et al., 2011; Robins, Keng, Ekblad, & Brantley, 2012; Taylor et al., 2011). In mindful awareness, one is able to step back and observe, rather than be controlled and carried away by emotions and thoughts (Shapiro et al., 2006). Gaining distance from negative thoughts and emotions can support the use of positive coping strategies rather than simply reacting. An analogy is standing on the bank of a flooded river watching the torrent flow by as opposed to falling in and being swept away with the current. Mindfulness allows the recognition of being carried away by autopilot/SIT and subsequently moving into mindful awareness. Traditionally from the Buddhist perspective, the aim of mindfulness is to spend all of one's time in mindful awareness (an awakened state). However, secular mindfulness practices typically start with a more modest goal of developing the ability to recognize autopilot-/SIT-based thinking and shift into mindfulness when appropriate. This is particularly important when experiencing symptoms of depression, such as dysphoria. A longer-term goal is to spend as much time as possible in a state of mindful awareness.

Another important effect of mindfulness is the development of an increased ability to tolerate uncomfortable emotions or sensations. In other words, practitioners develop the ability to stay present with physical or emotional pain. This avoids falling into autopilot/SIT thinking patterns that may worsen the experience of depression. Being present with emotional symptoms, such as sadness, may result in greater exposure to the discomfort and thus eventual desensitization.

The material discussed above may be best understood with an example. The dysphoria of depression is a very unpleasant emotion. The natural tendency of the mind is to avoid pain and discomfort, as discussed above. The mechanism to relieve the discomfort often involves autopilot-/SIT-based thinking about how to get rid of the pain. This is similar to a reflex like the automatic jerking back of a hand after accidently touching something hot. Sometimes autopilot/SIT may lead to adaptive behavioral responses. Often however, narrative rumination ensues about the symptoms and the self. For example, one might think, "Oh no, another bout of depression.

The last time this happened it lasted for weeks." Another example could be, "Now I won't be able to enjoy the party tonight." Or, "My antidepressant must have stopped working." It is readily apparent that these thoughts are not helpful and may lead to a vicious cycle of dysphoria leading to negative thoughts, leading to increased dysphoria, and so on. An important point is that the autopilot-/SIT-based thinking is not recognized; one is simply carried away with the thoughts and emotions.

Mindfulness facilitates the recognition of the autopilot/SIT cycle and provides a way to move out of it through meditation. For example, in MBCT (Segal et al., 2002), a short meditation practice is taught called the 3-min breathing space. Practitioners use this when they notice autopilot/SIT and/or uncomfortable emotions. After the short meditation, one may see reality more clearly (be more awake in Buddhist terms) and be able to take positive action to feel better rather than being stuck in a cycle of negative rumination.

In summary, mindfulness practices are thought to benefit depression as a result of changes in thinking patterns. Practitioners develop the ability to spend time in experiential self-reference with attention focused on the here and now. This decreases attachment to the idea of self in general and also decreases narrative self-referential thinking, which contributes to depression and negative thinking.

Neural Mechanisms of Depression and Mindfulness

In this section, neural process underlying the etiology of depression will be discussed first. This will be limited to a discussion of those regions impacted by a mindfulness practice. This will be followed by evidence from neuroimaging studies that indicate how mindfulness works at a systems neuroscience level. While there is considerable evidence in regard to the general effects of mindfulness, this author is not aware of any published neuroimaging studies investigating the mechanisms of mindfulness in unipolar illness. This section will provide evidence that mindfulness impacts brain regions known to exhibit aberrant function in individuals with depression. However, additional research will be required to demonstrate a direct link between symptom improvement and functional changes in these regions among individuals with unipolar depression.

Neural Mechanisms of Depression

Depressive spectrum disorders are complex conditions that likely have multiple etiologies. Nonetheless, some neural mechanisms thought to underlie these disorders may help elucidate the effects of mindfulness.

The medial surface of the cortex is an area of particular interest for understanding neural processes impacted by mindfulness. Most of the anterior and posterior midline cortex can be characterized as an anatomical and functional unit known collectively as the cortical midline structures (Northoff & Bermpohl, 2004). The cortical midline structures (CMS) are components of the default mode network (Gusnard & Raichle, 2001; Raichle et al., 2001), have connectivity with the amygdala (Amaral & Price, 1984; Barbas & De Olmos, 1990; Buckwalter, Schumann, & Van Hoesen, 2008; Carmichael & Price, 1995; Porrino, Crane, & Goldman-Rakic, 1981), and play a key role in both self-referential and emotional processing (Grimm, Boesiger et al. 2009; Heinzel et al., 2005; Northoff & Bermpohl, 2004; Northoff et al., 2006).

Many studies (Brooks et al., 2009; Drevets et al., 1997; Dunn et al., 2002; Grimm, Ernst et al. 2009; Johnson, Nolen-Hoeksema, Mitchell, & Levin, 2009; Kegeles et al., 2003; Liotti, Mayberg, McGinnis, Brannan, & Jerabek, 2002; Mayberg et al., 2000; Osuch et al., 2009; Pizzagalli et al., 2009; Ritchey, Dolcos, Eddington, Strauman, & Cabeza, 2010; Scheuerecker et al., 2010; Smith et al., 2009; Smoski et al., 2009; Wu et al., 1999) suggest functional alterations of CMS in unipolar illness. Specifically there is evidence that the CMS play a role in mediating the relationship between aberrant self-referential thinking and negative affect in mood disorders (Altshuler et al., 2008; Altshuler et al., 2005; Chen et al., 2006; Cooney, Joormann, Eugene, Dennis, & Gotlib, 2010; Elliott et al., 2004; Grimm, Boesiger et al. 2009; Grimm, Ernst et al. 2009; Lagopoulos & Malhi, 2011; Lemogne et al., 2010; Lennox, Jacob, Calder, Lupson, & Bullmore, 2004; Malhi et al., 2004; Marchand et al., 2011; Yoshimura et al., 2010).

The above studies tell us that the CMS is the area of the brain where self-referential thinking and emotional regulation intersect. This provides a neural explanation of why disruptions in thinking about the self and the emotional dysregulation of depression may be linked. The fact that the CMS has key nodes in the default mode network (DMN) is also important. The DMN (Gusnard & Raichle, 2001; Raichle et al., 2001) is the brain area that becomes active when an individual is not engaged in a task. Thus, it is thought of as the default mode of brain functioning or the area that automatically becomes active if the brain is not otherwise engaged. When attention involuntarily drifts away from an object of attention, the DMN is engaged (Mason et al., 2007). This may explain why SIT (described above) is an automatic process as well as why SIT often involves self-referential thinking.

As discussed above, there is compelling evidence that self-perception and processing of self-referent information are abnormal in affective disorders, of both bipolar and unipolar spectrum (Blairy et al., 2004; Gara et al., 1993; Nilsson et al., 2010; Shestyuk & Deldin, 2010). A key point (discussed above) is that unipolar illness is associated with increased self-focus (Ingram, 1990; Northoff, 2007). Importantly, evidence indicates that self-referential processing activates the CMS and that this neural response is associated with negative affectivity in healthy controls (Lemogne et al., 2010). Also, studies indicate that abnormal self-referential processing in unipolar illness is mediated by neural response in cortical and subcortical midline structures (Grimm, Ernst et al., 2009; Yoshimura et al., 2010). Finally, CMS circuit dysfunction persists in the euthymic state of recurrent major depression and thus may represent trait pathology (Marchand, Lee, Johnson, Thatcher, & Gale, 2013).

Within the CMS, the precuneus, cingulate, and neighboring medial parietal cortex are interconnected areas sometimes referred to as posterior medial cortex (Parvizi, Van Hoesen, Buckwalter, & Damasio, 2006), and this region has been specifically implicated as playing a role in self-reflection/self-awareness (Gusnard & Raichle, 2001; Johnson et al., 2002). The posterior CMS is densely connected with the hippocampus and implicated in encoding and retrieving autobiographical memory and therefore may play a role in putting self-referential stimuli within a temporal context linking them to past self-referential stimuli (Northoff & Bermpohl, 2004). The posterior CMS may also be more specifically engaged in self-reflection related to duties and obligations (Johnson et al., 2009). Studies suggest specific functional alterations in the posterior CMS in unipolar illness (Brooks et al., 2009; Grimm, Ernst et al., 2009; Johnson et al., 2009; Scheuerecker et al., 2010; Smith et al., 2009). Thus, it may be that the posterior CMS is particularly relevant for self-identification in general and the negative thoughts about self frequently associated with depressive disorders.

Taken together, these studies provide compelling evidence that the CMS plays a major role in aberrant self-referential thinking of depressive disorders.

The striatal circuits can be divided into three basic components. These are input (cortex to striatum), subcortical (striatum to thalamus), and output (thalamus to cortex) segments. Output of the striatal (corticobasal ganglia) circuitry is associated with the experience of pleasure and motivation; for extensive review, see Marchand (2010). The striatum, like the CMS, is extensively involved in emotional regulation (Marchand, 2010). Also, the striatum and CMS have extensive anatomical (Ferry, Ongur, An, & Price, 2000; Haber, Kunishio, Mizobuchi, & Lynd-Balta, 1995) and functional (Marchand et al., 2008) connectivity.

There is considerable evidence that the function of the striatum and associated corticobasal ganglia circuitry plays a role in the neuropathology of affective disorders; for reviews, see Marchand (2010) and Marchand and Yurgelun-Todd (2010). Studies suggest that corticobasal ganglia circuitry is likely a locus of primary pathology in major depression (Marchand, Lee, Suchy et al. 2012; Marchand et al., 2013). Our group found that a network involving the bilateral striatum and anterior CMS was associated with depressive symptom severity (Marchand, Lee, Johnson et al. 2012). Thus, striatal circuit dysfunction is thought to play a key role in the neurobiology of depression, and aberrant connectivity between the striatal and CMS regions may specifically contribute to symptom expression.

Research indicated that dysfunction of the lateral prefrontal cortex is associated with unipolar illness, for example (Halari et al., 2009; Harvey et al., 2005; Walter, Wolf, Spitzer, & Vasic, 2007). Areas in the lateral frontal cortex are generally associated with many processes generally associated with higher executive functioning. These regions are also components of some of the neural networks involved in the attention process, often labeled as alerting and executive attention circuits (Posner & Rothbart, 2007; Raz & Buhle, 2006). The alerting network modulates task-specific alertness as well as attention engagement and involves the right lateral frontal cortex (dorsolateral prefrontal cortex), CMS, and right parietal cortex (Raz & Buhle, 2006). The executive control network, including CMS, lateral frontal cortex, and basal ganglia (Posner & Rothbart, 2007), is involved with attention control, which includes top-down control as well as resolution of conflict between computations involving planning, error detection, and regulation of thoughts and feelings (Raz & Buhle, 2006).

Neural Mechanisms of Mindfulness and Meditation

There is substantial literature suggesting some of the neural mechanisms underlying the effects of practicing mindfulness and meditation in general. Many investigators have studied individuals who had completed mindfulness training, for example (Allen et al., 2012; Desbordes et al., 2012; Farb et al., 2010; Farb, Segal, & Anderson, 2013; Farb et al., 2007; Goldin, Ziv, Jazaieri, & Gross, 2012; Goldin, Ziv, Jazaieri, Hahn, & Gross, 2013;. Goldin & Gross, 2010; Holzel et al., 2013; Ives-Deliperi, Howells, Stein, Meintjes, & Horn, 2013; Kilpatrick et al., 2011; Wells et al., 2013; Zeidan et al., 2011; Zeidan, Martucci, Kraft, McHaffie, & Coghill, 2013). Investigations have focused specifically on experienced meditators (Baerentsen et al., 2010; Gard et al., 2012; Garrison, Santoyo et al. 2013; Garrison, Scheinost et al. 2013; Hasenkamp & Barsalou, 2012; Hasenkamp, Wilson-Mendenhall, Duncan, & Barsalou, 2012; Holzel et al., 2007; Kirk, Downar, & Montague, 2011; Kozasa et al., 2012; Lutz, McFarlin, Perlman, Salomons, & Davidson, 2013; Pagnoni, 2012; Pagnoni, Cekic, & Guo, 2008; Taylor et al., 2011, 2013) and brief mindfulness training (Dickenson, Berkman, Arch, & Lieberman, 2013; Lutz, McFarlin et al. 2013), as well as state (Ives-Deliperi, Solms, & Meintjes, 2011) and trait (Creswell, Way, Eisenberger, & Lieberman, 2007; Paul, Stanton, Greeson, Smoski, & Wang, 2013; Shaurya Prakash et al. 2013) mindfulness. At least one study has compared expert and novice meditators (Brefczynski-Lewis, Lutz, Schaefer, Levinson, & Davidson, 2007).

The studies listed above have evaluated mindfulness mechanisms in healthy subjects. Recently, some investigations have focused on using mindfulness interventions for psychiatric illness. There have been studies of individuals with social anxiety disorder (Goldin et al., 2012; Goldin et al., 2013; Goldin & Gross, 2010), generalized anxiety disorder (Holzel et al., 2013), and bipolar disorder (Ives-Deliperi et al., 2013).

Functional imaging studies indicate that mindfulness is associated with neural mechanisms involving several brain areas in healthy subjects. A large number of studies indicate mechanisms involving frontal cortex, for example (Allen et al., 2012; Creswell et al., 2007; Dickenson et al., 2013; Farb et al., 2007, 2013; Gard et al., 2012; Holzel et al., 2007, 2013; Ives-Deliperi et al., 2011, 2013; Kozasa et al., 2012; Lutz, Herwig et al. 2013; Lutz, McFarlin et al. 2013; Taylor et al., 2013; Zeidan et al., 2011, 2013). Some of these investigations suggest mechanisms involving lateral frontal regions (Allen et al., 2012; Gard et al., 2012; Holzel et al., 2013), such as ventrolateral prefrontal cortex (Holzel et al., 2013) and dorsolateral prefrontal cortex (Allen et al., 2012).

In contrast to lateral frontal regions, many studies suggest that mindfulness impacts the CMS (Farb et al., 2013; Farb et al., 2007; Gard et al., 2012; Goldin et al., 2012; Hasenkamp & Barsalou, 2012; Holzel et al., 2007; Ives-Deliperi et al., 2013; Ives-Deliperi et al., 2011; Kozasa et al., 2012; Taylor et al., 2013; Zeidan et al., 2011; Zeidan et al., 2013). Findings implicate anterior medial cortex, such as anterior cingulate cortex (Gard et al., 2012; Holzel et al., 2007; Ives-Deliperi et al., 2011; Zeidan et al., 2011; Zeidan et al., 2013) as well as posterior CMS (Baerentsen et al., 2010; Garrison, Santoyo, et al., 2013; Garrison, Scheinost, et al., 2013; Goldin et al., 2012; Ives-Deliperi et al., 2011; Pagnoni, 2012; Shaurya Prakash et al., 2013; Taylor et al., 2013). In particular, evidence suggests that mindfulness impacts the posterior cingulate cortex and precuneus (Baerentsen et al., 2010; Garrison, Santoyo, et al., 2013; Garrison, Scheinost, et al., 2013; Goldin et al., 2012; Ives-Deliperi et al., 2011; Shaurya Prakash et al., 2013; Taylor et al., 2013).

Additionally, some studies have specifically focused on the DMN (Garrison, Santoyo, et al., 2013; Hasenkamp et al., 2012; Pagnoni et al., 2008; Shaurya Prakash et al., 2013; Taylor et al., 2011, 2013) described above. These investigations indicate that mindfulness impacts DMN function.

Finally, there is evidence that mindfulness impacts the insula (Farb et al., 2007, 2013; Gard et al., 2012; Kirk et al., 2011; Lutz, Herwig et al. 2013; Lutz, McFarlin et al. 2013; Paul et al., 2013; Zeidan et al., 2011, 2013), amygdala (Creswell et al., 2007; Desbordes et al., 2012; Goldin & Gross, 2010; Holzel et al., 2013; Lutz, Herwig et al. 2013; Lutz, McFarlin et al. 2013; Taylor et al., 2011), basal ganglia (Baerentsen et al., 2010; Kozasa et al., 2012), and thalamus (Zeidan et al., 2011). Thus, mindfulness likely impacts the perception of physical sensations of emotion (insula), the fear response (amygdala), and motor, emotional, and cognitive processing as well as the experience of pleasure (basal ganglia).

These investigations indicate that mindfulness impacts several brain regions associated with depressive disorders as outlined above. Specifically, these areas are the CMS, DMN, basal ganglia, and lateral prefrontal cortex.

The studies reviewed above indicate brain regions for which there is strong evidence of functional changes associated with mindfulness and meditation. However, it is also possible to interpret studies in terms of functional specialization of brain regions.

A number of investigations suggest that mindfulness and meditation result in enhanced attention, which is associated with neural mechanisms involving the parietal cortex (Goldin et al., 2013), CMS (Kozasa et al., 2012), temporal cortex (Kozasa et al., 2012), sensorimotor cortex, (Kozasa et al., 2012), and basal ganglia (Kozasa et al., 2012).

Lastly, mindfulness also facilitates the enhancement of interoceptive attention to visceral bodily sensations as they occur in the present moment. One fMRI study (Farb et al., 2013) found that mindfulness training predicted greater interoceptive attention-related activity in anterior insula regions as well as decreased recruitment of CMS. This finding indicates that mindfulness appears to rewire the brain such that interoceptive attention is enhanced and attention to self-referential thinking based in the CMS may be decreased.

Mindfulness impacts DMN neural processes (Garrison, Santoyo, et al., 2013; Hasenkamp et al., 2012; Pagnoni et al., 2008; Shaurya Prakash et al., 2013; Taylor et al., 2011, 2013). Modification of this network likely plays a significant role in the objectification of the experience of automatic thoughts. Objective awareness of DMN-based autopilot/SIT is understood to be a primary mechanism by which mindfulness decreases symptoms of depression; for review, see Marchand (2012). Objective awareness allows one to interpret thoughts as "just thoughts" and prevents experiencing irrational negative thinking as fact.

Finally, studies indicate that mindfulness enhances emotional regulation. This involves modification of processing in lateral frontal regions (Holzel et al., 2013), CMS/DMN (Farb et al., 2010; Ives-Deliperi et al., 2013; Taylor et al., 2011), regions involved with interoception (Farb et al., 2010), and amygdala (Desbordes et al., 2012; Goldin & Gross, 2010; Holzel et al., 2013; Lutz, McFarlin et al. 2013; Taylor et al., 2011).

Evidence for Effectiveness of Mindfulness Interventions for Depression

There are limitations of the literature regarding the effectiveness of mindfulness. For example, some authors have pointed out (Chiesa & Malinowski, 2011; Chiesa & Serretti 2010a) that some studies have substantial methodological limitations. Of these, perhaps the most significant criticism concerns the lack of high-quality, randomized controlled studies (Chiesa & Malinowski, 2011). Other limitations include absence of follow-up measures as well as small sample size, reliance on self-report instruments, and a variety of differences across interventions (Chiesa & Malinowski, 2011; Fjorback, Arendt, Ornbol, Fink, & Walach, 2011).

In regard to the two most studied interventions, MBSR and MBCT, there is considerable evidence of benefit for depression and other psychiatric conditions. As reviewed elsewhere (Marchand, 2012), studies indicate effectiveness of MBSR for depressive and anxiety symptoms. For MBCT, the strongest evidence is for relapse prevention in unipolar illness (Bondolfi et al., 2010; Chiesa & Serretti, 2010a; Godfrin & van Heeringen, 2010a, 2010b; Kuyken et al., 2008; Manicavasgar, Parker, & Perich, 2010; Mathew, Whitford, Kenny, & Denson, 2010; Piet & Hougaard, 2011; Segal et al., 2010) particularly among those with three or more prior episodes. Furthermore, MBCT offers protection against relapse equal to that of maintenance antidepressant pharmacotherapy (Marchand, 2012; Segal et al., 2010). Evidence also suggests efficacy for those experiencing a current episode as well as for those in remission (Finucane & Mercer, 2006; van Aalderen et al., 2011), and one study indicates that MBCT is as effective as CBT in the treatment of current depression (Manicavasgar, Parker, & Perich, 2011).

Conclusions

Mindfulness is practiced with the objective of maintaining attention in the present moment rather than allowing thought patterns and emotional responses to be carried away by automatic thought processes (autopilot/SIT). Mindfulness is based upon Buddhist practices aimed at the reduction of suffering. Secular mindfulness interventions attempt to relieve suffering associated with psychiatric conditions, stress, and physical illness. The foundation of a mindfulness practice is meditation. By practicing mindfulness meditation, one may develop the skill of decreasing autopilot/SIT thought patterns, which contribute to depressive symptoms.

The main psychological mechanism of mindfulness is known as reperceiving, which is a perspective shift such that one sees thoughts and emotions as passing and frequently insignificant phenomena rather than as representing fact. This shift causes thought patterns associated with depressive symptoms to lose power. Thus, one is able to break the repetitive autopilot/SIT cycle of pessimistic thoughts leading to dysphoria, leading to more negative thoughts, resulting in more negative affect and so on.

Neuroimaging studies indicate that mindfulness induces neuroplasticity such that the brain is more likely to engage in moment-by-moment awareness than DMN-mediated autopilot/SIT.

Finally, compelling evidence indicates that two secular mindfulness-based interventions, MBSR and MBCT, have antidepressant benefits. Very strong evidence supports the use of MBCT as an adjunctive intervention for depressive spectrum illness.

References

Allen, M., Dietz, M., Blair, K. S., van Beek, M., Rees, G., Vestergaard-Poulsen, P., et al. (2012). Cognitive-affective neural plasticity following active-controlled mindfulness intervention. *The Journal of Neuroscience, 32*(44), 15601–15610. doi:10.1523/JNEUROSCI.2957-12.2012.

Altshuler, L. L., Bookheimer, S. Y., Townsend, J., Proenza, M. A., Eisenberger, N., Sabb, F., et al. (2005). Blunted activation in orbitofrontal cortex during mania: A functional magnetic resonance imaging study. *Biological Psychiatry, 58*(10), 763–769. doi:10.1016/j.biopsych.2005.09.012. S0006-3223(05)01208-4 [pii].

Altshuler, L., Bookheimer, S., Townsend, J., Proenza, M. A., Sabb, F., Mintz, J., et al. (2008). Regional brain changes in bipolar I depression: A functional magnetic resonance imaging study. *Bipolar Disorders, 10*, 708–717.

Amaral, D. G., & Price, J. L. (1984). Amygdalo-cortical projections in the monkey (Macaca fascicularis). *Journal of Comparative Neurology, 230*(4), 465–496. doi:10.1002/cne.902300402.

Baerentsen, K. B., Stodkilde-Jorgensen, H., Sommerlund, B., Hartmann, T., Damsgaard-Madsen, J., Fosnaes, M., et al. (2010). An investigation of brain processes supporting meditation. *Cognitive Processing, 11*(1), 57–84. doi:10.1007/s10339-009-0342-3.

Barbas, H., & De Olmos, J. (1990). Projections from the amygdala to basoventral and mediodorsal prefrontal regions in the rhesus monkey. *Journal of Comparative Neurology, 300*(4), 549–571. doi:10.1002/cne.903000409.

Beck, A. T. (1967). *Depression: Clinical, experimental, and theoretical aspects*. New York: Harper & Row.

Bishop, S. R., Lau, M., Shapiro, S., Carlson, L., Anderson, N. D., Carmody, J., et al. (2004). Mindfulness: A proposed operational definition. *Clinical Psychology-Science and Practice, 11*(3), 230–241. doi:10.1093/Clipsy/Bph077.

Blairy, S., Linotte, S., Souery, D., Papadimitriou, G. N., Dikeos, D., Lerer, B., et al. (2004). Social adjustment and self-esteem of bipolar patients: A multicentric study. *Journal of Affective Disorders, 79*(1–3), 97–103. doi:10.1016/S0165-0327(02)00347-6. S0165032702003476 [pii].

Bondolfi, G., Jermann, F., der Linden, M. V., Gex-Fabry, M., Bizzini, L., Rouget, B. W., et al. (2010). Depression relapse prophylaxis with Mindfulness-Based Cognitive Therapy: Replication and extension in the Swiss health care system. *Journal of Affective Disorders, 122*(3), 224–231. doi:10.1016/j.jad.2009.07.007. S0165-0327(09)00312-7 [pii].

Brefczynski-Lewis, J. A., Lutz, A., Schaefer, H. S., Levinson, D. B., & Davidson, R. J. (2007). Neural correlates of attentional expertise in long-term meditation practitioners. *Proceedings of the National Academy of Sciences United States of America, 104*(27), 11483–11488. doi:10.1073/pnas.0606552104.

Brooks, J. O., 3rd, Wang, P. W., Bonner, J. C., Rosen, A. C., Hoblyn, J. C., Hill, S. J., et al. (2009). Decreased prefrontal, anterior cingulate, insula, and ventral striatal metabolism in medication-free depressed outpatients with bipolar disorder. *Journal of Psychiatric Research, 43*(3), 181–188. doi:10.1016/j.jpsychires.2008.04.015. S0022-3956(08)00099-X [pii].

Brown, G. W., Andrews, B., Harris, T., Adler, Z., & Bridge, L. (1986). Social support, self-esteem and depression. *Psychological Medicine, 16*(4), 813–831.

Brown, K. W., Goodman, R. J., & Inzlicht, M. (2012). Dispositional mindfulness and the attenuation of neural responses to emotional stimuli. *Social Cognitive and Affective Neuroscience*. doi:10.1093/scan/nss004.

Buckwalter, J. A., Schumann, C. M., & Van Hoesen, G. W. (2008). Evidence for direct projections from the basal nucleus of the amygdala to retrosplenial cortex in the Macaque monkey. *Experimental Brain Research, 186*(1), 47–57. doi:10.1007/s00221-007-1203-x.

Burwell, R. A., & Shirk, S. R. (2007). Subtypes of rumination in adolescence: Associations between brooding, reflection, depressive symptoms, and coping. *Journal of Clinical Child & Adolescent Psychology, 36*(1), 56–65. doi:10.1207/s15374424jccp3601_6.

Carmichael, S. T., & Price, J. L. (1995). Limbic connections of the orbital and medial prefrontal cortex in macaque monkeys. *Journal of Comparative Neurology, 363*(4), 615–641. doi:10.1002/cne.903630408.

Chen, C. H., Lennox, B., Jacob, R., Calder, A., Lupson, V., Bisbrown-Chippendale, R., et al. (2006). Explicit and implicit facial affect recognition in manic and depressed States of bipolar disorder: A functional magnetic resonance imaging study. *Biological Psychiatry, 59*(1), 31–39. doi:10.1016/j.biopsych.2005.06.008. S0006-3223(05)00714-6 [pii].

Chiesa, A., & Malinowski, P. (2011). Mindfulness-based approaches: Are they all the same? *Journal of Clinical Psychology, 67*(4), 404–424. doi:10.1002/jclp.20776.

Chiesa, A., & Serretti, A. (2010a). Mindfulness based cognitive therapy for psychiatric disorders: A systematic review and meta-analysis. *Psychiatry Research*. doi:10.1016/j.psychres.2010.08.011. S0165-1781(10)00519-6 [pii].

Chiesa, A., & Serretti, A. (2010b). A systematic review of neurobiological and clinical features of mindfulness meditations. *Psychological Medicine, 40*(8), 1239–1252. doi:10.1017/S0033291709991747.

Cooney, R. E., Joormann, J., Eugene, F., Dennis, E. L., & Gotlib, I. H. (2010). Neural correlates of rumination in depression. *Cognitive, Affective, & Behavioral Neuroscience, 10*(4), 470–478. doi:10.3758/CABN.10.4.470. 10/4/470 [pii].

Creswell, J. D., Way, B. M., Eisenberger, N. I., & Lieberman, M. D. (2007). Neural correlates of dispositional mindfulness during affect labeling. *Psychosomatic Medicine, 69*(6), 560–565. doi:10.1097/PSY.0b013e3180f6171f.

Delgado, L. C., Guerra, P., Perakakis, P., Vera, M. N., Reyes del Paso, G., & Vila, J. (2010). Treating chronic worry: Psychological and physiological effects of a training programme based on mindfulness. *Behavior Research and Therapy, 48*(9), 873–882. doi:10.1016/j.brat.2010.05.012. S0005-7967(10)00108-7 [pii].

Desbordes, G., Negi, L. T., Pace, T. W., Wallace, B. A., Raison, C. L., & Schwartz, E. L. (2012). Effects of mindful-attention and compassion meditation training on amygdala response to emotional stimuli in an ordinary, non-meditative state. *Frontiers in Human Neuroscience, 6*, 292. doi:10.3389/fnhum.2012.00292.

Dickenson, J., Berkman, E. T., Arch, J., & Lieberman, M. D. (2013). Neural correlates of focused attention during a brief mindfulness induction. *Social Cognitive and Affective Neuroscience, 8*(1), 40–47. doi:10.1093/scan/nss030.

Drevets, W. C., Price, J. L., Simpson, J. R., Jr., Todd, R. D., Reich, T., Vannier, M., et al. (1997). Subgenual prefrontal cortex abnormalities in mood disorders. *Nature, 386*(6627), 824–827. doi:10.1038/386824a0.

Dunn, R. T., Kimbrell, T. A., Ketter, T. A., Frye, M. A., Willis, M. W., Luckenbaugh, D. A., et al. (2002). Principal components of the Beck depression inventory and regional cerebral metabolism in unipolar and bipolar depression. *Biological Psychiatry, 51*(5), 387–399. doi: S0006322301012446 [pii].

Elliott, R., Ogilvie, A., Rubinsztein, J. S., Calderon, G., Dolan, R. J., & Sahakian, B. J. (2004). Abnormal ventral frontal response during performance of an affective go/no go task in patients with mania. *Biological Psychiatry, 55*(12), 1163–1170. doi:10.1016/j.biopsych.2004.03.007. S0006322304003944 [pii].

Evans, J., Heron, J., Lewis, G., Araya, R., & Wolke, D. (2005). Negative self-schemas and the onset of depression in women: Longitudinal study. *British Journal of Psychiatry, 186*, 302–307. doi:10.1192/bjp.186.4.302. 186/4/302 [pii].

Farb, N. A., Anderson, A. K., Mayberg, H., Bean, J., McKeon, D., & Segal, Z. V. (2010). Minding one's emotions: Mindfulness training alters the neural expression of sadness. *Emotion, 10*(1), 25–33. doi:10.1037/a0017151.

Farb, N. A., Segal, Z. V., Mayberg, H., Bean, J., McKeon, D., Fatima, Z., et al. (2007). Attending to the present: Mindfulness meditation reveals distinct neural modes of self-reference. *Social Cognitive and Affective Neuroscience, 2*(4), 313–322. doi:10.1093/scan/nsm030.

Farb, N. A., Segal, Z. V., & Anderson, A. K. (2013). Mindfulness meditation training alters cortical representations of interoceptive attention. *Social Cognitive and Affective Neuroscience, 8*(1), 15–26. doi:10.1093/scan/nss066.

Ferry, A. T., Ongur, D., An, X., & Price, J. L. (2000). Prefrontal cortical projections to the striatum in macaque monkeys: Evidence for an organization related to prefrontal networks. *Journal of Comparative Neurology, 425*(3), 447–470. doi:10.1002/1096-9861(20000925)425:3<447::AID-CNE9>3.0.CO;2-V [pii].

Finucane, A., & Mercer, S. W. (2006). An exploratory mixed methods study of the acceptability and effectiveness of mindfulness-based cognitive therapy for patients with active depression and anxiety in primary care. *BMC Psychiatry, 6*, 14. doi:10.1186/1471-244X-6-14.

Fischer-Schreiber, I., Ehrhard, F.-K., & Diener, M. S. (1991). *The Shambhala dictionary of Buddhism and Zen* (M. H. Kohn, Trans.). Boston, MA: Shambhala.

Fjorback, L. O., Arendt, M., Ornbol, E., Fink, P., & Walach, H. (2011). Mindfulness-based stress reduction and mindfulness-based cognitive therapy - a systematic review of randomized controlled trials. *Acta Psychiatrica Scandinavica, 124*(2), 102–119. doi:10.1111/j.1600-0447.2011.01704.x.

Gallagher, I. I. (2000). Philosophical conceptions of the self: Implications for cognitive science. *Trends in Cognitive Sciences, 4*(1), 14–21.

Gara, M. A., Woolfolk, R. L., Cohen, B. D., Goldston, R. B., Allen, L. A., & Novalany, J. (1993). Perception of self and other in major depression. *Journal of Abnormal Psychology, 102*(1), 93–100.

Gard, T., Holzel, B. K., Sack, A. T., Hempel, H., Lazar, S. W., Vaitl, D., et al. (2012). Pain attenuation through mindfulness is associated with decreased cognitive control and increased sensory processing in the brain. *Cerebral Cortex, 22*(11), 2692–2702. doi:10.1093/cercor/bhr352.

Garrison, K. A., Santoyo, J. F., Davis, J. H., Thornhill, T. A. T., Kerr, C. E., & Brewer, J. A. (2013). Effortless awareness: Using real time neurofeedback to investigate correlates of posterior cingulate cortex activity in meditators' self-report. *Frontiers in Human Neuroscience, 7*, 440. doi:10.3389/fnhum.2013.00440.

Garrison, K. A., Scheinost, D., Worhunsky, P. D., Elwafi, H. M., Thornhill, T. A. T., Thompson, E., et al. (2013). Real-time fMRI links subjective experience with brain activity during focused attention. *NeuroImage, 81*, 110–118. doi:10.1016/j.neuroimage.2013.05.030.

Gibbons, C. J., Fournier, J. C., Stirman, S. W., DeRubeis, R. J., Crits-Christoph, P., & Beck, A. T. (2010). The clinical effectiveness of cognitive therapy for depression in an outpatient clinic. *Journal of Affective Disorders, 125*(1–3), 169–176. doi:10.1016/j.jad.2009.12.030. S0165-0327(10)00009-1 [pii].

Godfrin, K. A., & van Heeringen, C. (2010a). The effects of mindfulness-based cognitive therapy on recurrence of depressive episodes, mental health and quality of life: A randomized controlled study. *Behaviour Research and Therapy, 48*(8), 738–746. doi:10.1016/j.brat.2010.04.006.

Godfrin, K. A., & van Heeringen, C. (2010b). The effects of mindfulness-based cognitive therapy on recurrence of depressive episodes, mental health and quality of life: A randomized controlled study. *Behavior Research and Therapy, 48*(8), 738–746. doi:10.1016/j.brat.2010.04.006. S0005-7967(10)00071-9 [pii].

Goldin, P. R., & Gross, J. J. (2010). Effects of mindfulness-based stress reduction (MBSR) on emotion regulation in social anxiety disorder. *Emotion, 10*(1), 83–91. doi:10.1037/a0018441.

Goldin, P., Ziv, M., Jazaieri, H., Hahn, K., & Gross, J. J. (2013). MBSR vs aerobic exercise in social anxiety: fMRI of emotion regulation of negative self-beliefs. *Social Cognitive and Affective Neuroscience, 8*(1), 65–72. doi:10.1093/scan/nss054.

Goldin, P., Ziv, M., Jazaieri, H., & Gross, J. J. (2012). Randomized controlled trial of mindfulness-based stress reduction versus aerobic exercise: Effects on the self-referential brain network in social anxiety disorder. *Frontiers in Human Neuroscience, 6*, 295. doi:10.3389/fnhum.2012.00295.

Grimm, S., Boesiger, P., Beck, J., Schuepbach, D., Bermpohl, F., Walter, M., et al. (2009). Altered negative BOLD responses in the default-mode network during emotion processing in depressed subjects. *Neuropsychopharmacology, 34*(4), 932–943. doi:10.1038/npp.2008.81. npp200881 [pii].

Grimm, S., Ernst, J., Boesiger, P., Schuepbach, D., Hell, D., Boeker, H., et al. (2009). Increased self-focus in major depressive disorder is related to neural abnormalities in subcortical-cortical midline structures. *Human Brain Mapping, 30*(8), 2617–2627. doi:10.1002/hbm.20693.

Gusnard, D. A., & Raichle, M. E. (2001). Searching for a baseline: Functional imaging and the resting human brain. *Nature Reviews Neuroscience, 2*(10), 685–694. doi:10.1038/35094500.

Haber, S. N., Kunishio, K., Mizobuchi, M., & Lynd-Balta, E. (1995). The orbital and medial prefrontal circuit through the primate basal ganglia. *The Journal of Neuroscience, 15*(7 Pt 1), 4851–4867.

Halari, R., Simic, M., Pariante, C. M., Papadopoulos, A., Cleare, A., Brammer, M., et al. (2009). Reduced activation in lateral prefrontal cortex and anterior cingulate during attention and cognitive control functions in medication-naive adolescents with depression compared to controls. *Journal of Child Psychology and Psychiatry, and Allied Disciplines, 50*(3), 307–316. doi:10.1111/j.1469-7610.2008.01972.x.

Harvey, P. O., Fossati, P., Pochon, J. B., Levy, R., Lebastard, G., Lehericy, S., et al. (2005). Cognitive control and brain resources in major depression: An fMRI study using the n-back task. *NeuroImage, 26*(3), 860–869. doi:10.1016/j.neuroimage.2005.02.048.

Hasenkamp, W., & Barsalou, L. W. (2012). Effects of meditation experience on functional connectivity of distributed brain networks. *Frontiers in Human Neuroscience, 6*, 38. doi:10.3389/fnhum.2012.00038.

Hasenkamp, W., Wilson-Mendenhall, C. D., Duncan, E., & Barsalou, L. W. (2012). Mind wandering and attention during focused meditation: A fine-grained temporal analysis of fluctuating cognitive states. *NeuroImage, 59*(1), 750–760. doi:10.1016/j.neuroimage.2011.07.008.

Heinzel, A., Bermpohl, F., Niese, R., Pfennig, A., Pascual-Leone, A., Schlaug, G., et al. (2005). How do we modulate our emotions? Parametric fMRI reveals cortical midline structures as regions specifically involved in the processing of emotional valences. *Brain Research. Cognitive Brain Research, 25*(1), 348–358. doi:10.1016/j.cogbrainres.2005.06.009. S0926-6410(05)00191-6 [pii].

Hill, C. L., & Updegraff, J. A. (2011). Mindfulness and its relationship to emotional regulation. *Emotion*. doi:10.1037/a0026355.

Holzel, B. K., Hoge, E. A., Greve, D. N., Gard, T., Creswell, J. D., Brown, K. W., et al. (2013). Neural mechanisms of symptom improvements in generalized anxiety disorder following mindfulness training. *Neuroimage: Clinical, 2*, 448–458. doi:10.1016/j.nicl.2013.03.011.

Holzel, B. K., Ott, U., Hempel, H., Hackl, A., Wolf, K., Stark, R., et al. (2007). Differential engagement of anterior cingulate and adjacent medial frontal cortex in adept meditators and non-meditators. *Neuroscience Letters, 421*(1), 16–21. doi:10.1016/j.neulet.2007.04.074.

Ingram, R. E. (1990). Self-focused attention in clinical disorders: Review and a conceptual model. *Psychological Bulletin, 107*(2), 156–176.

Ives-Deliperi, V. L., Howells, F., Stein, D. J., Meintjes, E. M., & Horn, N. (2013). The effects of mindfulness-based cognitive therapy in patients with bipolar disorder: A controlled functional MRI investigation. *Journal of Affective Disorders, 150*(3), 1152–1157. doi:10.1016/j.jad.2013.05.074.

Ives-Deliperi, V. L., Solms, M., & Meintjes, E. M. (2011). The neural substrates of mindfulness: An fMRI investigation. *Social Neuroscience, 6*(3), 231–242. doi:10.1080/17470919.2010.513495.

Johnson, S. C., Baxter, L. C., Wilder, L. S., Pipe, J. G., Heiserman, J. E., & Prigatano, G. P. (2002). Neural correlates of self-reflection. *Brain, 125*(Pt 8), 1808–1814.

Johnson, M. K., Nolen-Hoeksema, S., Mitchell, K. J., & Levin, Y. (2009). Medial cortex activity, self-reflection and depression. *Social Cognitive and Affective Neuroscience, 4*(4), 313–327. doi:10.1093/scan/nsp022. nsp022 [pii].

Jones, S. (2004). Psychotherapy of bipolar disorder: A review. *Journal of Affective Disorders, 80*(2–3), 101–114. doi:10.1016/S0165-0327(03)00111-3. S0165032703001113 [pii].

Kabat-Zinn, J. (2005). *Full catastrophe living: Using the wisdom of your body and mind to face stress, pain, and illness* (Fifteenth Anniversary ed.). New York: Bantam Dell.

Kegeles, L. S., Malone, K. M., Slifstein, M., Ellis, S. P., Xanthopoulos, E., Keilp, J. G., et al. (2003). Response of cortical metabolic deficits to serotonergic challenge in familial mood disorders. *American Journal of Psychiatry, 160*(1), 76–82.

Kemeny, M. E., Foltz, C., Cavanagh, J. F., Cullen, M., Giese-Davis, J., Jennings, P., et al. (2011). Contemplative/emotion training reduces negative emotional behavior and promotes prosocial responses. *Emotion*. doi:10.1037/a0026118.

Kilpatrick, L. A., Suyenobu, B. Y., Smith, S. R., Bueller, J. A., Goodman, T., Creswell, J. D., et al. (2011). Impact of mindfulness-based stress reduction training on intrinsic brain connectivity. *NeuroImage, 56*(1), 290–298. doi:10.1016/j.neuroimage.2011.02.034.

King, C. A., Naylor, M. W., Segal, H. G., Evans, T., & Shain, B. N. (1993). Global self-worth, specific self-perceptions of competence, and depression in adolescents. *Journal of the American Academy of Child & Adolescent Psychiatry, 32*(4), 745–752. doi:10.1097/00004583-199307000-00007. S0890-8567(09)64863-2 [pii].

Kirk, U., Downar, J., & Montague, P. R. (2011). Interoception drives increased rational decision-making in meditators playing the ultimatum game. *Frontiers in Neuroscience, 5*, 49. doi:10.3389/fnins.2011.00049.

Kozasa, E. H., Sato, J. R., Lacerda, S. S., Barreiros, M. A., Radvany, J., Russell, T. A., et al. (2012). Meditation training increases brain efficiency in an attention task. *NeuroImage, 59*(1), 745–749. doi:10.1016/j.neuroimage.2011.06.088.

Kuyken, W., Byford, S., Taylor, R. S., Watkins, E., Holden, E., White, K., et al. (2008). Mindfulness-based cognitive therapy to prevent relapse in recurrent depression. *Journal of Consulting and Clinical Psychology, 76*(6), 966–978. doi:10.1037/a0013786. 2008-16943-016 [pii].

Lagopoulos, J., & Malhi, G. (2011). Impairments in "top-down" processing in bipolar disorder: A simultaneous fMRI-GSR study. *Psychiatry Research, 192*(2), 100–108. doi:10.1016/j.pscychresns.2010.11.011. S0925-4927(10)00397-5 [pii].

Lauder, S. D., Berk, M., Castle, D. J., Dodd, S., & Berk, L. (2010). The role of psychotherapy in bipolar disorder. *The Medical Journal of Australia, 193*(4 Suppl), S31–S35. doi: lau11471_fm [pii].

Lemogne, C., Gorwood, P., Bergouignan, L., Pelissolo, A., Lehericy, S., & Fossati, P. (2010). Negative affectivity, self-referential processing and the cortical midline structures. *Social Cognitive and Affective Neuroscience*. doi:10.1093/scan/nsq049. nsq049 [pii].

Lennox, B. R., Jacob, R., Calder, A. J., Lupson, V., & Bullmore, E. T. (2004). Behavioural and neurocognitive responses to sad facial affect are attenuated in patients with mania. *Psychological Medicine, 34*(5), 795–802.
Liotti, M., Mayberg, H. S., McGinnis, S., Brannan, S. L., & Jerabek, P. (2002). Unmasking disease-specific cerebral blood flow abnormalities: Mood challenge in patients with remitted unipolar depression. *American Journal of Psychiatry, 159*(11), 1830–1840.
Lo, C. S., Ho, S. M., & Hollon, S. D. (2010). The effects of rumination and depressive symptoms on the prediction of negative attributional style among college students. *Cognitive Therapy and Research, 34*(2), 116–123. doi:10.1007/s10608-009-9233-2.
Lutz, J., Herwig, U., Opialla, S., Hittmeyer, A., Jancke, L., Rufer, M., et al. (2013). Mindfulness and emotion regulation–an fMRI study. *Social Cognitive and Affective Neuroscience*. doi:10.1093/scan/nst043.
Lutz, A., McFarlin, D. R., Perlman, D. M., Salomons, T. V., & Davidson, R. J. (2013). Altered anterior insula activation during anticipation and experience of painful stimuli in expert meditators. *NeuroImage, 64*, 538–546. doi:10.1016/j.neuroimage.2012.09.030.
Lutz, A., Slagter, H. A., Dunne, J. D., & Davidson, R. J. (2008). Attention regulation and monitoring in meditation. *Trends in Cognitive Sciences, 12*(4), 163–169. doi:10.1016/j.tics.2008.01.005.
Malhi, G. S., Lagopoulos, J., Ward, P. B., Kumari, V., Mitchell, P. B., Parker, G. B., et al. (2004). Cognitive generation of affect in bipolar depression: An fMRI study. *European Journal of Neuroscience, 19*(3), 741–754. doi: 3159 [pii].
Manicavasgar, V., Parker, G., & Perich, T. (2010). Mindfulness-based cognitive therapy vs cognitive behaviour therapy as a treatment for non-melancholic depression. *Journal of Affective Disorders*. doi:10.1016/j.jad.2010.09.027. S0165-0327(10)00608-7 [pii].
Manicavasgar, V., Parker, G., & Perich, T. (2011). Mindfulness-based cognitive therapy vs cognitive behaviour therapy as a treatment for non-melancholic depression. *Journal of Affective Disorders, 130*(1–2), 138–144. doi:10.1016/j.jad.2010.09.027.
Marchand, W. R. (2010). Cortico-basal ganglia circuitry: A review of key research and implications for functional connectivity studies of mood and anxiety disorders. *Brain Structure and Function, 215*(2), 73–96. doi:10.1007/s00429-010-0280-y.
Marchand, W. R. (2012). Mindfulness-based stress reduction, mindfulness-based cognitive therapy, and Zen meditation for depression, anxiety, pain, and psychological distress. *Journal of Psychiatric Practice, 18*(4), 233–252. doi:10.1097/01.pra.0000416014.53215.86.
Marchand, W. R., Lee, J. N., Garn, C., Thatcher, J., Gale, P., Kreitschitz, S., et al. (2011). Aberrant emotional processing in posterior cortical midline structures in bipolar II depression. *Progress in Neuropsychopharmacology & Biological Psychiatry*. doi:10.1016/j.pnpbp.2011.05.017. S0278-5846(11)00187-4 [pii].
Marchand, W. R., Lee, J. N., Johnson, S., Thatcher, J., Gale, P., Wood, N., et al. (2012). Striatal and cortical midline circuits in major depression: Implications for suicide and symptom expression. *Progress in Neuropsychopharmacology & Biological Psychiatry, 36*(2), 290–299. doi:10.1016/j.pnpbp.2011.10.016.
Marchand, W. R., Lee, J. N., Johnson, S., Thatcher, J., & Gale, P. (2013). Striatal circuit function is associated with prior self-harm in remitted major depression. *Neuroscience Letters, 557*(Pt B), 154–158. doi:10.1016/j.neulet.2013.10.053.
Marchand, W. R., Lee, J. N., Suchy, Y., Johnson, S., Thatcher, J., & Gale, P. (2012). Aberrant functional connectivity of cortico-basal ganglia circuits in major depression. *Neuroscience Letters, 514*(1), 86–90. doi:10.1016/j.neulet.2012.02.063.
Marchand, W. R., Lee, J. N., Thatcher, J. W., Hsu, E. W., Rashkin, E., Suchy, Y., et al. (2008). Putamen coactivation during motor task execution. *Neuroreport, 19*(9), 957–960. doi:10.1097/WNR.0b013e328302c87300001756-200806110-00011 [pii].
Marchand, W. R., & Yurgelun-Todd, D. (2010). Striatal structure and function in mood disorders: A comprehensive review. *Bipolar Disorders, 12*(8), 764–785. doi:10.1111/j.1399-5618.2010.00874.x.
Mason, M. F., Norton, M. I., Van Horn, J. D., Wegner, D. M., Grafton, S. T., & Macrae, C. N. (2007). Wandering minds: The default network and stimulus-independent thought. *Science, 315*(5810), 393–395. doi:10.1126/science.1131295.

Mathew, K. L., Whitford, H. S., Kenny, M. A., & Denson, L. A. (2010). The long-term effects of mindfulness-based cognitive therapy as a relapse prevention treatment for major depressive disorder. *Behavioral and Cognitive Psychotherapy, 38*(5), 561–576. doi:10.1017/S135246581000010X. S135246581000010X [pii].

Mayberg, H. S., Brannan, S. K., Tekell, J. L., Silva, J. A., Mahurin, R. K., McGinnis, S., et al. (2000). Regional metabolic effects of fluoxetine in major depression: Serial changes and relationship to clinical response. *Biological Psychiatry, 48*(8), 830–843. doi: S0006-3223(00)01036-2 [pii].

McKiernan, K. A., D'Angelo, B. R., Kaufman, J. N., & Binder, J. R. (2006). Interrupting the "stream of consciousness": An fMRI investigation. *NeuroImage, 29*(4), 1185–1191. doi:10.1016/j.neuroimage.2005.09.030.

Michalak, J., Holz, A., & Teismann, T. (2010). Rumination as a predictor of relapse in mindfulness-based cognitive therapy for depression. *Psychology & Psychotherapy*. doi:10.1348/147608310X520166. pptrp580 [pii].

Miller, L., Warner, V., Wickramaratne, P., & Weissman, M. (1999). Self-esteem and depression: Ten year follow-up of mothers and offspring. *Journal of Affective Disorders, 52*(1–3), 41–49.

Mor, N., & Winquist, J. (2002). Self-focused attention and negative affect: A meta-analysis. *Psychological Bulletin, 128*(4), 638–662.

Nilsson, K. K., Jorgensen, C. R., Craig, T. K., Straarup, K. N., & Licht, R. W. (2010). Self-esteem in remitted bipolar disorder patients: A meta-analysis. *Bipolar Disorders, 12*(6), 585–592. doi:10.1111/j.1399-5618.2010.00856.x.

Northoff, G. (2007). Psychopathology and pathophysiology of the self in depression - neuropsychiatric hypothesis. *Journal of Affective Disorders, 104*(1–3), 1–14. doi:10.1016/j.jad.2007.02.012. S0165-0327(07)00084-5 [pii].

Northoff, G., & Bermpohl, F. (2004). Cortical midline structures and the self. *Trends in Cognitive Sciences, 8*(3), 102–107. doi:10.1016/j.tics.2004.01.004S136466130400021X [pii].

Northoff, G., Heinzel, A., de Greck, M., Bermpohl, F., Dobrowolny, H., & Panksepp, J. (2006). Self-referential processing in our brain–a meta-analysis of imaging studies on the self. *NeuroImage, 31*(1), 440–457. doi:10.1016/j.neuroimage.2005.12.002. S1053-8119(05)02515-2 [pii].

Osuch, E. A., Bluhm, R. L., Williamson, P. C., Theberge, J., Densmore, M., & Neufeld, R. W. (2009). Brain activation to favorite music in healthy controls and depressed patients. *Neuroreport, 20*(13), 1204–1208. doi:10.1097/WNR.0b013e32832f4da3.

Pagnoni, G. (2012). Dynamical properties of BOLD activity from the ventral posteromedial cortex associated with meditation and attentional skills. *The Journal of Neuroscience, 32*(15), 5242–5249. doi:10.1523/JNEUROSCI.4135-11.2012.

Pagnoni, G., Cekic, M., & Guo, Y. (2008). "Thinking about not-thinking": Neural correlates of conceptual processing during Zen meditation. *PLoS ONE, 3*(9), e3083. doi:10.1371/journal.pone.0003083.

Parvizi, J., Van Hoesen, G. W., Buckwalter, J., & Damasio, A. (2006). Neural connections of the posteromedial cortex in the macaque. *Proceedings of the National Academy of Sciences United States of America, 103*(5), 1563–1568. doi:10.1073/pnas.0507729103. 0507729103 [pii].

Paul, N. A., Stanton, S. J., Greeson, J. M., Smoski, M. J., & Wang, L. (2013). Psychological and neural mechanisms of trait mindfulness in reducing depression vulnerability. *Social Cognitive and Affective Neuroscience, 8*(1), 56–64. doi:10.1093/scan/nss070.

Piet, J., & Hougaard, E. (2011). The effect of mindfulness-based cognitive therapy for prevention of relapse in recurrent major depressive disorder: A systematic review and meta-analysis. *Clinical Psychology Review, 31*(6), 1032–1040. doi:10.1016/j.cpr.2011.05.002.

Pizzagalli, D. A., Holmes, A. J., Dillon, D. G., Goetz, E. L., Birk, J. L., Bogdan, R., et al. (2009). Reduced caudate and nucleus accumbens response to rewards in unmedicated individuals with major depressive disorder. *American Journal of Psychiatry, 166*(6), 702–710. doi:10.1176/appi.ajp.2008.08081201. appi.ajp.2008.08081201 [pii].

Porrino, L. J., Crane, A. M., & Goldman-Rakic, P. S. (1981). Direct and indirect pathways from the amygdala to the frontal lobe in rhesus monkeys. *Journal of Comparative Neurology, 198*(1), 121–136. doi:10.1002/cne.901980111.

Posner, M. I., & Rothbart, M. K. (2007). Research on attention networks as a model for the integration of psychological science. *Annual Review of Psychology, 58*, 1–23. doi:10.1146/annurev.psych.58.110405.085516.

Raichle, M. E., MacLeod, A. M., Snyder, A. Z., Powers, W. J., Gusnard, D. A., & Shulman, G. L. (2001). A default mode of brain function. *Proceedings of the National Academy of Sciences United States of America, 98*(2), 676–682. doi:10.1073/pnas.98.2.67698/2/676 [pii].

Raz, A., & Buhle, J. (2006). Typologies of attentional networks. *Nature Reviews Neuroscience, 7*(5), 367–379. doi:10.1038/nrn1903.

Rimes, K. A., & Watkins, E. (2005). The effects of self-focused rumination on global negative self-judgements in depression. *Behavior Research and Therapy, 43*(12), 1673–1681. doi:10.1016/j.brat.2004.12.002. S0005-7967(05)00018-5 [pii].

Ritchey, M., Dolcos, F., Eddington, K. M., Strauman, T. J., & Cabeza, R. (2010). Neural correlates of emotional processing in depression: Changes with cognitive behavioral therapy and predictors of treatment response. *Journal of Psychiatric Research*. doi:10.1016/j.jpsychires.2010.09.007. S0022-3956(10)00274-8 [pii].

Robins, C. J., Keng, S. L., Ekblad, A. G., & Brantley, J. G. (2012). Effects of mindfulness-based stress reduction on emotional experience and expression: A randomized controlled trial. *Journal of Clinical Psychology, 68*(1), 117–131. doi:10.1002/jclp.20857.

Sakamoto, S. (1999). A longitudinal study of the relationship of self-preoccupation with depression. *Journal of Clinical Psychology, 55*(1), 109–116. doi:10.1002/(SICI)1097-4679(199901)55:1<109::AID-JCLP11>3.0.CO;2–8 [pii].

Salmon, P., Sephton, S., Weissbecker, I., Hoover, K., Ulmer, C., & Studts, J. L. (2004). Mindfulness meditation in clinical practice. *Cognitive and Behavioral Practice, 11*(4), 434–446.

Schafer, R. B., & Keith, P. M. (1981). Self-esteem discrepancies and depression. *Journal of Psychology, 109*(1st Half), 43–49.

Scheuerecker, J., Meisenzahl, E. M., Koutsouleris, N., Roesner, M., Schopf, V., Linn, J., et al. (2010). Orbitofrontal volume reductions during emotion recognition in patients with major depression. *Journal of Psychiatry and Neuroscience, 35*(5), 311–320. doi:10.1503/jpn.090076 [pii]10.1503/jpn.090076.

Segal, Z. V., Bieling, P., Young, T., MacQueen, G., Cooke, R., Martin, L., et al. (2010). Antidepressant monotherapy vs sequential pharmacotherapy and mindfulness-based cognitive therapy, or placebo, for relapse prophylaxis in recurrent depression. *Archives of Genera, Psychiatry, 67*(12), 1256–1264. doi:10.1001/archgenpsychiatry.2010.168.

Segal, Z. V., Williams, J. M. G., & Teasdale, J. D. (2002). *Mindfulness-based cognitive therapy for depression: A new approach to preventing relapse*. New York: Guilford.

Shambhala Dragon Editions. (1991). *The shambhala dictionary of Buddhism and zen.* Boston: Shambhala.

Shapiro, D. H. (1992). A preliminary study of long term meditators: Goals, effects, religious orientation, cognitions. *Journal of Transpersonal Psychology, 24*, 23–39.

Shapiro, S. L., Carlson, L. E., Astin, J. A., & Freedman, B. (2006). Mechanisms of mindfulness. *Journal of Clinical Psychology, 62*(3), 373–386. doi:10.1002/jclp.20237.

Shaurya Prakash, R., De Leon, A. A., Klatt, M., Malarkey, W., & Patterson, B. (2013). Mindfulness disposition and default-mode network connectivity in older adults. *Social Cognitive and Affective Neuroscience, 8*(1), 112–117. doi:10.1093/scan/nss115.

Shestyuk, A. Y., & Deldin, P. J. (2010). Automatic and strategic representation of the self in major depression: Trait and state abnormalities. *American Journal of Psychiatry, 167*(5), 536–544. doi:10.1176/appi.ajp.2009.06091444. appi.ajp.2009.06091444 [pii].

Smallwood, J., & Schooler, J. W. (2006). The restless mind. *Psychological Bulletin, 132*(6), 946–958. doi:10.1037/0033-2909.132.6.946.

Smith, G. S., Kramer, E., Ma, Y., Kingsley, P., Dhawan, V., Chaly, T., et al. (2009). The functional neuroanatomy of geriatric depression. *International Journal of Geriatric Psychiatry, 24*(8), 798–808. doi:10.1002/gps.2185.

Smoski, M. J., Felder, J., Bizzell, J., Green, S. R., Ernst, M., Lynch, T. R., et al. (2009). fMRI of alterations in reward selection, anticipation, and feedback in major depressive disorder.

Journal of Affective Disorders, 118(1–3), 69–78. doi:10.1016/j.jad.2009.01.034. S0165-0327(09)00044-5 [pii].
Spasojevic, J., & Alloy, L. B. (2001). Rumination as a common mechanism relating depressive risk factors to depression. *Emotion, 1*(1), 25–37.
Taylor, V. A., Daneault, V., Grant, J., Scavone, G., Breton, E., Roffe-Vidal, S., et al. (2013). Impact of meditation training on the default mode network during a restful state. *Social Cognitive and Affective Neuroscience, 8*(1), 4–14. doi:10.1093/scan/nsr087.
Taylor, V. A., Grant, J., Daneault, V., Scavone, G., Breton, E., Roffe-Vidal, S., et al. (2011). Impact of mindfulness on the neural responses to emotional pictures in experienced and beginner meditators. *NeuroImage, 57*(4), 1524–1533. doi:10.1016/j.neuroimage.2011.06.001.
Teasdale, J. D. (1999). Emotional processing, three modes of mind and the prevention of relapse in depression. *Behavior Research and Therapy, 37*(Suppl 1), S53–S77.
van Aalderen, J. R., Donders, A. R., Giommi, F., Spinhoven, P., Barendregt, H. P., & Speckens, A. E. (2011). The efficacy of mindfulness-based cognitive therapy in recurrent depressed patients with and without a current depressive episode: A randomized controlled trial. *Psychological Medicine, 1–13*. doi: 10.1017/S0033291711002054
Walsh, R., & Shapiro, S. L. (2006). The meeting of meditative disciplines and Western psychology: A mutually enriching dialogue. *American Psychologist, 61*(3), 227–239. doi:10.1037/0003-066X.61.3.227. 2006-03947-004 [pii].
Walter, H., Wolf, R. C., Spitzer, M., & Vasic, N. (2007). Increased left prefrontal activation in patients with unipolar depression: An event-related, parametric, performance-controlled fMRI study. *Journal of Affective Disorders, 101*(1–3), 175–185. doi:10.1016/j.jad.2006.11.017.
Watkins, E. (2004). Adaptive and maladaptive ruminative self-focus during emotional processing. *Behavior Research and Therapy, 42*(9), 1037–1052. doi:10.1016/j.brat.2004.01.009 S0005796704001172 [pii].
Watkins, E., & Teasdale, J. D. (2004). Adaptive and maladaptive self-focus in depression. *Journal of Affective Disorders, 82*(1), 1–8. doi:10.1016/j.jad.2003.10.006. S016503270300288X [pii].
Wells, R. E., Yeh, G. Y., Kerr, C. E., Wolkin, J., Davis, R. B., Tan, Y., et al. (2013). Meditation's impact on default mode network and hippocampus in mild cognitive impairment: A pilot study. *Neuroscience Letters, 556*, 15–19. doi:10.1016/j.neulet.2013.10.001.
Williams, A. D., & Moulds, M. L. (2010). The impact of ruminative processing on the experience of self-referent intrusive memories in dysphoria. *Behavior Therapy, 41*(1), 38–45. doi:10.1016/j.beth.2008.12.003. S0005-7894(09)00042-2 [pii].
Work Group on Major Depressive Disorder. (2010). *American psychiatric association practice guideline for the treatment of patients with major depressive disorder* (3rd ed.). Arlington, VA: American Psychiatric.
Wright, J. H., Beck, A. T., & Thase, M. E. (2003). Cognitive therapy. In R. E. Hales & S. C. Yudofsky (Eds.), *Textbook of clinical psychiatry* (4th ed., pp. 1245–1284). Washington, DC: American Psychiatric.
Wu, J., Buchsbaum, M. S., Gillin, J. C., Tang, C., Cadwell, S., Wiegand, M., et al. (1999). Prediction of antidepressant effects of sleep deprivation by metabolic rates in the ventral anterior cingulate and medial prefrontal cortex. *American Journal of Psychiatry, 156*(8), 1149–1158.
Yoshimura, S., Okamoto, Y., Onoda, K., Matsunaga, M., Ueda, K., Suzuki, S., et al. (2010). Rostral anterior cingulate cortex activity mediates the relationship between the depressive symptoms and the medial prefrontal cortex activity. *Journal of Affective Disorders, 122*(1–2), 76–85. doi:10.1016/j.jad.2009.06.017. S0165-0327(09)00277-8 [pii].
Zeidan, F., Martucci, K. T., Kraft, R. A., Gordon, N. S., McHaffie, J. G., & Coghill, R. C. (2011). Brain mechanisms supporting the modulation of pain by mindfulness meditation. *The Journal of Neuroscience, 31*(14), 5540–5548. doi:10.1523/JNEUROSCI.5791-10.2011.
Zeidan, F., Martucci, K. T., Kraft, R. A., McHaffie, J. G., & Coghill, R. C. (2013). Neural correlates of mindfulness meditation-related anxiety relief. *Social Cognitive and Affective Neuroscience*. doi:10.1093/scan/nst041.

Chapter 8
Mindfulness for the Treatment of Stress Disorders

Karen Johanne Pallesen, Jesper Dahlgaard, and Lone Fjorback

Stress and Allostasis

In order to understand stress-related disorders, we need to consider stress against the background of evolution. We experience stress because our body runs a sequence of physiological reactions that evolved across animal species on a timescale of hundreds of millions of years. The stress response is automatic and instantaneous, because it is a survival mechanism that prepares the body for "fight or flight". In an evolutionary perspective, this makes sense: better to be prepared to take action than to stay calm and risk getting injured or killed.

As it turns out, the automaticity of the stress response is often not beneficial to humans. We become stressed out despite the absence of anything obviously "threatening". One reason for this is that our human intellectual capabilities have a drawback when it comes to stress; our brain can activate the stress response even when merely *imagining* unpleasant or dangerous situations. Furthermore, we have managed to develop a society that tricks our brains into falsely perceiving the presence of threat, even when there is none. Indications of danger, from an evolutionary perspective, are closely related to unpredictability. In our stimulus-packed societies, our brains are continuously bombarded with new information, making unpredictability abundant. Hence, in modern society, the innate stress response may keep our bodies and minds on high alert, while our rational knowledge about the basic

K.J. Pallesen, Ph.D. (✉) • L. Fjorback, Ph.D.
The Research Clinic for Functional Disorders and Psychosomatics,
Aarhus University Hospital, Nørrebrogade 44, Aarhus C 8000, Denmark
e-mail: karepall@rm.dk

J. Dahlgaard, Ph.D.
Unit for Psychooncology and Health Psychology, Aarhus University,
Bartholins Allé 9, Aarhus C 8000, Denmark

E. Shonin et al. (eds.), *Mindfulness and Buddhist-Derived Approaches in Mental Health and Addiction*, Advances in Mental Health and Addiction,
DOI 10.1007/978-3-319-22255-4_8

harmlessness of the surrounding environment has little to say. As a consequence, people may suffer from stress even in their normal, relatively safe, everyday life.

It is often posited that stress leads our bodies away from equilibrium or homeostasis, i.e. the physiological state in which metabolic processes function at their best. While it is true that stress has the potential to disrupt homeostasis, this says little about the nature of the processes involved in the stress response. As a remedy to the lack of an appropriate descriptive terminology, the term *allostasis*, has subsequently been adopted in stress research. Allostasis tags the physiological state in which processes in the body may be tilted between relatively wide-ranging states, for example, when the heart beat speeds up or when the bronchia dilate. Hence, whereas homeostasis and allostasis serve the common goal of keeping the body stable (i.e. "stasis"), the underlying processes differ. During ongoing stress, allostasis results in wear and tear on the body, and the organism enters a risk zone, in which physiological functions may go awry, a state coined by McEwen and Stellar as *allostatic load* (McEwen & Stellar, 1993). At some point, when the individual has become predisposed to develop disease, the term *allostatic overload* can be applied (McEwen & Wingfield, 2003). Allostatic load has been described as "the biological costs of a long-term or chronically activated stress response" (Zachariae 2009) or "a pathophysiological process in which multisystem biological dysregulation caused by chronic stress synergizes with unhealthy behaviours" (Picard, Juster, & McEwen, 2014).

The stress response is initiated by the brain on the basis of information from the senses or from internally driven thoughts and memories. In terms of brain structures, the hippocampus, critically involved in memory; the amygdala, essential to emotion processing; the prefrontal cortex, central in top-down regulation; and the hypothalamus are critically involved in triggering the stress response. The hypothalamus communicates to the body via the sympathetic nervous system (SNS; a branch of the autonomous nervous system) and the "HPA axis" (hypothalamus-pituitary-adrenal axis). SNS and its major stress hormone adrenalin are in charge of the first phase of the stress response, pushing the release of adrenalin by the inner organs and to the blood stream from the adrenal glands. Adrenalin makes the heart beat faster, causes the airways to expand, and stimulates the release of easily accessible energy (glucose and fatty acids) to the blood. The HPA axis, slightly delayed compared to SNS, initiates a range of additional processes via the secretion of hormones to the blood stream. The adrenals are stimulated to release glucocorticoids, including cortisol, by adrenocorticotropic hormone (ACTH) from the pituitary gland, which in turn is stimulated by corticotrophin-releasing factor (CRF) from the hypothalamus.

Allostasis involves multiple immune/inflammatory and metabolic mediators that respond to the signals from ANS and the HPA axis. Corticosteroids, primarily cortisol, work by binding to glucocorticoid receptors on cell surfaces throughout the body. During short-term stress, cortisol stimulates the storage of glucose into glycogen through the stimulation of enzymes in the liver, upregulates the expression of anti-inflammatory proteins, and stimulates the immune system. In the brain, cortisol, together with glutamate and noradrenaline, strengthens memory encoding

(Cahill & McGaugh, 1998; Roozendaal, Portillo-Marquez, & McGaugh, 1996) (O'Carroll, Drysdale, Cahill, Shajahan, & Ebmeier, 1999). An important function of cortisol is to enable the body to return to normal after a stressful event. This happens via a feedback signal to the brain.

The mediators of allostasis interact non-linearly and promote adaptation in the short run as long as they are turned on efficiently when needed and turned off when not needed (McEwen, Gray, & Nasca, 2015). During allostasis, processes controlled by the parasympathetic branch of ANS and sometimes referred to as "rest-and-digest", i.e. processes that serve maintenance and repair, are temporarily dampened. These processes return to normal as the stress response declines, due to downregulation of the HPA axis.

Allostatic Load

When the body's energy resources are becoming drained and parasympathetic functions are no longer being sufficiently maintained, we have entered a state of allostatic load. At some point, physiological processes that originally served in favour of beneficial adaptation start to change. Recent theories have abandoned the long-standing idea that long-term stress acts through the direct effects of elevated levels of stress hormones, as this idea has failed to comply, e.g. with observations of flattened or lowered cortisol levels in PTSD (Wingenfeld, Whooley, Neylan, Otte, & Cohen, 2015). Instead, it seems that receptor tissues change their willingness to respond normally to stress hormones (Cohen et al., 2012). Subsequently intracellular changes occur resulting in up- or downregulation of gene expression and a new transcriptional pattern that may fuel pathophysiological changes and cause diseases such as atherosclerosis (Schnall et al., 1990) and type 2 diabetes (Kelly & Ismail, 2015).

Allostatic Load in the Brain

The brain is the initiator, as well as the target of the stress response. Brain functions that we rely on every day in order to navigate efficiently in life are at risk in long-term stress. The ability to regulate the stress response to our own benefit critically depends on the proper feedback regulation of the HPA axis. During long-term stress, this mechanism is perturbed. The perturbation involves decreasing numbers of corticosteroid receptors in the hippocampus, with the result that its impact on the HPA axis changes. Ultimately, the secretion of corticosteroids from the adrenals is no longer regulated in an optimal manner. Studies show that this regulatory mechanism, once perturbed, may remain so for years, hence offering an explanation to why people who suffered from stress or depression feel "stress sensitive" for a long time afterwards. Numerous studies show that childhood adversity such as being exposed to bad parenting can lead to lifelong problems with stress regulation (Felitti et al., 1998) and that a dysfunctional HPA axis is a central part of the problem (McGowan et al., 2009; Meaney, 2001; Weaver et al., 2004). Early life adversity and cumulative stress exposure leading to decreased stress resilience is also linked to smaller amygdala and hippocampal volumes (Hanson et al., 2015).

During long-term stress, we no longer benefit from the strengthened memory encoding, which is present during short-term stress. The hippocampus appears partly to shut down during stress, and a hippocampal volume decrease has been observed in brain images in stress-related (or cortisol-related) disorders including Cushing's syndrome (Starkman, Gebarski, Berent, & Schteingart, 1992), PTSD (Bremner et al., 1995), depression (Sheline, Wang, Gado, Csernansky, & Vannier, 1996), and type 2 diabetes (Gold et al., 2007). Hippocampal volume decreases significantly in only 3 days (Brown et al., 2014), and just a single stress event modulates gene expression in rat hippocampus (Hunter, Gagnidze, McEwen, & Pfaff, 2014). These observations corroborate earlier studies of modulated synaptic plasticity (involved in the formation of new memories) following mild behavioural naturalistic stress (Xu, Anwyl, & Rowan, 1997).

Elevated levels of glucocorticoids were observed in relation to deterioration of memory functions (de Quervain, Roozendaal, & McGaugh, 1998; de Quervain, Roozendaal, Nitsch, McGaugh, & Hock, 2000). Prescribed medications such as prednisone were related to decreased long-term memory or "steroid dementia" and even confusion or delirium (Fardet et al, 2012). Severe cognitive disturbances were reported to persist after discontinuation of treatment (Ancelin et al., 2012). The detailed mechanistic explanation of how cognitive benefits turn into cognitive decline during severe stress also involves the neurotransmitter glutamate, which is stimulated by cortisol and which becomes toxic at high levels (Armanini, Hutchins, Stein, & Sapolsky, 1990; Choi, 1988). Apparently to avoid these negative effects, the hippocampus halts the production of new cells in the dentate gyrus of the hippocampus and reorganizes nerve cell structure, as dendrites are shortened and the production of transmitter molecules involved in communication is decreased (Magarinos & McEwen, 1995; Pham, Nacher, Hof, & McEwen, 2003). A recent study in rats indicated that blocking glutamate receptors during stress improves spatial working memory and modifies hippocampal synaptic plasticity (Amin, El-Aidi, Ali, Attia, & Rashed, 2015). Noradrenalin, in a manner similar to corticosteroids also loses its beneficial effect during long-term stress (Ramos & Arnsten, 2007; Rao, Williams, & Goldman-Rakic, 2000).

Glucocorticoids are also involved in the association between stress and the development of mood disorders (Heim & Nemeroff, 2001). Glucocorticoid treatment is associated with a sevenfold higher risk of suicide and suicide attempts and markedly higher risks of other severe neuropsychiatric conditions including depression, mania, panic disorder, and delirium, confusion, or disorientation (Bender, Lerner, & Kollasch, 1988; Fardet, Petersen, & Nazareth, 2012). Another neurotransmitter strongly linked to depression is serotonin. Recent findings suggest a link between glucocorticoid and serotonergic abnormalities (van der Doelen et al., 2014). Serotonin deficits were also linked to reductions in neurotrophic activity and smaller hippocampal volume (Coplan et al., 2014). Increased amygdala activity

(Drevets & Raichle, 1992) and volume (Lupien et al., 2011) has also been related to mood disorders, and threat-related amygdala reactivity is a predictor of psychological vulnerability to commonly experienced stressors (Swartz, Knodt, Radtke, & Hariri, 2015). Another study has related the link between stress and development of anxiety to a single neural circuit, initially involved in adaptive threat biases under stress and, subsequently, in anxiety disorders in the absence of the stressor (O. J. Robinson et al., 2014).

Sleep is normally a healthy response following stress exposure. Poor sleep quality often results from allostatic load and is also a characteristic sign of depression. Sleep is essential for restorative processes, and poor sleep may give rise to a range of dysfunctions and even to pain, e.g. in fibromyalgia (Moldofsky, 1995).

Normally a protective response to injury and normally downregulated via feedback corticosteroid effects, inflammation in tissues throughout the body results from long-term stress. Cohen and colleagues (2012) presented a plausible model suggesting that prolonged stressors result in glucocorticoid receptor resistance, which, in turn, interferes with appropriate regulation of inflammation (Cohen et al., 2012). Inflammation is likely to play a key role in the onset of psychopathology induced by stress. Neuroinflammation has been associated with Parkinson's disease (PD) (Epel et al., 2004) and major depressive disorder (Berk et al., 2013).

Allostatic Load in the Immune System

During a stress reaction, the immune system, in itself a complex system of processes that protects against disease, responds to signals from the brain communicated via the HPA axis. In accordance with the biopsychosocial model, effects of stress on the immune system show great interindividual variation (Kemeny & Laudenslager, 1999).

The possibility that stress modulates immune function emerged in the context of studies of social isolation and viral activity, e.g. herpes simplex viruses, HIV-1, Epstein-Barr virus, and cytomegalovirus. These are latent viruses that remain present in the cells of the body after the primary infection. The host remains free of symptoms as long as the immune system is able to control the infection. Weakening of the immune system by stress can reactivate the virus and lead to development of symptoms (Cole, 2013).

Prolonged stress can result in some immune system components being downregulated, with consequent increases in susceptibility to infections—and increased risk of cancer. Other components of the immune system may be upregulated, for example, an increased release of pro-inflammatory cytokines may result in increased risk of cardiovascular diseases, autoimmune diseases, cancer, and depression (Korte, Koolhaas, & Wingfield, 2005).

Some studies report that short-term and acute stressors (e.g. emotional stress) are associated with upregulation of the innate immune system, being the first line of defence against bacterial and viral infection resulting from, e.g. wounding. On the other hand, the acquired immunity, which may be considered as a second line of defence, appears to be downregulated (Segerstrom & Miller, 2004). For the acquired immune response, studies have found a downregulation of cellular immunity (e.g. the T cell response), whereas humoral immunity (i.e. antibody production) on the other hand is relatively unaffected. Prolonged stressors, e.g. grief from losing a spouse or persistent stress associated with caring for a family member with dementia, are associated with a general downregulation of both cellular and humoral immunity. In an evolutionary perspective, it may be meaningful that short-term stress sometimes leads to an upregulation of our innate immunity. This may prepare the organism to respond more effectively to potential infections in threatening situations with a risk of being wounded. Loneliness is also considered a stress factor, which may increase the risk of experiencing health problems. In two different populations, Jaremka and colleagues (Jaremka et al., 2013) demonstrated that the blood cells of lonely participants produced more cytokines in response to stress than less lonely participants.

Stress can also increase susceptibility to infection (Pedersen, Zachariae, & Bovbjerg, 2010). This may occur because prolonged stress results in a downregulation of acquired immunity (both cellular and humoral immunity). Stress can also weaken the response to influenza vaccination (Pedersen, Zachariae, & Bovbjerg, 2009). Many people, mainly elderly and other vulnerable people, die every year from influenza. These groups are therefore offered vaccination. Stress, however, can affect the efficacy of vaccinations, causing a lack of increase in the number of antibodies, and thus can pose a serious health hazard for these particularly weakened groups. Finally, other health-related processes, such as wound healing, autoimmune diseases, and allergic processes, have been found to be susceptible to stress (Zachariae 2009).

Allostatic Load Alters Gene Expression

Cellular receptors throughout the body translate the binding of signal molecules, such as cortisol, into activation of transcription factors that regulate the activity of hundreds of genes. When receptors no longer respond as usual to extracellular signals, such as observed during allostatic load, the intracellular sequence of events also changes, and ultimately the gene expression pattern changes. It is becoming increasingly clear that gene expression changes associated with severe stress can affect cellular mechanisms (Epel et al., 2004; Irie, Asami, Nagata, Miyata, & Kasai, 2002; Zieker et al. 2007),and that the consequence may be a wide range of physical and mental diseases.

In response to adversity, the mammalian immune system appears to have developed a conserved response in terms of decreasing transcription of some groups of immune response genes such as type I interferons and specific immunoglobulin genes. The transcription of other genes, including genes for pro-inflammatory cytokines, is simultaneously upregulated (Irwin & Cole, 2011).

A stressful life may lead to shortening of leucocyte telomeres (Epel et al., 2004), which in turn is linked to the development of Parkinson's diseases (Maeda, Guan, Koyanagi, Higuchi, & Makino, 2012).

Looking at blood cells, the mechanisms by which stress (e.g. traumatic stress, social isolation, or low socioeconomic status) induces genome wide expression changes involve peripheral blood mononuclear cells that stimulate inflammatory processes in tissues (Cole, 2013). Gene expression changes following long-term stress are associated with (a) decreased mitochondrial functioning, (b) increased oxidative stress, (c) a pro-inflammatory environment, (d) cellular ageing, and (e) increased NF-kB pathway activity (Epel et al., 2004; O'Donovan et al., 2011; Zieker et al. 2007). Such expression changes, during severe or prolonged stress, affect both the intra- and extracellular environment of the body. For example, studies on mitochondrial dysfunction reveal changes in the cellular environment including inflammatory-, immune-, and oxidative stress pathways (Maes & Twisk, 2010; Zolkipli, Pedersen, Lamhonwah, Gregersen, & Tein, 2011) that resemble the pathological phenotype in neurodegenerative (Chaturvedi & Beal, 2013) and psychiatric diseases (Manji et al., 2012).

Mindfulness: Allostatic Load Reversed?

The growing realization of the complex nature of the damaging consequences of allostatic load justifies the question: "Can allostatic load be reversed?" At present, we still need more knowledge to answer this question. However, increasing amounts of evidence indicate that, given the right conditions, the body seems to be capable of producing stress-compensation mechanisms (McEwen et al., 2015). Mindfulness-based therapies (MBT) have become a popular way to deal with stress and were shown by an increasing number of studies to mediate improvements by targeting stress perception and stress regulation mechanisms.

The perception of potential stressors is an early and critical stage in which the body decides whether or not to enter fight or flight mode. Studies show that MBT has the potential to alter the way we categorize events as stressful or non-stressful (Krusche, Cyhlarova, & Williams, 2013), indicating that the brain becomes less prone to engage in allostatic processes. This implies enhanced resilience, i.e. more optimal ways of handling adverse experiences. There is growing evidence that mindfulness training improves emotion or self-regulation skills as demonstrated through a range of self-report, physiological, and neuroimaging methods (Vago & Silbersweig, 2012). MBT results in neuroplastic changes, including reduced amygdala activation, increased hippocampal activity and growth, increased activity in the prefrontal cortex, and increased insula volume (Hölzel et al., 2010; Holzel et al., 2011; Lazar et al., 2005; Lutz et al., 2014). It was recently found that amygdala reactivity predicts psychological vulnerability to commonly experienced stressors, and hence reduced amygdala activity is a discrete target for intervention (Swartz et al., 2015).

As a consequence of altered stress perception, processes that mediate stress effects on, e.g. immune responses may be altered. Considering viral infections, MBSR has been found to reduce CD4 + T lymphocyte declines in HIV-1-infected adults (Creswell, Myers, Cole, & Irwin, 2009). Mindfulness may also affect susceptibility to infectious diseases, reducing the acute respiratory infection illness burden

(Barrett et al., 2012). Davidson, Kabat-Zinn, and co-workers found significant increases in antibody titres to influenza vaccine among subjects in a MBSR group compared with those in a waiting list control group (R. Davidson et al., 2003). MBSR may thus change immune function in positive ways increasing the capacity to react to influenza vaccination. Furthermore, the rate of healing or clearing of psoriatic lesions in patients with psoriasis was improved following body scan meditation during light treatment when compared to a waiting list control group receiving light treatment without body scan meditation (Kabat-Zinn et al., 1998).

Several studies have associated MBT with gene expression changes (Black et al., 2013; Irwin & Olmstead, 2012; Lavretsky et al., 2011, 2013; Pace et al., 2009). In a recent review, MBT effects were reported to involve gene expression changes resembling molecular antistress effects characterized by (a) increased mitochondrial functioning, (b) improved capacity to respond to oxidative stress and the associated molecular and cellular damages, (c) decreased pro-inflammatory environment, (d) a slowing down of cellular ageing, and (e) reduced NF-kB pathway activity (Dahlgaard & Zachariae, 2014). Reduced expression of the glutamate receptor GRM7A was also found and may be associated with a recent study in rats which indicated that blocking glutamate receptors during stress improves spatial working memory and modifies hippocampal synaptic plasticity (Amin et al., 2015). Hence, beneficial effects of MBT on hippocampal function could be associated with reduced GRM7 expression.

Compassion training mediates some of the positive health effects of mindfulness (Velden et al., 2015). Not surprisingly, self-compassion is positively associated with the practice of four key health-promoting behaviours: eating better, exercising more, getting more restful sleep, and stressing less (Sirois et al., 2014). By improving our health behaviour as well as psychological and social well-being, mindfulness may positively impact our immune system and our physical and mental health. Based on a small, randomized control trial, it was found that MBSR might be a novel treatment approach for reducing loneliness and related pro-inflammatory gene expression in older adults (Creswell et al., 2012).

In summary, evidence supports the theory that mindfulness practice has the potential to reverse physiological processes that go awry during allostatic load. In other words, mindfulness may represent a sophisticated way to overcome the instinctive responses of our own body.

Stress Disorders: A Clinical Perspective

There is an ongoing debate about the classification and the diagnostic criteria for "stress disorders". In modern terms, "allostatic load" could be the pivotal link between psychological processes and somatic illness. However, as matters stand today, the plausible categorization of severe somatic symptoms as "allostatic overload" continues to pose a challenge to traditional Descartes-inspired medical thinking.

The Psychosomatic Link

Stress disorders have existed since ancient times and were often categorized as psychosomatic and "somatization". These phenomena have caused stigmatization as evidenced by such concepts as "hysteria", which dates back to about 1900 BC. Although the medical profession has gained much ground since ancient times, somatization remains a puzzle. Medical professionals may find somatization difficult, and patients may be told that "it's all in your mind" and "you just have to live with it" or they may be told that if they coped better, they would not experience all these symptoms and use time and money in the healthcare system (Carson, Stone, Warlow, & Sharpe, 2004; Chew-Graham & May, 1999; Sharpe, Mayou, & Seagroatt, 1994; Wileman, May, & Chew-Graham, 2002). The "understanding" of the concept of somatization disclosed by such utterances may be rooted in the mind/body dualism deeply embedded in modern medicine, which tends to classify symptoms and diseases as either physical or mental. Illnesses without organ pathology are a source of confusion for physicians, who were often taught, "if it is not organic, it must be psychiatric": the prevailing paradigm simply makes it difficult to believe in the reality of an illness without organ pathology (McWhinney, Epstein, & Freeman, 2001). The physicians may think that the patients are faking and are untreatable, especially if they decline psychosocial treatment. The patients, on their part, may also believe that they can only be helped by means of medication prescribed to treat a biomedical problem. Furthermore, psychological or psychiatric treatment may seem inappropriate for a person with somatic complaints, and it may be perceived as unnecessarily stigmatizing. Thus, the sharp division of a healthcare system into "mental" and "physical" domains is problematic in the light of current research, which argues that the problem of stress disorders is one that encompasses both the body and the mind.

Bodily Distress Syndrome

The accumulation of detailed knowledge about the harmful effects of stress and allostatic load offers a new explanatory model and new ways to investigate a range of complex and poorly understood disorders and diseases, often labelled as "medically unexplained symptoms", "functional somatic syndromes", or "functional disorders". Characteristically in these disorders, patients present with various "functional symptoms", i.e. symptoms that impair normal everyday functions, and that cannot be ascribed to other well-known illness (Fink, Toft, Hansen, Ornbol, & Olesen, 2007). Certain symptom clusters are defined as functional somatic syndromes, including fibromyalgia, chronic fatigue syndrome, and irritable bowel syndrome.

Although functional symptoms/syndromes are often considered in the light of the biopsychosocial model (Engel, 1980), the respective roles of biological, psychological, and social factors in the pathogenesis are intensely debated in an often opinionated manner. Biological factors may, e.g. be "hard-wired" dispositions such as genes for hypertension but may also be a more general sensitivity which may manifest in behavioural patterns in early infancy (Rask, Ornbol, Olsen, Fink, & Skovgaard, 2013). Psychological and social factors that predispose to functional disorders include personality (Escolas & Escolas, 2015; Oswald et al., 2006), psychological distress (Carstensen et al., 2008), sexual abuse (Paras et al., 2009), dilemmas (Hatcher & House, 2003), negative events, traumatic events and infections (Afari et al., 2014; Theorell, Blomkvist, Lindh, & Evengard, 1999), as well as acquired attitudes and illness beliefs (Frostholm, Petrie, Ornbol, & Fink, 2014).

Functional symptoms are systemic, appearing throughout the body, including abnormal bodily sensations, chronic pain, and a range of neuropsychological abnormalities (Creed, Barsky, & Leiknes, 2011; Fink, Rosendal, & Toft, 2002; Henningsen, Zipfel, & Herzog, 2007; Rief & Broadbent, 2007). Once a functional symptom is present, the likelihood of acquiring another symptom increases; alas the strongest predictor of acquiring a functional symptom is already to have one (Fink & Schroder, 2010). These aspects strongly indicate a common aetiology. Schroder and Fink (2010) have suggested the research diagnosis "bodily distress syndrome" (BDS) conceptualized as "a (patho)physiologic response to prolonged or severe mental and/or physical stress in genetically susceptible individuals" (Schroder & Fink, 2011).

BDS is divided into subtypes referring to the bodily system(s) that produce the symptoms. The "multi-organ-type BDS" requires functional somatic symptoms from at least three out of the four bodily systems—cardiopulmonary, gastrointestinal, musculoskeletal, or general symptoms—as well as moderate to severe impairment in daily living and at least 6 months of duration (Fink & Schroder, 2010; Fink et al., 2007; Schroder & Fink, 2010) (Table 8.1).

It is estimated that functional disorders occur in approximately 6 % of the general population in Western countries, 16 % of primary care attendees, and up to 33 % of

Table 8.1 Diagnostic criteria for bodily distress syndrome (Fink et al., 2007)

Musculoskeletal	Gastrointestinal
Muscular ache or pain	Abdominal pain
Pain in the joints	Nausea
Feelings of paresis or localized weakness	Frequent loose bowel movements, diarrhoea
Backache	Feeling bloated/full of gas/distended
Pain moving from one place to another	Regurgitations, burning sensation in the chest
Unpleasant numbness or tingling sensations	Constipation
Pain in arms or legs	Vomiting

General symptoms	Heart and lung
Concentration difficulties	Palpitations/heart pounding
Impairment of memory	Hot or cold sweats
Excessive fatigue	Breathlessness without exertion
Headache	Hyperventilation, dry mouth
Dizziness	Trembling/shaking, churning in the stomach, flushing, or blushing

patients in secondary care clinics (Creed et al., 2011; de Waal, Arnold, Eekhof, & van Hemert, 2004; Fink, Sorensen, Engberg, Holm, & Munk-Jorgensen, 1999; Kirmayer & Robbins, 1991; Kringlen, Torgersen, & Cramer, 2006; Kroenke & Price, 1993). The impairments of BDS are comparable with those of depressive disorders or a general medical disease. Due to these impairments and the numerous investigations made to rule out any medical conditions, BDS is expensive in terms of healthcare use and time missed from work (Akehurst et al., 2002; Barsky, Ettner, Horsky, & Bates, 2001; Fink & Schroder, 2010; Fink et al., 1999; Kolk, Schagen, & Hanewald, 2004; Reynolds, Vernon, Bouchery, & Reeves, 2004; Robinson et al., 2003). In the Netherlands, medically unexplained symptoms and somatoform disorders form the fifth most expensive diagnostic category (Dunlop, Jenkins, & Spiller, 2003; Meerding, Bonneux, Polder, Koopmanschap, & van der Maas, 1998). The costs appear to be higher than those incurred by stroke and cancer. The high healthcare costs do not include time lost from work and reduced productivity or the time of carers. The money is spent on medical consultations and expensive investigations, which lead to little or no health gain (Creed et al., 2011). The greater societal costs are evidenced by the fact that these diagnoses account for 6–10 % of early retirement pensions in Denmark (Fink et al., 2007).

Allostatic Load in the Functional Disorders

The relationship between mental and/or physical stress and functional somatic syndromes is a long-standing theory, which has gradually developed into a theoretical framework. In particular, the absence of peripheral pathology and the systemic nature of the symptoms suggest that the central nervous system is involved in the pathophysiology. Currently, modern examination techniques are increasingly being employed to explore signs of allostatic load in the functional disorders.

Central nervous system abnormalities have been observed in several studies. The three most frequent functional syndromes (fibromyalgia, chronic fatigue syndrome, and irritable bowel syndrome) were consistently associated with alterations in the HPA axis (Bohmelt, Nater, Franke, Hellhammer, & Ehlert, 2005; Chang et al., 2009; Dinan et al., 2006; Macedo et al., 2008; Papadopoulos & Cleare, 2012). Both fibromyalgia and chronic fatigue syndrome are considered as hypocortisol disorders, whereas this tendency is not found in irritable bowel syndrome (Tak et al., 2011). Increased activation of the amygdala, facilitating activation of the hypothalamic-pituitary-adrenal (HPA) axis and enhancing symptomology, was observed in irritable bowel syndrome (Tillisch, Mayer, & Labus, 2011). Inflammation and altered cytokine profiles were also frequently observed in functional somatic syndromes (Clauw, 2001; Ford & Talley, 2011; Geiss, Rohleder, & Anton, 2012; Maes, 2009; Rosenkranz, 2007; Russell et al., 1994; Vaeroy, Helle, Forre, Kass, & Terenius, 1988), and elevated levels of pro-inflammatory markers were linked to abnormal glucocorticoid receptor function (Geiss et al., 2012). Several studies indicate that the aetiological factors include mitochondrial changes and oxidative stress

(Iqbal, Mughal, Arshad, & Arshad, 2011; Meeus, Nijs, Hermans, Goubert, & Calders, 2013; Oran et al., 2014).

Poor sleep quality, fatigue, and diffuse pains, all general symptoms in the functional disorders, were linked to CNS abnormalities and inflammation. In chronic fatigue syndrome, pain sensitivity increases with sleep disturbance (Agargun et al., 1999), and hypocortisolism has been related to the amount of sleep (Nijhof et al., 2014). Abnormal brain activity during the restorative (non-REM) sleep phase (Moldofsky, 1995) and a pattern of non-restful sleep and pain (Nicassio, Moxham, Schuman, & Gevirtz, 2002) were observed in fibromyalgia. In irritable bowel syndrome, a relationship between circulating inflammatory markers and poor sleep has been reported (Wilson et al., 2015).

Pain perception is strongly influenced by emotional and cognitive processes: in particular the co-occurrence of negative affect and pain is well recognized (Lapate et al., 2012; Price, 2000), and some studies point towards a deficiency in the cognitive regulation of pain perception in patients suffering from functional disorders (Kuzminskyte, Kupers, Videbech, Gjedde, & Fink, 2010). In irritable bowel syndrome, brain regions involved in the processing of visceral afferent information show normal activation, whereas the downregulation of emotional arousal circuitry appears to be less effective than in healthy controls (Tillisch et al., 2011). Indeed, acceptance commitment therapy led to modulation of cortical control mechanisms as well as improvement of symptoms and also improved depression and anxiety symptoms in fibromyalgia patients (Jensen et al., 2012).

Cognitive changes such as decreased attention and working memory function in functional disorders are linked to enhanced activity in several cortical and subcortical regions during cognitive tasks compared to healthy controls (Cockshella & Mathiasa 2010; Cook, O'Connor, Lange, & Steffener, 2007; Kennedy et al., 2014; Lange et al., 2005). Somatoform disorders were particularly associated with increased activity of limbic regions in response to painful stimuli and a generalized decrease in grey matter density (Browning, Fletcher, & Sharpe, 2011). Reductions in global grey matter volume are linked to a reduction in physical activity in chronic fatigue syndrome (de Lange et al., 2005). The high comorbidity of functional disorders and affective disorders (Creed et al., 2011; Fjorback et al., 2013; Schroder, Rehfeld, & Ornbol, 2012; Wingenfeld, Nutzinger, Kauth, Hellhammer, & Lautenbacher, 2010) appears further to be in line with the hypothesis that allostatic load underlies the functional disorders.

In addition to psychological and social factors, the multifactorial aetiology of the functional somatic syndromes involves innate factors. In the light of the allostatic load hypothesis, it is relevant to consider that abnormal cortisol levels are not due to allostatic load but may also be due to normal genetic variance, e.g. in the amount or affinity of glucocorticoid receptors (Gagliardi, Ho, & Torpy, 2010; Lin, Muller, & Hammond, 2010). Hence, HPA axis perturbations and associated symptoms may appear independently of exposure to long-term or severe stress.

The application of different treatment regimes has provided further evidence in support of the relevance of allostatic load-related illness mechanisms in the functional disorders. In particular, cognitive behavioural therapy can boost cortisol levels

(Papadopoulos & Cleare, 2012), and normalization of hypocortisolism is associated with treatment success in chronic fatigue syndrome (Nijhof et al., 2014), addressing the need for treatment strategies that target the HPA axis (Tomas, Newton, & Watson, 2013).

At present, accumulating evidence supports the theory that allostatic load is a central actor in symptom formation in the functional disorders. However, there is a lack of studies that directly compare the different functional syndromes on the same markers, including longitudinal studies that investigate the gradual appearance of these markers in connection with symptom development.

Mindfulness Treatment

The Buddhist Backdrop

From a traditional Buddhist point of view and as reflected in the four noble truths, suffering is a basic premise of life that we all share (Bhikkhu, 2010). The principal underlying cause of suffering is assumed to be attachment/clinging, which is also the basis of all destructive emotions. It is a central premise of mindfulness that if we investigate our emotions, analyse them, and look at their effects, we can attenuate negative emotions and cultivate positive emotions (Sauer, Walach, & Kohls, 2011). BDS patients are suffering, and mindfulness attempts to work with the very stress and pain that cause suffering (Kabat-Zinn, 1990).

According to some practice modalities, mindfulness starts by observing the body and holding the awareness of the body with a friendly, non-judgmental attitude. Daniel Siegel has proposed that the ability to observe the body enhances stress regulation or "bodily regulation" (Siegel, 2007). The next step is to observe the mind and to notice when thoughts and emotions arise. The point is not to try to block arising thoughts but not to allow them to invade the mind. What people do in meditation is to familiarize themselves with a new way of dealing with thoughts that come to their minds (Goleman, 2003). When a powerful thought of strong attraction or anger arises, you recognize it: "Oh that thought is coming". An example often given is that of a thief coming into an empty house. There is nothing to lose for the owner and nothing to gain for the thief. This is an experience of freedom. You do not become apathetic, but you gain mastery over your thoughts. This can only happen through sustained training and genuine experience (Goleman, 2003). Daniel Siegel has proposed that the ability to observe the mind is a seventh sense that may enhance attention and emotion regulation. The last step is to move towards acceptance and to observe relationships: your relationship towards yourself, the situation you are in, and your connection with others. Daniel Siegel has proposed that the ability to observe a relationship may enhance communication skills and enable one to feel part of a larger whole (Siegel, 2007).

Regulation of stress and emotions are well-documented effects of mindfulness (R. J. Davidson, 2000, 2004). Some of the active elements of mindfulness are

(1) connection to the body, (2) connection to the mind, and (3) connection to self and others. The yoga practices—body scan (yoga nidra) and hatha yoga— are the tools systematically used to enhance the connection with the body. The meditation practices systematically used to discipline the mind consist of concentration on the breath, the body as a whole, pain, sounds, thoughts, and emotions. These practices are used to keep the attention in the present, observing and embracing whatever comes up in awareness with a friendly, non-judgmental attitude. Connections to the self and others are practised through deep listening. From a mindfulness perspective, deep listening is one of the greatest gifts a person can offer: it is not just being silent, but it is being fully present with the patient. This presence may be explained as compassion in action or as an ethical action that is believed to be the outcome and expression of a clear mind and an open heart.

Mindfulness-Based Stress Reduction in the Treatment of BDS

BDS patients do not come to the hospital saying: "I am suffering", but they do come with a body they want to have fixed. It is beyond question that physical training has an impact on physical and mental health. Now, it is becoming increasingly acknowledged that the same mechanisms hold true for mental training, and since 2007, we have included MBSR in the treatment of patients suffering from BDS in our research clinic.

A Randomized Controlled Trial

We designed a project that could develop and evaluate a mindfulness treatment approach for those most severely disabled patients who suffer from multi-organ BDS (Fjorback, 2012). The results of the project indicate that mindfulness therapy is feasible and is acceptable to patients with multi-organ BDS, producing improvements within the range of those improvements that are reported by CBT. To evaluate the economic effectiveness of mindfulness therapy, it was compared with enhanced conventional treatment, and the 119 included BDS patients were compared with 5950 matched controls. Register data were analysed from 10 years before their inclusion to the 15-month follow-up. The main outcome measures were disability pension at the 15-month follow-up and reduction in total healthcare costs. Unemployment and sickness benefits prior to inclusion were tested as possible risk factors.

Mindfulness therapy had substantial socioeconomic benefits compared with enhanced conventional treatment. The costs related to permanently health-related benefits in general and disability pension in particular were significantly lower in the mindfulness therapy group than in the enhanced conventional treatment group over a 15-month follow-up period. Mindfulness therapy was significantly more expensive than enhanced conventional treatment. Despite these additional costs, mindfulness therapy appears to reduce overall healthcare costs within the range of enhanced conventional treatment. The reduction in costs observed due to primary care is equivalent to a reduction of four visits per year in both groups. Furthermore, the reduction in costs observed due to utilization of hospital facilities corresponds to a reduction of nine outpatient visits per year in the mindfulness therapy group. Five and ten years before their inclusion, the BDS patients were less self-supporting than an age-, gender-, and ethnicity-matched population control group; the BDS patients accumulated more weeks of sickness benefit and unemployment. Thus, the included BDS patients may have been ill and at high risk for social decline even 5 and 10 years before they received a proper diagnosis and treatment. For the year of inclusion, the BDS patients had a lower yearly income than the population controls, although the two groups had identical fractions of members with a higher education. This indicates that the social and economic consequences of BDS are significant and that mindfulness therapy is a cost-effective treatment.

In conclusion, preliminary evidence suggests that mindfulness therapy may prevent disability pension at 15-month follow-up and may reduce healthcare costs. Thus, mindfulness therapy may have a potential to significantly reduce societal costs, improve function, and increase effectiveness of care. The project also showed that even socially marginalized patients suffering from BDS are willing to participate and engage in a treatment that requires a high level of patient involvement.

Perspective

Mindfulness is not a cure, which can be used when nothing else is working, but it may very well be the right treatment if the body is distressed to a level where it is no longer functioning. In mindfulness therapy, the core focus is on observing what is present in the body, and by doing so insights may arise, for example: "I noticed that I am able to regulate the level of stress in my body", "I noticed that I hate myself", "I noticed that I feel isolated most of the time, but in class it is as if everything is okay, as if I am okay", "Now, I have tools so I can work without becoming ill", "I never believed in any of this, but experiencing a body without a simple symptom totally blew me away", "Not much happened, but I quit the painkillers", "I realized that I am not the only one suffering, but that it is a human condition just like happiness", and "I realized that by keeping my focus on the pain, humour suddenly arrived" .

Conclusion

Long-term or severe mental and physical stress can create a state of allostatic load in the body that induces a risk of pathological processes. At present, as these processes are becoming increasingly understood, the list of stress-related disorders appears to be growing. In particular, functional disorders including fibromyalgia, chronic fatigue syndrome, and more may eventually be found to share a common pathological basis, appropriately encompassed by the term "bodily distress syndrome".

The traditional tools offered by medicine, including psychiatry, are intended to fix or attack patients' symptoms not to release suffering or promote flourishing. Accumulating evidence supports the view that MBT represents a realistic and sophisticated approach to deal with stress via mechanisms that induce enhanced body awareness and self-empowerment.

The term mindfulness, which derives from the pāli word *sati*, means to "remember": remember the body, the mind (intelligence), and the heart (kindness). This is obvious and trivial, but it may, nevertheless, be exactly what is called for in modern medicine. Teaching how to feel whole, physically present, mentally clear, and emotionally balanced may, indeed, be an integrated part of modern medical practice.

References

Afari, N., Ahumada, S. M., Wright, L. J., Mostoufi, S., Golnari, G., Reis, V., et al. (2014). Psychological trauma and functional somatic syndromes: A systematic review and meta-analysis. *Psychosomatic Medicine, 76*(1), 2–11.

Agargun, M. Y., Tekeoglu, I., Gunes, A., Adak, B., Kara, H., & Ercan, M. (1999). Sleep quality and pain threshold in patients with fibromyalgia. *Comprehensive Psychiatry, 40*(3), 226–228. doi: S0010-440X(99)90008-1 [pii].

Akehurst, R. L., Brazier, J. E., Mathers, N., O'Keefe, C., Kaltenthaler, E., Morgan, A., et al. (2002). Health-related quality of life and cost impact of irritable bowel syndrome in a UK primary care setting. *PharmacoEconomics, 20*(7), 455–462. doi: 200703 [pii].

Amin, S. N., El-Aidi, A. A., Ali, M. M., Attia, Y. M., & Rashed, L. A. (2015). Modification of hippocampal markers of synaptic plasticity by memantine in animal models of acute and repeated restraint stress: implications for memory and behavior. *Neuromolecular Med.* doi:10.1007/s12017-015-8343-0.

Ancelin, M. L., Carriere, I., Helmer, C., Rouaud, O., Pasquier, F., Berr, C., et al. (2012). Steroid and nonsteroidal anti-inflammatory drugs, cognitive decline, and dementia. *Neurobiology of Aging, 33*(9), 2082–2090. doi:10.1016/j.neurobiolaging.2011.09.038. S0197-4580(11)00392-7 [pii].

Armanini, M. P., Hutchins, C., Stein, B. A., & Sapolsky, R. M. (1990). Glucocorticoid endangerment of hippocampal neurons is NMDA-receptor dependent. *Brain Research, 532*(1–2), 7–12. doi: 0006-8993(90)91734-X [pii].

Barrett, B., Hayney, M. S., Muller, D., Rakel, D., Ward, A., Obasi, C. N., et al. (2012). Meditation or exercise for preventing acute respiratory infection: a randomized. *Annals of Family Medicine, 10*, 337–346. doi:10.1370/afm.1376.INTRODUCTION.

Barsky, A. J., Ettner, S. L., Horsky, J., & Bates, D. W. (2001). Resource utilization of patients with hypochondriacal health anxiety and somatization. *Medical Care, 39*(7), 705–715.

Bender, B. G., Lerner, J. A., & Kollasch, E. (1988). Mood and memory changes in asthmatic children receiving corticosteroids. *Journal of the American Academy of Child and Adolescent Psychiatry, 27*(6), 720–725. doi:10.1097/00004583-198811000-00010. S0890-8567(09)65853-6 [pii].

Berk, M., Williams, L., Jacka, F., O'Neil, A., Pasco, J., Moylan, S., et al. (2013). So depression is an inflammatory disease, but where does the inflammation come from? *BMC Medicine, 11*.

Bhikkhu, A. (2010). *The earliest recorded discourses of the Buddha (translated) (from Lalitavistara, Mahākhandhaka & Mahāvastu*. Kuala Lumpur: Sukhi Hotu.

Black, D. S., Cole, S. W., Irwin, M. R., Breen, E., Cyr, S., Nazarian, N. M., et al. (2013). Yogic meditation reverses NF-kappaB and IRF-related transcriptome dynamics in leukocytes of family dementia caregivers in a randomized controlled trial. *Psychoneuroendocrinology, 38*(3), 348–355. doi:10.1016/j.psyneuen.2012.06.011. S0306-4530(12)00226-0 [pii].

Bohmelt, A. H., Nater, U. M., Franke, S., Hellhammer, D. H., & Ehlert, U. (2005). Basal and stimulated hypothalamic-pituitary-adrenal axis activity in patients with functional gastrointestinal disorders and healthy controls. *Psychosomatic Medicine, 67*(2), 288–294. doi:10.1097/01.psy.0000157064.72831.ba. 67/2/288 [pii].

Bremner, J. D., Randall, P., Scott, T. M., Bronen, R. A., Seibyl, J. P., Southwick, S. M., et al. (1995). MRI-based measurement of hippocampal volume in patients with combat-related posttraumatic stress disorder. *The American Journal of Psychiatry, 152*(7), 973–981.

Brown, E. S., Jeon-Slaughter, H., Lu, H., Jamadar, R., Issac, S., Shad, M., et al. (2014). Hippocampal volume in healthy controls given 3-day stress doses of hydrocortisone. *Neuropsychopharmacology, 40*, 1216–1221. doi:10.1038/npp.2014.307. npp2014307 [pii].

Browning, M., Fletcher, P., & Sharpe, M. (2011). Can neuroimaging help us to understand and classify somatoform disorders? A systematic and critical review. *Psychosomatic Medicine, 73*(2), 173–184. doi:10.1097/PSY.0b013e31820824f6. PSY.0b013e31820824f6 [pii].

Cahill, L., & McGaugh, J. L. (1998). Mechanisms of emotional arousal and lasting declarative memory. *Trends in Neurosciences, 21*(7), 294–299. doi: S0166-2236(97)01214-9 [pii].

Carson, A. J., Stone, J., Warlow, C., & Sharpe, M. (2004). Patients whom neurologists find difficult to help. *Journal of Neurology, Neurosurgery and Psychiatry, 75*(12), 1776–1778. doi:10.1136/jnnp.2003.032169. 75/12/1776 [pii].

Carstensen, T. B., Frostholm, L., Oernboel, E., Kongsted, A., Kasch, H., Jensen, T. S., et al. (2008). Post-trauma ratings of pre-collision pain and psychological distress predict poor outcome following acute whiplash trauma: A 12-month follow-up study. *Pain, 139*(2), 248–259. doi:10.1016/j.pain.2008.04.008. S0304-3959(08)00196-6 [pii].

Chang, L., Sundaresh, S., Elliott, J., Anton, P. A., Baldi, P., Licudine, A., et al. (2009). Dysregulation of the hypothalamic-pituitary-adrenal (HPA) axis in irritable bowel syndrome. *Neurogastroenterology and Motility, 21*(2), 149–159. doi:10.1111/j.1365-2982.2008.01171.x. NMO1171 [pii].

Chaturvedi, R. K., & Beal, M. F. (2013). Molecular and cellular neuroscience mitochondria targeted therapeutic approaches in Parkinson's and Huntington's diseases. *Molecular and Cellular Neurosciences, 55*, 101–114.

Chew-Graham, C., & May, C. (1999). Chronic low back pain in general practice: The challenge of the consultation. *Family Practice, 16*(1), 46–49.

Choi, D. W. (1988). Calcium-mediated neurotoxicity: Relationship to specific channel types and role in ischemic damage. *Trends in Neurosciences, 11*(10), 465–469. doi:0166-2236(88)90200-7 [pii].

Clauw, D. J. (2001). Potential mechanisms in chemical intolerance and related conditions. *The Annals of the New York Academy of Sciences, 933*, 235–253.

Cockshella, S. J., & Mathiasa, J. L. (2010). Cognitive functioning in chronic fatigue syndrome: A meta-analysis. *Psychological Medicine, 40*, 1253–1267.

Cohen, S., Janicki-Deverts, D., Doyle, W. J., Miller, G. E., Frank, E., Rabin, B. S., et al. (2012). Chronic stress, glucocorticoid receptor resistance, inflammation, and disease risk. *Proceedings of the National Academy of Sciences of the United States of America, 109*(16), 5995–5999. doi:10.1073/pnas.1118355109. 1118355109 [pii].

Cole, S. W. (2013). Social regulation of human gene expression: Mechanisms and implications for public health. *American Journal of Public Health, 103*, 84–93. doi:10.2105/AJPH.2012.301183.

Cook, D. B., O'Connor, P. J., Lange, G., & Steffener, J. (2007). Functional neuroimaging correlates of mental fatigue induced by cognition among chronic fatigue syndrome patients and controls. *NeuroImage, 36*(1), 108–122. doi:10.1016/j.neuroimage.2007.02.033. S1053-8119(07)00127-9 [pii].

Coplan, J. D., Fulton, S. L., Reiner, W., Jackowski, A., Panthangi, V., Perera, T. D., et al. (2014). Elevated cerebrospinal fluid 5-hydroxyindoleacetic acid in macaques following early life stress and inverse association with hippocampal volume: Preliminary implications for serotonin-related function in mood and anxiety disorders. *Frontiers in Behavioral Neuroscience, 8*, 440. doi:10.3389/fnbeh.2014.00440.

Creed, F., Barsky, A. J., & Leiknes, K. A. (2011). Epidemiology: Prevalence, causes and consequences. In F. Creed, P. Henningsen, & P. Fink (Eds.), *Medically unexplained symptoms, somatization and bodily distress. Developing better clinical services* (pp. 1–42). New York: Cambridge University Press.

Creswell, J. D., Irwin, M. R., Burklund, L. J., Lieberman, M. D., Arevalo, J. M. G., Ma, J., et al. (2012). Mindfulness-based stress reduction training reduces loneliness and pro-inflammatory gene expression in older adults: A small randomized controlled trial. *Brain, Behavior, and Immunity, 26*, 1095–1101. doi:10.1016/j.bbi.2012.07.006.

Creswell, J. D., Myers, H. F., Cole, S. W., & Irwin, M. R. (2009). Mindfulness meditation training effects on CD4+ T lymphocytes in HIV-1 infected adults: A small randomized controlled trial. *Brain, Behavior, and Immunity, 23*, 184–188. doi:10.1016/j.bbi.2008.07.004.

Dahlgaard, J., & Zachariae, R. (2014). *Gene expression anti-stress effects following a mind-body intervention.* Paper presented at the 72nd annual scientific meeting of the American Psychosomatic Society, San Francisco, CA.

Davidson, R. J. (2000). Affective style, psychopathology, and resilience: Brain mechanisms and plasticity. *The American Psychologist, 55*(11), 1196–1214.

Davidson, R. J. (2004). Well-being and affective style: Neural substrates and biobehavioural correlates. *Philosophical Transactions of the Royal Society of London. Series B, Biological Sciences, 359*(1449), 1395–1411. doi:10.1098/rstb.2004.1510 MCADFWA2B7X1KJAW [pii].

Davidson, R., Kabat-Zinn, J., Schumacher, J., Rosenkranz, M., Muller, D., Santorelli, S., et al. (2003). Alterations in brain and immune function produced by mindfulness meditation. *Psychosomatic Medicine, 65*, 564–570. doi:10.1097/01.PSY.0000077505.67574.E3.

de Lange, F. P., Kalkman, J. S., Bleijenberg, G., Hagoort, P., van der Meer, J. W., & Toni, I. (2005). Gray matter volume reduction in the chronic fatigue syndrome. *NeuroImage, 26*(3), 777–781. doi:10.1016/j.neuroimage.2005.02.037. S1053-8119(05)00139-4 [pii].

de Quervain, D. J., Roozendaal, B., Nitsch, R. M., McGaugh, J. L., & Hock, C. (2000). Acute cortisone administration impairs retrieval of long-term declarative memory in humans. *Nature Neuroscience, 3*(4), 313–314. doi:10.1038/73873.

de Quervain, D. J., Roozendaal, B., & McGaugh, J. L. (1998). Stress and glucocorticoids impair retrieval of long-term spatial memory. *Nature, 394*(6695), 787–790. doi:10.1038/29542.

de Waal, M. W., Arnold, I. A., Eekhof, J. A., & van Hemert, A. M. (2004). Somatoform disorders in general practice: Prevalence, functional impairment and comorbidity with anxiety and depressive disorders. *British Journal of Psychiatry, 184*, 470–476.

Dinan, T. G., Quigley, E. M., Ahmed, S. M., Scully, P., O'Brien, S., O'Mahony, L., et al. (2006). Hypothalamic-pituitary-gut axis dysregulation in irritable bowel syndrome: Plasma cytokines as a potential biomarker? *Gastroenterology, 130*(2), 304–311. doi:10.1053/j.gastro.2005.11.033. S0016-5085(05)02394-2 [pii].

Drevets, W. C., & Raichle, M. E. (1992). Neuroanatomical circuits in depression: Implications for treatment mechanisms. *Psychopharmacology Bulletin, 28*(3), 261–274.

Dunlop, S. P., Jenkins, D., & Spiller, R. C. (2003). Distinctive clinical, psychological, and histological features of postinfective irritable bowel syndrome. *American Journal of Gastroenterology, 98*(7), 1578–1583. doi:10.1111/j.1572-0241.2003.07542.x. S0002927003003757 [pii].

Engel, G. L. (1980). The clinical application of the biopsychosocial model. *The American Journal of Psychiatry, 137*(5), 535–544. doi:10.1176/ajp.137.5.535.

Epel, E. S., Blackburn, E. H., Lin, J., Dhabhar, F. S., Adler, N. E., Morrow, J. D., et al. (2004). Accelerated telomere shortening in response to life stress. *Proceedings of the National Academy of Sciences of the United States of America, 101*(49), 17312–17315. doi:10.1073/pnas.0407162101. 0407162101 [pii].

Escolas, S. M., & Escolas, H. D. (2015). Temperament dimensions and posttraumatic stress symptoms in a previously deployed military sample. *US Army Medical Department Journal, Jan-Mar*, 79–85.

Fardet, L., Petersen, I., & Nazareth, I. (2012). Suicidal behavior and severe neuropsychiatric disorders following glucocorticoid therapy in primary care. *The American Journal of Psychiatry, 169*(5), 491–497.

Felitti, V. J., Anda, R. F., Nordenberg, D., Williamson, D. F., Spitz, A. M., Edwards, V., et al. (1998). Relationship of childhood abuse and household dysfunction to many of the leading causes of death in adults. The Adverse Childhood Experiences (ACE) Study. *American Journal of Preventive Medicine, 14*(4), 245–258. doi: S0749379798000178 [pii].

Fink, P., Rosendal, M., & Toft, T. (2002). Assessment and treatment of functional disorders in general practice: The extended reattribution and management model--an advanced educational program for nonpsychiatric doctors. *Psychosomatics, 43*(2), 93–131. doi:10.1176/appi.psy.43.2.93. S0033-3182(02)70423-4 [pii].

Fink, P., & Schroder, A. (2010). One single diagnosis, bodily distress syndrome, succeeded to capture 10 diagnostic categories of functional somatic syndromes and somatoform disorders. *Journal of Psychosomatic Research, 68*(5), 415–426. doi:10.1016/j.jpsychores.2010.02.004. S0022-3999(10)00075-9 [pii].

Fink, P., Sorensen, L., Engberg, M., Holm, M., & Munk-Jorgensen, P. (1999). Somatization in primary care. Prevalence, health care utilization, and general practitioner recognition. *Psychosomatics, 40*(4), 330–338. doi:10.1016/S0033-3182(99)71228-4. S0033-3182(99)71228-4 [pii].

Fink, P., Toft, T., Hansen, M. S., Ornbol, E., & Olesen, F. (2007). Symptoms and syndromes of bodily distress: An exploratory study of 978 internal medical, neurological, and primary care patients. *Psychosomatic Medicine, 69*(1), 30–39. doi:10.1097/PSY.0b013e31802e46eb. 69/1/30 [pii].

Fjorback, L. O. (2012). *Mindfulness and Bodily Distress.* Ph.D. dissertation, Aarhus University, Aarhus.

Fjorback, L. O., Arendt, M., Ornbol, E., Walach, H., Rehfeld, E., Schroder, A., et al. (2013). Mindfulness therapy for somatization disorder and functional somatic syndromes: Randomized trial with one-year follow-up. *Journal of Psychosomatic Research, 74*(1), 31–40. doi:10.1016/j.jpsychores.2012.09.006. S0022-3999(12)00244-9 [pii].

Ford, A. C., & Talley, N. J. (2011). Mucosal inflammation as a potential etiological factor in irritable bowel syndrome: A systematic review. *Journal of Gastroenterology, 46*(4), 421–431. doi:10.1007/s00535-011-0379-9.

Frostholm, L., Petrie, K. J., Ornbol, E., & Fink, P. (2014). Are illness perceptions related to future healthcare expenditure in patients with somatoform disorders? *Psychological Medicine, 44*(13), 2903–2911. doi:10.1017/S003329171400035X. S003329171400035X [pii].

Gagliardi, L., Ho, J. T., & Torpy, D. J. (2010). Corticosteroid-binding globulin: The clinical significance of altered levels and heritable mutations. *Molecular and Cellular Endocrinology, 316*(1), 24–34. doi:10.1016/j.mce.2009.07.015. S0303-7207(09)00375-X [pii].

Geiss, A., Rohleder, N., & Anton, F. (2012). Evidence for an association between an enhanced reactivity of interleukin-6 levels and reduced glucocorticoid sensitivity in patients with fibromyalgia. *Psychoneuroendocrinology, 37*(5), 671–684. doi:10.1016/j.psyneuen.2011.07.021. S0306-4530(11)00263-0 [pii].

Gold, S. M., Dziobek, I., Sweat, V., Tirsi, A., Rogers, K., Bruehl, H., et al. (2007). Hippocampal damage and memory impairments as possible early brain complications of type 2 diabetes. *Diabetologia, 50*(4), 711–719. doi:10.1007/s00125-007-0602-7.

Goleman, D. (2003). *Destructive emotions: How can we overcome them? A scientific dialogue with the Dalai Lama.* New York: Bantam Dell. A Division of the Random House, Inc.

Hanson, J. L., Nacewicz, B. M., Sutterer, M. J., Cayo, A. A., Schaefer, S. M., Rudolph, K. D., et al. (2015). Behavioral problems after early life stress: Contributions of the hippocampus and amygdala. *Biological Psychiatry, 77*(4), 314–323. doi:10.1016/j.biopsych.2014.04.020. S0006-3223(14)00351-5 [pii].

Hatcher, S., & House, A. (2003). Life events, difficulties and dilemmas in the onset of chronic fatigue syndrome: A case–control study. *Psychological Medicine, 33*(7), 1185–1192.

Heim, C., & Nemeroff, C. B. (2001). The role of childhood trauma in the neurobiology of mood and anxiety disorders: Preclinical and clinical studies. *Biological Psychiatry, 49*(12), 1023–1039. doi: S000632230101157X [pii].

Henningsen, P., Zipfel, S., & Herzog, W. (2007). Management of functional somatic syndromes. *Lancet, 369*(9565), 946–955. doi:10.1016/S0140-6736(07)60159-7. S0140-6736(07)60159-7 [pii].

Hölzel, B. K., Carmody, J., Evans, K. C., Hoge, E. A., Dusek, J. A., Morgan, L., et al. (2010). Stress reduction correlates with structural changes in the amygdala. *Social Cognitive and Affective Neuroscience, 5*, 11–17. doi:10.1093/scan/nsp034.

Holzel, B. K., Carmody, J., Vangel, M., Congleton, C., Yerramsetti, S. M., Gard, T., et al. (2011). Mindfulness practice leads to increases in regional brain gray matter density. *Psychiatry Research, 191*(1), 36–43. doi:10.1016/j.pscychresns.2010.08.006. S0925-4927(10)00288-X [pii].

Hunter, R. G., Gagnidze, K., McEwen, B. S., & Pfaff, D. W. (2014). Stress and the dynamic genome: Steroids, epigenetics, and the transposome. *Proceedings of the National Academy of Sciences of the United States of America, 11*(22), 6828–6833. doi:10.1073/pnas.1411260111. 1411260111 [pii].

Iqbal, R., Mughal, M. S., Arshad, N., & Arshad, M. (2011). Pathophysiology and antioxidant status of patients with fibromyalgia. *Rheumatology International, 31*(2), 149–152. doi:10.1007/s00296-010-1470-x.

Irie, M., Asami, S., Nagata, S., Miyata, M., & Kasai, H. (2002). Psychological mediation of a type of oxidative DNA damage, 8-hydroxydeoxyguanosine, in peripheral blood leukocytes of non-smoking and non-drinking workers. *Psychotherapy and Psychosomatics, 71*(2), 90–96. doi: 49351 [pii] 49351.

Irwin, M. R., & Cole, S. W. (2011). Reciprocal regulation of the neural and innate immune systems. *Nature Reviews Immunology, 11*, 625–632.

Irwin, M. R., & Olmstead, R. (2012). Mitigating cellular inflammation in older adults: A randomized controlled trial of Tai Chi Chih. *The American Journal of Geriatric Psychiatry, 20*(9), 764–772. doi:10.1097/JGP.0b013e3182330fd3.

Jaremka, M., Fagundes, C., Peng, J., Bennett, J., Glaser, R., Malarkey, W., et al. (2013). Loneliness promotes inflammation during acute stress. *Psychological Science, 24*. doi: 10.1177/0956797612464059

Jensen, K. B., Kosek, E., Wicksell, R., Kemani, M., Olsson, G., Merle, J. V., et al. (2012). Cognitive behavioral therapy increases pain-evoked activation of the prefrontal cortex in patients with fibromyalgia. *Pain, 153*(7), 1495–1503. doi:10.1016/j.pain.2012.04.010. S0304-3959(12)00238-2 [pii].

Kabat-Zinn, J. (1990). *Full catastrophe living: Using the wisdom of your body and mind to face stress, pain, and illness*. New York: Delacorte.

Kabat-Zinn, J., Wheeler, E., Light, T., Skillings, A., Scharf, M. J., Cropley, T. G., et al. (1998). Influence of a mindfulness meditation-based stress reduction intervention on rates of skin clearing in patients with moderate to severe psoriasis undergoing phototherapy (UVB) and photochemotherapy (PUVA). *Psychosomatic Medicine, 60*, 625–632.

Kelly, S. J., & Ismail, M. (2015). Stress and type 2 diabetes: A review of how stress contributes to the development of type 2 diabetes. *Annual Review of Public Health*. doi:10.1146/annurev-publhealth-031914-122921.

Kemeny, M. E., & Laudenslager, M. L. (1999). Introduction beyond stress: The role of individual difference factors in psychoneuroimmunology. *Brain, Behavior, and Immunity, 13*(2), 73–75. doi:10.1006/brbi.1999.0562. S0889-1591(99)90562-7 [pii].

Kennedy, P. J., Clarke, G., O'Neill, A., Groeger, J. A., Quigley, E. M., Shanahan, F., et al. (2014). Cognitive performance in irritable bowel syndrome: Evidence of a stress-related impairment in visuospatial memory. *Psychological Medicine, 44*(7), 1553–1566. doi:10.1017/S0033291713002171. S0033291713002171 [pii].

Kirmayer, L. J., & Robbins, J. M. (1991). Three forms of somatization in primary care: Prevalence, co-occurrence, and sociodemographic characteristics. *Journal of Nervous and Mental Disease, 179*(11), 647–655.

Kolk, A. M., Schagen, S., & Hanewald, G. J. (2004). Multiple medically unexplained physical symptoms and health care utilization: Outcome of psychological intervention and patient-related predictors of change. *Journal of Psychosomatic Research, 57*(4), 379–389. doi:10.1016/j.jpsychores.2004.02.012. S0022399904000364 [pii].

Korte, S., Koolhaas, J., & Wingfield, J. (2005). The Darwinian concept of stress: Benefits of allostasis and costs of allostatic load and the trade-offs in health and disease. *Neuroscience & Biobehavioral Reviews, 29*, 3–38.

Kringlen, E., Torgersen, S., & Cramer, V. (2006). Mental illness in a rural area: A Norwegian psychiatric epidemiological study. *Social Psychiatry and Psychiatric Epidemiology, 41*(9), 713–719. doi:10.1007/s00127-006-0080-0.

Kroenke, K., & Price, R. K. (1993). Symptoms in the community. Prevalence, classification, and psychiatric comorbidity. *Archives of Internal Medicine, 153*(21), 2474–2480.

Krusche, A., Cyhlarova, E., & Williams, J. M. G. (2013). Mindfulness online: An evaluation of the feasibility of a web-based mindfulness course for stress, anxiety and depression. *BMJ Open, 3*, e003498. doi:10.1136/bmjopen-2013-003498.

Kuzminskyte, R., Kupers, R., Videbech, P., Gjedde, A., & Fink, P. (2010). Increased sensitivity to supra-threshold painful stimuli in patients with multiple functional somatic symptoms (MFS). *Brain Research Bulletin, 82*(1–2), 135–140. doi:10.1016/j.brainresbull.2010.03.002. S0361-9230(10)00062-6 [pii].

Lange, G., Steffener, J., Cook, D. B., Bly, B. M., Christodoulou, C., Liu, W. C., et al. (2005). Objective evidence of cognitive complaints in Chronic Fatigue Syndrome: A BOLD fMRI study of verbal working memory. *NeuroImage, 26*(2), 513–524. doi:10.1016/j.neuroimage.2005.02.011. S1053-8119(05)00104-7 [pii].

Lapate, R. C., Lee, H., Salomons, T. V., van Reekum, C. M., Greischar, L. L., & Davidson, R. J. (2012). Amygdalar function reflects common individual differences in emotion and pain regulation success. *Journal of Cognitive Neuroscience, 24*(1), 148–158. doi:10.1162/jocn_a_00125.

Lavretsky, H., Altstein, L., Olmstead, R., Ercoli, L., Riparetti-Brown, M., Cyr, N., et al. (2011). Complementary use of tai chi chih augments escitalopram treatment of geriatric depression: A randomized controlled trial. *The American Journal of Geriatric Psychiatry, 19*, 839–850. doi:10.1097/JGP.0b013e31820ee9ef.Complementary.

Lavretsky, H., Epel, E. S., Siddarth, P., Nazarian, N., Cyr, N. S., Khalsa, D. S., et al. (2013). A pilot study of yogic meditation for family dementia caregivers with depressive symptoms: Effects on mental health, cognition, and telomerase activity. *International Journal of Geriatric Psychiatry, 28*(1), 57–65. doi:10.1002/gps.3790.

Lazar, S. W., Kerr, C. E., Wasserman, R. H., Gray, J. R., Greve, D. N., Treadway, M. T., et al. (2005). Meditation experience is associated with increased cortical thickness. *Neuroreport, 16*(17), 1893–1897. doi: 00001756-200511280-00005 [pii].

Lin, H. Y., Muller, Y. A., & Hammond, G. L. (2010). Molecular and structural basis of steroid hormone binding and release from corticosteroid-binding globulin. *Molecular and Cellular Endocrinology, 316*(1), 3–12. doi:10.1016/j.mce.2009.06.015. S0303-7207(09)00374-8 [pii].

Lupien, S. J., Parent, S., Evans, A. C., Tremblay, R. E., Zelazo, P. D., Corbo, V., et al. (2011). Larger amygdala but no change in hippocampal volume in 10-year-old children exposed to maternal depressive symptomatology since birth. *Proceedings of the National Academy of Sciences of the United States of America, 108*(34), 14324–14329. doi:10.1073/pnas.1105371108. 1105371108 [pii].

Lutz, J., Herwig, U., Opialla, S., Hittmeyer, A., Jäncke, L., Rufer, M., et al. (2014). Mindfulness and emotion regulation–an fMRI study. *Social Cognitive and Affective Neuroscience, 9*, 776–785. doi:10.1093/scan/nst043.

Macedo, J. A., Hesse, J., Turner, J. D., Meyer, J., Hellhammer, D. H., & Muller, C. P. (2008). Glucocorticoid sensitivity in fibromyalgia patients: Decreased expression of corticosteroid receptors and glucocorticoid-induced leucine zipper. *Psychoneuroendocrinology, 33*(6), 799–809. doi:10.1016/j.psyneuen.2008.03.012. S0306-4530(08)00070-X [pii].

Maeda, T., Guan, J. Z., Koyanagi, M., Higuchi, Y., & Makino, N. (2012). Aging-associated alteration of telomere length and subtelomeric status in female patients with Parkinson's disease. *Journal of Neurogenetics, 26*, 245–251. doi:10.3109/01677063.2011.651665.

Maes, M. (2009). Inflammatory and oxidative and nitrosative stress pathways underpinning chronic fatigue, somatization and psychosomatic symptoms. *Current Opinion in Psychiatry, 22*(1), 75–83.

Maes, M., & Twisk, F. N. (2010). Chronic fatigue syndrome: Harvey and Wessely's (bio)psychosocial model versus a bio(psychosocial) model based on inflammatory and oxidative and nitrosative stress pathways. *BMC Medicine, 8*, 35. doi:10.1186/1741-7015-8-35. 1741-7015-8-35 [pii].

Magarinos, A. M., & McEwen, B. S. (1995). Stress-induced atrophy of apical dendrites of hippocampal CA3c neurons: Involvement of glucocorticoid secretion and excitatory amino acid receptors. *Neuroscience, 69*(1), 89–98. doi: 030645229500259L [pii].

Manji, H., Kato, T., Di Prospero, N. A., Ness, S., Beal, M. F., Krams, M., et al. (2012). Impaired mitochondrial function in psychiatric disorders. *Nature Reviews Neuroscience, 13*, 293–307. doi:10.1038/nrn3229.

McEwen, B. S., Gray, J., & Nasca, C. (2015). Recognizing resilience: Learning from the effects of stress on the brain. *Neurobiology Stress, 1*, 1–11. doi:10.1016/j.ynstr.2014.09.001.

McEwen, B. S., & Stellar, E. (1993). Stress and the individual. Mechanisms leading to disease. *Archives of Internal Medicine, 153*(18), 2093–2101.

McEwen, B. S., & Wingfield, J. C. (2003). The concept of allostasis in biology and biomedicine. *Hormones and Behavior, 43*(1), 2–15. doi: S0018506X02000247 [pii].

McGowan, P. O., Sasaki, A., D'Alessio, A. C., Dymov, S., Labonte, B., Szyf, M., et al. (2009). Epigenetic regulation of the glucocorticoid receptor in human brain associates with childhood abuse. *Nature Neuroscience, 12*(3), 342–348. doi:10.1038/nn.2270. nn.2270 [pii].

McWhinney, I. R., Epstein, R. M., & Freeman, T. R. (2001). Rethinking somatization. *Advances in Mind-Body Medicine, 17*(4), 232–239.

Meaney, M. J. (2001). Maternal care, gene expression, and the transmission of individual differences in stress reactivity across generations. *Annual Review of Neuroscience, 24*, 1161–1192. doi:10.1146/annurev.neuro.24.1.1161. 24/1/1161 [pii].

Meerding, W. J., Bonneux, L., Polder, J. J., Koopmanschap, M. A., & van der Maas, P. J. (1998). Demographic and epidemiological determinants of healthcare costs in Netherlands: Cost of illness study. *BMJ, 317*(7151), 111–115.

Meeus, M., Nijs, J., Hermans, L., Goubert, D., & Calders, P. (2013). The role of mitochondrial dysfunctions due to oxidative and nitrosative stress in the chronic pain or chronic fatigue syndromes and fibromyalgia patients: Peripheral and central mechanisms as therapeutic targets? *Expert Opinion on Therapeutic Targets, 17*(9), 1081–1089. doi:10.1517/14728222.2013.818657.

Moldofsky, H. (1995). Sleep, neuroimmune and neuroendocrine functions in fibromyalgia and chronic fatigue syndrome. *Advances in Neuroimmunology, 5*(1), 39–56.

Nicassio, P. M., Moxham, E. G., Schuman, C. E., & Gevirtz, R. N. (2002). The contribution of pain, reported sleep quality, and depressive symptoms to fatigue in fibromyalgia. *Pain, 100*(3), 271–279. doi: S0304395902003007 [pii].

Nijhof, S. L., Rutten, J. M., Uiterwaal, C. S., Bleijenberg, G., Kimpen, J. L., & Putte, E. M. (2014). The role of hypocortisolism in chronic fatigue syndrome. *Psychoneuroendocrinology, 42*, 199–206. doi:10.1016/j.psyneuen.2014.01.017. S0306-4530(14)00042-0 [pii].

O'Carroll, R. E., Drysdale, E., Cahill, L., Shajahan, P., & Ebmeier, K. P. (1999). Stimulation of the noradrenergic system enhances and blockade reduces memory for emotional material in man. *Psychological Medicine, 29*(5), 1083–1088.

O'Donovan, A., Sun, B., Cole, S., Rempel, H., Lenoci, M., Pulliam, L., et al. (2011). Transcriptional control of monocyte gene expression in post-traumatic stress disorder. *Disease Markers, 30*(2–3), 123–132. doi:10.3233/DMA-2011-0768. W1L2343430776467 [pii].

Oran, M., Tulubas, F., Mete, R., Aydin, M., Sarikaya, H. G., & Gurel, A. (2014). Evaluation of paraoxonase and arylesterase activities in patients with irritable bowel syndrome. *Journal of the Pakistan Medical Association, 64*(7), 820–822.

Oswald, L. M., Zandi, P., Nestadt, G., Potash, J. B., Kalaydjian, A. E., & Wand, G. S. (2006). Relationship between cortisol responses to stress and personality. *Neuropsychopharmacology, 31*(7), 1583–1591. doi:10.1038/sj.npp.1301012. 1301012 [pii].

Pace, T. W., Negi, L. T., Adame, D. D., Cole, S. P., Sivilli, T. I., Brown, T. D., et al. (2009). Effect of compassion meditation on neuroendocrine, innate immune and behavioral responses to psychosocial stress. *Psychoneuroendocrinology, 34*(1), 87–98. doi:10.1016/j.psyneuen.2008.08.011. S0306-4530(08)00219-9 [pii].

Papadopoulos, A. S., & Cleare, A. J. (2012). Hypothalamic-pituitary-adrenal axis dysfunction in chronic fatigue syndrome. *Nature Reviews Endocrinology, 8*(1), 22–32. doi:10.1038/nrendo.2011.153. nrendo.2011.153 [pii].

Paras, M. L., Murad, M. H., Chen, L. P., Goranson, E. N., Sattler, A. L., Colbenson, K. M., et al. (2009). Sexual abuse and lifetime diagnosis of somatic disorders: A systematic review and meta-analysis. *JAMA, 302*(5), 550–561. doi:10.1001/jama.2009.1091. 302/5/550 [pii].

Pedersen, A. F., Zachariae, R., & Bovbjerg, D. H. (2009). Psychological stress and antibody response to influenza vaccination: A meta-analysis. *Brain, Behavior, and Immunity, 23*, 427–433. doi:10.1016/j.bbi.2009.01.004.

Pedersen, A., Zachariae, R., & Bovbjerg, D. H. (2010). Influence of psychological stress on upper respiratory infection–a meta-analysis of prospective studies. *Psychosomatic Medicine, 72*, 823–832. doi:10.1097/PSY.0b013e3181f1d003.

Pham, K., Nacher, J., Hof, P. R., & McEwen, B. S. (2003). Repeated restraint stress suppresses neurogenesis and induces biphasic PSA-NCAM expression in the adult rat dentate gyrus. *European Journal of Neuroscience, 17*(4), 879–886. doi: 2513 [pii].

Picard, M., Juster, R. P., & McEwen, B. S. (2014). Mitochondrial allostatic load puts the 'gluc' back in glucocorticoids. *Nature Reviews Endocrinology, 10*(5), 303–310. doi:10.1038/nrendo.2014.22. nrendo.2014.22 [pii].

Price, D. D. (2000). Psychological and neural mechanisms of the affective dimension of pain. *Science, 288*(5472), 1769–1772. doi: 8580 [pii].

Ramos, B. P., & Arnsten, A. F. (2007). Adrenergic pharmacology and cognition: Focus on the prefrontal cortex. *Pharmacology and Therapeutics, 113*(3), 523–536. doi:10.1016/j.pharmthera.2006.11.006. S0163-7258(06)00202-6 [pii].

Rao, S. G., Williams, G. V., & Goldman-Rakic, P. S. (2000). Destruction and creation of spatial tuning by disinhibition: GABA(A) blockade of prefrontal cortical neurons engaged by working memory. *Journal of Neuroscience, 20*(1), 485–494.

Rask, C. U., Ornbol, E., Olsen, E. M., Fink, P., & Skovgaard, A. M. (2013). Infant behaviors are predictive of functional somatic symptoms at ages 5–7 years: Results from the Copenhagen Child Cohort CCC2000. *Journal of Pediatrics, 162*(2), 335–342. doi:10.1016/j.jpeds.2012.08.001. S0022-3476(12)00905-5 [pii].

Reynolds, K. J., Vernon, S. D., Bouchery, E., & Reeves, W. C. (2004). The economic impact of chronic fatigue syndrome. *Cost Effectiveness and Resource Allocation, 2*(1), 4. doi:10.1186/1478-7547-2-4. 1478-7547-2-4 [pii].

Rief, W., & Broadbent, E. (2007). Explaining medically unexplained symptoms-models and mechanisms. *Clinical Psychology Review, 27*(7), 821–841. doi:10.1016/j.cpr.2007.07.005. S0272-7358(07)00126-2 [pii].

Robinson, R. L., Birnbaum, H. G., Morley, M. A., Sisitsky, T., Greenberg, P. E., & Claxton, A. J. (2003). Economic cost and epidemiological characteristics of patients with fibromyalgia claims. *Journal of Rheumatology, 30*(6), 1318–1325. doi: 0315162X-30-1318 [pii].

Robinson, O. J., Krimsky, M., Lieberman, L., Allen, P., Vytal, K., & Grillon, C. (2014). Towards a mechanistic understanding of pathological anxiety: The dorsal medial prefrontal-amygdala 'aversive amplification' circuit in unmedicated generalized and social anxiety disorders. *Lancet Psychiatry, 1*(4), 294–302. doi:10.1016/S2215-0366(14)70305-0.

Roozendaal, B., Portillo-Marquez, G., & McGaugh, J. L. (1996). Basolateral amygdala lesions block glucocorticoid-induced modulation of memory for spatial learning. *Behavioral Neuroscience, 110*(5), 1074–1083.

Rosenkranz, M. A. (2007). Substance P at the nexus of mind and body in chronic inflammation and affective disorders. *Psychological Bulletin, 133*(6), 1007–1037. doi:10.1037/0033-2909.133.6.1007. 2007-15350-008 [pii].

Russell, I. J., Orr, M. D., Littman, B., Vipraio, G. A., Alboukrek, D., Michalek, J. E., et al. (1994). Elevated cerebrospinal fluid levels of substance P in patients with the fibromyalgia syndrome. *Arthritis and Rheumatism, 37*(11), 1593–1601.

Sauer, S., Walach, H., & Kohls, N. (2011). Gray's behavioural inhibition system as a mediator of mindfulness towards well-being. *Personality and Individual Differences, 50*, 506–511.

Schnall, P. L., Pieper, C., Schwartz, J. E., Karasek, R. A., Schlussel, Y., Devereux, R. B., et al. (1990). The relationship between 'job strain', workplace diastolic blood pressure, and left ventricular mass index. Results of a case–control study. *JAMA, 263*(14), 1929–1935.

Schroder, A., & Fink, P. (2010). The proposed diagnosis of somatic symptom disorders in DSM-V: Two steps forward and one step backward? *Journal of Psychosomatic Research, 68*(1), 95–96. doi:10.1016/j.jpsychores.2009.06.013. author reply 99–100. S0022-3999(09)00266-9 [pii].

Schroder, A., & Fink, P. (2011). Functional somatic syndromes and somatoform disorders in special psychosomatic units: Organizational aspects and evidence-based treatment. *The Psychiatric Clinics of North America, 34*(3), 673–687. doi:10.1016/j.psc.2011.05.008. S0193-953X(11)00053-0 [pii].

Schroder, A., Rehfeld, E., & Ornbol, E. (2012). Cognitive-behavioural group treatment for a range of functional somatic syndromes: Randomized trial. *British Journal of Psychiatry, 26*(4).

Segerstrom, S., & Miller, G. (2004). Psychological stress and the human immune system: A meta-analytic study of 30 years of inquiry. *Psychological Bulletin, 130*, 601–630.

Sharpe, M., Mayou, R., & Seagroatt, V. (1994). Why do doctors find some patients difficult to help? *QJM, 87*, 187–193.

Sheline, Y. I., Wang, P. W., Gado, M. H., Csernansky, J. G., & Vannier, M. W. (1996). Hippocampal atrophy in recurrent major depression. *Proceedings of the National Academy of Sciences of the United States of America, 93*(9), 3908–3913.

Siegel, D. J. (2007). *The mindful brain. Reflection and attunement in the cultivation of well-being*. New York: W. W. Norton & Company.

Sirois, F. M., Kitner, R., Hirsch, J. K., Behaviors, H.-P., Kitner, R., & Hirsch, J. K. (2014). Self-compassion, affect, and health-promoting behaviors. *Health Psychology, 2015 June; 34*(6): 661–669.

Starkman, M. N., Gebarski, S. S., Berent, S., & Schteingart, D. E. (1992). Hippocampal formation volume, memory dysfunction, and cortisol levels in patients with Cushing's syndrome. *Biological Psychiatry, 32*(9), 756–765. doi: 0006-3223(92)90079-F [pii].

Swartz, J. R., Knodt, A. R., Radtke, S. R., & Hariri, A. R. (2015). A neural biomarker of psychological vulnerability to future life stress. *Neuron, 85*(3), 505–511. doi:10.1016/j.neuron.2014.12.055. S0896-6273(14)01164-7 [pii].

Tak, L. M., Cleare, A. J., Ormel, J., Manoharan, A., Kok, I. C., Wessely, S., et al. (2011). Meta-analysis and meta-regression of hypothalamic-pituitary-adrenal axis activity in functional somatic disorders. *Biological Psychology, 87*(2), 183–194. doi:10.1016/j.biopsycho.2011.02.002. S0301-0511(11)00032-9 [pii].

Theorell, T., Blomkvist, V., Lindh, G., & Evengard, B. (1999). Critical life events, infections, and symptoms during the year preceding chronic fatigue syndrome (CFS): An examination of CFS patients and subjects with a nonspecific life crisis. *Psychosomatic Medicine, 61*(3), 304–310.

Tillisch, K., Mayer, E. A., & Labus, J. S. (2011). Quantitative meta-analysis identifies brain regions activated during rectal distension in irritable bowel syndrome. *Gastroenterology, 140*(1), 91–100. doi:10.1053/j.gastro.2010.07.053. S0016-5085(10)01151-0 [pii].

Tomas, C., Newton, J., & Watson, S. (2013). A review of hypothalamic-pituitary-adrenal axis function in chronic fatigue syndrome. *ISRN Neuroscience, 2013*, 784520. doi:10.1155/2013/784520.

Vaeroy, H., Helle, R., Forre, O., Kass, E., & Terenius, L. (1988). Elevated CSF levels of substance P and high incidence of Raynaud phenomenon in patients with fibromyalgia: New features for diagnosis. *Pain, 32*(1), 21–26. doi: 0304-3959(88)90019-X [pii].

Vago, D. R., & Silbersweig, D. A. (2012). Self-awareness, self-regulation, and self-transcendence (S-ART): A framework for understanding the neurobiological mechanisms of mindfulness. *Frontiers in Human Neuroscience, 6*, 296. doi:10.3389/fnhum.2012.00296.

van der Doelen, R. H., Calabrese, F., Guidotti, G., Geenen, B., Riva, M. A., Kozicz, T., et al. (2014). Early life stress and serotonin transporter gene variation interact to affect the transcription of the glucocorticoid and mineralocorticoid receptors, and the co-chaperone FKBP5, in the adult rat brain. *Frontiers in Behavioral Neuroscience, 8*, 355. doi:10.3389/fnbeh.2014.00355.

Velden, A. M. V., Kuyken, D., Wattar, W., Crane, U., Pallesen, C., Dahlgaard, K. J., et al. (2015). A systematic review of mechanisms of change in mindfulness-based cognitive therapy in the treatment of recurrent major depressive disorder. *Clinical Psychology Review, 37*, 26–39. doi:10.1016/j.cpr.2015.02.001.

Weaver, I. C., Cervoni, N., Champagne, F. A., D'Alessio, A. C., Sharma, S., Seckl, J. R., et al. (2004). Epigenetic programming by maternal behavior. *Nature Neuroscience, 7*(8), 847–854. doi:10.1038/nn1276 nn1276 [pii].

Wileman, L., May, C., & Chew-Graham, C. A. (2002). Medically unexplained symptoms and the problem of power in the primary care consultation: A qualitative study. *Family Practice, 19*(2), 178–182.

Wilson, R. G., Stevens, B. W., Guo, A. Y., Russell, C. N., Thornton, A., Cohen, M. A., et al. (2015). High C-reactive protein is associated with poor sleep quality independent of nocturnal symptoms in patients with inflammatory bowel disease. *Digestive Diseases and Sciences*. doi:10.1007/s10620-015-3580-5.

Wingenfeld, K., Nutzinger, D., Kauth, J., Hellhammer, D. H., & Lautenbacher, S. (2010). Salivary cortisol release and hypothalamic pituitary adrenal axis feedback sensitivity in fibromyalgia is associated with depression but not with pain. *The Journal of Pain, 11*(11), 1195–1202. doi:10.1016/j.jpain.2010.02.011. S1526-5900(10)00350-0 [pii].

Wingenfeld, K., Whooley, M. A., Neylan, T. C., Otte, C., & Cohen, B. E. (2015). Effect of current and lifetime posttraumatic stress disorder on 24-h urinary catecholamines and cortisol: Results from the mind your heart study. *Psychoneuroendocrinology, 52*, 83–91. doi:10.1016/j.psyneuen.2014.10.023. S0306-4530(14)00407-7 [pii].

Xu, L., Anwyl, R., & Rowan, M. J. (1997). Behavioural stress facilitates the induction of long-term depression in the hippocampus. *Nature, 387*(6632), 497–500. doi:10.1038/387497a0.

Zachariae, R. (2009). Psychoneuroimmunology: A bio-psycho-social approach to health and disease. *Scandinavian Journal of Psychology, 50*, 645–651.

Zieker, J., Zieker, D., Jatzko, A., Dietzsch, J., Nieselt, K., Schmitt, A., et al. (2007). Differential gene expression in peripheral blood of patients suffering from post-traumatic stress disorder. *Molecular Psychiatry, 12*(2), 116–118. doi:10.1038/sj.mp.4001905. 4001905 [pii].

Zolkipli, Z., Pedersen, C. B., Lamhonwah, A.-M., Gregersen, N., & Tein, I. (2011). Vulnerability to oxidative stress in vitro in pathophysiology of mitochondrial short-chain acyl-CoA dehydrogenase deficiency: Response to antioxidants. *PLoS ONE, 6*, e17534. doi:10.1371/journal.pone.0017534.

Chapter 9
The Emerging Science of Mindfulness as a Treatment for Addiction

Sean Dae Houlihan and Judson A. Brewer

Introduction

There are few conditions that cause as much suffering on a personal and societal level as addictions. Extensive strides have been made in understanding the neurobiological circuitry that drives various substance addictions in both animal models and humans, but these insights have yet to produce comparable advances in treatment methods. Mindfulness trainings, which are based on ancient Buddhist psychological models, have recently been tested as addiction treatments and have yielded promising results. Fascinatingly, these Buddhist models revolve around the elimination of suffering, which is thought to be the inevitable product of craving. Further, there are considerable overlaps between these ancient ideas and modern models of behavioral reinforcement. The early Buddhist models may even offer a more sophisticated understanding of the psychological mechanisms of addiction and ways to improve current treatment strategies. Since mindfulness itself has recently become the subject of psychological and neurobiology study, this chapter will consider the overlaps between the early Buddhist and contemporary models of the addictive process, review studies of mindfulness-based addiction treatments, and discuss recent neuroimaging studies to further inform our understanding of the neurological mechanisms and potential effects of mindfulness-based addiction treatments.

When people think of addiction, it is often the debilitating drug addictions that first spring to mind such as heroin and alcohol dependence. Indeed, drug addictions are one of the costliest human conditions, having significant effects on mental, physical, and economic health. As a whole, substance abuse in the United States

S.D. Houlihan • J.A. Brewer, MD, PhD (✉)
Department of Medicine, Center for Mindfulness, University of Massachusetts Medical School, Shrewsbury, MA, 01545, USA
e-mail: Judson.Brewer@umassmed.edu

E. Shonin et al. (eds.), *Mindfulness and Buddhist-Derived Approaches in Mental Health and Addiction*, Advances in Mental Health and Addiction,
DOI 10.1007/978-3-319-22255-4_9

cost approximately $193 billion in 2007, primarily as a result of lost productivity (Office of National Drug Control Policy, 2007). While many salient examples of addictive behavior are associated with drug use, addictive tendencies take many (often subtler) forms, and an exogenous chemical dependency is not requisite for an addiction to exist. Compulsive gamblers can be helplessly ensnared by a slot-machine in much the same way as someone else is by cocaine. If a drug dependency does manifest, however, the physical effects of withdrawal reinforce the addiction and add momentum to an already powerful feedback loop (Baker, Piper, McCarthy, Majeskie, & Fiore, 2004).

Acquisition of an addictive behavior is a complex process with a basis in operant conditioning: the pairing of actions with "effects," which alters future behaviors. Behavioral modification occurs via induction of positive (pleasant) and negative (unpleasant) affective states linked to action patterns. This sets up positive and negative loops by reinforcing the associative memories between these affective states and behaviors. The consequence is the formation of associative memories that pair actions with "affects." Subsequently, stimuli cue associative memories and are interpreted as positive or negative in light of prior experiences, which induces positive or negative affective states. The affective states in turn trigger cravings to either maintain the state if it is positive or alleviate the state if it is negative. The cravings incite behaviors that are rewarded or punished by the subsequent affective state, thus encoding more associative memories and fueling a feedback loop. In this way, craving drives the repetition of behavior patterns (Baker et al., 2004).

In some cases, the associative loops are strengthened, modified, and eventually molded into an addiction that takes on a life of its own. This automatization of the loop leads to a habitual cue-induced behavior that is largely outside of consciousness, let alone conscious control (Bargh & Chartrand, 1999; Curtin, McCarthy, Piper, & Baker, 2006). Additionally, neutral cues that have been classically conditioned may directly trigger craving (Lazev et al., 1999). These associative learning processes may then lead to increased motivational salience of future cues, fortifying the addictive loop (Robinson & Berridge, 2008).

There are limitless variations of the circumstances that initiate addictive tendencies, and addictions can seem quite dissimilar—addictive loops might similarly develop around the euphoria and dysphoria cycle of cocaine use, the passion and comfort of a romantic relationship, or the excitement of receiving facebook likes for a witty post about an ill-suited presidential candidate. Seemingly innocuous behaviors such as eating or checking one's cell phone can also become objects of addiction. The expanding understanding of brain function has partially illuminated what common neurological features underlie seemingly disparate behaviors such as cocaine use, romantic infatuation, rich food, and posting selfies to Facebook, when they turn addictive (Aron et al., 2005; Bartels & Zeki, 2004; Tang, Fellows, Small, & Dagher, 2012; Meshi, Morawetz, & Heekeren, 2013). The range of behaviors that can be incorporated into addictive loops suggests that the effects of associative learning are widespread, underlie many of our cognitive functions, and are probably, from an evolutionary perspective, quite ancient.

The neural circuitry permitting this type of associative learning has extensively influenced the evolution of our species, shaping behaviors critical to our survival by enabling learned associations between actions and the consequences of those actions (e.g., learning where a food source is or where danger is lurking). The mechanisms underlying associative learning can be observed not only in our species and our close relatives but even in the most primitive nervous systems, for instance, those of sea slugs (Aplysia). The near ubiquity of associative learning among animals suggests that the process is evolutionarily conserved. This is relevant for our consideration of addiction because like other primitive nervous system functions, associative learning is likely resistant to cognitive manipulation (Nargeot & Simmers, 2011; Treat, Viken, Kruschke, & McFall, 2011). This may provide some explanatory power for the relative strengths and weaknesses of current treatment paradigms.

To recapitulate: the addictive loop model is noteworthy for several reasons. First, its general and ubiquitous nature blurs the line between addictions and habitual reactivity, indicating that addictive process might be more of a norm and less an exception. Second, each link in the chain is supported by convergent findings from both nonhuman animal and human studies, suggesting an evolutionarily conserved process. Third, its self-propagating nature aligns surprisingly well with Buddhist psychological models of human suffering, which the next section of this chapter will explore.

Early Buddhist Models of Addiction

Mindfulness endeavors to help reduce the experience of suffering, which is understood to be ultimately derived from attachment to particular experiences and fear of other experiences. The early Buddhist texts present a therapeutic model that explicates the pervasiveness of suffering, its cause, the possibility for a cure, and the methods for achieving that cure. The method prescribed revolves around understanding the cause of suffering and the way to interrupt the positive feedback loops that perpetuate it. External objects are not considered the origin of these loops nor are our spontaneously arising internal experiences. Rather, it is our reactions to our own sensoria that drive the process. In Pali, the language of these early texts, the critical juncture between sensory perception and the cycle of suffering is called *taṇhā* (N.B. there are six senses in Buddhist psychology: the five that we are accustomed to, plus the experience of mental thought activity). *Taṇhā* is commonly translated as "craving,"' though it more literally means "thirst," and can be understood in some contexts as habitual reactivity. Mindfulness aims to teach the "relinquishment, release, and letting go" of this reactive craving, such that suffering is cured (SN.56.11 in Thanissaro, 2010).

The early Buddhist texts that articulate the model are understood to be the teachings of a North Indian prince named Siddhartha Gautama who, as an adolescent, abdicated his royal title to single-mindedly investigate the nature of suffering.

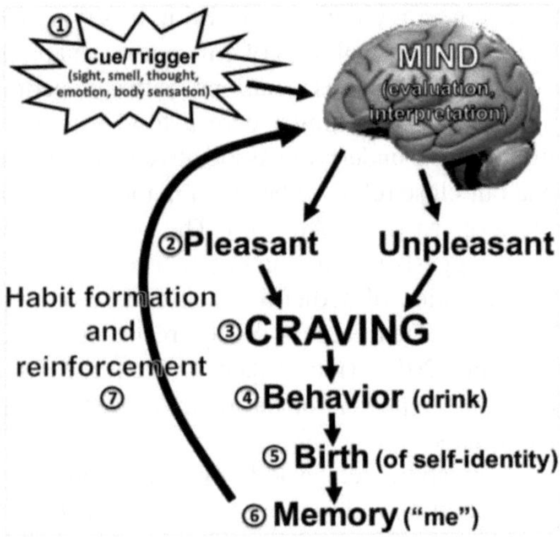

Fig. 9.1 Early models of addiction: dependent origination (Copyright 2011 Judson Brewer. Reprinted with permission of author)

Gautama's campaign led him to study with the premiere teachers of his time, but he found their methods to be unsatisfactory. Their approaches largely dealt with the objects of temptation (sex, drugs, physical comfort, etc.) by avoiding them and the objects of aversion (pain, fear, not getting what we want, etc.) by building extreme tolerances to them (SN.56.11 in Thanissaro, 2010). Finding that these methods did not fully accomplish what they intended to, Gautama isolated himself and set about investigating his own mental processes. By way of his intensive introspection, it is said that Gautama brought about the ultimate fruition of his mind: Buddhahood, which is marked by the cessation of suffering caused by craving (movement toward objects of desire) and aversion (movement away from objects of dislike).

Gautama Buddha's central discovery was how the human mind processes information, i.e., the sequence of causal links by which our minds construct experience. Interestingly, this shows major overlaps with modern-day models of operant conditioning (Brewer, Elwafi, & Davis, 2013). This model, called "dependent [co-]origination," posits that at any given moment, our minds exist in a state preconditioned by our prior experiences (For this brief illustration of dependent origination, consider the example of Sally in the adjoining text box.). When Sally encounters sensory input (cf. #1 in Fig. 9.1), her mind interprets the input based on her mind's prior experiences (conditioning; #2). Registration of the incoming information rapidly and automatically generates somatic information, an "affective tone," which can be felt as pleasant or unpleasant. That is, the valence of the affective tone arises from the interaction of the current state of the mind with the sensory input. Subsequently, an impulse arises as a psychological urge (craving; #3) to perform some behavior that will continue the pleasant or discontinue the unpleasant feeling. The craving motivates action (#4) and fuels the birth of what is referred to in Buddhist psychology as "self-identity" (#5; Brewer et al., 2013). The outcomes of that action are recorded in memory (#6), resulting in the formation of a new associative link, which updates the conditioning of Sally's mind, leading to subsequent rounds of this process (#7).

Consider Sally, a junior at Hypothetical High School, who is invited to drink with a group of older students that she looks up to (see #1, "positive cue" in Fig. 9.1). She learns to associate drinking with social disinhibition, peer-group bonding, and excitement. When she is drinking at a party with her friends, she feels good (#2). In fact, even when she is not so happy, she finds that she can still go and have fun at a party, and the tribulations of her life at Hypothetical High fade into the background (#2–6). As Sally grows up and the thrill of underage drinking dissipates, the adrenaline rush gives way to a subtle sense of relief that she can come home from work and relax with a bottle of wine. When her boss yells at her or she feels stressed out (#2), she finds herself thinking, "I could use a drink" (#3). The more Sally drinks in these situations, the more she reinforces her behavioral pattern and the deeper she engrains the sense of release and escape from unpleasantness with the act of drinking (#5–7). At times, she may even find herself "waking up" en route to a bar she occasionally stops at on the way home, before knowing that she decided to go there. At other times, she may find that she notices the urge to drink before noticing that something is actually bothering her, stimulating the craving.

In this way, an individual learns that some action (mental or physical) decreases unpleasant feelings and begins to form a behavior pattern around these affective reactions. The perception of any object is influenced by a person's prior experiences. One's mind interprets and filters incoming sensory stimuli according to its current state of conditioning. The present encounter, which is now a composite of present and past, is then consolidated with related memories, leading to the formation of a habit pattern. These patterns do not need to be complicated and drawn out but can be nearly instantaneous reactions. Thus, the current experience modifies the perception of future experiences. The recursive nature of these loops means that they can fortify and fuel themselves via positive feedback. Further, since the states of craving and aversion are themselves unpleasant, individuals often develop aversive reactions toward their own reactions. Fortunately, the iterative nature of this cyclic process also means that it can be disrupted at each new round.

From this Buddhist perspective, clinically defined addictions can be thought of as dependent origination loops that have developed in such a way that they no longer fit with societal norms to the point of causing concern. However, the associative loops that fall within a given culture's criteria for addiction are themselves not categorically different than the many other associative loops that we have all developed over the course of our lives. If Buddhist methods are effective at uprooting craving from a person's mind, we might reasonably expect that the same methods could also have clinical utility as treatments for addiction. The pervasiveness of associative learning and its capacity to form addictive feedback loops set up an important caveat for traditional addiction treatment strategies. Without understanding the fundamental structure of the addictive process, it is all too easy to unwittingly perpetuate it. Many treatment regimes utilize the transferability of addictive tendencies through behavioral substitution. For example, someone might "will" themselves to exercise when the urge to smoke a cigarette arises, thereby diminishing smoking behavior by building a new link between the urge to smoke and an exercise. This approach can meet with moderate success in treating the targeted addictive behavior, but it does not address the person's underlying addictive tendencies, which can lead to relapses (and other problems) down the road. The difficulty with treating people's addictions is that many treatments attempt to treat a specific addictive behavior instead of treating the fundamental cause of addiction: craving itself.

Since the English word "craving" only partially maps onto the Pali term, it is important to understand that *taṇhā* encompasses both wanting to gain and maintain desirable things (craving), as well as wanting to avoid undesirable things (aversion). Furthermore, the psychological process in question occurs rapidly and automatically in most cases, such that people are frequently only conscious of its downstream effects. It is through the practice of closely observing one's experiences that the sequence of these events becomes readily apparent. Further, the rapidity with which *taṇhā* forms then subsequently generates the next step in the process, which may pose a problem for cognitive interventions. Cognition is a comparatively slow process. This inherently forces cognitive interventions to contend not with the ephemeral reactivity at the core of the process but rather with the cascade of self-reinforcing loops that the initial craving begat. Thus, cognitive-behavioral and/or control-based treatments focus on building willpower—"mental muscle" to avoid, think through, and substitute behaviors—essentially putting individuals at odds with their unruly minds. Further, this willpower may be "depleted" precisely at times when individuals are most susceptible to relapse, such as when they are mentally and physically tired (Muraven & Baumeister, 2000). Mindfulness training teaches us to see more clearly the nature of our addictions, rather than avoiding or trying to change them. When we can perceive the mental processes, we feel and know more clearly the pain of perpetuating emotional craving and aversion, and we naturally begin to become disenchanted with the cycle, which begins the process of letting go. Conversely, blindness to this process leads to proliferation of craving through the iterative reinforcement of these cycles (This process is referred to as *avijjā* in Pali. It is commonly translated as *ignorance* and literally means "to not see."). Buddhist texts call this repetitive proliferation *saṇsāra*, or endless wandering, as there is no obvious way out of it when propagated.

The central point of the early Buddhist model is that craving and aversion arise in response to an affective tone that is associated with perceptual representations of a sensory object (Grabovac, Lau, & Willett, 2011). This provides a critical entry point for therapeutic interventions. By paying careful attention to present-moment experience, the Buddhist model claims that one can see that perceptions and the associated affective reactions (affective tone) are separate from—and indeed separable from—craving and aversion, as well as the elaborative thought processes that these can initiate. In theory, the potential of mindfulness practice is to prevent the associative loop from beginning. However, since it can require substantial practice to develop the mental acuity required to clearly perceive and modify dependent origination, it is important to note that even when craving has already arisen, mindful awareness can prevent further cycles of aversive reaction by helping an individual disengage from the loop. In this way, mindfulness practice can immediately begin deconstructing these links. By overcoming the habitual reactions of craving and aversion that biases attention and memory, mindfulness allows individuals to feel and know more clearly the pain of perpetuating emotional craving and aversion. Being fully present with the pain of this emotional reactivity may be sufficient to motivate individuals not to perpetuate it (Brewer, Davis, & Goldstein, 2012).

Another concept that bears consideration is the birth of "self-identity" (#5). The sense of self that is generated in the process of dependent origination is composed of one's habitual reactions of clinging to pleasant aspects of experience and to the absence of unpleasant aspects. Imagine how, in a moment of desperate craving for something, the mind can collapse into a singular want. It seems as if appeasing this particular desire will bring all that one needs, even if one knows better. This is a distorted perception (i.e., ignorance); sense pleasures are fleeting and incapable of resolving the core distress that fuels the cycle of searching for gratification. As one discourse relates it, *"Indeed, I have long been tricked, cheated, and defrauded by this mind. For when clinging, I have been clinging just to material form... feeling... perception... formations, consciousness... With my clinging as condition, being... birth... aging and death, sorrow, lamentation, pain, grief, and despair come to be. Such is the origin of this whole mass of suffering"* (MN.75 in Ñāṇamoli & Bodhi, 1995). In this model, a sense of self is born by craving and clinging to any kind of experience. This sense of self is very basic, being dependent only on grasping after experiences, and it does not depend on an explicit narrative of self-identity to exist. As long as there is craving for any aspect of experience, this affectively constructed sense of self continues. Even a person with complete retrograde amnesia (a common cliché in soap operas) who does not remember anything about his past still has a felt sense of self, although he cannot say who that is. When the sense of self is threatened by the inability to prevent the loss of what is grasped after, or to prevent the occurrence of what is pushed away, then one suffers. We postulate that mindfulness does not prevent the cognitive construction of self-identity necessary for functioning in the world but instead targets previously developed affective biases that bring about internal conflict and limit perspective (Elliott, Zahn, Deakin, & Anderson, 2011). The reactive impulses produced when the sense of self is threatened prevent one from accurately assessing what is happening in the present moment and acting accordingly. Through deconstructing the habitual process by which we generate a reactive nonconceptual self-identity, the self does not go away, it simply loses the ability to obscure (i.e., ignorance is no longer at play). That is to say, mindfulness does not stop one from being a person but rather from taking things personally.

Given that one's self-identity stems largely from memory, the Buddhist description of dependent origination is remarkably similar to the contemporary model of the addictive loop (Brewer et al., 2013). When Sally, who has learned to associate drinking with the reduction of stress and/or the temporary abatement of withdrawal (#6), encounters a stressful situation or alcohol withdrawal symptoms such as irritability, restlessness, or agitation (#1), her neural conditioning interprets these as unpleasant (#2). She wants the unpleasant feeling to go away and consequently experiences a craving to drink (#3). When she drinks, she reinforces the habituated reaction to affective experience (e.g., "if I drink, I will feel better"; #4–6).

While Sally might take this personally, having thoughts such as "I am a drinker," it is not these particular self-related thoughts but rather the affective bias underlying the reaction of taking things personally that fuels the birth of self-identity (i.e., habituated reactions to affective experience). Sally may even begin to ruminate about drinking and start planning her day around access to alcohol, which, as we will see later, likely engages brain circuits involved in self-referential processing, thus further fueling this process. An addictive loop appears remarkably similar to the endless wandering characterized by Buddhist psychology. However, the psychological terms and links employed in dependent origination will need careful refinement and empirical validation to determine their relative explanatory and predictive power in contemporary models of addiction.

Conventional and Mindfulness-Based Treatments for Addiction

Mainstay addiction treatments have focussed on manipulating addiction behavior by teaching afflicted individuals to avoid cues, divert attention from cravings, substitute healthy activities for deleterious ones, foster positive affective states (e.g., practicing relaxation), and develop social support structures (Fiore et al., 2008). Such cognitively based treatments typically yield abstinence rates between 20 and 30 % (Law & Tang, 1995). From the view of Buddhist psychology, these methods of treatment are unlikely to have more than a limited effect on addictive loops because they do not sufficiently address the critical links of dependent origination but rather upstream and downstream elements (Niaura & Abrams, 2002). Avoiding cues that lead to temptation limits input to the addictive loop but does not dismantle it, and substitutive behaviors (e.g., eating carrot sticks in lieu of candy or doing pushups when the urge to smoke arises) only reorients the craving impulse to a different object. Acute treatments can work as short-term fixes but leave the individual to contend with the same addictive tendencies as before. It is even possible that cue-induced cravings increase with the duration of abstinence, suggesting that avoiding cues or substituting behaviors might do little to target the core processes driving addictive behaviors (Bedi et al., 2011). These methods also require recruitment of substantial mental effort (willpower) to enact, which undermines their efficacy since self-control is impaired by stress and strong affective states (Muraven & Baumeister, 2000). The experimental evidence for common addictive circuitry and the modest long-term success rates of existing treatment options suggests that treating addictive behavior may be insufficient. Innovative treatments that directly target the core networks underlying addiction may be able to produce substantially improved results. The early Buddhist model of suffering claims to do precisely this, and the clinical therapeutic interventions it has inspired have gained support from recent studies.

The meditation practices taught by Siddhartha Gautama emerged out of a vastly different cultural milieu than Western modernity. Many aspects of his basic teachings were practiced in ways best suited to his historical context and should be reexamined in light of a different culture's psychological background, the aims of a specific application, and the availability of new teaching tools. Mindfulness and the associated concepts are adaptations of Buddhist practice and philosophy (Shonin, Van Gordon, & Griffiths, 2014), which have taken forms such as Mindfulness-Based Stress Reduction (MBSR), Mindfulness-Based Cognitive Therapy (MBCT; combined with Cognitive Therapy for depression relapse prevention), and Mindfulness-Based Relapse Prevention (MBRP; combined with Relapse Prevention for addiction treatment). The framing of Buddhist practices by MBSR and the related mindfulness adaptations reflects the values of the adoptive culture, namely scientific empiricism. Mindfulness-based treatments incorporate multiple elements, most with origins in techniques taught by Gautama, but from its inception, MBSR was designed to interface with the scientific tools employed by Western medicine to assess the efficacy of medical treatments. Common features of these mindfulness-based treatments include, for instance, the training of equanimous attention in order to detect and modify automatic patterns of thought and reactivity (Desbordes, Gard, Hoge, Holzel, & Kerr, 2014). Mindfulness trainings have been evaluated in the treatment of a number of ailments including pain, anxiety, and depression (see Goyal et al., 2014 for meta-analysis). These data are promising, but additional work is needed as many of the studies to date have used small sample sizes, wait-lists, and other suboptimal control conditions.

The use of mindfulness in addiction treatments has been a more recent adaptation (Bowen et al., 2009; Brewer et al., 2009; Zgierska et al., 2008). The training has been operationalized to deploy two distinct components: (1) maintaining attention on immediate experience and (2) maintaining an attitude of acceptance toward this experience (Bishop et al., 2004). For example, when the desire for a cigarette comes on, a smoker might choose to bring mindful awareness to the sensations that constitute the craving. A key point of this practice is to begin to dissect the composite sensations that make up an experience. By heading straight into an aversive feeling like an intense craving, the surprising discovery that practitioners can make is that the overwhelming intensity breaks up into a manageable flow of simple sensory input (heat, tingling, tightness, etc.). By training the ability to directly and closely examine the somatic manifestation of an experience such as craving, one discovers that the horrific, ghastly figure lumbering through one's mind is actually only the shadow of a mouse. Paradoxically, the intensity is much greater when an experience is viewed at a distance, or out of the corner of one's eye, so to speak. Skillful application of this technique turns even judgment of the craving into an object for nonreactive examination rather than a driving force for subsequent behavior.

As such, mindfulness training may specifically target the associative learning process with an emphasis on the critical link between affect and craving (Nyanaponika, 2000). According to the early Buddhist model, this process of close, nonreactive observation has the potential to dismantle not only the associative links of the targeted addiction but the reactive tendencies of the mind in general.

Mindfulness has been packaged into several addiction treatments, such as Acceptance and Commitment Therapy (ACT) and MBRP (Bowen et al., 2009; Brewer et al., 2009). Assessment of these treatment regimes has yielded preliminary success. For example, Gifford et al. (2004) randomized 76 participants to receive either nicotine replacement treatment or ACT. The regimes performed comparably by the end of the treatment period, with 33 % of the nicotine replacement group and 35 % of the ACT group showing 24-h abstinence. At a 1-year follow-up, however, the abstinence within the nicotine replacement group had diminished to 15 % while the ACT group maintained 35 %. Other studies have not found evidence that mindfulness treatments are more effective than comparison conditions (Zgierska et al., 2009). A study by Bowen and colleagues comparing MBRP to Relapse Prevention (RP) or Treatment as Usual (TAU) as aftercare to standard treatment and found that both MBRP and RP showed significantly lower risks of relapse to substance use and heavy drinking compared to TAU at 6-month follow-up. Where RP showed an advantage in increasing the time to first drug use, MBRP showed fewer days of use and less heavy drinking at a 12-month follow-up (Bowen et al., 2014). There are several major confounds in assessing the efficacy of mindfulness treatments for addictions. Until 2009, of the 22 published studies that included mindfulness training, none tested mindfulness training as a stand-alone treatment and only one was randomized. There is also a lack of standardization between treatment regimes, and fidelity in the delivery of those regimes can be an issue. Further, since mindfulness-based trainings are often an amalgamation of multiple elements (some Buddhist, some not), there is currently little mechanistic understanding of what components at what dosages produce what effects.

With regard to smoking, mindfulness training has shown preliminary utility for reducing cigarette cravings and withdrawal symptoms (Cropley, Ussher, & Charitou, 2007), as well as for smoking cessation (Davis, Fleming, Bonus, & Baker, 2007). Bowen et al. (2009) provided college students with brief mindfulness-based instructions and found that they smoked significantly fewer cigarettes 1-week after the intervention compared to those that did not receive instructions. Brewer, Mallik et al. (2011)) studied the effects of stand-alone mindfulness training for smoking cessation. This study randomized 88 subjects to receive a tailored mindfulness training or the American Lung Association's Freedom from Smoking (FFS) program—a gold standard smoking cessation treatment. The mindfulness groups smoked significantly fewer cigarettes during the program and upon completion showed twofold greater abstinence rates (36 % compared with 15 % in the Freedom from Smoking Program). At a 4-month follow-up, the abstinence rate of the mindfulness group had largely maintained (31 %), whereas over half of the FFS group had relapsed, bringing the 4-month success rate for the FFS group to 6 % ($p=0.01$). Similar to previous studies of psychological health and mindfulness training

(Carmody & Baer, 2008), this study observed that the more individuals in the mindfulness training group practiced, the more favorable their outcomes: increased home practice was correlated with decreased cigarette use for both formal ($r=-0.44$, $p<0.02$) and informal practice ($r=-0.48$, $p<0.01$). The FFS group performed home practices such as relaxation, but these did not show any correlations with smoking cessation outcomes.

Through attentional focus, individuals learn to become more aware of habit-linked, minimally conscious affective states and bodily sensations (e.g., low-level craving), thus "de-automating" this largely habitual process (Brewer, Bowen, Smith, Marlatt, & Potenza, 2010). Effective implementation of mindfulness training may, over time, lead to the attenuation and eventual dismantling of addictive loops that perpetuate smoking, drug use, and other deleterious behaviors. In the absence of an intact associative loop, subsequent addiction-related cues will fail to elicit cravings. If the underlying craving is uprooted, it would be consistent with Buddhist theory that even recalcitrant addictions, which can lay dormant only to reemerge years later, can be eradicated through the sustained application of nonreactive attention to subjective somatic experience. Of course, it will take many years of longitudinal addiction studies to assess if this claim is borne out. There is, however, evidence that mindfulness practice alters the way the brain processes interoceptive cues. Bornemann, Herbert, and Mehling (2015) found that following a 3-month mindfulness training, participants reported significantly greater awareness of bodily sensations, including increased awareness of emotions and mind–body interactions and a higher propensity to listen to their bodies for insight about their emotional state, particularly under stress. Another study showed that relative to a relaxation control group, mindfulness training decreased emotional interference on a cognitive processing task and lead to significant changes in a psychophysiological measure of arousal while viewing pleasant and unpleasant images (Ortner, Kilner, & Zelazo, 2007). These findings may suggest that mindfulness practice leads not only to greater emotional stability at a physiological level but also that this emotional stability is paired with better neural monitoring of the body and association of its states with the external environment; in essence, helping individuals to "see things as they are." For example, women who are distracted by emotionally driven self-evaluative thoughts were shown to be much slower in registering bodily reactions to emotionally charged images, an effect that is reversed by meditation training (Silverstein, Brown, Roth, & Britton, 2011).

Simply by teaching individuals to observe aversive body and mind states (e.g., negative affect) rather than reacting to them, mindfulness training may foster the replacement of stress- and affect-induced habitual reactions with more adaptive responses (e.g., enhancing self-control; Curtin et al., 2006). Additionally, mindfulness training may help individuals change their relationships to negative affective or physically unpleasant states and thoughts (i.e., "not taking them personally"). To be clear, we postulate that the mechanism of action here is the attenuation of affective bias underlying the reaction of "taking things personally," rather than a change in self-related thoughts or cognitive attributions. Since it is the habitual affective bias underlying emotional reactivity that fuels further rounds of craving and habituation, attenuation of this affective bias diminishes momentum of the feedback loop and ultimately leads to smoking cessation (Bowen et al., 2009; Bowen & Marlatt, 2009; Brewer et al., 2010). However, studies that directly test these hypotheses are needed.

Craving at the Core

Mindfulness training teaches that rather than running away from unpleasantness, one can learn to accept what is happening right now and, paradoxically, move "into" the experience and explore what it actually feels like in the body, no matter how unpleasant it might be at the moment. In this way, mindfulness training may help individuals sit with or "ride out" their cravings. In drugs that produce physical dependencies, sitting with a craving can be overwhelming; the longer a craving goes unsatisfied, the more it may intensify as it becomes fueled by further reactions to the symptoms of withdrawal and the unpleasantness of the wanting itself. In a study of treatment-seeking smokers, for each standard deviation increase in craving scores on the target quit date, the risk of lapsing rose by 43 % on that day and 65 % on the following day (Ferguson, Shiffman, & Gwaltney, 2006). Mindful dissection of these intense experiences can lead people to see two aspects clearly. First, that cravings are physical sensations in their bodies, not moral imperatives that must be acted on. Second, that each time they successfully ride out a craving—experiencing its physicality without acting on it—cravings naturally subside on their own, even if not satiated. Through repeated and sustained application of this introspective observation, individuals learn "from experience" that cravings are inherently impermanent and that the intense experiences are not as overwhelming as they first seemed.

Through the practice of "befriending" all of one's experiences as they arise and pass, one strengthens one's cognitive capacity for equanimity (nonjudgmental awareness), attenuates one's habitual emotional reactivity, and begins to build insight into the mechanisms of dependent origination. Cravings may continue to arise (often with a vengeance, especially at the beginning), but literally sitting with these urges and becoming curious about their nature (rather than immediately reacting to them) disrupt both the automaticity and the strength of the associative loop. If mindfulness is a causative agent in the success of these addiction treatments, one might predict that it would decouple the traditional observation that smoking and craving are positively correlated.

In a follow-up to their smoking cessation trial of mindfulness training, Brewer and colleagues examined the relationship between craving and smoking behavior during treatment (Elwafi, Witkiewitz, Mallik, Thornhill, & Brewer, 2013). At the beginning of treatment, subjects showed strong positive correlations between average daily cigarette use and their self-reported craving for cigarettes, as measured by the Questionnaire on Smoking Urges ($r=0.58, p<0.001$). At the end of the 4-week treatment period, the relationship between self-reported cigarette cravings and smoking had decoupled to the point of statistical nonsignificance ($r=0.13, p=0.49$).

In fact, the individuals who quit smoking showed no difference in craving scores compared to those who continued to smoke and instead demonstrated a delayed reduction in reported craving, while those who did not quit reported an increase in craving concomitant with increases in smoking. Further, the observed decoupling was itself moderated by mindfulness practice—the more that individuals practiced during treatment, the less their craving correlated with the number of cigarettes they smoked at the end of treatment. These results suggest that after just 4 weeks of outpatient mindfulness training, individuals were no longer reacting to their cravings by smoking. This finding is consistent with the hypothesis that mindfulness decouples the relationship between craving and smoking. In other words, mindfulness practice may help individuals stop adding fuel to the fire (craving) so that while the fire still continues to burn off of the fuel already present, the heat is no longer intolerable. Over time, without continued sustenance (smoking), the fire burns out by itself.

The capacity of mindfulness training to attenuate the relationship between craving and substance use has been observed in other studies as well. Witkiewitz and Bowen (2010) examined the relationship between craving, substance use, and depression following a randomized clinical trial of Mindfulness-Based Relapse Prevention. They found that craving mediated the relationship between depressive symptoms and substance use in the group that received a conventional treatment but not in the group that received MBRP. These results further support the Buddhist claim that mindfulness training targets craving itself. The Buddhist model goes on to claim that when the craving is attenuated, over time the addictive loop will become dismantled through a dis-identification with the object (or dismantling of self-identity; Brewer et al., 2013). The next logical steps will be to determine how these map onto current psychological models of behavior. For example, do tolerance of craving and dismantling of self-identity equate to reappraisal and extinction, respectively, or to other skills, or constitute unique processes unto themselves?

Neurobiological Underpinnings of Addiction as Related to Mindfulness

Mindfulness meditation integrates multiple neurological systems, including networks that regulate attention, working memory, somatic perception, and emotion (for a more detailed review see Hölzel et al., 2011). Brain systems that show commonality between a number of different maladies and have also been theoretically and functionally linked to mindfulness training may provide a logical starting point for assaying the neurobiological mechanisms by which mindfulness impacts disease progression and for identifying promising targets for clinical interventions. The default mode network (DMN; a collection of brain regions that show robust functional correlation when one's mind is otherwise unoccupied) may be one such point of convergence (see Andrews-Hanna, Reidler, Sepulcre, Poulin, & Buckner, 2010; Buckner, Andrews-Hanna, & Schacter, 2008; Fox & Raichle, 2007).

The DMN was originally identified as a conserved pattern of regional activations that the participants in fMRI studies "defaulted" to while laying in a neuroimaging scanner and waiting for experiments to begin (Raichle et al., 2001). The DMN is strongly associated with off-task ideation (mind-wandering), self-referential processing, and with a number of psychiatric disorders ranging from anxiety to addiction (Buckner et al., 2008; Whitfield-Gabrieli et al., 2011; Whitfield-Gabrieli & Ford, 2012). Two primary nodes of the DMN, the medial prefrontal cortex (MPFC)and the posterior cingulate cortex (PCC), show temporally correlated activity with multiple peripheral nodes and anticorrelated activity with brain regions involved in self-monitoring and cognitive control (including the anterior insula, AI; dorsal anterior cingulate cortex, dACC; and dorsolateral prefrontal cortex, DLPFC; Andrews-Hanna et al., 2010). Though self-referential processing is a complex area of investigation in itself, on first approximation, this may be where models of self-identity formation at least partially overlap with cognitive disorders; memory retrieval and the "self across time" are linked by PCC activity (Andrews-Hanna et al., 2010; Buckner et al., 2008). Mindfulness practices generate marked deactivation of the DMN and have also been shown to increase functional connectivity between the DMN and regions associated with cognitive control (the DLPFC and dACC). Long-term meditators show these differences both during meditation and at rest compared to controls, suggesting that the functional connectivity alterations associated with active meditation practice may become stably integrated as trait changes in these individuals. Given the primacy of the DMN in numerous psychiatric disorders and contribution to self-referential processing and mind-wandering, the DMN appears a biologically plausible target for mindfulness training, which retrains the mind's tendency for discursive thought activity and for developing pathological self-constructs. Of course, the exact patterns and functions of these networks should be interpreted with some caution as there are limitations to our current analytic methods; we are only just beginning to understand the various causal factors that lead to the observed patterns (e.g., see Fan et al., 2012).

The DMN, and in particular the PCC, are also implicated specifically in addiction. PCC activity has been positively correlated with the severity of alcohol addiction (Claus, Ewing, Filbey, Sabbineni, & Hutchison, 2011; Tapert et al., 2003) and with the likelihood of relapse following treatment for cocaine and nicotine addiction (Kosten et al., 2006; Janes et al., 2010). In cocaine users, a relatively higher PCC response to cocaine-related cues during a 2-week treatment program distinguished patients who used again from those that did not in the 10-week following treatment (Kosten et al., 2006). Similarly, Janes et al. (2010) found that smokers who slipped after attaining abstinence had shown greater activations in response to smoking cues in brain regions including the PCC during the treatment. The PCC is only one of many brain regions implicated in the progression of addiction, yet it may be a central player. A meta-analysis of the neural substrates of reactivity to smoking-related cues found that the most reliably activated regions were the PCC and adjacent areas (Engelmann, Versace, Robinson, & Minnix, 2012). Other meta-analyses have similarly found that cue reactivity in nicotine addiction positively correlated with PCC activation (Tang et al., 2012). Importantly, in a direct comparison of cigarette smokers currently undergoing treatment who were shown smoking cues and instructed to either allow themselves to crave smoking or resist their cravings, Brody et al. (2007) found that resisting craving was associated with increased activity in the MPFC and PCC. It may seem counterintuitive that increased PCC activity correlates with addiction severity and relapse, but also with resisting cravings during treatment. After all, it could be reasonably presumed that patients who are committed to quitting smoking "should" be resisting their cravings. From the dependent origination model, however, it is clear that resistance reengages the addictive cycle, rather than dismantling it, ultimately undermining the intention of the effort.

In this chapter alone, we have seen that PCCactivity correlates with multiple attributes of addiction, self reference, internal resistance, and mind-wandering and that PCC deactivation is seen across multiple types of meditation. While still preliminary, there are some converging lines of evidence that while the function of mindfulness practice may be to disassemble pathological habit patterns, the unskillful use of self-identified effort to accomplish this may itself be a pathological loop. To better understand the contribution of PCC function to conscious experience, Garrison et al. (2013) used real-time fMRI neurofeedback for PCC activity in the context of mindfulness meditation. Activation of this structure tracked with the experience of being "caught up" in one's experience, whereas PCC deactivation corresponded with the sense of "effortless awareness" (being nonreactively aware of one's present experience). Farb et al. (2007) found that participants of an 8-week MBSR course showed less DMN (including PCC and MPFC) activation when mindfully viewing self-referential adjectives. Another group found that experienced meditators exhibited deactivation of DMN structures (including the PCC and MPFC) during mindful viewing of emotionally evocative pictures whereas novice meditators did not (Taylor et al., 2011). These findings suggest that the success of mindfulness training for addictions may be due to the disengagement from self-identified habitual response patterns and that the sense of "effort" during enacting control might actually be part of the problem.

Since DMN activity is tightly coupled with mind-wandering, the possibility that in the above studies, mindful viewing of the images and the self-referential words simply suppressed mental elaboration should be considered. Indeed some elements of mindfulness training are intended to develop the practitioner's capacity to direct attention and focus uninterruptedly on a specified object (commonly the somatic perception of breath). As the skill of the practitioner increases, this type of concentration practice progressively eliminates mind-wandering during the meditation period and elicits pronounced DMN deactivations, as one might expect (Brewer, Worhunsky et al., 2011; Hasenkamp, Wilson-Mendenhall, Duncan, & Barsalou, 2012). However, other mindfulness practices that do not aim to alter the prevalence of mind-wandering, but rather the practitioner's relationship to it, also elicit MPFC and PCC deactivation (Brewer, Worhunsky et al., 2011). In these "choiceless awareness" practices, the intent is to bring nonreactive observation to one's experience, which includes unrestricted spontaneous thought. In the same study, the very experienced meditators (having on average over 10,000 h of practice) showed greater functional connectivity than controls between the PCC and regions associated with self-monitoring and cognitive control (namely the dACC and DLPFC). In the vast majority of contexts, the PCC and these regions are anticorrelated (Fox & Raichle, 2007). In this case, the control subjects showed typical anticorrelation patterns between these structures at baseline, which decreased during meditation, suggesting a state-dependent connectivity pattern in untrained individuals. However, the observed increased connectivity patterns seen in experienced meditators were present both at baseline and during meditation, suggesting that diligent meditation practice may have established a "new" default mode of intrinsic brain activity and connectivity. These neurological findings are consistent with the notion that awareness and affective control are being coupled with spontaneous mental activity, not suppressing it. These findings should be interpreted with caution, however, as this study was cross-sectional and could be influenced by self-selection bias.

Action-monitoring/prediction (e.g., dACC) and cognitive control regions (e.g., DLPFC) have been shown to be important in self-control, addictions, and treatment outcomes (Brewer, Worhunsky, Carroll, Rounsaville, & Potenza, 2008). The above findings from Brewer, Worhunsky et al. (2011), showing that experienced meditators exhibited altered resting-state networks, suggest that mindfulness practice may fundamentally alter brain activity and connectivity patterns in networks important for the perpetuation of addictive behaviors. In essence, mindfulness may help to integrate the capacity to monitor internal and external environments (AI/dACC; see Farb, Segal, & Anderson, 2013), especially when craving or self-referential states arise (likely activating the DMN and its major nodes, the MPFC and PCC), and to utilize self-control (likely activating the DLPFC) when needed. Over time, as the ability to meta-cognitively monitor one's experience strengthens and the processes of craving weaken due to a lack of sustenance, effortful self-control may not be needed as much.

In theory, the more Sally develops her capability to pay attention to her internal and external environments while maintaining affective equipoise, the less fuel she would add to her habitual "coping" strategies of drinking to deal with stress and withdrawal states, leading to the winding-down of her habituated affective self-identity and its eventual cessation. However, prospective studies of individuals receiving mindfulness training for addictions that measure changes in brain activity and connectivity over time are needed to test such hypotheses. We focused mainly on the DMN in this chapter, but studies assessing other possible brain regions/networks that may emerge as prominent players in the neural mechanisms of mindfulness will also be important.

Conclusions and Future Directions

The past century has seen a great leap forward in the understanding of the psychology and neurobiology of behavioral change mechanisms and addiction mechanisms (Goldstein et al., 2009; Kalivas & Volkow, 2005). This impressive body of work has shown remarkable similarities to the ancient Buddhist model, which is aimed at describing the causes and cure of human suffering. Modern treatments that have reframed Buddhist practices for use in addiction treatment have shown preliminary utility. While longitudinal studies will be needed to assess the long-term efficacy of mindfulness-based trainings compared to conventional treatments, it is possible that mindfulness-based approaches offer substantial improvements in the durability of addiction cessation rates. If the Buddhist theory holds, it may also be that mindfulness treatments are able to induce fundamental modifications to neural networks so as to act nonspecifically on the root of craving, rather than on targeted behaviors. Neuroimaging data are beginning to inform the neural mechanisms of mindfulness and how mindfulness practices specifically interface with active addictions. Insight into the functional, structural, and network changes brought about by mindfulness may open the door for improved therapies and therapeutic tools. The initial evidence indicates that meditation practice grants one deeper access to one's own cognitive functions and present-moment experience. With practice, this may lead to more adaptive choices with concomitant decreases in stress and suffering. It is particularly interesting that there are fundamental similarities between the methods of Western empiricism and the methods of Buddhist insight meditation. While the practice of meditation takes many years to master, at essence, all that is required is to simply observe one's experience without preconception and see what one discovers.

References

Andrews-Hanna, J. R., Reidler, J. S., Sepulcre, J., Poulin, R., & Buckner, R. L. (2010). Functional-anatomic fractionation of the brain's default network. *Neuron, 65*, 550–562.

Aron, A., Fisher, H., Mashek, D. J., Strong, G., Li, H., & Brown, L. L. (2005). Reward, motivation, and emotion systems associated with early-stage intense romantic love. *Journal of Neurophysiology, 94*(1), 327–337.

Baker, T. B., Piper, M. E., McCarthy, D. E., Majeskie, M. R., & Fiore, M. C. (2004). Addiction motivation reformulated: An affective processing model of negative reinforcement. *Psychological Review, 111*, 33–51.

Bargh, J. A., & Chartrand, T. L. (1999). The unbearable automaticity of being. *American Psychologist, 54*, 462–479.

Bartels, A., & Zeki, S. (2004). The neural correlates of maternal and romantic love. *NeuroImage, 21*(3), 1155–1166.

Bedi, G., Preston, K. L., Epstein, D. H., Heishman, S. J., Marrone, G. F., Shaham, Y., et al. (2011). Incubation of cue-induced cigarette craving during abstinence in human smokers. *Biological Psychiatry, 69*, 708–711.

Bishop, S. R., Lau, M., Shapiro, S., Carlson, L., Anderson, N. D., Carmody, J., et al. (2004). Mindfulness: A proposed operational definition. *Clinical Psychology: Science and Practice, 11*, 230–241.

Bornemann, B., Herbert, B. M., & Mehling, W. E. (2015). Differential changes in self-reported aspects of interoceptive awareness through 3 months of contemplative training. *Frontiers in Psychology, 5*, 1–13.

Bowen, S., Chawla, N., Collins, S. E., Witkiewitz, K., Hsu, S., Grow, J., et al. (2009). Mindfulness-based relapse prevention for substance use disorders: A pilot efficacy trial. *Substance Abuse, 30*, 295–305.

Bowen, S., & Marlatt, A. (2009). Surfing the urge: Brief mindfulness-based intervention for college student smokers. *Psychology of Addictive Behaviors, 23*, 666–671.

Bowen, S., Witkiewitz, K., Clifasefi, S. L., Grow, J., Chawla, N., Hsu, S. H., et al. (2014). Relative efficacy of mindfulness-based relapse prevention, standard relapse prevention, and treatment as usual for substance use disorders: A randomized clinical trial. *JAMA Psychiatry, 71*(5), 547–556.

Brewer, J. A., Bowen, S., Smith, J. T., Marlatt, G. A., & Potenza, M. N. (2010). Mindfulness-based treatments for co-occurring depression and substance use disorders: What can we learn from the brain? *Addiction, 105*, 1698–1706.

Brewer, J. A., Davis, J. H., & Goldstein, J. (2012). Why is it so hard to pay attention, or is it? Mindfulness, the factors of awakening and reward-based learning. *Mindfulness, 1–6*.

Brewer, J. A., Elwafi, H. M., & Davis, J. H. (2013). Craving to Quit: Psychological models and neurobiological mechanisms of mindfulness training as treatment for addictions. *Psychology of Addictive Behaviors, 27*(2), 366–379.

Brewer, J. A., Mallik, S., Babuscio, T. A., Nich, C., Johnson, H. E., Deleone, C. M., et al. (2011). Mindfulness training for smoking cessation: Results from a randomized controlled trial. *Drug and Alcohol Dependence, 119*, 72–80.

Brewer, J. A., Sinha, R., Chen, J. A., Michalsen, R. N., Babuscio, T. A., Nich, C., et al. (2009). Mindfulness training and stress reactivity in substance abuse: Results from a randomized, controlled stage I pilot study. *Substance Abuse, 30*, 306–317.

Brewer, J. A., Worhunsky, P. D., Carroll, K. M., Rounsaville, B. J., & Potenza, M. N. (2008). Pretreatment brain activation during stroop task is associated with outcomes in cocaine-dependent patients. *Biological Psychiatry, 64*, 998–1004.

Brewer, J. A., Worhunsky, P. D., Gray, J. R., Tang, Y. Y., Weber, J., & Kober, H. (2011). Meditation experience is associated with differences in default mode network activity and connectivity. *Proceedings of the National Academy of Sciences of the United States of America, 108*, 20254–20259.

Brody, A. L., Mandelkern, M. A., Olmstead, R. E., Jou, J., Tiongson, E., Allen, V., et al. (2007). Neural substrates of resisting craving during cigarette cue exposure. *Biological Psychiatry, 62*(6), 642–651.

Buckner, R. L., Andrews-Hanna, J. R., & Schacter, D. L. (2008). The brain's default network: Anatomy, function, and relevance to disease. In A. Kingstone & M. B. Miller (Eds.), *The year in cognitive neuroscience 2008* (pp. 1–38). Malden, MA: Blackwell.

Carmody, J., & Baer, R. (2008). Relationships between mindfulness practice and levels of mindfulness, medical and psychological symptoms and well-being in a mindfulness-based stress reduction program. *Journal of Behavioral Medicine, 31*, 23–33.

Claus, E. D., Ewing, S. W. F., Filbey, F. M., Sabbineni, A., & Hutchison, K. E. (2011). Identifying neurobiological phenotypes associated with alcohol use disorder severity. *Neuropsychopharmacology, 36*(10), 2086–2096.

Cropley, M., Ussher, M., & Charitou, E. (2007). Acute effects of a guided relaxation routine (body scan) on tobacco withdrawal symptoms and cravings in abstinent smokers. *Addiction, 102*, 989–993.

Curtin, J. J., McCarthy, D. E., Piper, M. E., & Baker, T. B. (2006). Implicit and explicit drug motivational processes: A model of boundary conditions. In R. W. Wiers & A. W. Stacy (Eds.), *Handbook of implicit cognition and addiction* (pp. 233–250). Thousand Oaks, CA: Sage.

Davis, J. M., Fleming, M. F., Bonus, K. A., & Baker, T. B. (2007). A pilot study on mindfulness based stress reduction for smokers. *BMC Complementary and Alternative Medicine, 7*, 2.

Desbordes, G., Gard, T., Hoge, E. A., Holzel, B. K., & Kerr, C. (2014). Moving beyond mindfulness: Defining equanimity as an outcome measure in meditation and contemplative research. *Mindfulness, 6*, 356–372.

Elliott, R., Zahn, R., Deakin, J. F., & Anderson, I. M. (2011). Affective cognition and its disruption in mood disorders. *Neuropsychopharmacology, 36*, 153–182.

Elwafi, H. M., Witkiewitz, K., Mallik, S., Thornhill, T. A., 4th, & Brewer, J. A. (2013). Mindfulness training for smoking cessation: Moderation of the relationship between craving and cigarette use. *Drug and Alcohol Dependence, 130*, 222–229.

Engelmann, J. M., Versace, F., Robinson, J. D., & Minnix, J. A. (2012). Neural substrates of smoking cue reactivity: A meta-analysis of fMRI studies. *NeuroImage, 60*, 252–262.

Fan, J., Xu, P., Van Dam, N. T., Eilam, T., Gu, X., Luo, Y., et al. (2012). Spontaneous brain fluctuations relate to autonomic arousal. *Journal of Neurosicence, 15*, 11176–11186.

Farb, N. A., Segal, Z. V., Mayberg, H., Bean, J., McKeon, D., Fatima, Z., et al. (2007). Attending to the present: Mindfulness meditation reveals distinct neural modes of self-reference. *Social, Cognitive, and Affective Neuroscience, 2*, 313–322.

Farb, N. A., Segal, Z. V., & Anderson, A. K. (2013). Mindfulness meditation training alters cortical representations of interoceptive attention. *Social, Cognitive, and Affective Neuroscience, 8*, 15–26.

Ferguson, S. G., Shiffman, S., & Gwaltney, C. J. (2006). Does reducing withdrawal severity mediate nicotine patch efficacy? A randomized clinical trial. *Journal of Consulting and Clinical Psychology, 74*, 1153–1161.

Fiore, M. C., Jaen, C. R., Baker, T. B., Bailey, W. C., Bennowitz, N. L., Curry, S. J., et al. (2008). *Treating tobacco use and dependence: 2008 update*. Washington, DC: U.S. Department of Health and Human Services.

Fox, M. D., & Raichle, M. E. (2007). Spontaneous fluctuations in brain activity observed with functional magnetic resonance imaging. *Nature Reviews Neuroscience, 8*, 700–711.

Garrison, K. A., Scheinost, D., Worhunsky, P. D., Elwafi, H. M., Thornhill, T. A., 4th, Thompson, E., et al. (2013). Real-time fMRI links subjective experience with brain activity during focused attention. *NeuroImage, 81*(C), 110–118.

Gifford, E. V., Kohlenberg, B. S., Hayes, S. C., Antonuccio, D. O., Piasecki, M. M., Rasmussen-Hall, M. L., et al. (2004). Acceptance-based treatment for smoking cessation. *Behavior Therapy, 35*, 689–705.

Goldstein, R. Z., Craig, A. D., Bechara, A., Garavan, H., Childress, A. R., Paulus, M. P., et al. (2009). The neurocircuitry of impaired insight in drug addiction. *Trends in Cognitive Sciences, 13*, 372–380.

Goyal, M., Singh, S., Sibinga, E. M. S., Gould, N. F., Rowland-Seymour, A., Sharma, R., et al. (2014). Meditation programs for psychological stress and well-being: A systematic review and meta-analysis. *JAMA Internal Medicine, 174*(3), 357–368.

Grabovac, A., Lau, M., & Willett, B. (2011). Mechanisms of mindfulness: A Buddhist psychological model. *Mindfulness, 2*, 154–166.

Hasenkamp, W., Wilson-Mendenhall, C. D., Duncan, E., & Barsalou, L. W. (2012). Mind wandering and attention during focused meditation: A fine-grained temporal analysis of fluctuating cognitive states. *NeuroImage, 59*(1), 750–760.

Hölzel, B. K., Lazar, S. W., Gard, T., Schuman-Olivier, Z., Vago, D. R., & Ott, U. (2011). How does mindfulness meditation work? Proposing mechanisms of action from a conceptual and neural perspective. *Perspectives on Psychological Science, 6*, 537–559.

Janes, A. C., Pizzagalli, D. A., Richardt, S., de Frederick, B., Chuzi, S., Pachas, G., et al. (2010). Brain reactivity to smoking cues prior to smoking cessation predicts ability to maintain tobacco abstinence. *Biological Psychiatry, 67*(8), 722–729.

Kalivas, P. W., & Volkow, N. D. (2005). The neural basis of addiction: A pathology of motivation and choice. *American Journal of Psychiatry, 162*, 1403–1413.

Kosten, T. R., Scanley, B. E., Tucker, K. A., Oliveto, A., Prince, C., Sinha, R., et al. (2006). Cue-induced brain activity changes and relapse in cocaine-dependent patients. *Neuropsychopharmacology, 31*(3), 644–650.

Law, M., & Tang, J. L. (1995). An analysis of the effectiveness of interventions intended to help people stop smoking. *Archives of Internal Medicine, 155*, 1933–1941.

Lazev, A. B., Herzog, T. A., & Brandon, T. H. (1999). Classical conditions of environmental cues to cigarette smoking. *Experimental and Clinical Psychopharmacology, 7*, 56–63.

Meshi, D., Morawetz, C., & Heekeren, H. R. (2013). Nucleus accumbens response to gains in reputation for the self relative to gains for others predicts social media use. *Frontiers in Human Neuroscience, 7*, 1–11.

Muraven, M., & Baumeister, R. F. (2000). Self-regulation and depletion of limited resources: Does self-control resemble a muscle? *Psychological Bulletin, 126*, 247–259.

Ñāṇamoli, B., & Bodhi, B. (trans). (1995). *The middle length discourses of the Buddha: A translation of the Majjhima Nikāya*. Boston: Wisdom.

Nargeot, R., & Simmers, J. (2011). Neural mechanisms of operant conditioning and learning-induced behavioral plasticity in Aplysia. *Cellular and Molecular Life Sciences, 68*(5), 803–816.

Niaura, R., & Abrams, D. B. (2002). Smoking cessation: Progress, priorities, and prospectus. *Journal of Consulting and Clinical Psychology, 70*, 494–509.

Nyanaponika, T. (2000). *The vision of Dhamma: Buddhist writings of Nyanponika Thera* (2nd ed.). Seattle: Buddhist Publication Society.

Office of National Drug Control Policy. (2007). *The economic costs of drug abuse in the United States*. Retrieved January 25, 2015, from http://www.whitehouse.gov/ondcp

Ortner, C. N. M., Kilner, S. J., & Zelazo, P. D. (2007). Mindfulness meditation and reduced emotional interference on a cognitive task. *Motivation and Emotion, 31*, 271–283.

Raichle, M. E., MacLeod, A. M., Snyder, A. Z., Powers, W. J., Gusnard, D. A., & Shulman, G. L. (2001). A default mode of brain function. *Proceedings of the National Academy of Sciences of the United States of America, 98*(2), 676–682.

Robinson, T. E., & Berridge, K. C. (2008). The incentive sensitization theory of addiction: Some current issues. *Philosophical Transactions of the Royal Society, B: Biological Sciences, 363*, 3137–3146.

Shonin, E., Van Gordon, W., & Griffiths, M. D. (2014). The emerging role of Buddhism in clinical psychology: Toward effective integration. *Psychology of Religion and Spirituality, 6*(2), 123–137.

Silverstein, R. G., Brown, A. H., Roth, H. D., & Britton, W. B. (2011). Effects of mindfulness training on body awareness to sexual stimuli: Implications for female sexual dysfunction. *Psychosomatic Medicine, 73*, 817–825.

Tang, D. W., Fellows, L. K., Small, D. M., & Dagher, A. (2012). Food and drug cues activate similar brain regions: A meta-analysis of functional MRI studies. *Physiology & Behavior, 106*(3), 317–324.

Tapert, S. F., Cheung, E. H., Brown, G. G., Frank, L. R., Paulus, M. P., Schweinsburg, A. D., et al. (2003). Neural response to alcohol stimuli in adolescents with alcohol use disorder. *Archives of General Psychiatry, 60*(7), 727–735.

Taylor, V. A., Grant, J., Daneault, V., Scavone, G., Breton, E., Roffe-Vidal, S., et al. (2011). Impact of mindfulness on the neural responses to emotional pictures in experienced and beginner meditators. *NeuroImage, 57*, 1524–1533.

Thanissaro, B., trans. (2010). *Dhammacakkappavattana Sutta: Setting in motion the wheel of truth (SN 56.11)*. Retrieved October 7, 2011, from http://www.accesstoinsight.org/tipitaka/sn/sn56/sn56.011.than.html

Treat, T. A., Viken, R. J., Kruschke, J. K., & McFall, R. M. (2011). Men's memory for women's sexual-interest and rejection cues. *Applied Cognitive Psychology, 25*(1), 802–810.

Whitfield-Gabrieli, S., & Ford, J. M. (2012). Default mode network activity and connectivity in psychopathology. *Annual Review of Clinical Psychology, 8*(1), 49–76.

Whitfield-Gabrieli, S., Moran, J. M., Nieto-Castañón, A., Triantafyllou, C., Saxe, R., & Gabrieli, J. D. E. (2011). Associations and dissociations between default and self-reference networks in the human brain. *NeuroImage, 55*(1), 225–232.

Witkiewitz, K., & Bowen, S. (2010). Depression, craving, and substance use following a randomized trial of mindfulness-based relapse prevention. *Journal of Consulting and Clinical Psychology, 78*, 362–374.

Zgierska, A., Rabago, D., Chawla, N., Kushner, K., Koehler, R., & Marlatt, A. (2009). Mindfulness meditation for substance use disorders: A systematic review. *Substance Abuse, 30*, 266–294.

Zgierska, A., Rabago, D., Zuelsdorff, M., Coe, C., Miller, M., & Fleming, M. (2008). Mindfulness meditation for alcohol relapse prevention: A feasibility pilot study. *Journal of Addiction Medicine, 2*, 165–173.

Chapter 10
Mindfulness for the Treatment of Psychosis: State of the Art and Future Developments

Álvaro I. Langer, José A. Carmona-Torres, William Van Gordon, and Edo Shonin

Introduction

In conjunction with competencies such as ethical awareness, compassion, and loving-kindness, mindfulness is a key component of the Buddhist path to spiritual awakening (Brito, 2013). In the late 1970s, Jon Kabat-Zinn extracted and synthesised aspects of the Buddhist mindfulness teachings into a secular group intervention, called Mindfulness-Based Stress Reduction (MBSR). Mindfulness has positioned itself in the last decade as a key area of scientific development, and recent meta-analyses indicate that mindfulness can be effective for treating various psychopathologies, particularly anxiety and depression (Hofmann, Sawyer, Witt, & Oh, 2010). There is also growing evidence suggesting that mindfulness leads to immune system improvements and neuroplastic changes in the brain (Hölzel et al., 2011). However, despite growing scientific interest into the health benefits of mindfulness, there is limited research examining the suitability of mindfulness as a treatment for psychosis.

Á.I. Langer (✉)
Millennium Institute for the Study of Depression and Personality,
School of Psychology, Pontifical Catholic University of Chile, Santiago, Chile
e-mail: alvaro.langer@gmail.com

J.A. Carmona-Torres
Department of Psychology, University of Almeria, Almeria, Spain

W. Van Gordon • E. Shonin
Awake to Wisdom, Centre for Meditation and Mindfulness Research, Nottingham, UK

Bodhayati School of Buddhism, Nottingham, UK

Division of Psychology, Chaucer Building, Nottingham Trent University,
Burton Street, Nottingham, UK
e-mail: e.shonin@awaketowisdom.co.uk

E. Shonin et al. (eds.), *Mindfulness and Buddhist-Derived Approaches in Mental Health and Addiction*, Advances in Mental Health and Addiction,
DOI 10.1007/978-3-319-22255-4_10

While current diagnostic manuals of mental disorders, such as ICD-10 or DSM-5, present psychosis as a specific set of symptoms (e.g., hallucinations or delusions), based on the subjective experiences of individuals who have experienced psychosis, the condition can be characterised by the presence of: (1) a deep state of personal confusion regarding what is real in the individual's inner and external world and (2) stress and conflict for both the individual and their families (Hayward, Awenat, McCarthy Jones, Paulik, & Berry, 2014; British Psychological Society Division of Clinical Psychology, 2014). The National Institute for Health and Care Excellence (NICE) advocates the use of cognitive behavioural therapy (CBT) for treating individuals with psychosis and schizophrenia (NICE, 2014). However, given the functional consequences and complexity of the condition, CBT is not an effective treatment for all individuals with psychosis, and relapse is not uncommon (Shonin, Van Gordon, & Griffiths, 2014a).

Consequently, a key direction in treatment-related psychosis research has been the formulation and empirical validation of interventions that advocate and impart new ways of relating to psychotic experiences. Mindfulness-based interventions (MBIs) have assumed an important role in this respect due to the manner in which they target reducing the sources of stress (i.e., rather than eliminate symptoms such as hallucinations) and promote healthy engagement (or reengagement) with meaningful experiences and interpersonal interactions (Chadwick, Taylor, & Abba, 2005; Gaudiano & Herbert, 2006).

However, despite encouraging findings concerning the application of MBIs in psychosis, some clinicians are of the view that mindfulness (and/or meditation) can trigger an increase in psychotic symptoms and that it is thus an inappropriate treatment for this target group (Chadwick, 2014). The present chapter focuses on these issues and undertakes a timely appraisal of the role of MBIs in the treatment of psychosis. We evaluate key quantitative and qualitative research findings and make recommendations relating to future research directions and the effective use of mindfulness in psychosis treatment settings.

Mindfulness in the Field of Psychosis

Overview of Key Findings from Quantitative Studies

In one of the first studies investigating the role of mindfulness in the treatment of psychosis, Chadwick et al. (2005) conducted an uncontrolled study in which mindfulness was taught to individuals with current, subjectively distressing psychosis. During the six-session (each of 90-min duration) group intervention, participants practised a range of mindfulness techniques including: (1) a brief body scan, (2) mindfulness of breathing, and (3) 'choiceless awareness'. Prolonged periods of silence were avoided and participants received an audiotape of guided meditations to facilitate at-home practice. The results showed an improvement in ability to regulate distressing thoughts and images, and participants' levels of general well-being and mindfulness also improved. The same mindfulness techniques were subsequently employed in a small ($n=22$) randomised controlled trial (RCT) in which participants' (all of whom were experiencing psychosis-related distress) levels of subjective well-being and mindfulness skills were improved following the intervention (i.e., relative to participants in the wait-list control group) (Chadwick, Hughes, Russell, Russell, & Dagnan, 2009).

Dannahy et al. (2011) conducted an uncontrolled study to investigate the effects of person-based cognitive therapy (PBCT) on individuals experiencing distressing voices. PBCT incorporates mindfulness and is based on the principle of acceptance of both voices and self in order to enhance well-being and reduce distress. At the end of the treatment, participants demonstrated improvements in general quality of life as well as in their ability to accept and regulate auditory hallucinations. These interventional gains were maintained at 1-month follow-up.

A further uncontrolled study involved 16 patients recovering from a first episode of psychosis (van der Valk, van de Waerdt, Meijer, van den Hout, & de Haan, 2013). Participants were offered mindfulness-based therapy consisting of eight 1-h sessions that were conducted within a 4-week time span. No significant increase in psychotic symptoms was observed, and participants demonstrated a decrease in agoraphobic and psycho-neuroticism symptoms.

In a small RCT, 23 patients with a schizophrenia-spectrum disorder participated in a mindfulness intervention for 8 weeks (weekly sessions of 60-min duration). Participants received a CD of guided meditations in order to facilitate daily self-practice. Compared to the control group, participants demonstrated significant improvements in their ability to accept distressing thoughts and to regulate stressful internal events (Langer, Cangas, Salcedo, & Fuentes, 2012).

A further RCT assessed the effects of a mindfulness-based psychoeducational programme (MBPP) on Chinese outpatients ($n=96$) with schizophrenia. MBPP includes guided awareness exercises and homework practice within a psychoeducational framework (e.g., in order to increase participants' insight into their illness and symptoms). The results showed significant improvements in the intervention group (i.e., compared to the treatment-as-usual control group) in illness insight, severity of symptoms, adaptive psychosocial functioning, and the number and length of re-hospitalisations at 18 months post-treatment (Chien & Lee, 2013).

Although the abovementioned studies suggest that mindfulness appears to ameliorate psychotic symptoms, the generalisability of findings is limited by factors such as: (1) small sample sizes, (2) inadequately defined and inactive control conditions (i.e., not controlling for potential confounding factors such as therapeutic alliance, group interaction, etc.), (3) heterogeneity between intervention types (i.e., differences in treatment duration, facilitator contact hours, use of non-meditative techniques, etc.), (4) fidelity of implementation not assessed (i.e., the extent to which facilitators deviated from the planned delivery format), and (5) adherence to practice not assessed (Shonin, Van Gordon, & Griffiths, 2014b). See Table10.1 for an overview of key study characteristics and outcomes.

Table 10.1 Characteristics of quantitative studies of mindfulness-based interventions in Psychosis (MBIp)

Study	Sample	Intervention: type and length	Group experimental (dropout) (n)	Study Design (follow-up)	Measures	Statistical significance or effect size
Chien and Lee (2013)	$n=96$ Schizophrenia Mean age: 29.4 years	MBPP 12 sessions, twice a week, 120 min	48 (3)	RCT Control: Usual Care (18 months follow-up)	– ITAQ – BPRS – SSQ-6 – SLOF – Rehospitalisation (number/duration)	[B]ITAQ $F=5.80$** BPRS $F=4.00$** SLOF $F=3.73$* Rehospitalisation Number $F=4.03$** Duration $F=5.75$**
Chadwick et al. (2009)	$n=22$ Schizophrenia spectrum disorders with distressing voices Mean age: 41.6 years	MBIp 5 weeks of group plus home practice (twice a week) and 5 further weeks of home practice	11 (2)	RCT Control: Wait list (no follow-up)	– CORE – SMQ – PSYRATS – SMVQ – BAVQ-r	Within-groups comparison CORE $p=0.013$ SMQ (thoughts and images) $p=0.037$
Chadwick et al. (2005)	$n=14$ Schizophrenia spectrum disorders Mean age: 33.1 years	MBIp 6 sessions, once a week, 90 min	14 (3)	Non-controlled (no follow-up)	– CORE – SMQ	CORE $p=0.008$ SMQ For distressing thoughts/images, all participants scored higher post group: mean increase of 36.6 %

Dannahy et al. (2011)	$n=62$ Schizophrenia spectrum disorders with distressing voices Mean age: 41.1 years	PBCT 8–12 sessions, twice a week, 90 min	62 (12)	Non-controlled (1-month follow-up)	– CORE-OM – Voice distress – Voice control – VAY Voice Intrusiveness – VAY Voice dominance – VAY Hearer Distance – VAY Hearer Dependence	CORE Total: $d=0.57$ $d=0.63$ (follow-up) Voice distress: $d=0.75$ $d=0.95$ (follow-up) Voice control $d=0.62$ $d=0.52$ (follow-up)
Langer et al. (2012)	$n=23$ Schizophrenia spectrum disorders Mean age of experimental group: 34.7 years	MBIp 8 sessions, once a week, 60 min	11 (4)	RCT Control: wait list (no follow-up)	– CGI-SCH – AAQII – SMQ	SMQ $p=0.028$
van der Valk et al. (2013)	$n=16$ Schizophrenia spectrum disorders patients recovery from a first psychotic episode Mean age: 31.8 years	MBIp 4 sessions, once a week, 60 min	16 (3)	Non-controlled (1-month follow-up)	– PANSS – SCL-90 – SMQ – CSQ-8	Agoraphobic symptoms: $p=0.028$ Psychoneuroticism: $p=0.025$ Satisfied with therapy: 62 % good 23 % excellent

Notes by study: *MBPP* mindfulness-based psychoeducation programme, *ITAQ* insight and treatment attitudes questionnaire, *BPRS* brief psychiatric rating scale, *SSQ-6* social support questionnaire, *SLOF* specific level of functioning scale, [B] 18 months follow-up results, *MBIp* mindfulness-based intervention for psychosis, *CORE* clinical outcomes in routine evaluation, *SMQ* southampton mindfulness questionnaire, *PSYRATS* psychiatric symptom rating scale, *SMVQ* southampton mindfulness voices questionnaire, *BAVQ-r* beliefs about voices questionnaire revised, *PBCT* person-based cognitive psychotherapy, *VAY* voice and you, *CGI-SCH* clinical global impression-schizophrenia scale, *AAQ II* acceptance and action scale, *PANSS* the positive and negative syndrome scale, *SCL-90* the symptoms checklist 90, *CSQ-8* the client satisfaction questionnaire

Overview of Key Findings from Qualitative Studies

Abba, Chadwick, and Stevenson (2008) utilised grounded theory analysis (Glaser & Strauss, 1967) in order to cast light on the process of how people with distressing psychosis learn to respond mindfully to unpleasant experiences. The sample comprised 16 participants (4 women and 12 men; age range 22–58) with chronic, treatment-resistant positive symptoms (including paranoia and hallucinations). The questions administered during the semi-structured interviews addressed the following topics: (1) how participants experienced the group, (2) experience of practising mindfulness, (3) how participants would describe mindfulness, (4) aspects of the programme that could be improved, and (5) general comments about their experiences. Following the mindfulness intervention, findings demonstrated that participants were able to relate differently to psychosis. The authors proposed a key shift, through a three-stage process, wherein participants changed their relationship with their symptoms: (1) centering in awareness of psychosis, (2) allowing voices, thoughts, and images to come and go without reacting or struggle, and (3) reclaiming autonomy through acceptance of psychosis and the self.

In order to address the paucity of research relating to how people with early psychosis respond to mindfulness-based therapy, Ashcroft, Barrow, Lee, and MacKinnon (2012) employed grounded theory to explore the experiences of nine participants recruited from an early intervention for psychosis service. Participants received a group mindfulness intervention based on person-centred therapy. Seventeen themes emerged from the coded data, which were grouped into four categories: (1) making use of mindfulness, (2) making sense of mindfulness (i.e., in the context of improving coping skills), (3) relating to people differently, and (4) greater self-understanding and acceptance. Although participants initially found mindfulness a difficult concept to come to terms with, the learning process and associated salutary outcomes were facilitated by the group-based delivery format.

The specific effects of mindfulness on anxiety in people with schizophrenia were investigated by Brown, Davis, LaRocco, and Strasburger (2010). The qualitative study comprised 15 males (age range, 45–58; mean age, 51 [$SD = 4.78$]) with a diagnosis of schizophrenia ($n = 5$) or schizoaffective disorder ($n = 10$). An inclusion criterion was the presence of anxiety symptoms whilst being in a stable, post-acute phase of schizophrenia. Examples of questions posed during the semi-structured interviews are: *'Have you noticed any ways in which you have benefited from practising mindfulness?'*; *'Has anything about the program caused you to feel uncomfortable in any way?'*; and *'What keeps you coming back to classes?'* The four most frequent themes to emerge from the data analysis were: (1) relaxation, (2) symptom reduction, (3) ability to focus on the present moment, and (4) cognitive changes. All participants reported relief from hallucinations (and ten reported relief from delusions) following completion of the intervention. Participants also reported improvements with regard to anxiety, depression, paranoia, memory problems, sleep problems, and somatic pain.

Dennick, Fox, and Walter-Brice (2013) utilised interpretative phenomenological analysis (IPA) (Smith, Flowers, & Larkin, 2009) in order to explore participants' 'lived experiences' of mindfulness group practice. The sample comprised three adults (age range, 30–40) who were experiencing distressing psychosis. Four primary themes emerged from the dataset: (1) experiencing distress (i.e., associated with experiences of psychosis), (2) the group as a safe environment to explore experiences of hearing voices (and of practising mindfulness), (3) mindfulness as beneficial (i.e., changing the way participants relate to distressing experiences, including reacting mindfully to voices instead of struggling), and (4) group interaction as part of the process of recovery (involving re-establishing or re-affirming a sense of self).

Consistent with a number of other studies, including that of Abba et al. (2008), mindfulness provided the participants with an 'open space' where they could explore concerns and fears such as societal labelling and feelings of ostracisation. This creation of 'shared meanings' through interaction with others proved to be constructive and positive. The participants of this study also described experiencing a greater intuitive awareness of self, thus developing a sense of agency and a desire to respond mindfully to feelings of distress. It appears that taking part in the mindfulness groups helped participants to cultivate 'metacognitive awareness', allowing them to change how they respond to experiences such as hearing voices. Participants reported being able to make use of mindfulness in various life situations including family struggles and stressful situations. None of the participants reported experiencing difficulty in learning or practising mindfulness (Dennick et al., 2013).

Using a thematic analysis approach, May, Strauss, Coyle, and Hayward (2014) evaluated the experiences of individuals who had enrolled in person-based cognitive therapy in order to alleviate distressing voices. Ten individuals (age range, 36–55; mean age, 47.2) diagnosed with schizophrenia ($n = 8$), post-traumatic stress disorder ($n = 1$), and non-specified personality disorder ($n = 1$) participated in this study. The interview explored participants' experiences across six broad areas: (1) reasons for attending the group, (2) expectations of the group therapy interactions, (3) experience and understanding of the therapeutic process, (4) understanding auditory hallucinations, (5) sense of self, and (6) levels of well-being following the intervention.

The analysis of the data generated three themes that corresponded to how participants changed the way they relate to: (1) voices (i.e., through developing mindfulness skills), (2) the self (i.e., developing a separate and positive identity compared to one dominated and defined by voices), and (3) other people (i.e., empowerment in societal roles and social relationships). Participants reported that they found mindfulness practice to be beneficial, and participants spoke of the voices becoming 'quieter' and 'more distant'. Most participants reported practising and making use of mindfulness outside of the group therapy sessions. These outcomes support Abba et al.'s (2008) earlier finding that mindfulness can change the relationship that individuals with psychosis have with their internal experiences (i.e., by observing and relating to their symptoms with greater perceptual distance).

What Do We Know About the Iatrogenic Effects of Mindfulness?

There is some small-scale clinical evidence to suggest that over-intensive meditation practice can induce psychotic episodes—including in people who do not have a history of psychiatric illness. A summary of the cases extant in the peer-reviewed clinical and scientific literature are as follows:

1. Three individuals with a history of schizophrenia who experienced acute psychotic episodes whilst engaging in meditation retreats (Walsh & Roche, 1979).
2. Two individuals previously diagnosed with schizotypal personality disorder who experienced acute psychosis following meditation (Garcia-Trujillo, Monterrey, & Gonzalez de Riviera, 1992).
3. Three individuals with a psychiatric history who experienced psychotic symptoms following meditation practice (Chan-ob & Boonyanaruthee, 1999).
4. A 25-year-old female graduate student in whom delusional episodes accompanied by violent outbursts and inappropriate laughter were induced by meditation (Yorston, 2001).
5. Two individuals without a history of psychiatric illness who experienced psychotic experiences following meditation practice (Sethi & Subhash, 2003).
6. A male patient who experienced an acute and transient psychotic episode following meditation (Kuijpers, van der Heijden, Tuinier, & Verhoeven, 2007)

Although the above-mentioned studies indicate that meditation can induce psychotic episodes, it is important to examine the quality and reliability of this evidence. In other words, these findings should be considered in light of their many limitations, including the fact that all of these studies: (1) utilised very low participant numbers, (2) did not employ a control condition, and (3) involved participants who in some cases had a history of psychiatric illness (Shonin et al., 2014b).

It is also important to note that in the majority of the studies outlined above, participants were invariably engaging in very intensive meditation retreats (in some cases, this involved 18 h of meditation practice per day that was accompanied by lengthy periods of fasting and/or silence). For these participants, practising meditation for up to 18 h per day—under conditions of silence and/or fasting—most probably reflected a sudden change to their normal daily routine. Within Buddhism, a philosophy of quality as opposed to quantity of meditation is widely advocated, and practising meditation in an extreme and potentially stressful manner is discouraged (Shonin et al., 2014b). This is consistent with the view in Western psychology that stress is a key risk factor for psychosis. Therefore, even for those individuals who did not have a history of psychiatric illness, it is perhaps unsurprising that engaging in intensive meditation retreats led to psychotic episodes.

A further consideration when evaluating the above evidence is that most of the studies provided insufficient information in terms of the exact modality of meditation that was employed (Shonin et al., 2014b). Therefore, it is very difficult to conclusively isolate mindfulness (i.e., as opposed to other forms of meditation) as the source of the psychotic episodes. This is a particularly important consideration because numerous reports of adverse effects exist for non-mindfulness variants of meditation such as Transcendental Meditation and Qigong. Examples of such adverse effects reported for these types of meditation include panic attacks, musculoskeletal pain, anti-social behaviour, impaired reality testing, dissociation, guilt, uncomfortable kinaesthetic sensations, despair, suicidal feelings, and exhaustion (Perez-De-Albeniz & Holmes, 2000; Shonin et al., 2014b). Thus, although techniques such as mindfulness meditation, Transcendental Meditation, and Qigong can be broadly grouped together as modalities of 'meditation', it is important to note that these techniques represent fundamentally different approaches. For instance, Transcendental Meditation is a commercial technique introduced in the 1950s by Maharishi Mahesh Yogi—it includes mantra recitation and derives from Hinduism. Conversely, mindfulness is a 2500-year-old Buddhist practice and does not include chanting or mantra recitation—it primarily focuses on breath and present-moment awareness (Shonin et al., 2014b).

Another related factor that limits the generalisability of findings from the above-mentioned studies is that little or no information was provided on the levels of experience or competency of the meditation instructor. The extent to which a meditation instructor is able to impart an 'authentic embodied transmission' of the meditation teachings is a factor that considerably affects outcomes (Van Gordon, Shonin, Griffiths, & Singh, 2015). Indeed, poorly administered meditation training can lead to adverse health effects including: (1) asociality, (2) nihilistic and/or defeatist outlooks, (3) dependency on meditative 'bliss' (Sanskrit:*prīti*), (4) a more generalised addiction to meditation, (5) engaging in compassionate activity beyond one's spiritual capacity (and at the expense of psychological well-being), and (6) spiritual materialism (a form of self-deception in which rather than potentiating spiritual development and subduing selfish or egotistical tendencies, meditation practice serves only to increase ego-attachment and narcissistic behaviour) (Shonin, Van Gordon, & Griffiths, 2015).

Discussion

In the words of the British Psychological Society Division of Clinical Psychology (2014):

> It is vital that mental health workers are open to different ways of understanding experiences, and do not insist that people see their difficulties in terms of an illness. This simple change will have a profound and transformative effect on our mental health services (p. 72).

To be in touch with the inner world of people with psychosis is challenging for clinicians, and both skill and experience are required in order to avoid anxiety being introduced into the therapeutic relationship (Fromm-Reichmann, 1960). In the treatment of psychosis, clinician competencies of acceptance, patience, and letting go should be driven by an understanding of the 'worldview' of the individual with psychotic experiences and by an appreciation of how these experiences could be an attempt to make sense and cope—albeit in a maladaptive manner—with significant events in their life. Thus, for treating individuals with psychosis, the importance of establishing a strong therapeutic alliance cannot be over-emphasised (Pinto, 2009). Learning to objectify distressing thoughts and voices is a key objective of psychotherapy, and shorter (i.e., 15 min) rather than prolonged periods of formal seated meditation practice are preferred (Wyatt, Harper, & Weatherhead, 2014).

By practising mindfulness themselves, clinicians can improve their capacity to be fully present, thereby creating an atmosphere that allows the client to freely express their world. Although some therapists have undoubtedly acquired this skill without necessarily engaging in mindfulness practice, mindfulness is likely to help clinicians cope with transferrable emotional distress as well as the various psychological demands placed on the therapist (Siegel, 2010).

Based on an overview of key empirical findings, mindfulness appears to be an effective treatment for individuals with psychosis. Findings demonstrate that mindfulness can lead to improvements in: (1) general psychological functioning, (2) ability to regulate positive and negative symptoms, (3) non-psychotic symptoms (e.g., agoraphobia), and (4) diminution of re-hospitalisations (both number and duration). Qualitative studies demonstrate that mindfulness can help participants relate differently to symptoms and exert greater 'control' over how they respond to unpleasant experiences (e.g., Abba et al., 2008). Mindfulness appears to help individuals with psychosis by allowing them to mindfully notice their internal experiences—no matter if these are pleasant or unpleasant—in the context of cultivating a more adaptive sense of self (Dennick et al., 2013; May et al., 2014). Thus, instead of being 'paralysed' by voices, hallucinations, or undesirable thoughts, individuals with psychosis can objectify such experiences and use them to foster greater self-understanding and ultimately greater levels of well-being (Ashcroft et al., 2012). Findings indicate that mindfulness taught in the contexts of a group setting is a particularly effective means for eliciting such well-being and for helping participants to successfully integrate mindfulness into everyday life situations (e.g., family, job, etc.).

However, despite promising outcomes, further RCTs that use larger sample sizes are required in order to replicate findings (Shonin et al., 2014b). In addition to addressing this issue, future studies should focus not only on individuals currently experiencing psychosis (either first episode or chronic) but also on individuals: (1) deemed to be 'at risk mental state' (ARMS) for psychosis, (2) with distressing psychotic-like experiences (Langer, Cangas, & Gallego, 2010), and (3) those that provide a supporting role in the context of a family member or caregiver (Carmona-Torres & García-Montes, 2010). Future research could also assess the possible impact of mindfulness on cognitive impairments as well as structural and functional brain abnormalities reported in psychosis (Smieskova et al., 2013).

In terms of adverse effects, there is some small-scale clinical evidence that suggesting that meditation can induce psychotic episodes in individuals with or without a psychiatric history. However, the quality of this evidence is highly questionable—especially when viewed in light of the abundance of more methodologically robust evidence indicating that mindfulness and meditation improve somatic, psychological, and spiritual well-being (Shonin et al., 2014b). Thus, although poorly practiced or poorly taught meditation can actually be harmful to a person's health, where mindfulness and meditation are taught by an experienced and authentic teacher who is aware of all of the risks, we conclude that adverse side effects are unlikely.

Acknowledgments AIL is supported by the Chilean National Fund for Scientific and Technological Development, PAI, Project N° 8213005 and by the Fund for Innovation and Competitiveness (FIC) of the Chilean Ministry of Economy, Development and Tourism, through the Millennium Scientific Initiative, Grant N° IS130005.

References

Abba, N., Chadwick, P., & Stevenson, C. (2008). Responding mindfully to distressing psychosis: A grounded theory analysis. *Psychotherapy Research, 18*, 77–87. doi:10.1080/10503300701367992.

Ashcroft, K., Barrow, F., Lee, R., & MacKinnon, K. (2012). Mindfulness groups for early psychosis: A qualitative study. *Psychology and Psychotherapy: Theory, Research and Practice, 85*, 327–334. doi:10.1111/j.2044-8341.2011.02031.

British Psychological Society Division of Clinical Psychology. (2014). *Understanding psychosis and schizophrenia*. Available from URL: http://www.bps.org.uk

Brito, G. (2013). Rethinking mindfulness in the therapeutic relationship. *Mindfulness, 5*, 351–359.

Brown, L. F., Davis, L. W., LaRocco, V. A., & Strasburger, A. (2010). Participant perspectives on mindfulness meditation training for anxiety in schizophrenia. *American Journal of Psychiatric Rehabilitation, 13*, 224–242. doi:10.1080/15487768.2010.501302.

Carmona-Torres, J. A., & García-Montes, J. M. (2010). Terapia de Aceptación y Compromiso (ACT) para el tratamiento de los síntomas psicóticos. In A. J. Cangas & V. Ibañez (Eds.), *Nuevas Perspectivas en el Tratamiento del Trastorno Mental Grave* (pp. 133–160). Granada: Alborán Editores.

Chadwick, P. (2014). Mindfulness for psychosis. *British Journal of Psychiatry, 204*, 333–334.

Chadwick, P., Hughes, S., Russell, D., Russell, I., & Dagnan, D. (2009). Mindfulness groups for distressing voices and paranoia: A replication and randomized feasibility trial. *Behavioural and Cognitive Psychotherapy, 37*, 403–412.

Chadwick, P., Taylor, K. N., & Abba, N. (2005). Mindfulness groups for people with psychosis. *Behavioural and Cognitive Psychotherapy, 33*, 351–359.

Chan-ob, T., & Boonyanaruthee, V. (1999). Meditation in association with psychosis. *Journal of Medical Association of Thailand, 82*, 925–929.

Chien, W. T., & Lee, I. Y. M. (2013). The mindfulness-based psychoeducation program for Chinese patients with schizophrenia. *Psychiatric Services, 64*, 376–379.

Dannahy, L., Hayward, M., Strauss, C., Turton, W., Harding, E., & Chadwick, P. (2011). Group person-based cognitive therapy for distressing voices: Pilot data from nine groups. *Journal of Behavior Therapy and Experimental Psychiatry, 42*, 111–116.

Dennick, L., Fox, A. P., & Walter-Brice, A. (2013). Mindfulness groups for people experiencing distressing psychosis: An interpretative phenomenological analysis. *Mental Health Review Journal, 18*, 32–43. doi:10.1108/13619321311310009.

Fromm-Reichmann, F. (1960). *Principles of intensive psychotherapy*. Chicago: University of Chicago Press.

Garcia-Trujillo, R., Monterrey, A. L., & Gonzalez de Riviera, J. L. (1992). Meditación y psicosis. *Psiquis Revista de Psiquiatría Psicología y Psicosomática, 13*, 39–43.

Gaudiano, B. A., & Herbert, J. D. (2006). Acute treatment of inpatients with psychotic symptoms using acceptance and commitment therapy: Pilot results. *Behaviour Research and Therapy, 44*, 415–437.

Glaser, B. G., & Strauss, A. L. (1967). *Discovery of grounded theory*. Chicago, IL: Aldine.

Hayward, M., Awenat, Y., McCarthy Jones, S., Paulik, G., & Berry, K. (2014). Beyond beliefs: A qualitative study of people's opinions about their changing relations with their voices. *Psychosis, 12*, doi:10.1080/17522439.2014.926388

Hofmann, S. G., Sawyer, A. T., Witt, A. A., & Oh, D. (2010). The effect of mindfulness-based therapy on anxiety and depression: A meta-analytic review. *Journal of Consulting and Clinical Psychology, 78*, 169–183. doi:10.1037/a0018555.

Hölzel, B. K., Carmody, J., Vangel, M., Congleton, C., Yerramsetti, S. M., Gard, T., et al. (2011). Mindfulness practice leads to increases in regional brain gray matter density. *Psychiatry Research: Neuroimaging, 191*, 36–43.

Kuijpers, H. J. H., van der Heijden, F. M. M. A., Tuinier, S., & Verhoeven, W. M. A. (2007). Meditation-induced psychosis. *Psychopathology, 40*, 461–464.

Langer, Á. I., Cangas, A. J., Salcedo, E., & Fuentes, B. (2012). Applying mindfulness therapy in a group of psychotic individuals: A controlled study. *Behavioural and Cognitive Psychotherapy, 40*, 105–109.

Langer, Á. I., Cangas, A. J., & Gallego, J. (2010). Mindfulness-based intervention on distressing hallucination-like experiences in a nonclinical sample. *Behaviour Change, 27*, 176–183.

May, K., Strauss, C., Coyle, A., & Hayward, M. (2014). Person-based cognitive therapy groups for distressing voices: A thematic analysis of participant experiences of the therapy. *Psychosis: Psychological, Social and Integrative Approaches, 6*, 16–26. doi:10.1080/17522439.2012.708775.

National Institute for Health and Clinical Excellence (NICE). (2014). *Psychosis and schizophrenia in adults: treatment and management.* Available from URL: http://www.nice.org.uk/guidance/cg178

Perez-De-Albeniz, A., & Holmes, J. (2000). Meditation: Concepts, effects and uses in therapy. *International Journal of Psychotherapy, 5*, 49–59.

Pinto, A. (2009). Mindfulness and psychosis. In F. Didonna (Ed.), *Clinical handbook of mindfulness* (pp. 339–368). New York: Springer.

Sethi, S., & Subhash, C. (2003). Relationship of meditation and psychosis: Case studies. *Australian and New Zealand Journal of Psychiatry, 37*, 382.

Shonin, E., Van Gordon, W., & Griffiths, M. D. (2014a). Cognitive behavioral therapy (CBT) and meditation awareness training (MAT) for the treatment of co-occurring schizophrenia with pathological gambling: A case study. *International Journal of Mental Health and Addiction, 12*, 181–196.

Shonin, E., Van Gordon, W., & Griffiths, M. D. (2014b). Do mindfulness-based therapies have a role in the treatment of psychosis*? Australia and New Zealand Journal of Psychiatry, 48*, 124–127.

Shonin, E., Van Gordon, W., & Griffiths, M. D. (2015). Are there risks associated with using mindfulness for the treatment of psychopathology? *Clinical Practice, 11*, 389–392.

Siegel, D. J. (2010). *The mindful therapist: A clinician's guide to mindsight and neural integration*. New York: W.W. Norton.

Smieskova, R., Marmy, J., Schmidt, A., Bendfeldt, K., Riecher-Rössler, A., Walter, M., et al. (2013). Do subjects at clinical high risk for psychosis differ from those with a genetic high risk? A systematic review of structural and functional brain abnormalities. *Current Medicinal Chemistry, 20*, 467–481. doi:10.2174/0929867311320030018.

Smith, J. A., Flowers, P., & Larkin, M. (2009). *Interpretative phenomenological analysis: Theory, method and research*. London: Sage.

van der Valk, R., van de Waerdt, S., Meijer, C. J., van den Hout, I., & de Haan, L. (2013). Feasibility of mindfulness-based therapy in patients recovering from a first psychotic episode: A pilot study. *Early Intervention in Psychiatry, 7*, 64–70.

Van Gordon, W., Shonin, E., Griffiths, M. D., & Singh, N. N. (2015). There is only one mindfulness: Why science and Buddhism need to work together. *Mindfulness, 6*, 49–56.

Walsh, R., & Roche, L. (1979). Precipitation of acute psychotic episodes by intensive meditation in individuals with a history of schizophrenia. *American Psychiatry Association, 136*, 1085–1086.

Wyatt, C., Harper, B., & Weatherhead, S. (2014). The experience of group mindfulness-based interventions for individuals with mental health difficulties: A meta-synthesis. *Psychotherapy Research, 24*, 214–228.

Yorston, G. (2001). Mania precipitated by meditation: A case report and literature review. *Mental Health, Religion and Culture, 4*, 209–213.

Chapter 11
Mindfulness and Meditation in the Conceptualization and Treatment of Posttraumatic Stress Disorder

Anka A. Vujanovic, Barbara L. Niles, and Jocelyn L. Abrams

Introduction

In recent years, mindfulness and meditation have received increasing scholarly attention in the traumatic stress field due to their potential theoretical and clinical relevance to the etiology, maintenance, and treatment of posttraumatic stress disorder (PTSD; Kim, Schneider, Bevans et al., 2013; Lang et al., 2012; Vujanovic, Niles, Pietrefasa, Schmertz, & Potter, 2011). High levels of mindfulness may serve as a protective factor in the context of trauma recovery (e.g., Thompson, Arnkoff, & Glass, 2011), while lower levels of mindfulness may be a risk factor following trauma exposure. In addition, interventions that increase levels of present-centered attention, awareness, and/or acceptance (e.g., mindfulness skills, meditation) have great promise in terms of improving treatment outcomes for individuals with PTSD.

Indeed, the increased interest in mindfulness and/or meditation is driven largely by its noted potential as a target for intervention in clinical problems when emotional avoidance is prominent (e.g., Linehan, 1993), such as with PTSD. Although well-established evidence-based treatments for PTSD, namely, prolonged exposure therapy (PE; Foa, Hembree, & Rothbaum, 2007) and cognitive processing therapy (CPT; Resick & Schnicke, 1993), are available, a substantial proportion of individuals with PTSD do not seek treatment, drop out of treatment prematurely, refuse treatment, or do not manifest significant improvements (Imel, Laska, Jakupcak, & Simpson, 2013;

A.A. Vujanovic (✉) • J.L. Abrams
Department of Psychiatry and Behavioral Sciences, University of Texas Health Science Center at Houston, 1941 East Road, Houston, TX, 77054, USA
e-mail: Anka.A.Vujanovic@uth.tmc.edu

B.L. Niles
National Center for PTSD—Behavioral Science Division, VA Boston Healthcare System, and Department of Psychiatry, Boston University School of Medicine, 150 South Huntington Avenue (116B-2), Boston, MA, 02130, USA

E. Shonin et al. (eds.), *Mindfulness and Buddhist-Derived Approaches in Mental Health and Addiction*, Advances in Mental Health and Addiction,
DOI 10.1007/978-3-319-22255-4_11

Schottenbauer, Glass, Arnkoff, Tendick, & Gray, 2008). Furthermore, individuals with PTSD may not feel "ready" to engage in trauma-focused treatment and/or may benefit more from an alternative treatment approach. Currently, such individuals are typically referred to skills-based group treatment programs, including mindfulness- or meditation-based programs, as a precursor or adjunct intervention. However, the extent to which targeting present-centered attention, awareness, or acceptance skill deficits in adjunctive treatments for PTSD improves outcomes is still worthy of empirical exploration. Questions remain as to whether mindfulness or meditation programs should be offered as stand-alone interventions or as precursor programs to improve retention and outcomes for evidence-based PTSD treatments, such as PE or CPT.

Indeed, mindfulness- and meditation-based interventions have significant clinical implications for ultimately functioning as either stand-alone or adjunctive interventions for PTSD. Furthermore, enhancing mindfulness or meditation skills may be a successful avenue for primary or secondary prevention of PTSD for populations with a high probability of exposure to intense or chronic potentially traumatizing events (PTEs), such as police or military personnel. Offering mindfulness skill-building or meditation-based interventions to such populations in advance of their service—or shortly following exposure to PTE if PTSD symptoms are emergent—might serve to preclude the development of PTSD in a significant proportion of cases.

Chapter Overview

The goal of this chapter is to further elucidate the construct of mindfulness in terms of its potential utility in conceptualizing, preventing, and treating PTSD so as to stimulate further scholarly and clinical thought in this domain. Notably, distinct, though related, practices such as meditation are included as well so as to provide a broad-based picture of relevant clinical and empirical landscapes. Given the theoretical and clinical utility of gaining further understanding of mindfulness and meditation in the context of trauma, the most salient research relevant to PTE exposure, posttraumatic stress/PTSD, and mindfulness and meditation is reviewed. This chapter is not meant to serve as a systematic literature review, but instead as a review of highlights of current theoretical and clinical work. The clinical implications of mindfulness and meditation for the treatment of PTSD are also discussed. In order to provide a comprehensive view of this literature, all forms of mindfulness- and meditation-based interventions studied in the context of PTSD are highlighted, including approaches such as mindfulness-based stress reduction (MBSR), mindfulness-based cognitive therapy (MBCT), mindfulness-based stretching and deep breathing, as well as yoga. In addition, related practices, such as transcendental meditation (TM) and Mantram Repetition, are included in order to provide an overly inclusive picture of the empirical landscape. Finally, a discussion of limitations of extant research is presented along with several future research directions with the potential of informing both clinical and research efforts.

Defining Mindfulness

Mindfulness is most commonly conceptualized as involving two key components: (1) intentional regulation of attention to and "awareness" of the present moment and (2) nonjudgmental "acceptance" of the ongoing flow of sensations, thoughts, and/or emotional states (Baer, Smith, Hopkins, Krietemeyer, & Toney, 2006; Bishop et al., 2004). "Awareness" is cultivated through intentional regulation of attention to present experience. While attending to the present, mindfulness also entails a stance of "acceptance" or willingness to experience the array of one's thoughts and emotions without judgment. Awareness of one's present-centered experience might be considered a necessary first step toward nonjudgmental acceptance of that experience. For the purposes of this chapter, we refer to mindfulness according to this most common operational definition, which emphasizes the two factors of awareness and acceptance. We include meditation-based interventions as well, as meditation practice ostensibly may be related to at least the cultivation of attention and awareness.

Defining PTSD

PTSD, historically conceptualized as an anxiety disorder, is currently categorized as a "trauma-related disorder" (American Psychiatric Association [APA], 2013). PTSD may result from a traumatic event, defined as exposure to actual or threatened death, serious injury, or sexual violence via directly experiencing or witnessing the traumatic event, learning that the trauma (violent or accidental) occurred to a close family member or close friend, or experiencing exposure to repeated or extreme details of the trauma (APA, 2013). Notably, PTSD can result from many different types of trauma, including—but not limited to—sexual assault, military combat, natural disasters, motor vehicle accidents, and childhood sexual or physical abuse. Recent epidemiological estimates indicate that up to 89.7 % of the general population is exposed to a traumatic event during their lifetimes, while approximately 7–8 % will develop PTSD (APA, 2013; Kilpatrick et al., 2013). Prevalence rates of PTSD in populations chronically exposed to trauma, such as military personnel, are estimated at up to 20 % (Ramchand et al., 2010).

Four symptom clusters define PTSD: (1) trauma-related intrusion symptom (e.g., distressing memories, nightmares), (2) trauma-related avoidance symptoms (e.g., avoidance of memories or reminders of the trauma), (3) negative alterations in cognitions and mood associated with the trauma (e.g., negative beliefs or expectations about oneself, others, or the world), and (4) alterations in arousal or reactivity associated with the trauma (e.g., irritability, reckless or self-destructive behavior, sleep disturbance). For a diagnosis of PTSD to be considered, symptoms need to last more than 1 month and cause clinically significant distress or functional impairment (APA, 2013). The public health burden associated with PTSD is significant, as it is associated with high rates of comorbidity with other mental health conditions (e.g., Brady, Killeen, Brewerton, & Lucerini, 2000), significant functional impairment (e.g., Sareen et al., 2007), deleterious health outcomes (e.g., Schnurr & Jankowski, 1999), and increased healthcare utilization (e.g., Kartha et al., 2008).

Posttraumatic Stress and Mindfulness: A Theoretical Framework

Given the beneficial effects of mindfulness and meditation practice on enhancing emotion regulation as well as decreasing anxiety and depressive symptoms, these practices have been increasingly discussed in the context of PTSD and its treatment (see Orsillo and Batten, 2005). During the past 5–7 years, there has been an exponential proliferation of work on this topic, and the theoretical and empirical literature suggests that mindfulness and/or meditation may serve at least five clinically meaningful functions in terms of alleviating PTSD symptoms.

First, regular mindfulness or meditation practice can enhance or create a greater present-centered awareness and nonjudgmental acceptance of distressing internal states as well as trauma-related triggers (e.g., Walser & Westrup, 2007). Indeed, mindfulness may serve as an indirect mechanism of cognitive-affective exposure, as it involves an intrinsic willingness to approach, rather than to avoid, distressing thoughts and feelings. Mindfulness and meditation practice may increase an individual's ability to attend to thoughts and emotions as they arise and to tolerate distressing internal experiences by observing their transient nature, thus increasing meta-cognitive and meta-emotional awareness. Mindfulness or meditation may serve as a protective, or resilience, factor for some individuals exposed to PTE, thus preventing the development of PTSD. Mindfulness also may be an especially useful skill for individuals with PTSD, as it may help facilitate approach-oriented coping with trauma-related internal or external cues and decrease experiential avoidance. Through mindfulness or meditation practice, an individual with PTSD may become more willing to confront trauma-related triggers, including cognitions and emotions but also people, places, and activities. Consistent engagement in these exercises may decrease PTSD avoidance symptoms over time, thus targeting the core maintenance factor of the disorder (Foa, Riggs, Massie, & Yarczower, 1995).

Second, individuals who are more aware of present experience may be better able to effectively engage in various forms of treatment. For example, greater levels of present-centered awareness might facilitate client-therapist communication via enhanced openness. Clients who are more keenly aware of their thoughts and emotions may be better able to talk about them in treatment. Furthermore, greater levels of nonjudgmental acceptance of internal experience might decrease shame, guilt, and difficulties in self-acceptance, core issues for many individuals with PTSD (e.g., Henning & Frueh, 1997).

Third, regular mindfulness or meditation practice has been shown to decrease physiological arousal and stress reactivity (e.g., Delizonna, Williams, & Langer,

2009), perhaps via greater awareness and acceptance of such symptoms. In this manner, mindfulness might have a beneficial effect on symptoms of PTSD-related hyperarousal over time. As one example, mindfulness, indexed with the Mindful Attention Awareness Scale (MAAS; Brown & Ryan, 2003), has been associated with more adaptive sleep functioning (Howell, Digdon, & Buro, 2010). It is thought that mindfulness may foster a greater sensitization to bodily cues (e.g., breathing rate, heart rate), thereby providing individuals with the necessary awareness to self-regulate in a more adaptive manner (e.g., Brown & Ryan, 2003). The cultivation of greater interoceptive awareness and acceptance may also serve indirectly as exposure to uncomfortable physical sensations (e.g., chest tightness), thus increasing tolerance to such sensations over time. Furthermore, with ongoing attention to bodily processes, individuals are thought to become more attuned to their intrinsic needs and thus better able to tend to those needs.

Fourth, both dispositional mindfulness and mindfulness practice have demonstrated associations with greater empathy and compassion (e.g., Birnie, Speca, & Carlson, 2010; Tirch, 2010). Furthermore, self-compassion has shown inverse associations with both symptom severity and quality of life in distressed samples with anxiety and depressive symptoms, even over and beyond the effects of mindfulness (Van Dam, Sheppard, Forsyth, & Earleywine, 2011). Indeed, compassion might serve as a mediating function in associations between mindfulness and a variety of adaptive psychological outcomes (Hollis-Walker, & Colosimo, 2011). As individuals with PTSD are often plagued by excessive and maladaptive degrees of self-blame, fear, and anger, a mindfulness or meditation practice with the potential to cultivate greater levels of self-empathy and self-compassion and empathy and compassion for others could serve a meaningful purpose in healing from psychological trauma (e.g., Gilbert & Tirch, 2009; Tesh, Learman, & Pulliam, 2015). Compassion and empathy thus might serve as potential mechanisms of change in the alleviation of PTSD symptoms in mindfulness- and meditation-based interventions.

Finally, "mindful distraction" exercises (e.g., grounding; Batten, Orsillo, & Walser, 2005) can be used to foster psychological flexibility, such that individuals might learn (a) when it is appropriate and beneficial to sit with distressing internal experience and (b) when it might be more constructive to shift attention away from ruminative thoughts and prevent dissociation. Psychological flexibility has been defined as the ability to adopt a present-centered stance and to act in accordance with one's values in a given situation (Hayes, Strosahl, Bunting, Twohig, & Wilson, 2005). Indeed, mindfulness training has been associated with the cultivation of sustained attention and attention switching (e.g., Jha, Krompinger, & Baime, 2007) or the increased ability to selectively direct attention from one stimulus (e.g., internal experience) to another. Relatedly, mindfulness training has also been associated with an increased ability to inhibit secondary elaborative processing of thoughts, feelings, and sensations (e.g., Jha et al., 2007). Thus, with increased mindfulness training, individuals might be better able to notice repetitive negative thinking and to prevent extensive engagement with maladaptive ruminative processes by attending to feelings and sensations in the present moment.

Mindfulness and Posttraumatic Stress: Review of Non-treatment Studies

Cross-Sectional Studies

Several published cross-sectional studies have examined associations between mindfulness and PTSD symptoms across a variety of populations, including community samples, police personnel, firefighters, military veterans, and undergraduate students. Most of these studies operationalized mindfulness as a multifaceted construct and included self-report instruments that measured various facets of mindfulness. To promote clarity in the operationalization of the mindfulness construct, the specific instruments utilized across studies are delineated along with the specific mindfulness facets measured.

For instance, Vujanovic, Youngwirth, Johnson, and Zvolensky (2009) found a significant negative association between both the "acting with awareness" and "accepting without judgment" subscales of the Kentucky Inventory of Mindfulness Skills (KIMS; Baer, Smith, & Allen, 2004) and posttraumatic stress symptoms in a community sample of adults exposed to PTE. This association remained statistically significant even after controlling for the variance accounted for by negative affectivity and number of trauma exposure types. "Accepting without judgment" emerged as the most robust mindfulness factor, demonstrating incremental negative associations with each of the posttraumatic stress symptom clusters, while "acting with awareness" was incrementally negatively associated with only the reexperiencing symptom cluster (Vujanovic et al., 2009).

Chopko and Schwartz (2013) partially replicated the findings of Vujanovic et al. (2009) with a sample of active-duty police officers, documenting an inverse (negative) association between "accepting without judgment," also measured via the KIMS, and posttraumatic stress avoidance and intrusion symptoms and an inverse association between both "describing" and "accepting without judgment" and posttraumatic stress hyperarousal symptoms. Wahbeh, Lu, and Oken (2011) extended this line of work to military veterans and conducted a cross-sectional study comparing levels of mindfulness, measured with the MAAS (Brown & Ryan, 2003) and the "accepting without judgment" subscale of the KIMS (Baer et al., 2004), across three groups: 15 combat veterans with PTSD, 15 combat veterans without PTSD, and 15 noncombat veterans without PTSD. Groups were matched on age, gender, depression, other trauma histories, and other demographic characteristics. No group differences in MAAS scores were documented. However, in terms of "accepting without judgment," the group of combat veterans without PTSD reported the highest levels. In addition, mindfulness accounted for up to 32 % of unique variance in PTSD symptoms; and only "accepting without judgment" was significant in the model.

In a sample of undergraduate students, Thompson and Waltz (2010) found incremental negative relations between "non-judging of inner experience"—as indexed via the Five Facet Mindfulness Questionnaire (FFMQ; Baer et al., 2008)—and posttraumatic stress avoidance symptoms, even after controlling for various indices of experiential avoidance. In a follow-up study also employing an undergraduate student sample and using the FFMQ, Kalill, Treanor, and Roemer (2014) found somewhat discrepant findings from Thompson and Waltz (2010). Kalill et al. (2014) documented incremental negative associations between "describing," also measured via the FFMQ, and posttraumatic stress hyperarousal symptoms and between "non-reactivity to inner experience" and posttraumatic stress symptom severity and severity of reexperiencing and hyperarousal symptoms. Notably, effects were established even after controlling for negative affect, age, number of traumas, and years since the trauma.

Furthermore, in an adult community sample reporting exposure to PTE, Bernstein, Tanay, and Vujanovic (2011) found that levels of mindful attention and awareness—as measured with the MAAS (Brown & Ryan, 2003)—were significantly and negatively associated with posttraumatic stress symptom severity, psychiatric multi-morbidity, anxious arousal, and anhedonic depression symptoms, above and beyond the number of traumatic event types. Relatedly, Smith et al. (2011) extended these findings to urban firefighters, documenting significant (negative) associations between mindful attention and awareness, indexed via the MAAS, and PTSD symptoms, depressive symptoms, physical symptoms, and alcohol problems. Mindful attention and awareness were incrementally (negatively) associated with PTSD symptoms, depressive symptoms, physical symptoms, and alcohol problems, when controlling for demographic characteristics and firefighter stress.

Taken together, these studies support the clinical utility of mindfulness, as higher levels of mindfulness were related to lower posttraumatic stress and related symptoms and vice versa. However, these studies are limited in their exclusive reliance on a cross-sectional design, self-report measures of mindfulness and posttraumatic stress, and mostly nonclinical samples of adults exposed to PTE. Discrepancies in findings might be attributed to several factors, including differences in the populations studied (e.g., undergraduates, police personnel), in the measures of PTSD symptomatology implemented, and in the covariates employed in statistical models.

Mindfulness in Residential PTSD Treatment

At least two studies have documented relations between mindfulness and changes in PTSD and relevant symptomatology in the context of residential PTSD treatment. Although not treatment studies, these publications documented the associations of mindfulness with relevant symptom outcomes in residential PTSD treatment programs for military veterans. First, Owens, Walter, Chard, and Davis (2012) documented significant associations between three KIMS subscales—"acting with awareness," "describing," and "accepting without judgment" and self-reported PTSD symptoms at posttreatment among military veterans in residential treatment for PTSD. Improvements on the "acting with awareness" subscale of the KIMS were significantly associated with lower interview-based PTSD symptoms at posttreatment. Changes in the "describing," "acting with awareness," and "accepting without judgment" subscales of the KIMS were significantly associated with self-reported PTSD symptoms at posttreatment. Furthermore, changes in the "describing" subscale of the KIMS were associated with lower self-reported depressive symptoms at posttreatment, while changes in the "acting with awareness" subscale were associated with major depressive disorder diagnostic status at posttreatment. Similarly, Boden et al. (2012) investigated pre- to posttreatment changes in various facets of mindfulness, as measured via the KIMS, and relations to posttreatment PTSD and depression symptoms in 48 military veterans enrolled in residential PTSD treatment. The residential program adhered to a cognitive-behavioral treatment framework, which included group CPT, psychoeducation, communication skills, and non-trauma cognitive therapy. Boden et al. (2012) documented that elements of mindfulness, specifically self-reported levels of "acting with awareness" and "accepting without judgment," increased during the course of treatment. Furthermore, changes in "acting with awareness" explained unique variance in posttreatment PTSD symptom severity, and changes in "accepting without judgment" explained unique variance in posttreatment depression symptom severity.

Taken together, these studies suggest at least two important postulations worthy of further study. Firstly, cognitive-behavioral treatment programming for PTSD might indirectly improve levels of mindfulness and acceptance. Secondly, perhaps greater baseline levels of mindfulness might predict the extent of symptom change in PTSD treatment. These lines of inquiry necessitate further empirical exploration.

Mindfulness Interventions for Posttraumatic Stress

Review of Clinical Trials

An overview of the clinical research literature on mindfulness and PTSD is presented here, and findings from both uncontrolled and randomized controlled trials (RCTs) are presented. Relevant distinctions are noted with regard to methodology, as necessary. Furthermore, in the interest of being overly inclusive of all literature broadly relevant to the cultivation of awareness and acceptance, published trials of meditation-based and mind-body interventions that incorporate meditation are included as well.

Transcendental Meditation

The first published study to examine the preliminary efficacy of a meditation-based intervention for PTSD was conducted by Brooks and Scarano (1985). This study was comprised of a group of 18 male Vietnam veterans and compared the efficacy of TM to eclectic psychotherapy for PTSD. The TM program consisted of 4 days of

1.5-h daily instruction and then weekly 1-h follow-up meetings for 3 months. Psychotherapy consisted of 1-h weekly sessions along with the option to participate in group or family therapy. Veterans randomly assigned to TM were instructed to meditate twice daily for 20 min. A significant positive treatment effect for TM, as compared to psychotherapy, was documented in terms of PTSD symptoms, anxiety and depressive symptoms, alcohol consumption, insomnia, and family problems. Furthermore, the TM group manifested a faster habituation response to a stressful stimulus. This study offered an important step in the study of mindfulness-based processes in trauma-exposed populations, but it was limited due to several factors, including loose inclusion/exclusion criteria (e.g., veterans were not required to meet criteria for PTSD to participate), small sample size, lack of standardization of the psychotherapy condition, and reliance on self-report measures for most outcomes.

Since the original Brooks and Scarano (1985) work, a more recent, albeit small, pilot study on the effects of TM in Operation Enduring Freedom (OEF)/Operation Iraqi Freedom (OIF) veterans with PTSD was conducted (Rosenthal, Grosswatd, Ross, & Rosenthal, 2011). In this study, TM was taught over 3 consecutive days, and participants were asked to meditate for 20 min twice a day for 12 weeks. A total of seven veterans were enrolled. Veterans reported positive effects including decreased stress and anxiety and sleep improvements. However, this study was limited due to the lack of a control group and the small sample size.

Mindfulness-Based Stress Reduction

To date, one of the most popular and well-researched mindfulness interventions to address both psychological and physical ailments is MBSR (Kabat-Zinn, 1990), an 8-week group treatment that introduces a meditative practice and cultivates present awareness of mental processes and physical states. MBSR has demonstrated efficacy for individuals with a wide range of medical and mental health diagnoses. In the first study to apply MBSR to the treatment of trauma survivors, Kimbrough, Magyari, Langenberg, Margaret, and Berman (2010) conducted an 8-week MBSR pilot program that is comprised of 2.5–3-h classes and a 5-h silent retreat, with 27 adult survivors of childhood sexual abuse. The authors concluded that this trial of MBSR was efficacious in significantly decreasing posttraumatic stress symptoms, with symptoms of avoidance/numbing most significantly reduced. This MBSR trial, though lacking a randomized controlled condition, demonstrated promising results with regard to the efficacy of a mindfulness-based intervention for reducing symptoms of posttraumatic stress among adult survivors of childhood trauma.

More recently, Kearney, McDermott, Malte, Martinez, and Simpson (2012) investigated the preliminary feasibility, acceptability, and initial efficacy of MBSR as an adjunct to military veterans' usual care. A total of 92 veterans participated in the MBSR course, and results demonstrated that participation in MBSR was associated with improvements in PTSD symptoms, depression, behavioral activation, acceptance, and mindfulness over a 6-month period. Inclusion criteria for this study were intentionally broad-based, and veterans were not required to meet criteria for PTSD.

In a follow-up study, Kearney, McDermott, Malte, Martinez, and Simpson (2013) investigated the efficacy of MBSR for veterans with PTSD in the context of an RCT, and the findings were mixed. Compared to treatment as usual (TAU), no reliable effect of MBSR plus TAU on PTSD or depression symptoms was found using intention-to-treat analyses. However, completer analyses of those veterans who attended at least half of the classes (4 or more) showed medium to large effects for depression, health-related quality of life, and mindfulness skills.

A mindfulness intervention that is consistent with the tenets of MBSR, though considerably less intensive, and delivered using telephone treatment was also done with military veterans (Niles et al., 2012). In this Niles et al. (2012) study, the mindfulness telehealth intervention was compared to a psychoeducation intervention and both treatments consisted of two individual in-person sessions and 6 telephone sessions. Completer analyses showed drops in self-reported and clinician-assessed PTSD symptoms at posttreatment with large effect sizes. However, symptoms returned to baseline at the 6-week follow-up. Notably, this mindfulness telehealth intervention was also associated with gains in self-reported mindfulness skills, as measured via the MAAS, and the "observing" and "describing" facets of the FFMQ (Niles, Vujanovic, Silberbogen, Seligowski, & Potter, 2013).

Omidi, Mohammadi, Zargar, and Akbari (2013) conducted a clinical trial of MBSR of male veterans with PTSD in Iran. In this study, veterans were randomized to either MBSR, consisting of 2-h weekly group sessions for 8 weeks, or TAU, described as "routine treatment" by a psychiatrist. A positive treatment effect for MBSR was documented, and those assigned to MBSR, as compared to those in TAU, reported significantly reduced rates of depression, dizziness, fatigue, and tension.

Mindfulness-Based Cognitive Therapy

King et al. (2013) adapted MBCT (group format), an intervention with demonstrated efficacy for prevention of depression relapse (Segal, Williams, & Teasdale, 2013) and for combat veterans with PTSD, and conducted a pilot study—comparing MBCT to TAU—to investigate feasibility, acceptability, and initial clinical outcomes. The TAU group interventions were comprised of either PTSD psychoeducation and skills group or imagery rehearsal therapy group. Group assignment was not randomized; consecutive patients were recruited from a PTSD outpatient clinic and assigned to one group at a time. Intent-to-treat analyses indicated a significant improvement in PTSD symptoms in the MBCT condition, as compared to TAU. In addition, veterans in the MBCT condition demonstrated good compliance with assigned exercises and clinically meaningful improvement in PTSD symptom severity, particularly avoidance/numbing symptoms and self-blame.

Mantram Repetition

Two studies by Bormann et al. (Bormann, Thorp, Wetherell, & Golshan, 2008; Bormann, Thorp, Wetherell, Golshan, & Lang, 2013) evaluated Mantram Repetition, a 6-session group meditation-based intervention that teaches three tools for training attention and regulating emotion, including the silent repetition of a typically spiritual or "sacred" word or phrase, called a mantram. The initial Bormann et al. (2008) study was a feasibility pilot trial indicating that this treatment is acceptable to veterans with PTSD, feasible to deliver, and associated with improvements in symptoms of PTSD, psychological distress, and quality of life compared to a delayed treatment control. The second larger RCT (Bormann et al., 2013) indicated that Mantram Repetition, as compared with TAU, was associated with improvements in PTSD symptoms with moderate posttreatment effect sizes reported for both self-reported and clinician-assessed symptoms.

Oman and Bormann (2015) then evaluated the Mantram Repetition program in terms of its effects on self-efficacy to manage PTSD symptoms in the same group of veterans with PTSD. The Mantram Repetition group evidenced approximately linear weekly increases, from baseline to post-intervention, in self-efficacy to manage PTSD symptoms. Furthermore, self-efficacy (to manage PTSD symptoms) partially mediated the effects of Mantram Repetition on depression and mental health and full mediated effects on PTSD symptoms.

Mindfulness-Based Stretching and Deep Breathing

Kim et al. (2013) delivered an intervention, in the context of an RCT, consisting of mindfulness-based stretching and deep breathing (MBX) to intensive care unit nurses with subclinical symptoms of PTSD. Completer analyses indicated that, compared to a waitlist control group, those randomized to the MBX condition showed greater drops in self-reported PTSD symptoms that were maintained at the 8-week follow-up. Serum cortisol concentrations also increased and moved toward the normal range for those in the MBX condition.

Yoga Interventions for Posttraumatic Stress

Yoga is a physical and contemplative practice commonly comprised of breath control, simple meditation, and the adoption of a series of specific body postures. Yoga is increasingly implemented in PTSD treatment centers, including those housed in the Veterans Affairs Healthcare System. Yet, until very recently, there were no RCTs supporting its use for PTSD, specifically.

Two clinical trials of yoga breath interventions have been published to date. First, in an uncontrolled study, Descilo et al. (2009) examined the effect of a yoga breath intervention, as compared to yoga breath intervention plus 3-h trauma reduction exposure techniques or waitlist control, on symptoms of PTSD and depression in survivors of the 2004 tsunami in Southeast Asia. The yoga breath intervention was comprised of 2-h sessions, administered on 4 consecutive days, covering four distinct breathing techniques. Here, significant treatment vs. waitlist control effects were found with regard to PTSD and depression symptoms. That is, both of the yoga breath intervention conditions performed better than the waitlist control condition with regard to symptom outcomes, as measured up to 24 weeks posttreatment. Second, Seppala et al. (2014) published an RCT of a breathing-based meditation for PTSD in military veterans. Seppala et al. (2014) evaluated the efficacy of Sudarshan Kriya yoga, a group-oriented, manualized controlled breathing meditation intervention that focuses on several types of breathing exercises interspersed with discussion and stretching. Compared to a waitlist control group ($n = 10$), the active group ($n = 11$) demonstrated significant reductions in PTSD symptoms, anxiety symptoms, and respiration rate. Reductions in startle responsivity were associated with reduction in hyperarousal symptoms at post-intervention and at 1-year follow-up.

Moreover, a recent RCT, conducted in Australia by Carter et al. (2013), provides important new evidence that yoga may be effective in the treatment of PTSD for male veterans. This study examined an intensive yoga intervention that consisted of 22-h guided group yoga instruction over 5 days followed by weekly 2-h group sessions for 5 months. Compared to a waitlist control, the yoga group showed a significant decrease in clinician-assessed PTSD 6 weeks following intervention completion, while the waitlist group had no decline. The waitlist group then received the yoga intervention and also improved significantly on clinician-assessed PTSD. For both groups, improvements were maintained at the 6-month follow-up.

To evaluate the efficacy of yoga for women with PTSD symptomatology, Mitchell et al. (2014) completed a pilot study with women using a much less intensive yoga intervention and a more active control condition. The yoga condition, consisting of twelve 75-min group sessions of yoga, was compared to a 12-session assessment control condition in which the participants completed questionnaires in a group format. The results showed that there was a significant drop in self-reported PTSD symptoms over time, but that there was no significant difference between the groups indicating no advantage for yoga over group assessment. Post hoc analyses indicated that PTSD symptoms decreased significantly for the yoga group and the effect size was small.

Also in 2014, van der Kolk et al. published a RCT of trauma-informed yoga, as compared to supportive women's health education, for 64 women with chronic, treatment-resistant PTSD. Both conditions were held as weekly 1-h classes for 10 weeks. While both conditions reported significant decreases in PTSD symptoms, decreases in the yoga group were in the large effect size range ($d = 1.07$), as compared to the medium to large effect size decreases in the control group ($d = 0.66$). Furthermore, while both conditions manifested significant decreases in PTSD symptoms during the first half of treatment, these improvements were maintained only by the yoga group; the control group relapsed after initial improvement.

Although these results are encouraging, given demonstrated reductions in PTSD symptoms for participants in the yoga conditions, these studies do not provide enough evidence to determine whether yoga is an effective treatment for PTSD. The considerable difference in the number of hours of yoga offered across studies, the sex of the participants (all men in the Carter et al. study and all women in the Mitchell et al. and van der Kolk et al. studies), or the comparison groups utilized (waitlist compared to assessment or health education controls) may account for the differences in results. Additional studies are needed to further investigate this popular form of therapy.

Summary of Clinical Trials

Taken together, the data are encouraging, indicating that mindfulness- and meditation-based interventions are acceptable and feasible for individuals with PTSD, can impact both clinical and subclinical levels of PTSD symptoms, and can be delivered in a group or telehealth format. Furthermore, effect sizes—when reported—are moderate, suggesting that the impact is more than minimal. However, most studies used a TAU or waitlist control group instead of an active treatment comparison. Sample sizes are small in most studies and intention-to-treat analyses were not consistently utilized. Although evidence is accumulating, additional RCTs are needed in order to establish mindfulness as an effective stand-alone treatment for PTSD.

Posttraumatic Stress and Mindfulness: The Substance Use Context

Posttraumatic stress and substance use disorders co-occur at exceptionally high rates, with up to 43 % of individuals with PTSD reporting a lifetime history of substance use disorders and up to 75 % of military combat veterans with lifetime PTSD also meeting criteria for alcohol use disorders (e.g., Jacobsen, Southwick, & Kosten, 2001). Evidence-based interventions for this highly prevalent comorbidity are limited, and examination of mechanisms underlying the comorbidity has great potential to inform specialized treatment approaches. Mindfulness has been identified as one such promising mechanism underlying the association between posttraumatic stress and substance use disorders and with potential as a significant target for integrated treatments for this difficult-to-treat comorbidity. In fact, mindfulness-based interventions have demonstrated preliminary efficacy in terms of decreasing substance use and craving (e.g., Bowen et al., 2014; Witkiewitz & Bowen, 2010; Witkiewitz, Bowen, Douglas, & Hsu, 2013; Witkiewitz, Greenfield, & Bowen, 2013). However, there are only a few studies to date that have explored the role of mindfulness-based processes in posttraumatic stress and substance use disorders.

For example, Vujanovic, Bonn-Miller, and Marlatt (2011) examined the role of nonjudgmental acceptance with regard to posttraumatic stress and alcohol use coping motives. Specifically, Vujanovic, Bonn-Miller, et al. (2011) found that "accepting without judgment," measured via the KIMS, partially mediated the association between posttraumatic stress symptom severity and alcohol use coping motives. Consistent with previous findings (Bowen & Marlatt, 2009; Ostafin & Marlatt, 2008), this study suggests that for alcohol users with exposure to PTE, a lower level of nonjudgmental acceptance may be a mechanism by which coping-oriented alcohol use is maintained.

Similarly, Bonn-Miller, Vujanovic, Twohig, Medina, and Huggins (2010) explored the role of nonjudgmental acceptance in the association between posttraumatic stress symptom severity and marijuana use coping motives. In a community-based sample of adults with a history of PTE exposure and recent marijuana use, Bonn-Miller et al. (2010) found that "accepting without judgment," measured via the KIMS, partially mediated the association between posttraumatic stress symptom severity and marijuana use coping motives. Taken together, these findings begin to suggest a potential clinically significant avenue for further empirical consideration: the role of "acceptance" in the prevalent association of posttraumatic stress and substance use disorders.

Furthermore, in a clinical sample of trauma-exposed adults in residential treatment for substance use, Garland and Roberts-Lewis (2013) investigated associations among dispositional mindfulness, measured via the FFMQ, thought suppression, posttraumatic stress symptoms, and substance craving. Here, dispositional mindfulness was significantly (negatively) associated with posttraumatic stress symptom severity and substance cravings, after controlling for extent of trauma history (i.e., number of traumatic event types experienced). Path analyses indicated that individuals reporting more extensive trauma histories also described greater tendencies to engage in thought suppression, which in turn was associated with more severe posttraumatic stress symptomatology. Thought suppression mediated the (negative) association between dispositional mindfulness and posttraumatic stress symptom severity.

Furthermore, the applicability of mindfulness-based interventions, such as MBSR, to the integrated treatment of PTSD and substance use disorders has been considered (e.g., Lange, 2011). However, there are no available published studies reporting upon the feasibility or efficacy of MBSR or other mindfulness- or meditation-based interventions for individuals suffering from PTSD and substance use disorders. This is a fruitful area for future exploration, given the need for more integrated treatments for this difficult-to-treat comorbidity and the mounting evidence in support of the efficacy of mindfulness-based approaches for PTSD and substance use disorders, respectively.

Mindfulness and Posttraumatic Stress in Children and Adolescents

In our review of the literature, a significant paucity of research on associations between mindfulness and posttraumatic stress in children and adolescents was revealed. Although treatments that include a significant mindfulness component, such as dialectical behavior therapy (Linehan, 1993), have been implemented with demonstrated efficacy in adolescent samples (e.g., Klein & Miller, 2011; Rathus & Miller, 2015; Wagner, Rathus, & Miller, 2006), no direct studies of mindfulness and posttraumatic stress in this population have been published to date. The studies reviewed here thus are meditation-based, largely mind-body skills group programs delivered to children *and* adolescents exposed to trauma.

In terms of trauma-exposed adolescents, Gordon, Staples, Blyta, Bytyqi, and Wilson (2008) evaluated the efficacy of a 6-week mind-body skills program in postwar Kosovar adolescents. This mind-body skills program was comprised of meditation, biofeedback, guided imagery, drawings, autogenic training, movement, and breathing techniques. In the context of an RCT, the mind-body skills group, as compared to a waitlist control group, reported significantly greater decreases in PTSD symptom severity in postwar Kosovar adolescents. These findings were consistent with results from their previous pilot study (Gordon, Staples, Blyta, & Bytqi, 2004). However, these adolescents manifested varying levels of PTSD symptomatology and were not screened for the PTSD diagnosis, but all were exposed to war-related trauma. A similar mind-body skills group was conducted with Palestinian children and adolescents in Gaza (Staples, Abdel Atti, & Gordon, 2011). This uncontrolled trial documented significant improvements in PTSD and depression symptoms and a significant decrease in hopelessness in these children, which was maintained for up to 7-months post-intervention.

With regard to children, Catani et al. (2009) conducted an RCT wherein Sri Lankan children, affected by civil war and the 2004 tsunami and diagnosed with PTSD, were randomly assigned to either 2-week (6 sessions) meditation-relaxation intervention or narrative exposure therapy for children. Children in both treatment conditions evidenced significant reductions in PTSD symptoms and functional impairment at 1-month posttreatment and at 6-month follow-up. Taken together, the study and application of meditation-based interventions to trauma-exposed children/adolescents certainly represent important areas of great clinical significance for further study.

Limitations of Current Research and Future Directions

The extant literature is limited in several key ways, each of which represents a pertinent avenue for future work. First, despite the recent proliferation of research on mindfulness and/or meditation and PTSD, there are still only a handful of clinical intervention studies, including RCTs in this area. Although findings are promising, there is a need for more extensive clinical examination of these phenomena, with attention to more diverse samples in terms of race/ethnicity, age, trauma exposure types, settings (e.g., inpatient vs. outpatient), and intervention types (e.g., individual vs. group).

Second, extant clinical trials on mindfulness and meditation interventions for PTSD have differed in the use of individual vs. group formats for the interventions.

It would be interesting for future studies to examine the possibility of differential effects of interventions simply based on the delivery platform. Relatedly, as some researchers have begun to do (Niles et al., 2012), it will be important to investigate telehealth, Internet-, or smartphone-based models of service delivery. Such technologies would allow for alleviation of disparities in access to care for underprivileged and/or rural populations.

Third, as the literature is in a nascent stage, most of the work has focused on determining associations or comparing symptom outcomes in treatment trials, and much less attention has been allotted to the examination of mechanisms of change. Both biological and psychological mechanisms would be important to study. Relatedly, the utilization of diverse paradigms to index mindfulness, PTSD, and related outcomes is important in order to more directly examine, manipulate, and control variables of interest. For instance, incorporating neurobiological (e.g., neurostructural, neuroendocrine, neurophysiological) and genetic/epigenetic perspectives and techniques would provide a methodologically rigorous biopsychosocial lens through which to better understand mindfulness and meditation-based processes and their role in the etiology, maintenance, and treatment of PTSD. These lines of inquiry will help us to gain a better understanding of the processes driving the noted gains yielded by mindfulness-based interventions.

Fourth, most extant studies have relied heavily on self-report measures to index factors of interest, both in cross-sectional and treatment studies. Furthermore, several studies have attempted to measure change in levels of mindfulness over time using available self-report measures, and yet, many such measures are not necessarily "state" measures with documented sensitivity to change. Future work should strive to incorporate multimodal assessments of the primary outcomes of interest (e.g., interview-based measures, experimental paradigms).

Fifth, no published studies to date have evaluated mindfulness- or meditation-based interventions in the context of PTSD prevention or early intervention postexposure to PTE. This type of application of mindfulness or meditation represents a potentially fruitful avenue for alleviating the suffering associated with psychological trauma. Mindfulness- or meditation-based interventions potentially could have transdiagnostic implications for individuals exposed to PTE.

Sixth, the applications of mindfulness to the study of PTSD-relevant comorbidity are just emerging. Very few studies have evaluated the role of mindfulness in posttraumatic stress and substance use disorders. While several of the published RCTs of mindfulness-based interventions for PTSD have included depression and other symptom outcomes, a more focused effort to evaluate the potential transdiagnostic efficacy of mindfulness or meditation in targeting several symptom clusters concurrently is imperative. Over 80 % of individuals with PTSD present with a comorbid diagnosis (e.g., Brady et al., 2000; Sareen et al., 2007), and thus, more attention to transdiagnostic implications is clinically imperative.

Finally, as aforementioned, there has been a relative dearth of research on the relevance of mindfulness- or meditation-based processes for trauma-exposed children and adolescents. However, several studies have documented the positive effects of mindfulness on social-emotional development in children, more generally (e.g., Schonert-Reichl et al., 2015). This is a highly relevant area for future study, especially given the promising results of the emerging literature on mindfulness in youth.

Summary and Conclusions

Our understanding of the therapeutic role of mindfulness and meditation in the treatment of PTSD is just beginning to take form. Available evidence suggests that mindfulness and meditation have significant clinical relevance to our understanding of the etiology and maintenance of PTSD as well as its prevention and treatment. However, given the nascent stage of this research literature, much more study is needed to solidify our theoretical and clinical conceptualization of the effects of mindfulness- and meditation-based practice on PTSD and the mechanisms implicated in such effects. Given the need for additional effective treatment avenues for PTSD and related disorders, and the solid empirical foundation that is forming relevant to mindfulness- and meditation-based processes, the study of these processes and interventions has the potential to change the landscape of PTSD treatment in the not-so-distant future.

References

American Psychiatric Association. (2013). *Diagnostic and statistical manual of mental disorders: DSM-5*. Washington, DC: American Psychiatric Association.

Baer, R. A., Smith, G. T., & Allen, K. B. (2004). Assessment of mindfulness by self-report: The Kentucky inventory of mindfulness skills. *Assessment, 11*, 191–203.

Baer, R. A., Smith, G. T., Hopkins, J., Krietemeyer, J., & Toney, L. (2006). Using self-report assessment methods to explore facets of mindfulness. *Assessment, 13*, 27–45.

Baer, R. A., Smith, G. T., Lykins, E., Button, D., Krietemeyer, J., Sauer, S., et al. (2008). Construct validity of the five facet mindfulness questionnaire in meditating and nonmeditating samples. *Assessment, 15*, 329–342.

Batten, S. V., Orsillo, S. M., & Walser, R. D. (2005). Acceptance and mindfulness-based approaches to the treatment of posttraumatic stress disorder. In S. M. Orsillo & L. Roemer (Eds.), *Acceptance and mindfulness-based approaches to anxiety: Conceptualization and treatment* (pp. 241–269). New York: Springer Science+Business Media.

Bernstein, A., Tanay, G., & Vujanovic, A. A. (2011). Concurrent relations between mindful attention and awareness and psychopathology among trauma-exposed adults: Preliminary evidence of transdiagnostic resilience. *Journal of Cognitive Psychotherapy, 25*, 99–113.

Birnie, K., Speca, M., & Carlson, L. E. (2010). Exploring self-compassion and empathy in the context of mindfulness-based stress reduction (MBSR). *Stress and Health, 26*, 359–371.

Bishop, S. R., Lau, M. A., Shapiro, S., Carlson, L., Anderson, N. D., Carmody, J., et al. (2004). Mindfulness: A proposed operational definition. *Clinical Psychology: Science and Practice, 11*, 230–241.

Boden, M. T., Bernstein, A., Walser, R. D., Bui, L., Alvarez, J., & Bonn-Miller, M. O. (2012). Changes in facets of mindfulness and posttraumatic stress disorder treatment outcome. *Psychiatry Research, 200*, 609–613.

Bonn-Miller, M. O., Vujanovic, A. A., Twohig, M. P., Medina, J. L., & Huggins, J. L. (2010). Posttraumatic stress symptom severity and marijuana use coping motives: A test of the mediating role of non-judgmental acceptance within a trauma-exposed community sample. *Mindfulness, 1*, 98–106.

Bormann, J. E., Thorp, S., Wetherell, J. L., & Golshan, S. (2008). A spiritually based group intervention for combat veterans with posttraumatic stress disorder: Feasibility study. *Journal of Holistic Nursing, 26*, 109–116.

Bormann, J. E., Thorp, S. R., Wetherell, J. L., Golshan, S., & Lang, A. J. (2013). Meditation-based mantram intervention for veterans with posttraumatic stress disorder: A randomized trial. *Psychological Trauma: Theory, Research, Practice, and Policy, 5*, 259–267.

Bowen, S., & Marlatt, G. A. (2009). Surfing the urge: Brief mindfulness-based intervention for college student smokers. *Psychology of Addictive Behaviors, 23*, 666–671.

Bowen, S., Witkiewitz, K., Clifasefi, S. L., Grow, J., Chawla, N., Hsu, S. H., et al. (2014). Relative efficacy of mindfulness-based relapse prevention, standard relapse prevention, and treatment as usual for substance use disorders: A randomized clinical trial. *JAMA Psychiatry, 71*, 547–556.

Brady, K. T., Killeen, T. K., Brewerton, T., & Lucerini, S. (2000). Comorbidity of psychiatric disorders and posttraumatic stress disorder. *Journal of Clinical Psychiatry, 61*(Suppl. 7), 22–32.

Brooks, J. S., & Scarano, T. (1985). Transcendental meditation in the treatment of post-Vietnam adjustment. *Journal of Counseling and Development, 64*, 212–215.

Brown, K. W., & Ryan, R. M. (2003). The benefits of being present: Mindfulness and its role in psychological well-being. *Journal of Personality and Social Psychology, 84*, 822–848.

Carter, J. J., Gerbarg, P. L., Brown, R. P., Ware, R. S., D'Ambrosio, C., Anand, L., et al. (2013). Multi-component yoga breath program for Vietnam veteran posttraumatic stress disorder: Randomized controlled trial. *Journal of Traumatic Stress Disorders and Treatment, 2*, 3.

Catani, C., Kohiladevy, M., Ruf, M., Schauer, E., Elbert, T., & Neuner, F. (2009). Treating children traumatized by war and Tsunami: A comparison between exposure therapy and meditation-relaxation in North-East Sri Lanka. *BMC Psychiatry, 9*, 22–33.

Chopko, B. A., & Schwartz, R. C. (2013). The relation between mindfulness and posttraumatic stress symptoms among police officers. *Journal of Loss and Trauma, 18*, 1–9.

Delizonna, L. L., Williams, R. P., & Langer, E. J. (2009). The effect of mindfulness on heart rate control. *Journal of Adult Development, 16*, 61–65.

Descilo, T., Vedamurtachar, A., Gerbarg, P. L., Nagaraja, D., Gangadhar, B. N., Damodaran, B., et al. (2009). Effects of a yoga breath intervention alone and in combination with an exposure therapy for posttraumatic stress disorder and depression in survivors of the 2004 South-East Asia tsunami. *Acta Psychiatrica Scandinavica, 121*, 289–300.

Foa, E. B., Hembree, E. A., & Rothbaum, B. O. (2007). *Prolonged exposure therapy for PTSD: Emotional processing of traumatic experiences. Therapist guide*. New York: Oxford University Press, Inc.

Foa, E. B., Riggs, D. S., Massie, E. D., & Yarczower, M. (1995). The impact of fear activation and anger on the efficacy of exposure treatment for posttraumatic stress disorder. *Behavior Therapy, 26*, 487–499.

Garland, E. L., & Roberts-Lewis, A. (2013). Differential roles of thought suppression and dispositional mindfulness in posttraumatic stress symptoms and cravings. *Addictive Behaviors, 38*, 1555–1562.

Gilbert, P., & Tirch, D. (2009). Emotional memory, mindfulness, and compassion. In F. Di Donna (Ed.), *Clinical handbook of mindfulness* (pp. 99–110). New York: Springer Science.

Gordon, J. S., Staples, J. K., Blyta, A., & Bytqi, M. (2004). Treatment of posttraumatic stress disorder in postwar Kosovo high school students using mind-body skills groups: A pilot study. *Journal of Traumatic Stress, 17*, 143–147.

Gordon, J. S., Staples, J. K., Blyta, A., Bytyqi, M., & Wilson, A. T. (2008). Treatment of posttraumatic stress disorder in postwar Kosovar adolescents using mind-body skills groups: A randomized controlled trial. *Journal of Clinical Psychiatry, 69*, 1469–1476.

Hayes, S. C., Strosahl, K. D., Bunting, K., Twohig, M., & Wilson, K. G. (2005). What is acceptance and commitment therapy? In S. C. Hayes & K. D. Strosahl (Eds.), *A practical guide to acceptance and commitment therapy* (pp. 3–29). New York: Springer Science+Business Media.

Henning, K. R., & Frueh, B. C. (1997). Combat guilt and its relationship to PTSD symptoms. *Journal of Clinical Psychology, 53*, 801–808.

Hollis-Walker, L., & Colosimo, K. (2011). Mindfulness, self-compassion, and happiness in non-meditators: A theoretical and empirical examination. *Personality and Individual Differences, 50*, 222–227.

Howell, A. J., Digdon, N. L., & Buro, K. (2010). Mindfulness predicts sleep-related self-regulation and well-being. *Personality and Individual Differences, 48*, 419–424.

Imel, Z. E., Laska, K., Jakupcak, M., & Simpson, T. L. (2013). Meta-analysis of dropout in treatments for posttraumatic stress disorder. *Journal of Consulting and Clinical Psychology, 81*, 394–404.

Jacobsen, L. K., Southwick, S. M., & Kosten, T. R. (2001). Substance use disorders in patients with posttraumatic stress disorder: A review of the literature. *American Journal of Psychiatry, 158*, 1184–1190.

Jha, A. P., Krompinger, J., & Baime, M. J. (2007). Mindfulness training modifies subsystems of attention. *Cognitive, Affective & Behavioral Neuroscience, 7*, 109–119.

Kabat-Zinn, J. (1990). *Full catastrophe living: Using the wisdom of your mind to face stress, pain and illness*. New York: Dell.

Kalill, K. S., Treanor, M., & Roemer, L. (2014). The importance of non-reactivity to posttraumatic stress symptoms: A case for mindfulness. *Mindfulness, 5*, 314–321.

Kartha, A., Brower, V., Saitz, R., Samet, J. H., Keane, T. M., & Liebschutz, J. (2008). The impact of trauma exposure and posttraumatic stress disorder on healthcare utilization among primary care patients. *Medical Care, 46*, 388–393.

Kearney, D. J., McDermott, K., Malte, C. A., Martinez, M., & Simpson, T. L. (2012). Association of participation in a mindfulness program with measures of PTSD, depression and quality of life in a veteran sample. *Journal of Clinical Psychology, 68*, 101–116.

Kearney, D. J., McDermott, K., Malte, C., Martinez, M., & Simpson, T. L. (2013). Effects of participation in a mindfulness program for veterans with posttraumatic stress disorder: A randomized controlled pilot study. *Journal of Clinical Psychology, 69*, 14–27.

Kilpatrick, D. G., Resnick, H. S., Milanak, M. E., Miller, M. W., Keyes, K. M., & Friedman, M. J. (2013). National estimates of exposure to traumatic events and PTSD prevalence using DSM-IV and DSM-5 criteria. *Journal of Traumatic Stress, 26*, 537–547.

Kim, S. H., Schneider, S. M., Bevans, M., Kravitz, L., Mermier, C., Qualls, C., et al. (2013). PTSD symptom reduction with mindfulness-based stretching and deep breathing exercise: Randomized controlled clinical trial of efficacy. *Journal of Clinical Endocrinology and Metabolism, 98*, 2984–2992.

Kim, S. H., Schneider, S. M., Kravitz, L., Mermier, C., & Burge, M. R. (2013). Mind-body practices for posttraumatic stress disorder. *Journal of Investigative Medicine, 61*, 827–834.

Kimbrough, E., Magyari, T., Langenberg, P., Margaret, C., & Berman, B. (2010). Mindfulness intervention for child abuse survivors. *Journal of Clinical Psychology, 66*, 17–33.

King, A. P., Erickson, T. M., Giardino, N. D., Favorite, T., Rauch, S. A., Robinson, E., et al. (2013). A pilot study of group mindfulness-based cognitive therapy (MBCT) for combat veterans with posttraumatic stress disorder. *Depression and Anxiety, 30*, 638–645.

Klein, D. A., & Miller, A. L. (2011). Dialectical behavior therapy for suicidal adolescents with borderline personality disorder. *Child and Adolescent Psychiatric Clinics of North America, 20*, 205–216.

Lang, A. J., Strauss, J. L., Bomyea, J., Bormann, J. E., Hickman, S. D., Good, R. C., et al. (2012). The theoretical and empirical basis for meditation as an intervention for PTSD. *Behavior Modification, 36*, 759–786.

Lange, B. (2011). Co-creating a communicative space to develop a mindfulness meditation manual for women in recovery from substance abuse disorders. *Advances in Nursing Science, 3*, 1–13.

Linehan, M. M. (1993). *Cognitive-behavioral treatment of borderline personality disorder*. New York: Guilford Press.

Mitchell, K. S., Dick, A. M., DiMartino, D. M., Smith, B. N., Niles, B. L., Koenen, K. C., et al. (2014). A pilot study of a randomized controlled trial of yoga for PTSD symptoms in women. *Journal of Traumatic Stress, 27*, 121–128.

Niles, B. L., Klunk-Gillis, J., Ryngala, D. J., Silberbogen, A. K., Paysnick, A., & Wolf, E. J. (2012). Comparing mindfulness and psychoeducation treatments for combat-related PTSD using a telehealth approach. *Psychological Trauma: Theory, Research, Practice, and Policy, 4*, 538–547.

Niles, B. L., Vujanovic, A. A., Silberbogen, A. K., Seligowski, A. V., & Potter, C. M. (2013). Changes in mindfulness following a mindfulness telehealth intervention. *Mindfulness, 4*, 301–310.

Oman, D., & Bormann, J. E. (2015). Mantram repetition fosters self-efficacy in veterans for managing PTSD: A randomized trial. *Psychology of Religion and Spirituality, 7*, 34–45.

Omidi, A., Mohammadi, A., Zargar, F., & Akbari, H. (2013). Efficacy of mindfulness-based stress reduction on mood states of veterans with posttraumatic stress disorder. *Archives of Trauma Research, 1*, 151–154.

Orsillo, S. M., & Batten, S. V. (2005). Acceptance and commitment therapy in the treatment of posttraumatic stress disorder. *Behavior Modification, 29*, 95–129.

Ostafin, B. D., & Marlatt, G. A. (2008). Surfing the urge: Experiential acceptance moderates the relation between automatic alcohol motivation and hazardous drinking. *Journal of Social and Clinical Psychology, 27*, 404–418.

Owens, G. P., Walter, K. H., Chard, K. M., & Davis, P. A. (2012). Changes in mindfulness skills and treatment response among veterans in residential PTSD treatment. *Psychological Trauma: Theory, Research, Practice, and Policy, 2*, 221–228.

Ramchand, R., Schell, T. L., Karney, B. R., Osilla, K. C., Burns, R. M., & Calderone, L. B. (2010). Disparate prevalence estimates of PTSD among service members who served in Iraq and Afghanistan: Possible explanations. *Journal of Traumatic Stress, 23*, 59–68.

Rathus, J. H., & Miller, A. L. (2015). *DBT Skills training manual for adolescents*. New York: Guilford Press.

Resick, P. A., & Schnicke, M. K. (1993). Cognitive processing therapy for sexual assault victims. *Journal of Consulting and Clinical Psychology, 60*, 748–756.

Rosenthal, J. Z., Grosswatd, S., Ross, R., & Rosenthal, N. (2011). Effects of transcendental meditation in veterans of operation enduring freedom and operation Iraqi freedom with posttraumatic stress disorder: A pilot study. *Military Medicine, 176*, 626.

Sareen, J., Cox, B. J., Stein, M. B., Afifi, T. O., Fleet, C., & Asmundson, G. J. G. (2007). Physical and mental comorbidity, disability, and suicidal behavior associated with posttraumatic stress disorder in a large community sample. *Psychosomatic Medicine, 69*, 242–248.

Schnurr, P. P., & Jankowski, M. K. (1999). Physical health and posttraumatic stress disorder. Review and synthesis. *Seminars in Clinical Neuropsychiatry, 4*, 295–304.

Schonert-Reichl, K. A., Oberle, E., Lawlor, M. S., Abbott, D., Thomson, K., Oberlander, T. F., et al. (2015). Enhancing cognitive and social-emotional development through a simple-to-administer mindfulness-based school program for elementary school children: A randomized controlled trial. *Developmental Psychology, 51*, 52–66. doi:10.1037/a0038454.

Schottenbauer, M. A., Glass, C. R., Arnkoff, D. B., Tendick, V., & Gray, S. H. (2008). Nonresponse and dropout rates in outcome studies on PTSD: Review and methodological considerations. *Psychiatry: Interpersonal and Biological Processes, 71*, 134–168.

Segal, Z. V., Williams, J. M. G., & Teasdale, J. D. (2013). *Mindfulness-based cognitive therapy for depression* (2nd ed.). New York: Springer Press.

Seppala, E. M., Nitschke, J. B., Tudorascu, D. L., Hayes, A., Goldstein, M. R., Nguyen, D. T., et al. (2014). Breathing-based meditation decreases posttraumatic stress disorder symptoms in U.S. military veterans: A randomized controlled longitudinal study. *Journal of Traumatic Stress, 27*, 397–405.

Smith, B. W., Ortiz, J. A., Steffen, L. E., Tooley, E. M., Wiggins, K. T., Yeater, E. A., et al. (2011). Mindfulness is associated with fewer PTSD symptoms, depressive symptoms, physical symptoms, and alcohol problems in urban firefighters. *Journal of Consulting and Clinical Psychology, 79*, 613–617.

Staples, J. K., Abdel Atti, J. A., & Gordon, J. S. (2011). Mind-body skills groups for posttraumatic stress disorder and depression symptoms in Palestinian children and adolescents in Gaza. *International Journal of Stress Management, 18*, 246–262.

Tesh, M., Learman, J., & Pulliam, R. M. (2015). Mindful self-compassion strategies for survivors of intimate partner abuse. *Mindfulness, 6*, 192–201.

Thompson, R. W., Arnkoff, D. B., & Glass, C. R. (2011). Conceptualizing mindfulness and acceptance as components of psychological resilience to trauma. *Trauma, Violence, and Abuse, 12*, 220–235.

Thompson, B. L., & Waltz, J. (2010). Mindfulness and experiential avoidance as predictors of posttraumatic stress disorder avoidance symptom severity. *Journal of Anxiety Disorders, 24*, 409–415.

Tirch, D. D. (2010). Mindfulness as a context for the cultivation of compassion. *International Journal of Cognitive Therapy, 3*, 113–123.

Van Dam, N. T., Sheppard, S. C., Forsyth, J. P., & Earleywine, M. (2011). Self-compassion is a better predictor than mindfulness of symptom severity and quality of life in mixed anxiety and depression. *Journal of Anxiety Disorders, 25*, 123–130.

van der Kolk, B. A., Stone, L., West, J., Rhodes, A., Emerson, D., Suvak, M., et al. (2014). Yoga as an adjunctive treatment for posttraumatic stress disorder: A randomized controlled trial. *Journal of Clinical Psychiatry, 75*, e559–e565.

Vujanovic, A. A., Bonn-Miller, M. O., & Marlatt, G. A. (2011). Posttraumatic stress and alcohol use coping motives among a trauma-exposed community sample: The mediating role of non-judgmental acceptance. *Addictive Behaviors, 36*, 707–712.

Vujanovic, A. A., Niles, B., Pietrefasa, A., Schmertz, S., & Potter, C. M. (2011). Mindfulness in the treatment of posttraumatic stress disorder among military veterans. *Professional Psychology: Research and Practice, 42*, 24–31.

Vujanovic, A. A., Youngwirth, N. E., Johnson, K. A., & Zvolensky, M. J. (2009). Mindfulness-based acceptance and posttraumatic stress symptoms among trauma-exposed adults without axis I psychopathology. *Journal of Anxiety Disorders, 23*(2), 297–303.

Wagner, E., Rathus, J. H., & Miller, A. L. (2006). Mindfulness in dialectical behavior therapy (DBT) for adolescents. In R. Baer (Ed.), *Mindfulness-based treatment approaches: Clinicians' guide to evidence base and applications* (pp. 167–189). Boston: Academic.

Wahbeh, H., Lu, M., & Oken, B. (2011). Mindful awareness and non-judging in relation to post-traumatic stress disorder symptoms. *Mindfulness, 2*, 219–227.

Walser, R. D., & Westrup, D. (2007). *Acceptance & commitment therapy for the treatment of post-traumatic stress disorder and trauma-related problems: A practitioner's guide to using mindfulness and acceptance strategies*. Oakland, CA: New Harbinger Publication.

Witkiewitz, K., & Bowen, S. (2010). Depression, craving, and substance use following a randomized trial of mindfulness-based relapse prevention. *Journal of Consulting and Clinical Psychology, 78*, 362–374.

Witkiewitz, K., Bowen, S., Douglas, H., & Hsu, S. H. (2013). Mindfulness-based relapse prevention for substance craving. *Addictive Behaviors, 38*, 1563–1571.

Witkiewitz, K., Greenfield, B. L., & Bowen, S. (2013). Mindfulness-based relapse prevention with racial and ethnic minority women. *Addictive Behaviors, 38*, 2821–2824.

Chapter 12
The Last of Human Desire: Grief, Death, and Mindfulness

Joanne Cacciatore and Jeffrey B. Rubin

The last of human desire: he grasps at the air.
Jin'yoku no saigo koku tsukamu nari

—Senryu poet

Introduction

Death has, for millennia, intrigued and terrified, preoccupied, and mesmerized human beings around the world. Even more mysterious and frightening is what faces those who survive the death of a loved one: grief. Some resist and avoid, some deny and repress, and yet others turn toward grief. Artists sculpt grief. Authors lament grief. Spiritual leaders preach about grief. Ethicists argue about grief. Counselors seek to provide solace to the grieving. Cultures ritualize grief. Physicians treat grief. As the post-industrialization era has taken death and grief out of personal tragedy and into the private sector, they remain largely unexplored territory in contemporary Western culture.

J. Cacciatore, Ph.D. (✉)
Arizona State University, 401 N Central Avenue, Phoenix, AZ 85004, USA
e-mail: Dr_Joanne@me.com

J.B. Rubin, Ph.D.
New York, NY, USA

Bedford Hills, NY, USA

E. Shonin et al. (eds.), *Mindfulness and Buddhist-Derived Approaches in Mental Health and Addiction*, Advances in Mental Health and Addiction,
DOI 10.1007/978-3-319-22255-4_12

Death and Grief and Suffering

There are more than 2000 published studies on death anxiety, perhaps ignited by the work of Ernest Becker (1973) in his landmark book *The Denial of Death*. Strack and Feifel (2003) found that the majority in the Western world report some fear of death and that most people are more concerned about potential pain, helplessness, dependency, and the well-being of loved ones after their death. This latter fear is reported as more significant than their own deaths, that is, the fear of grief and how their loved ones will survive their deaths.

Western culture tends to deny death, push away thoughts of mortality (Becker, 1973), and run away from grief. There are a great premium placed on youth, happiness, and hedonism and a pervasive avoidance of aging, grief, and discomfort. Thus, suffering and mourning are treated as something to avoid altogether or from which we "move on" rather expeditiously. We have witnessed, personally and professionally, a pervasive pattern: many people are disturbed and frightened by grief and approach it with clichés and pat slogans—"it's meant to be," "everything happens for a reason," "don't dwell on the past," "God has a plan for you," and "just let go and choose happiness." These empty platitudes leave the grief-stricken person feeling worse than before they shared their grief—often full of shame about their inability to "let go" of their agony.

For several thousand years, Eastern philosophy has recognized that suffering is a central part of the human condition. In the Buddhist parable about the mustard seed, for example, the Buddha tried to help a grieving mother see that no one was immune to loss and suffering, revealing the qualitative oneness of grief. And yet, despite the explicit recognition in Buddhism that suffering pervades human existence, Buddhist-inspired theories and practices, especially when taken out of context, may not be enough to help those struggling with grief. Furthermore, we have seen the way spiritual theories and practices all-too-often lead to spiritual bypassing, attempting to do an end-run around unavoidable human and existential challenges. As Wallace Stevens (1982) noted, "The way through the world/Is more difficult to find than the way beyond it" (p. 446). Authentic living is harder than creating illusory solutions. In spiritual bypassing, individuals adopt a "spiritual" perspective, either as a means to temporarily comfort self or others—such as "God has a plan," "the self is an illusion," "just trust in God," and "all things happen for a reason"—or pursues a spiritual practice (e.g., meditation, yoga, prayer) so as to, often unconsciously, avoid, rather than turn toward, confront, and explore, what afflicts them so profoundly. This transitory solution is brittle and rarely enduring, and, of course, the grief remains unexplored and unprocessed. Often, it then returns with a vengeance in the form of symptoms, physiological, emotional, and social, adding unnecessary suffering to necessary grieving.

Mindfulness Comes to the Contemporary West

In 1979, mindfulness-based stress reduction (MBSR) was developed by Jon Kabat-Zinn at the University of Massachusetts Medical Center. The program, a secular group-based curriculum, was designed primarily to treat patients with chronic pain (Ospina et al., 2007), typically administered over 8 weeks and including a daily home meditation practice. Then, in the 1990s, Teasdale, Segal, and Williams developed mindfulness-based cognitive therapy (MBCT) specifically to prevent and treat major depressive disorder (MDD) relapse, combining aspects of MBSR with aspects of cognitive therapy plus the introduction of the 3-min breathing space (Ospina et al., 2007). Their program emphasizes awareness and tolerance of thoughts, similar to the way in which exposure therapy might function (Shigaki, Glass, & Schopp, 2006).

Now, mindfulness-based interventions have demonstrated significant efficacy in reducing symptoms for a broad range of medical and psychological ailments including fibromyalgia, heart disease, chronic pain, obesity, eating disorders (Grossman, Niemann, Schmidt, & Walach, 2004), asthma, type II diabetes mellitus, hypertension, substance abuse (Ospina et al., 2007), epilepsy, psoriasis, HIV (Carlson et al., 2004), and multiple sclerosis (Shigaki et al., 2006). And yet, despite the extensive applicability of mindfulness, deeper understanding demands that we also examine areas that have been neglected.

Death, Grief, and Mindfulness

Several scholars have begun to explore the relationship between mortality salience, or "impermanence awareness," and posttraumatic growth (Kumar, 2005; Wada & Park, 2009). The cultivation of this state of mind is believed to ease the overwhelming burden of grief by understanding its normalcy and necessity while not avoiding, pathologizing, or medicalizing grief. Wada and Park (2009) suggest that the mindful approach to grief recognizes suffering and emotional vulnerability as essential forces to propel one forward into growth, when he or she is ready, rather than the view of grief as pathology which requires medical attention. The middle path through grief wherein one neither avoids, represses, nor numbs affects nor does one grasp, cling, or unnecessarily punish oneself in grief. Both extreme states, that is, "severing the bond with the deceased or rigidly holding on to the loss…will not lead one to cope with the loss in a wholesome way" (p. 665).

Very few scholars, and even fewer empirical studies, however, have focused on death, grief, and mindfulness practice, for client, provider, *and* the relationship. Cacciatore (2011) proposed the first mindfulness-based paradigm, its utility focused on the tripartite relationship. The model's utility and success have been demonstrated in several studies since its inception (Cacciatore & Flint, 2012; Cacciatore, Thieleman, Osborn, & Orlowski, 2014; Thieleman & Cacciatore, 2014; Thieleman,

Cacciatore, & Wonch, 2014). For example, using this model, Thieleman et al. (2014) found a reduction in trauma, depressive, and anxious symptoms in a population of the traumatically bereaved after an average of just 14 h in counseling. Still, the model does not tout a particular goal or objective, nor does it seek to reduce symptoms within a specific time period. Rather, this paradigm merely seeks to facilitate and bear witness to a process of being with, surrendering to, then, when ready, doing, or taking compassionate action, with grief (Cacciatore, 2014).

The model, known as ATTEND (**a**ttunement, **t**rust, **t**ouch, **e**galitarianism, **n**uance, and **d**eath education), built upon a foundation of self-care practices, encourages mindfulness practice for the provider, modeling for the client, and bringing such practice into the therapeutic relationship (attunement). Providers, themselves, are strongly encouraged to cultivate a meditation practice and grief/death education as part of the client's treatment. Particularly with traumatic grief, it is crucial that providers have high affect tolerance and radical acceptance of the client's painful memories and accompanying emotions. In so doing, this psychological environment fosters a sense of safety and nurturance for the bereaved client (trust). In the context of this model, once trust has been established, haptic feedback in the form of non-perfunctory touch, when appropriate and therapeutic, is encouraged rather than anathema (touch). Relational power is shared, provider humility is paramount, and the counselor or therapist recognizes the client as his or her own expert, acting more as a guide. The emphasis is not on pathologizing the client's experiences; rather, the provider meets the client wherever he or she is in the grief experience and allows what is, in that moment, to be (egalitarianism). Because of the inherent fluidity of this model, there isn't a standardized protocol. Rather, the provider recognizes the individuality of each family, every circumstance, and every presentation as unique, acting with sensitivity for his or her cultural identification (nuance). The model also encourages providers to contemplate and study mortality and grief (death education), shown to significantly increase both mindfulness and empathy in second-year graduate students (Cacciatore, Thieleman, Killian, & Tavasolli, 2014). This yields benefits to both the practitioner and to the client, and this, ultimately then, supports the therapeutic relationship.

Finally, this model is built upon a foundation of self-care and compassion. Practitioners using this model are strongly encouraged to engage in various strategies for self-care, empirically demonstrated to diminish compassion fatigue and vicarious trauma, not just for their own benefit but, also, to help the client. Compassion fatigue is defined in the literature as a reduction in a provider's capacity for empathy toward clients as a result of repeated trauma exposure (Adams, Boscarino, & Figley, 2006). Obviously, both compassion fatigue and vicarious trauma have profoundly negative effects on both providers and the clients they serve. Yet, there is some evidence to suggest that a mindfulness-model of practice may protect providers from compassion fatigue and vicarious trauma.

Thieleman and Cacciatore (2014) found that providers using the ATTEND model, despite working in one of the highest risk populations (the traumatically bereaved), were protected from vicarious trauma, provider burnout, and reported higher life satisfaction. No doubt, these protective variables yield a more helpful and compassionate environment for clients and thus they benefit from such a milieu (Thieleman & Cacciatore, 2014). Grepmair et al. (2007) conducted a double-blind randomized controlled trial wherein, indeed, the clients of "providers who meditated" had better therapeutic outcomes than clients of therapists who did not meditate. This is potent ethical motivation for provider mindfulness practices.

What Mindful Care Looks Like

Mindful care, vis-à-vis the ATTEND model, cannot be quantified, manualized, or put into a neat formula. Nevertheless, it has certain common ingredients including empathy and compassion, patience and humility, understanding, and flexibility. Deep self-awareness and attunement foster the development of all these states. Empathy, striving to understand someone from within their unique frame of reference (Kohut, 1977), is the foundation upon which the relationship is built because without it there is no safety or understanding. And compassion, ancillary to empathy, has been described as "empathic action" (Parr, 2002). Patience is crucial because the grieving person must have the time and space to experience the full range of their loss and agony. They cannot be rushed; nor can they follow someone else's timetable. Humility recognizes and respects the inherent wisdom of the client's pain, presenting "symptoms," and personal process. A humble provider fosters an environment of culturally appropriate care that is individualized for this particular person in his or her painful situation. Flexibility is crucial because each person is unique; and every therapeutic dyad must discover the best way to approach healing and transformation (Rubin, 1998).

We have found that there is always an emotional logic to the client's situation, even when we, as providers, don't necessarily understand initially. However, we strive to create an environment in which the client's feelings and experiences are not only fundamental but also revered—even if they clash with or are foreign to our own experiences. For example, we both believe in the transformative power of speaking about and witnessing what feels overwhelming and unbearable. But when a particular client needs to avoid talking about what afflicts them in order to protect against anticipated re-traumatization, their needs are more important than our models of helping.

We use the therapeutic relationship as an arena to gently explore, illuminate, and hopefully transform the client's struggles in coping with grief and trauma. Crucial to this process is our willingness to accompany them on their journey of mourning, witnessing, and validating their experience. They are our guide as together we struggle to understand and make meaning or sense of that which most haunts them.

Beyond Mindfulness: The Marriage of Mindful Care and Meaning

It's one thing to talk about mindfulness in treating traumatic grief. It's another thing to practice this unique type of caregiving. One of the greatest challenges facing clinicians who work in this field is how we, ourselves, process our own emotional reactions to traumatic loss, including feelings of vulnerability for ourselves and for our loved ones. Meditation and psychotherapy can be immensely helpful in doing this. And, also, each tradition has its blind spots and weaknesses, and the strength of each corrects for the limitations of the other (Rubin, 1996).

Meditation is a remarkable tool for cultivating heightened attention and presence, a wonderful asset to therapists and clients. But meditation tends to neglect meaning (Rubin, 2013). It features, for example, being aware of what arises, but that doesn't always lead to understanding its emotional significance. For example, noting anger while meditating is different than experiencing the disappointment and hurt that sometimes underlies it. The emphasis in certain meditative practices on investigating the causes and significance of experienced phenomena doesn't mean that meditators are illuminating the unconscious underpinnings of its meaning. Indeed, meditators, potentially, have greater access to their emotions; yet they often do not do enough with it. Western psychotherapy does a wonderful job of understanding meaning. Combining the meditative ability to develop refined concentration, equanimity, and self-compassion with the therapeutic capacity to illuminate human experience is an extraordinarily potent and often neglected means of helping people in pain. For example, when we are truly attentive and present, and then examine the emotional significance of what we are feeling—from anger and sadness to jealousy and grief—we are more likely to understand ourselves and be able to skillfully cope with our own feelings in the moment (Rubin, 2009).

[1]*Glenn, Client of JC*

Glenn is a first-time father in his early 30s of mixed ethnic descent. His son, Sean, died 2 years earlier during birth. Sean was 2 weeks over his due date when he died. Glenn and his partner discussed inducing labor but ultimately he discouraged the procedure, wanting to wait until Sean was "ready for birth." He blamed himself for Sean's death. So did his partner, Ann. Shortly after Sean's birth and death, Ann left Glenn. He began using alcohol, along with prescription drugs, to help him "cope with the grief of losing both his son and his partner." He began showing up late at work, personal hygiene declined, and his family expressed significant concern over his well-being. Glenn sought counseling at the urging of loved ones after being

[1]Clients' names have been changed to protect their anonymity and they have given permission to use their stories for this manuscript.

arrested while driving under the influence. He was reluctant to seek help because he "contributed to Sean's death" and felt "unworthy to live." I noticed, in my first few meetings with Glenn, that his affect was flat, inconsistent with what he reported verbally. His range of emotional expression felt stunted, frozen perhaps. While he could recount details of his experiences, much of the narrative was told in a rather detached manner. Once I felt Glenn trusted me, I asked him about the story he was telling. I inquired as to his degree of "deeply felt emotion" and asked if he felt he could share from a more authentic place. He said he'd felt this disconnect since he began using substances, and he reported a strong desire to stop the abuse. With the aid of his primary care physician, Glenn titrated off a low-dose anxiolytic and SSRI. Our weekly 2-h meetings continued. He shared more openly over time and eventually his emotional expression became increasingly more potent, congruent with the narrative of his story. It felt like a deeply trusting relationship, and I practiced being aware of my own sense of grief with and for Glenn, particularly when he would weep. My own meditation practice helped immensely in this regard. Within 9 months, Glenn was off his psychiatric medications and had restricted his alcohol consumption to two glasses of wine a week. Glenn still felt he was not ready to implement a mindfulness practice. He felt like there was a "truck sitting on [his] chest" and "breathing was hard." He also felt his discursive mind would interfere with his ability to be still. I invited him to a practice of mindful movement, which he embraced. He began walking every morning, in silence, paying careful attention to the placement of his feet, the cool air on his face, and the swing of his arms. Eventually, when he felt ready, we incorporated breath awareness to his mindful morning walk. He began to feel and express deeper sadness than ever, yet he had cultivated a practice wherein he trusted his ability to be with the pain—and the painful memories—without feeling overwhelmed, threatened, or paralyzed by it. Six months later, Glenn attended a meditation retreat for the first time. That was 5 years ago, and he continues his practice even today. He feels that his mindfulness practices help him to "both remember and cope with the inevitable suffering" and "lifelong grief" he will experience as a bereaved father.

Annie, Traumatic Grief Client of JC

Annie is a 38-year-old mother of three who lost her youngest child, Maggie, 8 years old, after a routine surgical procedure. She was given psychiatric medication 2 days after her daughter's death, both a benzodiazepine and an antidepressant which she had been taking, without adjunctive psychotherapy, for 2 years prior to seeking counseling. During Annie's first session, she lamented the loss of her primary social support system, friends who had children Maggie's age who she felt "now avoided" her because they were "too terrified to confront" her pain and grief. Annie was also experiencing marital discordance as she reported "no interest in sex or intimacy at all" and felt her "skin crawled" every time her husband tried to initiate intimate contact. When I asked her if she could share details of Maggie's death, she declined saying it felt "too hard to tell the story" and that "she hadn't told the story in years."

Of course, I did not push her; rather, I reengaged in exploring her experiences in the dyadic and social relationships which were so painful for her. When she spoke of her marital disharmony, she also said that she'd gained weight since Maggie's death and "felt unsexy and undesirable" noting a significant decline in sexual interest and arousal. She seemed to have some insight of this feeling "unfair" to her partner but was "uncertain how to change anything." Additionally, in recounting her feelings of isolation within her former social group, she noted that she "self-isolates," and despite being invited by her friends, she often "declines because of a lack of motivation" and "desire to be alone." We spent much of our first session building trust in the relationship and I listened deeply to not only the rare glimpses into her grief over Maggie's death but also her expression of isolation and loneliness. During our third session, Annie began to open up more fully, shared more detail about Maggie's death, and asked if I would be willing to look at photos of her, to which, of course, I replied an unequivocal assent. At one point while looking at photos, she began to divulge her sense of guilt: "I killed Maggie," she said with tears in her eyes. "Annie, tell me more, please?" I said softly and gently. She continued to explain that when they'd left the hospital, she had a "very specific feeling" that something wasn't "right with Maggie… that something bad, terrible, was going to happen." She began sobbing, uncontrollably, saying repeatedly how Maggie's death was her fault and how ashamed she felt for having "let her die." I noticed my own feelings of pain for and with Annie in this moment of abysmal suffering. I leaned into her pain and just sat closely with my head bowed: "I'm so sorry, Annie. I'm just so sorry." She continued to weep, audibly, for the next 10–15 min without pause. I remained silent but very present, holding space for her feelings of guilt and shame. I did not try to change her heart. I did not try to convince her otherwise. I just bore witness to the dark emotions that surfaced. By the end of that session, I could sense that something, inexplicable, had shifted. She hugged me before she left, thanked me profusely, and even sent a follow-up e-mail about how she'd never been able to share so honestly with anyone. It wasn't for a lack of trying. She'd tried to express her feelings of guilt and shame with others. But they couldn't bear to hear it and quickly dismissed her feelings as invalid, "ridiculous," and "outrageous." She stopped sharing her story, her feelings, and her thoughts shortly thereafter. By the tenth session, Annie began titrating off her psychiatric medications and we began to introduce brief breath meditation to her daily journaling practice. By the 15th session, she was off her psychiatric medication and "feeling much more depth and pain," but she also noted a renewed interest in sexual intimacy and social interaction. She attended a four-day meditation retreat, began a yoga practice, and lost 25 pounds. It's been 4 years since Annie walked through my door. The shift in her ability to cope has been extraordinary.

Beverly, Trauma Client of JR

Several years into treatment, Beverly, a middle-aged woman with a severe trauma history, began to unthaw from a horrendous history of abuse that left her feeling grief-stricken, demoralized, and self-doubting. While she was making significant progress understanding the causes and the impact of her uncle's sexual abuse, she still struggled with a difficulty tolerating feelings and a tendency to either retreat into protective isolation or pathologically accommodate the wishes of those people she interacted with. She informed me that Buddhist meditation was very helpful in trying to cope with distressing feelings that seemingly came out of nowhere and made her feel as if she was drowning. But she sheepishly admitted that she was resistant to meditating. As we explored what happened when she tried to meditate at home on her own, I asked her if meditating at home left her alone with extremely painful feelings and if she stayed away from meditating so that she was not alone with these feelings. Tears rolled down her face as she shook her head up and down in assent.

We meditated together in that session and some subsequent ones and then processed the feelings that arose. Her capacity to sit with and accept a fuller range of feelings—especially sadness and grief—slowly developed. Meditation helped her become more self-accepting and less self-judging.

In our own personal and clinical experience, mindful care entails the marriage of mindfulness and meaning (Rubin, 2013). Mindfulness practices, like psychotherapy, increase awareness of our experience in the present. It also lessens judgment and increases our—and our client's—tolerance of painful emotions. In other words, both participants in therapy can sit with and through a wider range of feelings without prematurely and reactively denying them, drowning in them, or attributing them to someone else. And this makes it possible to explore their meaning and cultivate experiential understanding of their significance. And this is crucial for the therapeutic process. Without that mindfulness of feelings by itself—knowing that we feel sad without understanding its full meaning and significance (that we, e.g., might blame ourselves or imagine we are bad for feeling what we are feeling)—may not lead to coming to terms with that which, consciously or unconsciously, haunts us so.

Conclusion

Grief is inevitable for us all. Yet, a culture which does not foster a compassionate response in the face of inevitable and universal grief simply adds to the suffering of its members. And we live in a world in which individuals—and even various therapeutic and spiritual systems—tend to minimize, if not outright neglect and ignore, afflictive emotions such as grief, anger, and shame. Instead, both implicit and explicit messages coercively focus only on positive feelings, which can create an increasingly painful social milieu for those who experience traumatic grief (Cacciatore & Devine, 2015; Welwood, 2002).

Mindfulness practices allow us to deepen the genuineness of our relationships with self and other, bringing us closer, even amidst tragedy, and can enhance the feeling of safety as we all seek solace for our experiences of unfathomable pain. As providers, our hearts can remain open to the other, without needing to self-protect or to erect unnecessary boundaries of fear and death anxiety. But mindfulness practices, while necessary, are often insufficient, for the grief-stricken mourner. They need to judiciously integrate mindfulness with developing and deepening meaning and understanding. And that provides something rare and vital in our fraught world—namely, an emotional home for the grief and trauma and death that permeate our lives.

References

Adams, R. E., Boscarino, J. A., & Figley, C. R. (2006). Compassion fatigue and psychological distress among social workers: A validation study. *American Journal of Orthopsychiatry, 76*, 103–108.

Becker, E. (1973). *The denial of death*. New York: Free Press.

Cacciatore, J. (2011). ATTEND: Toward a patient-centered model of psychosocial care. In C. Spong (Ed.), *Stillbirth: Prediction, prevention, and management 1e*. Wiley Blackwell Publishing. Hoboken, New Jersey.

Cacciatore, J. (2014). *Selah: A guide to fully inhabited grief.* Austin, TX: MISS Foundation.

Cacciatore, J., & Devine, M. (2015). To love or not to love: To grieve or not to grieve. In G. Warburton & H. Martins (Eds.), *The theory of love*. London: Portfolio Publishing.

Cacciatore, J., & Flint, M. (2012). ATTEND: A mindfulness-based bereavement care model. *Death studies, 36*, 61–82.

Cacciatore, J., Thieleman, K., Killian, M., & Tavasolli, K. (2014). Braving human suffering: Death education and its relationship to empathy and mindfulness. *Social Work Education, 34*, 91–109.

Cacciatore, J., Thieleman, K., Osborn, J., & Orlowski, K. (2014). Of the soul and suffering: Mindfulness based interventions and bereavement. *Clinical Social Work Journal, 42*, 269–281.

Carlson, L. E., Angen, M., Cullum, J., Goodey, E., Koopmans, J., Lamont, L., et al. (2004). High levels of untreated distress and fatigue in cancer patients. *Psycho-Oncology, 13*, S49–S50.

Grepmair, L., Mitterlehner, F., Loew, T., Bachler, E., Rother, W., & Nickel, M. (2007). Promoting mindfulness in psychotherapists in training influences the treatment results of their patients: A randomized, double-blind, controlled study. *Psychotherapy and Psychosomatics, 76*, 332–338.

Grossman, P., Niemann, L., Schmidt, S., & Walach, H. (2004). Mindfulness-based stress reduction and health benefits: A meta-analysis. *Journal of Psychosomatic Research, 57*, 35–43.

Kohut, H. (1977). *The restoration of the self.* Chicago: University of Chicago Press.

Kumar, S. M. (2005). *Grieving mindfully: A compassionate and spiritual guide to coping with loss*. Oakland, CA: New Harbinger.

Ospina M. B., Bond T. K., Karkhaneh M., Tjosvold, L., Vandermeer, B., Liang Y., et al. (2007). *Meditation practices for health: State of the research* (Evidence Report/Technology Assessment No. 155. Prepared by the University of Alberta Evidence-based Practice Center under Contract No. 290-02-0023.). Rockville, MD: Agency for Healthcare Research and Quality.

Parr, L. (2002). Understanding others' emotions: From empathic resonance to empathic action. *Behavioral and Brain Sciences, 25*(1), 44–45.

Rubin, J. B. (1996). *Psychotherapy and Buddhism: Toward an integration*. New York: Plenum.

Rubin, J. B. (1998). *A psychoanalysis for our time: Exploring the blindness of the seeing I*. New York: New York University Press.

Rubin, J. B. (2009). *The art of flourishing*. New York: Crown.

Rubin, J. B. (2013). *Meditative psychotherapy*. Kindle. New York: Abiding Change Press.

Shigaki, C. L., Glass, B., & Schopp, L. H. (2006). Mindfulness-based stress reduction in medical settings. *Journal of Clinical Psychology in Medical Settings, 13*, 209–215.

Stevens, W. (1982). Reply to Papini. In *The collected poems of Wallace Stevens*. New York: Vintage Books.

Strack, S., & Feifel, H. (2003). Psychology. In R. J. Kastenbaum (Eds.), *Macmillan encyclopedia of death and dying* (Vol. 2: L-Z). New York: Macmillan Reference USA, The Gale Group, 687.

Thieleman, K., & Cacciatore, J. (2014). A witness to suffering: Mindfulness and compassion fatigue amongst traumatic bereavement volunteers and professionals. *Social Work, 59*(1), 34–41.

Thieleman, K., Cacciatore, J., & Wonch, T. (2014). Traumatic bereavement and mindfulness: A preliminary study of mental health outcomes. *Clinical Social Work Journal, 42*, 260–268.

Wada, K., & Park, J. (2009). Integrating Buddhist psychology into grief counseling. *Death Studies, 33*, 657–683.

Welwood, J. (2002). *Toward a psychology of awakening*. Boston: Shambhala Press.

Chapter 13
Mindfulness for Cultivating Self-Esteem

Christopher A. Pepping, Penelope J. Davis, and Analise O'Donovan

Mindfulness for Cultivating Self-Esteem

Self-esteem is widely conceptualized as a fundamental and pervasive human need (Greenberg et al., 1992; Pyszczynski, Greenberg, Solomon, Arndt, & Schimel, 2004). In the present chapter, we argue that mindfulness may be associated with increased self-esteem and, in particular, with secure forms of self-esteem rather than fragile high self-esteem. We begin by providing an overview of self-esteem, including the benefits of healthy self-esteem and the costs of low self-esteem. Next, we differentiate between secure high self-esteem and fragile high self-esteem and argue that individuals high in dispositional mindfulness may have greater capacity for secure high self-esteem. We then review evidence from clinical and experimental studies examining causal associations between mindfulness and self-esteem. Finally, we conclude with a discussion of how mindfulness-based interventions may enhance healthy self-esteem and outline directions for future research.

Self-Esteem

Self-esteem refers to an individual's evaluation of his or her own self-worth, and it is considered to be a relatively stable personality trait that varies across individuals (Kernis, 2003; Waterman, 1992). Self-esteem is generally considered a fundamental

C.A. Pepping (✉)
School of Psychology and Public Health, La Trobe University, Melbourne, Australia
e-mail: c.pepping@latrobe.edu.au

P.J. Davis • A. O'Donovan
School of Applied Psychology, Behavioral Basis of Health, and Griffith Health Institute, Griffith University, Brisbane, Australia

E. Shonin et al. (eds.), *Mindfulness and Buddhist-Derived Approaches in Mental Health and Addiction*, Advances in Mental Health and Addiction,
DOI 10.1007/978-3-319-22255-4_13

human desire, and individuals are particularly motivated to maintain high self-esteem and engage in efforts to protect their self-esteem when it is threatened. Two main theories have been proposed to explain the human need for self-esteem, namely, sociometer theory (Leary, 1999; Leary, Tambor, Terdal, & Downs, 1995) and terror management theory (Greenberg, Pyszczynski, & Solomon, 1986). According to the sociometer theory of self-esteem (Leary, 1999; Leary et al., 1995), self-esteem is an evolved system that serves as a meter of social acceptance and relationship quality with others. From an evolutionary perspective, humans are driven to maintain connection with others and strive towards acceptance from peer groups. Thus, individuals are not necessarily motivated to maintain high self-esteem as the end goal but rather to maintain acceptance from other people. This then motivates behaviors designed to enhance the chances of being valued and accepted by others. Consistent with this proposition, Leary et al. (1995) found that individuals' self-esteem correlates with the extent to which they believe they are accepted or excluded, with self-esteem decreasing in response to social exclusion.

Terror management theory (TMT) offers a distinct though somewhat related explanation as to why humans desire self-esteem (Greenberg et al., 1986, 1992; Pyszczynski et al., 2004). Humans are in the unique position of being aware of their own mortality and the inevitability of death. This awareness generates significant existential anxiety and motivates individuals to engage in anxiety-buffering defensive strategies. TMT posits that humans are motivated to pursue self-esteem as it serves as a buffer to existential death anxiety. Specifically, self-esteem is derived from meeting the standards and expectations of one's particular culture and provides individuals with a sense that they are a valuable contributor to the world, and thus their life has meaning and importance (Pyszczynski et al., 2004). Consistent with the TMT perspective, experimental studies indicate that high self-esteem buffers death anxiety and that priming mortality leads individuals to engage in efforts to increase their self-esteem. However, when individuals are experimentally convinced of the existence of an afterlife, their efforts to increase self-esteem in response to mortality salience primes are diminished (Pyszczynski et al., 2004). In brief, self-esteem is a fundamental human desire, and individuals are particularly motivated to maintain high self-esteem and engage in efforts to protect self-esteem when it comes under threat.

Self-esteem is an important construct and is related to a variety of positive psychological and social outcomes, including general psychological adjustment, positive emotion, social confidence, prosocial behavior, work well-being, satisfying relationships, and overall life satisfaction (Diener, Emmons, Larsen, & Griffin, 1985; Leary & MacDonald, 2003; Orth & Robins, 2014). In addition, a meta-analysis of 77 longitudinal studies suggested that low self-esteem predicts depression; low self-esteem is not simply an outcome of depression (Sowislo & Orth, 2013). Finally, low self-esteem in adolescence prospectively predicts poorer mental and physical health and higher criminal behavior in adulthood, compared to those with high self-esteem (Trzesniewski et al., 2006). In brief, much evidence indicates that high self-esteem is a positive personal resource.

Despite the pervasive pursuit for high self-esteem and the widely documented positive outcomes associated with high self-esteem, several researchers have noted that high self-esteem is not always beneficial (e.g., Deci & Ryan, 1995; Jordan, Spencer, Zanna, Hoshino-Browne, & Correll, 2003; Kernis, 2003; Ryan & Brown, 2003). For example, some studies have found that high self-esteem is associated with increased prejudice (Verkuyten & Masson, 1995), defensive self-enhancement (Baumeister, Heatherton, & Tice, 1993), and heightened violence and aggression (Baumeister, Smart, & Boden, 1996). What might explain these somewhat counterintuitive findings? One possibility is that there are two forms of high self-esteem: one associated with positive outcomes and one with negative outcomes. Accordingly, several researchers have proposed that high self-esteem can indeed take two forms (Kernis, 2003; Ryan & Brown, 2003), namely, secure high self-esteem and fragile high self-esteem.

Secure high self-esteem refers to a positive self-view that is grounded in reality and is not easily threatened, whereas fragile high self-esteem reflects a positive self-view and feelings of self-worth that require frequent validation, are vulnerable to threat, and oftentimes reflect some form of self-deception or compensation for underlying feelings of low self-esteem (Zeigler-Hill, 2006). There are several ways in which secure and fragile high self-esteem have been conceptualized and distinguished. For example, defensive high self-esteem (Jordan et al., 2003; Kernis, 2003) refers to a defensive attempt to bolster or enhance explicit views of oneself, despite implicit or unconscious low self-esteem. Similarly, contingent high self-esteem is an additional conceptualization of fragile high self-esteem. Contingent high self-esteem refers to the tendency to base one's self-worth and self-value on achievements or meeting an ideal standard relative to others. Deci and Ryan (1995) note that when these achievements or standards on which this self-esteem is contingent upon cease, self-esteem also tends to decrease.

In summary, several terms have been used in the literature to differentiate between secure forms of self-esteem and fragile high self-esteem (i.e., defensive high self-esteem, contingent high self-esteem). Although there are differences between the various conceptualizations of self-esteem, for the purposes of the present review, we use the terms secure high self-esteem and fragile high self-esteem throughout the chapter and refer to the more specific forms of fragile high self-esteem, namely, defensive high self-esteem and contingent high self-esteem, only when reporting on individual studies using these specific conceptualizations. We propose here that mindfulness is likely to be associated with high self-esteem and, in particular, may facilitate the development of secure high self-esteem as opposed to fragile high self-esteem.

Dispositional Mindfulness and Self-Esteem

In the present chapter, we use the definition of mindfulness proposed by Kabat-Zinn whereby mindfulness is defined as "paying attention in a particular way: on purpose, in the present moment, non-judgmentally" (Kabat-Zinn, 1994, p. 4). Consistent with the definition outlined by Kabat-Zinn (1994), Bishop et al. (2004) propose that mindfulness includes two core components: (1) the self-regulation of attention and (2) a certain orientation to experience. Self-regulation of attention refers to the process of directing attention towards the present moment, coupled with the ability to observe and attend to the ever-changing stream of thoughts, emotions, and sensations that individuals experience at any moment. Bishop et al. (2004) argue that self-regulation of attention facilitates pure awareness of thoughts, feelings, and sensations based on direct experience rather than elaborative processing of these experiences or becoming involved in rumination about these experiences. The second component of the conceptualization outlined by Bishop et al. (2004) is a certain orientation to experiences, which refers to a nonjudgmental and curious stance directed towards experiences in the present moment, together with an attitude of openness and acceptance to whatever may arise in each moment.

There have been a number of measures of mindfulness developed (e.g., Baer, Smith, Hopkins, Krietemeyer, & Toney, 2006; Brown & Ryan, 2003; Lau et al., 2006; Walach, Buchheld, Buttenmuller, Kleinknecht, & Schmidt, 2006). To provide a more in-depth analysis of the construct of mindfulness, Baer et al. (2006) examined the underlying factor structure assessed by items from five measures of mindfulness and found a five-factor solution. The factors identified were "observing," which refers to the process of noticing internal and external experiences, including thoughts, physical sensations, and emotions; "non-judging of inner experiences," which refers to taking a nonjudgmental and accepting stance to internal experiences such as difficult thoughts, emotions, and physical sensations; "describing" which is the ability to label with words one's own internal experiences; "non-reactivity" to inner experiences refers to the capacity to remain present with thoughts and emotions without impulsively responding to them and without being either consumed by them or seeking to avoid these experiences; and, finally, "acting with awareness" refers to the process of paying attention to the present moment rather than being preoccupied with thoughts or emotions about the future or past (Baer et al., 2006, 2008). The five facets are moderately correlated with each other but differentially predict theoretically related outcomes. With regard to the association between mindfulness and self-esteem, identification of the relative importance of a range of facets of mindfulness in the prediction of self-esteem may be a useful focus with important clinical implications.

Why might high dispositional mindfulness enhance self-esteem? We have argued previously (Pepping, O'Donovan, & Davis, 2013) that individuals dispositionally high in mindfulness may be less consumed by the thoughts and emotions that characterize low self-esteem and thus have greater capacity to cope with these experiences. A key feature of mindfulness is a decentered stance towards thoughts. Further, individuals higher in mindfulness tend to possess a nonjudgmental, open, and receptive stance to their experiences and their thoughts and emotions (Baer et al., 2006), which may allow them to be less consumed by harsh, critical, and judgmental thoughts relating to the self. Although it may be that those high in mindfulness are less likely to generate harsh negative thoughts about the self in the first place, it is also likely that high mindfulness enables individuals to respond to harsh and self-critical thoughts, when they do occur, more adaptively.

Drawing from Ryan, Brown, and Creswell's (2007) discussion of attachment and mindfulness, individuals who have low self-esteem have cognitive biases that are based on past experiences and deeply held beliefs about the self that are oftentimes highly negative. However, mindfulness may allow an individual to transcend these cognitive biases and maladaptive schemas. Mindfulness facilitates nonjudgmental acceptance of the present moment, including thoughts and emotions, without being influenced or overwhelmed by cognitive biases relating to the past. Therefore, high dispositional mindfulness may act as a buffer to low self-esteem. Individuals who are high in dispositional mindfulness may have enhanced capacity to step back from, and cope with, negative thoughts relating to the self.

Consistent with the proposition that high dispositional mindfulness should be related to increased self-esteem, several studies have found a positive relationship between mindfulness and self-esteem (Brown & Ryan, 2003; Michalak, Teismann, Heidenreich, Strohle, & Vocks, 2011; Rajamaki, 2011; Rasmussen & Pidgeon, 2011; Thompson & Waltz, 2008). Very little research has examined which specific facets of mindfulness predict increased self-esteem. Michalak et al. (2011) found that "acceptance" (similar to non-judging of experiences) predicted increased mindfulness. However, the research focused only on the acceptance facet, and the other facets of mindfulness were therefore not examined. To extend prior research examining the association between mindfulness and self-esteem, we recently conducted two studies examining the association between mindfulness and self-esteem (Pepping et al., 2013). The research had two major aims: the first was to examine associations between individual facets of mindfulness and self-esteem (Study 1) and the second focus was to examine the effects of a brief experimental mindfulness induction on self-esteem (Study 2).

With regard to the association between specific facets of mindfulness and self-esteem, we argued that understanding the relative importance of various facets of mindfulness in the prediction of self-esteem may inform mindfulness-based clinical interventions to increase self-esteem. That is, understanding the specific components of mindfulness that relate to increased self-esteem would enable clinicians to tailor interventions, focusing in particular on the specific processes that predict self-esteem.

We predicted that four of the five mindfulness facets (*non-reactivity, awareness, labeling*, and *non-judging of inner experience*) would significantly predict self-esteem (Pepping et al., 2013, Study 1) as measured by the Rosenberg self-esteem scale (Rosenberg, 1965). Consistent with predictions, individuals scoring high on these four facets of mindfulness were higher in self-esteem. We argued that "non-judging" should facilitate increased self-esteem as individuals higher in this facet may be better able to take a nonjudgmental and less self critical stance towards themselves. In addition, they may be less prone to judging and evaluating specific thoughts themselves (Baer et al., 2006, 2008). That is, "non-judging" facilitates a nonjudgmental stance towards thoughts, emotions, and experiences, and these experiences are observed from a neutral, objective standpoint, as opposed to being judged as good or bad (Baer et al., 2006). With regard to self-esteem, those who are higher on the non-judging facet may be less likely to experience self-critical thoughts in the first place but may also display enhanced capacity to perceive these thoughts purely as thoughts, rather than evaluating them or becoming caught up in the content. Interestingly, "non-judging" was most strongly associated with increased self-esteem which suggests that the ability to maintain an open and non-judgmental approach to thoughts, feelings, and sensations has a particularly positive effect on self-esteem. Individuals high on this facet may be less likely to get caught up in harsh judgmental thoughts about the self.

The "labeling" subscale was also associated with higher self-esteem. Individuals with greater capacity to label, describe, and express cognitive and emotional experiences may be less likely to become mindlessly caught up in self-critical thoughts about themselves (Baer et al., 2006). Specifically, self-critical thoughts can be labeled, which we proposed might allow the individual to continue with other activities without becoming overwhelmed by these experiences. This may be why psychotherapies such as dialectical behavior therapy (DBT) encourage individuals to label and describe thoughts and emotions (Linehan, 1993). In brief, the ability to "label" thoughts and feelings with words appears to be associated with increased self-esteem, perhaps reflecting the beneficial effects of being able to identify self-critical thoughts.

Individuals high on the "non-reactivity" facet were also higher in self-esteem. It may be that these individuals are able to allow internal experiences such as thoughts and feelings relating to the self to enter and leave awareness, without engaging in efforts to avoid or get rid of these experiences but also without engaging in rumination (Baer et al., 2006, 2008). Rather than defensively trying to bolster self-esteem or reduce self-critical thoughts, individuals high on the "non-reactivity" facet may be better able to experience these thoughts and emotions without responding in maladaptive ways. It seems likely that "non-reactivity" enables individuals to treat harsh and self-critical thoughts associated simply as thoughts, rather than a true reflection of reality.

We also predicted that the "acting with awareness" subscale would be associated with increased self-esteem, as individuals high on this facet are able to attend to the present moment as opposed to being distracted by self-critical thoughts. Low "awareness," on the other hand, is associated with the tendency to get caught up in thoughts about the future or past. In line with this proposition, we found that individuals higher on the "acting with awareness" subscales were higher in self-esteem, suggesting that the capacity to maintain present-focused attention may assist with an individual's ability to transcend deep-seated negative beliefs relating to the self.

The "observe" facet did not predict self-esteem. It thus appears that noticing or observing self-critical thoughts and difficult emotions does not necessarily enhance self-esteem, but rather it is the attitude or stance taken towards these experiences that is important. It is probable that individuals with both high and low self-esteem may observe self-critical thoughts. However, it appears that the "relationship" one has with these experiences is more strongly related to increased self-esteem. The finding that "observe" did not predict increased self-esteem is consistent with this proposition.

The study described here (Pepping et al., 2013, Study 1) represented the first attempt to examine the "relative" importance of five facets of mindfulness in the prediction of healthy self-esteem. This level of analysis allows us to understand more specifically which aspects of mindfulness are associated with self-esteem. It appears that present-focused attention; a nonjudgmental, nonreactive, and accepting stance towards thoughts and emotions; and the ability to label thoughts and feelings all contribute to the development of healthy self-esteem. It is important to note, however, that the research reviewed above, although very useful with regard to providing insight into the specific factors of mindfulness relating to increased self-esteem, is cross-sectional. This limits the extent to which we can conclude that mindfulness actively enhances self-esteem. We therefore turn to the use of mindfulness-based clinical interventions and experimental studies examining causal associations between mindfulness and self-esteem.

Mindfulness-Based Interventions to Cultivate Healthy Self-Esteem

Mindfulness-Based Clinical Interventions

As mentioned previously, past research has demonstrated that mindfulness is associated with high self-esteem (Brown & Ryan, 2003; Michalak et al., 2011; Rajamaki, 2011; Rasmussen & Pidgeon, 2011; Thompson & Waltz, 2008) and that several specific facets of mindfulness each make unique contributions in the prediction of high self-esteem (Pepping et al., 2013, Study 1). To more fully understand the clinical applications of mindfulness for cultivating healthy self-esteem, however, it is necessary to examine the effects of mindfulness-based clinical interventions on self-esteem.

Several studies have shown that mindfulness-based clinical interventions have beneficial effects on self-esteem. Goldin and Gross (2010) and Goldin, Ramel, and Gross (2009) examined the efficacy of an 8-week mindfulness-based stress reduction intervention for the treatment of social anxiety disorder. The researchers also included measures of self-esteem. Consistent with the mindfulness-based stress reduction protocol, participants completed eight 2.5-h sessions and a half-day retreat. Further, daily practice of mindfulness skills between sessions was encouraged. Participants who completed the intervention displayed improvements not only in their symptoms of social anxiety but also displayed increased self-esteem. It is important to note, however, that the study did not utilize a control group which does limit the extent to which results can be attributed specifically to the intervention.

In a mindfulness-based stress reduction intervention for adolescents with depression, Biegel, Brown, Shapiro, and Schubert (2009) found that participants in the mindfulness intervention condition displayed a reduction in depression, and an increase in self-esteem, relative to a treatment as usual control condition.

Participants in the mindfulness intervention group received eight weekly 2-h group sessions of mindfulness that emphasized both formal mindfulness meditation training and informal mindfulness practice.

More recently, Rajamaki (2011) examined the effects of mindfulness-based stress reduction on different forms of self-esteem. Specifically, the authors examined whether an 8-week mindfulness intervention would increase basic self-esteem and reduce competence-based self-esteem, which is a more fragile form of self-esteem, characterized by the tendency to strive for achievement in order to counteract or compensate for underlying low self-esteem (Johnson & Blom, 2007). Interestingly, participants reported decreased competence-based self-esteem and increased basic self-esteem from pre- to post-intervention. Also of interest, increased mindfulness resulting from the intervention predicted decreased competence-based self-esteem. However, increased mindfulness across the intervention did not predict increased basic self-esteem. Although it is important to note that there was no control condition included in this study, results do suggest that enhancing mindfulness may facilitate the development of secure forms of self-esteem and reduce more fragile, insecure forms of self-esteem.

Results of the abovementioned studies clearly suggest that mindfulness-based interventions may be beneficial for cultivating self-esteem in a range of populations, including adolescents with depression (Biegel et al., 2009) and individuals with social anxiety disorder (Goldin et al., 2009; Goldin and Gross, 2010). Interestingly, enhancing mindfulness is also associated with a decrease in defensive forms of self-esteem (i.e., competence-based self-esteem) and an increase in basic self-esteem (Rajamaki, 2011). This is consistent with the proposition that mindfulness may facilitate the development of healthy, secure forms of self-esteem, as opposed to defensive or fragile high self-esteem, an issue that will be discussed in more depth below. We now turn to the use of experimental mindfulness inductions to examine causal associations between mindfulness and self-esteem.

Experimental Mindfulness Inductions

The results of the mindfulness-based clinical interventions reported above clearly demonstrate that mindfulness-based interventions lead to improved self-esteem. However, it is somewhat difficult to draw definitive conclusions here because of the nature of the interventions, the lack of control groups in some studies, and the nature of the samples used in the studies. It is unclear whether mindfulness itself was directly responsible for the improved self-esteem, or whether other factors associated with clinical interventions, such as the therapeutic relationship, group cohesion, or the alleviation of suffering associated with the presenting problem itself (i.e., depression and social anxiety), were more important in enhancing self-esteem. To examine direct, immediate causal associations between mindfulness and psychological outcomes, researchers are beginning to use brief experimental mindfulness inductions (e.g., Arch & Craske, 2006; Eifert & Heffner, 2003; Keng, Smoski, &

Robins, 2011). Researchers have examined the effects of experimental mindfulness inductions on dysphoric mood (Broderick, 2005), negative affect and emotional volatility (Arch & Craske, 2006), symptoms of panic attacks (Eifert & Heffner, 2003), self-reported physical pain (Braams, Blechert, Boden, & Gross, 2012), and pain tolerance (Liu, Wang, Chang, Chen, & Si, 2013).

We recently extended this research to investigate whether a brief mindfulness induction could lead to increased state self-esteem (Pepping et al., 2013, Study 2). We proposed that participants in the experimental mindfulness induction condition should increase not only in state mindfulness as a result of the mindfulness induction but also should display an increase in state self-esteem. No such effects were predicted for those in the control condition. Here, we briefly describe the experimental procedures used in the study and outline the findings.

Sixty-eight participants were randomly assigned to either a 15-min mindfulness induction condition or to a control condition. Participants in the mindfulness condition completed a mindfulness meditation of the breath that also included a focus on mindfulness of thoughts. The meditation script was read aloud to participants in groups of up to ten participants per session. The script is included in the Appendix of this chapter. Participants in the control condition were read a 15-min story about Venus flytrap plants. This control condition was chosen because it was unlikely to enhance mindfulness or self-esteem but was still an active condition whereby participants were required to listen to a story. All participants completed brief measures of state mindfulness and state self-esteem before and after the experimental manipulation.

Results revealed that state mindfulness significantly increased in the experimental condition (pre-post) and not in the control condition, which indicated that the manipulation (inducing a mindful state) was successful. With regard to whether inducing mindfulness led to change in self-esteem, we found that state self-esteem also increased in the experimental condition (pre-post) and not in the control condition, demonstrating that enhancing state mindfulness led to a positive change in state self-esteem. Although this experimental mindfulness induction was successful in enhancing both state mindfulness and state self-esteem, it is important to consider that the effects of this brief mindfulness induction are likely to be temporary. However, the findings are consistent with the cross-sectional evidence of a relationship between mindfulness and self-esteem and are also consistent with evidence from clinical studies that demonstrate that enhancing mindfulness leads to increased self-esteem. Importantly, results reported by Pepping et al. (2013, Study 2) demonstrate that mindfulness has a "direct" positive influence on self-esteem. In brief, systematically enhancing mindfulness leads to positive effects on self-esteem.

Mindfulness to Cultivate Secure as Opposed to Fragile High Self-Esteem

We propose that mindfulness should cultivate secure rather than fragile high self-esteem. Mindfulness emphasizes the importance of a nonjudgmental and accepting stance to difficult thoughts and emotions that arise moment to moment (Baer, 2003).

In the context of self-esteem, an individual high in dispositional mindfulness would therefore notice positive and negative thoughts about the self without getting "caught up" in these experiences and engaging in elaborative processing but also without engaging in efforts to avoid or change these experiences. This is consistent with the finding that individuals high in four facets of mindfulness, each of which involves mindful acceptance and awareness (non-reactivity, labeling, non-judging, and awareness), were higher in self-esteem (Pepping et al., 2013, Study 1).

Importantly, the processes of mindful acceptance and awareness are vastly different from the cognitive strategy of reappraisal, which refers to the process of cognitively reappraising the situation by changing the way one views the situation (Gross, 2011; Gross & John, 2003). Cognitive reappraisal is somewhat removed from, and even antithetical to, the concept of mindfulness (Chambers, Gullone, & Allen, 2009). Indeed, Chambers et al. (2009) argue that reappraisal may even reflect a form of experiential avoidance at its most extreme. Much evidence indicates that efforts to avoid or control difficult thoughts and emotions can have paradoxical effects by increasing or intensifying these experiences (e.g., Hayes, Luoma, Bond, Masuda, & Lillis, 2006; Salters-Pedneault, Tull, & Roemer, 2004; Wenzlaff & Wegner, 2000). Engaging in efforts to cognitively reappraise and bolster explicit views of oneself despite underlying low levels of self-esteem may represent defensive high self-esteem (a form of fragile high self-esteem) (Jordan et al., 2003; Kernis, 2003). Mindfulness, on the other hand, allows an individual to accept and transcend these thoughts relating to the self without reacting to them.

Similarly, reappraisal could lead to contingent high self-esteem, which is an additional conceptualization of fragile high self-esteem (Deci & Ryan, 1995). Contingent high self-esteem refers to the process of temporarily bolstering one's self-view based on achievements, successes, or adherence to some ideal standard (Deci & Ryan, 1995). However, as noted earlier, when the standards, achievements, or successes on which this form of self-esteem is contingent upon are threatened or ceased, self-esteem is likely to suffer as a result. We therefore propose that strategies used to cognitively reappraise and temporarily bolster views of the self may not lead to secure forms of self-esteem, whereas mindfulness may facilitate the ability to nonjudgmentally accept difficult thoughts and emotions without buying into them and without reacting to them impulsively.

Perhaps, the most compelling evidence that mindfulness may lead to secure forms of self-esteem comes from our recent experimental study described earlier whereby participants were induced with a mindful state, which resulted in increased state self-esteem (Pepping et al., 2013, Study 2). Interestingly, this experimental mindfulness induction did not explicitly target self-esteem. Participants in the mindfulness meditation condition were not asked to think more positively about themselves; no attempt was made to temporarily bolster self-esteem; and participants were also not asked to think about achievement or positive aspects of their lives. Instead, the focus of the induction (consistent with mindfulness) was to adopt a different "relationship" to thoughts and feelings (Baer et al., 2006; Kabat-Zinn, 1994). It appears that participants in the mindfulness induction condition were better able to let go of negative thoughts about the self and were more open to perceiving thoughts purely as events in the mind, rather than a true reflection of reality. The above description may reflect a form of secure high self-esteem as opposed to fragile high self-esteem.

Niemiec et al. (2010) recently reported on research pertaining to mindfulness and self-esteem from a terror management perspective. As mentioned earlier, according to terror management theory, humans attempt to regulate death anxiety by striving for self-esteem (Greenberg et al., 1986, 1992; Pyszczynski et al., 2004). Niemiec et al. (2010) found that individuals who were low in mindfulness were more likely to strive for self-esteem in response to experimental mortality salience inductions, which reflects an attempt to buffer death anxiety by bolstering self-esteem. Interestingly, the need to defensively bolster self-esteem was not observed in those high in mindfulness following the experimental mindfulness induction. Again, this is consistent with the notion that mindfulness is associated with enhanced self-esteem and, importantly, secure high self-esteem.

In summary, both cross-sectional and experimental research suggest that mindfulness may facilitate the development of secure high self-esteem as opposed to fragile forms of self-esteem. The finding that measures of mindfulness, which focuses on nonjudgmental acceptance as opposed to cognitive reappraisal, predicts increased self-esteem is consistent with this proposition (Brown & Ryan, 2003; Michalak et al., 2011; Rajamaki, 2011; Rasmussen & Pidgeon, 2011; Thompson & Waltz, 2008). Further, experimentally inducing a mindful state, without bolstering self-esteem or restructuring self-views, led to an increase in state self-esteem (Pepping et al., 2013, Study 2), again, consistent with a non-defensive, secure form of self-esteem resulting from increased mindfulness. Mindfulness may thus be a useful way to address the underlying processes associated with low self-esteem, without temporarily bolstering positive views of oneself by focusing on achievement or other transient factors.

Conclusions and Future Directions

The findings from the research reviewed in this chapter suggest that individuals high in dispositional mindfulness tend to be high in self-esteem and that mindfulness-based clinical interventions may assist in cultivating secure self-esteem. With regard to which specific components of mindfulness enhance self-esteem, results by Pepping et al. (2013, Study 1) indicate that the "non-judging" facet of mindfulness most strongly relates to high self-esteem, suggesting that mindfulness-based interventions that utilize strategies to foster a nonjudgmental stance towards the self, thoughts, and emotions may be particularly beneficial to individuals low in self-esteem. Further, "non-reactivity," "acting with awareness," and "describing" were also associated with high self-esteem, again, suggesting that mindfulness strategies focusing on these specific skills may also enhance self-esteem. Importantly, the proposition that mindfulness-based clinical interventions increase self-esteem has been supported by both intervention studies (Biegel et al., 2009; Goldin et al., 2009; Rajamaki, 2011) and experimental research (Pepping et al., 2013, Study 2).

Although this research is promising, the challenge for future research is to examine whether mindfulness-based interventions lead to enhanced self-esteem in samples specifically seeking assistance for low self-esteem and also in nonclinical populations. It would also be very useful for future research to explore potential mediators of the relationship between mindfulness and self-esteem and to examine the underlying mechanisms of the beneficial effects of mindfulness interventions on self-esteem. This would have particularly important clinical implications as it would elucidate the specific underlying processes responsible for any benefit from mindfulness interventions. In summary, the research reviewed in this chapter clearly demonstrates that mindfulness and self-esteem are related, that enhancing mindfulness increases self-esteem, and that specific components of mindfulness may be particularly important for cultivating self-esteem.

Appendix

Experimental Mindfulness Induction Script

I am now going to take you through a 15-min guided mindfulness meditation. The purpose of this meditation is not necessarily to feel more relaxed or calm or better than you did at the start of the meditation but to just simply practice mindfulness. So, taking a few moments now to settle into a comfortable position, wiggle into a position so that your back is straight but not rigid. Place your feet squarely on the ground. If you wear glasses, you may like to take them off, and gently close your eyes if you feel comfortable doing so. And if not, just find a spot on the floor to focus on.

Feel all the points of contact between your body and the chair and just settle into the stillness. Let's begin by just noticing that you can feel your feet on the ground. Notice that you can feel the bottom of your feet in your shoes. Just settle into this… bringing attention now to the feeling of the palms of your hands, and either paying attention to what you're touching or the feeling of contact or perhaps the feeling of the air or the temperature of the air on your palms. And just bring all your attention and awareness to this part of the body.

And now shift your attention to the sensation of breathing. We're not trying to change the breath in any way. It doesn't have to become deeper or slower or calmer. Just pay attention to the breath as it is in this moment. Throughout this meditation, we will be using the breath as an anchor. So, every time you find that your mind wanders, you start thinking or responding to sounds or thoughts as they arise; every time you notice this, just time and time again, bring your mind back to the breath, that is, your attention back to the breath. And so now for the next few moments, just sit and bring your attention to the feeling of the in-breath and the feeling of the out-breath. Hold in awareness that part of the body where the breath feels most vivid or strong for you. It might be your abdomen or your chest or nose or throat. Just bring all your attention and awareness to that part.

Every time you find your mind has wandered, just gently bring your attention back to the breath. You may already find that your mind has wandered, and your mind is just doing what minds do. You may be noticing thoughts about the meditation, whether you are doing it right or whether this is boring. You may have thoughts about how relaxing or calming this feels. No matter what your thoughts are, just know that they are thoughts; they're mental events that come into the mind, and just as easily, if you leave them well alone, they will also go out of your mind and be replaced by more. You may be noticing bizarre or random thoughts. You might be planning what you will do for the rest of the day or tomorrow.

The purpose of a mindfulness meditation is not to stop your thoughts or suppress them or resist them or get rid of them. It's just to know that you're thinking. And then shift your attention back to the breath. So, your thoughts become like background chatter—like a radio going in the background—they are there; your mind is chattering away, and you are just not getting caught up with it.

Just notice your breathing and what is happening in the present moment.

So, just bring your attention to where the mind is now. And if you need to come back to the breath, then gently bring your mind back. You may also like to notice the reactions when you find that your mind has wandered when you bring awareness to the focus of the thoughts. Perhaps, you have a reaction that you don't want to be having this thought or you shouldn't be having this thought at the moment. Perhaps, if you are finding it difficult for your mind to settle that it shouldn't be this way or that this is hard, just notice those thoughts as thoughts. Your mind is giving a commentary of what it is thinking at the moment, nothing more and nothing less. The thoughts are not necessarily true, are not necessarily things to be believed, and are not necessarily things to be acted upon. Just let the thoughts do their thing, and just bring your attention back to the breath, no matter what your thoughts are telling you.

So, breathe in and breathe out… just simply observe the breath, in this moment…. And now in this moment…. Just breathe in and just breathe out. Being aware of everything that is happening, in each moment, as it passes, your thoughts are going to be there whether you want them to be there or not. So, sometimes you may as well just let them. But bring your attention to the experience of breathing in and breathing out, and let your thoughts come and go as they will. And you may be noticing themes to your thoughts—these are the "hard and boring" thoughts. These are the "planning" thoughts. Just when you notice the theme of the thoughts, just remember they are just thoughts too, and bring your attention back to the breathing.

You may be also becoming aware of feelings and sensations as you're sitting for this amount of time. You may be noticing themes of discomfort or itches as you sit. See if you can experience these just as sensations. You may notice thoughts like this really hurt or this is unbearable or I have to scratch. And again, just because they're thoughts doesn't mean they are real or that you have to obey them. Just be willing to experience it—be open to allowing it to be there. Hold these sensations in one part of awareness and focus on the breath at the same time.

And observe your mind's reaction. Perhaps, your mind is irritated. Perhaps, your mind is telling you to scratch or to move. And if you do decide to move, or to itch, just do so mindfully. And then just come back to the breath, and allow things to be just as they are. Just breathe in, and just breathe out. Let thoughts and sensations just enter awareness and then leave awareness. And continue to focus on your breath. So, mindfulness is awareness of everything that is happening in the present moment. Just allow it to be there. Be willing to have the experience you are having. And just breathe in, and just breathe out.

Be aware of whatever is happening in the present moment. If you find you're lost in thoughts, just notice where your mind went, and bring your mind back to the breath. You might find that the background chatter gets less, or maybe it doesn't. Regardless of what's happening… just come back to the breath.

And now bring your attention and awareness to the feeling in your body on the chair and all the points of contact between you and the surface. And now, just notice that you can feel your feet on the ground. Notice that you can feel the bottom of your feet in your shoes.

Then bring your attention to the palms of your hands. Whether they are touching the chair or your body or whether you can just feel the temperature of the air on them… just bring your attention to the palms of your hands. Now, gently bring your attention and awareness of the room around you. And when you're ready, open your eyes, and come back to the room.

Script used in Study 2 reported by Pepping et al. (2013).

References

Arch, J. J., & Craske, M. G. (2006). Mechanisms of mindfulness: Emotion regulation following a focused breathing induction. *Behaviour Research and Therapy, 44*(12), 1849–1858. doi:10.1016/j.brat.2005.12.007.

Baer, R. A. (2003). Mindfulness training as a clinical intervention: A conceptual and empirical review. *Clinical Psychology: Science and Practice, 10*, 125–143. doi:10.1093/clipsy/bpg015.

Baer, R. A., Smith, G. T., Hopkins, J., Krietemeyer, J., & Toney, L. (2006). Using self-report assessment methods to explore facets of mindfulness. *Assessment, 13*, 27–45. doi:10.1177/1073191105283504.

Baer, R. A., Smith, G. T., Lykins, E., Button, D., Krietemeyer, J., Sauer, S., et al. (2008). Construct validity of the five facet mindfulness questionnaire in meditating and nonmeditating samples. *Assessment, 15*(3), 329–342. doi:10.1177/1073191107313003.

Baumeister, R. F., Heatherton, T. F., & Tice, D. M. (1993). When ego threats lead to self-regulation failure: Negative consequences of high self-esteem. *Journal of Personality and Social Psychology, 64*(1), 141–156. doi:10.1037/0022-3514.64.1.141.

Baumeister, R. F., Smart, L., & Boden, J. M. (1996). Relation of threatened egotism to violence and aggression: The dark side of high self-esteem. *Psychological Review, 103*(1), 5–33. doi:10.1037/0033-295X.103.1.5.

Biegel, G. M., Brown, K. W., Shapiro, S. L., & Schubert, C. M. (2009). Mindfulness-based stress reduction for the treatment of adolescent psychiatric outpatients: A randomized clinical trial. *Journal of Consulting and Clinical Psychology, 77*(5), 855–866. doi:10.1037/a0016241.

Bishop, S. R., Lau, M., Shapiro, S., Carlson, L., Anderson, N. D., Carmody, J., et al. (2004). Mindfulness: A proposed operational definition. *Clinical Psychology: Science and Practice, 11*(3), 230–241. doi:10.1093/clipsy.bph077.

Braams, B. R., Blechert, J., Boden, M. T., & Gross, J. J. (2012). The effects of acceptance and suppression on anticipation and receipt of painful stimulation. *Journal of Behavior Therapy and Experimental Psychiatry, 43*(4), 1014–1018. doi:10.1016/j.jbtep.2012.04.001.

Broderick, P. C. (2005). Mindfulness and coping with dysphoric mood: Contrasts with rumination and distraction. *Cognitive Therapy and Research, 29*(5), 501–510. doi:10.1007/s10608-005-3888-0.

Brown, K. W., & Ryan, R. M. (2003). The benefits of being present: Mindfulness and its role in psychological well-being. *Journal of Personality and Social Psychology, 84*(4), 822–848. doi:10.1037/0022-3514.84.4.822.

Chambers, R., Gullone, E., & Allen, N. B. (2009). Mindful emotion regulation: An integrative review. *Clinical Psychology Review, 29*(6), 560–572. doi:10.1016/j.cpr.2009.06.005.

Deci, E. L., & Ryan, R. M. (1995). Human autonomy: The basis for true self-esteem. In M. Kernis (Ed.), *Efficacy, agency, and self-esteem* (pp. 31–49). New York: Plenum.

Diener, E., Emmons, R. A., Larsen, R. J., & Griffin, S. (1985). The satisfaction with life scale. *Journal of Personality Assessment, 49*(1), 71–75. doi:10.1207/s15327752jpa4901_13.

Eifert, G. H., & Heffner, M. (2003). The effects of acceptance versus control contexts on avoidance of panic-related symptoms. *Journal of Behavior Therapy and Experimental Psychiatry, 34*, 293–312. doi:10.1016/j.jbtep.2003.11.001.

Goldin, P. R., & Gross, J. J. (2010). Effects of mindfulness-based stress reduction (MBSR) on emotion regulation in social anxiety disorder. *Emotion, 10*(1), 83–91. doi:10.1037/a0018441.

Goldin, P., Ramel, W., & Gross, J. (2009). Mindfulness meditation training and self-referential processing in social anxiety disorder: Behavioral and neural effects. *Journal of Cognitive Psychotherapy: An International Quarterly, 23*(3), 242–257. doi:10.1891/0889-8391.23.3.242.

Greenberg, J., Pyszczynski, T., & Solomon, S. (1986). The causes and consequences of a need for self-esteem: A terror management theory. In *Public Self and Private Self* (pp. 189–212). New York: Springer.

Greenberg, J., Solomon, S., Pyszczynski, T., Rosenblatt, A., Burling, J., Lyon, D., et al. (1992). Why do people need self-esteem? Converging evidence that self-esteem serves an anxiety-buffering function. *Journal of Personality and Social Psychology, 63*(6), 913–922. doi:10.1037/0022-3514.63.6.913.

Gross, J. J. (Ed.). (2011). *Handbook of emotion regulation*. New York: Guilford Press.

Gross, J. J., & John, O. P. (2003). Individual differences in two emotion regulation processes: Implications for affect, relationships, and well-being. *Journal of Personality and Social Psychology, 85*(2), 348–362. doi:10.1037/0022-3514.85.2.348.

Hayes, S. C., Luoma, J. B., Bond, F. W., Masuda, A., & Lillis, J. (2006). Acceptance and commitment therapy: Model, process and outcomes. *Behaviour Research and Therapy, 44*(1), 1–25. doi:10.1016/j.brat.2005.06.006.

Johnson, M., & Blom, V. (2007). Development and validation of two measures of contingent self-esteem. *Individual Differences Research, 5*(4), 300–328.

Jordan, C. H., Spencer, S. J., Zanna, M. P., Hoshino-Browne, E., & Correll, J. (2003). Secure and defensive high self-esteem. *Journal of Personality and Social Psychology, 85*(5), 969–978. doi:10.1037/0022-3514.85.5.969.

Kabat-Zinn, J. (1994). *Wherever you go, there you are: Mindfulness meditation in everyday life*. New York: Hyperion.

Keng, S.-L., Smoski, M. J., & Robins, C. J. (2011). Effects of mindfulness on psychological health: A review of empirical studies. *Clinical Psychology Review, 31*, 1041–1056. doi:10.1016/j.cpr.2011.04.006.

Kernis, M. H. (2003). Toward a conceptualization of optimal self-esteem. *Psychological Inquiry, 14*(1), 1–26. doi:10.1207/S15327965PLI1401_01.

Lau, M. A., Bishop, S. R., Segal, Z. V., Buis, T., Anderson, N. D., Carlson, L., et al. (2006). The Toronto mindfulness scale: Development and validation. *Journal of Clinical Psychology, 62*(12), 1445–1467. doi:10.1002/jclp.20326.

Leary, M. R. (1999). Making sense of self-esteem. *Current Directions in Psychological Science, 8*(1), 32–35. doi:10.1111/1467-8721.00008.

Leary, M. R., Tambor, E. S., Terdal, S. K., & Downs, D. L. (1995). Self-esteem as an interpersonal monitor: The sociometer hypothesis. *Journal of Personality and Social Psychology, 68*(3), 518–530. doi:10.1037/0022-3514.68.3.518.

Leary, M. R., & MacDonald, G. (2003). Individual differences in self-esteem: A review and theoretical integration. In M. R. Leary & J. P. Tangney (Eds.), *Handbook of self and identity* (pp. 401–418). New York: Guilford Press.

Linehan, M. M. (1993). *Cognitive-behavioral treatment of borderline personality disorder*. New York: Guilford Press.

Liu, X., Wang, S., Chang, S., Chen, W., & Si, M. (2013). Effect of brief mindfulness intervention on tolerance and distress of pain induced by cold-pressor task. *Stress and Health, 29*(3), 199–204. doi:10.1002/smi.2446.

Michalak, J., Teismann, T., Heidenreich, T., Strohle, G., & Vocks, S. (2011). Buffering low self-esteem: The effect of mindful acceptance on the relationship between self-esteem and depression. *Personality and Individual Differences, 50*, 751–754. doi:10.1016/j.paid.2010.11.029.

Niemiec, C. P., Brown, K. W., Kashdan, T. B., Cozzolino, P. J., Breen, W. E., Levesque-Bristol, C., et al. (2010). Being present in the face of existential threat: The role of trait mindfulness in reducing defensive responses to mortality salience. *Journal of Personality and Social Psychology, 99*(2), 344–365. doi:10.1037/a0019388.

Orth, U., & Robins, R. W. (2014). The development of self-esteem. *Current Directions in Psychological Science, 23*(5), 381–387. doi:10.1177/0963721414547414.

Pepping, C. A., O'Donovan, A., & Davis, P. (2013). The positive effects of mindfulness on self-esteem. *The Journal of Positive Psychology, 8*(5), 376–386. doi:10.1080/17439760.2013.807353.

Pyszczynski, T., Greenberg, J., Solomon, S., Arndt, J., & Schimel, J. (2004). Why do people need self-esteem? A theoretical and empirical review. *Psychological Bulletin, 130*(3), 435–468. doi:10.1037/0033-2909.130.3.435.

Rajamaki, S. (2011). *Mindfulness-based stress reduction: Does mindfulness training affect competence based self-esteem and burnout?* Unpublished Masters Dissertation, Stockholm University.

Rasmussen, M. K., & Pidgeon, A. M. (2011). The direct and indirect benefits of dispositional mindfulness on self-esteem and social anxiety. *Anxiety, Stress & Coping, 24*(2), 227–233. doi: 10.1080/10615806.2010.515681.

Rosenberg, M. (1965). *Society and the adolescent self-image*. Princeton, NJ: Princeton University Press.

Ryan, R. M., & Brown, K. W. (2003). Why we don't need self-esteem: On fundamental needs, contingent love, and mindfulness. *Psychological Inquiry, 14*(1), 71–76.

Ryan, R. M., Brown, K. W., & Creswell, J. D. (2007). How integrative is attachment theory? Unpacking the meaning and significance of felt security. *Psychological Inquiry, 18*(3), 177–182. doi:10.1080/10478400701512778.

Salters-Pedneault, K., Tull, M. T., & Roemer, L. (2004). The role of avoidance of emotional material in the anxiety disorders. *Applied and Preventative Psychology, 11*(2), 95–114. doi:10.1016/j.appsy.2004.09.001.

Sowislo, J. F., & Orth, U. (2013). Does low self-esteem predict depression and anxiety? A meta-analysis of longitudinal studies. *Psychological Bulletin, 139*(1), 213–240. doi:10.1037/a0028931.

Thompson, B. L., & Waltz, J. A. (2008). Mindfulness, self-esteem, and unconditional self-acceptance. *Journal of Rational-Emotive Cognitive-Behavior Therapy, 26*(2), 119–126. doi:10.1007/s10942-007-0059-0.

Trzesniewski, K. H., Donnellan, M. B., Moffitt, T. E., Robins, R. W., Poulton, R., & Caspi, A. (2006). Low self-esteem during adolescence predicts poor health, criminal behavior, and limited economic prospects during adulthood. *Developmental Psychology, 42*(2), 381–390. doi:10.1037/0012-1649.42.2.381.

Verkuyten, M., & Masson, K. (1995). 'New racism', self-esteem, and ethnic relations among minority and majority youth in the Netherlands. *Social Behavior and Personality: An International Journal, 23*(2), 137–154. doi:10.2224/sbp.1995.23.2.137.

Walach, H., Buchheld, N., Buttenmuller, V., Kleinknecht, N., & Schmidt, S. (2006). Measuring mindfulness—The Freiburg Mindfulness Inventory (FMI). *Personality and Individual Differences, 40*(8), 1543–1555. doi:10.1016/j.paid.2005.11.025.

Waterman, A. S. (1992). Identity as an aspect of optimal psychological functioning. In G. R. Adams, T. P. Gullotta, & R. Montemayor (Eds.), *Adolescent identity formation* (pp. 50–72). Newbury Park, CA: Sage.

Wenzlaff, R. M., & Wegner, D. M. (2000). Thought suppression. *Annual Review of Psychology, 51*(1), 59–91. doi:10.1146/annurev.psych.51.1.59.

Zeigler-Hill, V. (2006). Discrepancies between implicit and explicit self-esteem: Implications for narcissism and self-esteem instability. *Journal of Personality, 74*(1), 119–144. doi:10.1111/j.1467-6494.2005.00371.x.

Chapter 14
Beyond Deficit Reduction: Exploring the Positive Potentials of Mindfulness

Tim Lomas and Itai Ivtzan

Introduction

Mindfulness has travelled a long distance, in all kinds of ways. In historical terms, as we peer back through the mists of time from our current vantage point at the dawn of the twenty-first century, we can discern its origins in antiquity, over two and a half millennia ago. Geographically, as we sit in England writing this chapter, we can appreciate how, from its initial roots on the Indian subcontinent, mindfulness has slowly migrated across the world, finally reaching the West towards the close of the nineteenth century. Finally, in conceptual terms, it is fascinating to trace the way in which the idea of mindfulness has shifted and developed as it has journeyed through time and space, often changing shape to suit the needs, values, and worldviews of the various cultures that have embraced it. And so it is the case with the way mindfulness has been taken up in the West today. As this chapter will show, its main route of transmission has been through therapeutic interventions that were developed in a clinical context, most notably Jon Kabat-Zinn's (1982) seminal Mindfulness-Based Stress Reduction (MBSR) programme. Given their formative and influential role, these interventions have rightly been celebrated as making a hugely important contribution in bringing mindfulness to new Western audiences. However, at the same time, one can recognise that the type of clinical psychological context in which these interventions were formulated has had a definite influence on the way in which mindfulness has so far been appraised, understood, and utilised.

Unfortunately, it could be argued that, by being filtered through this clinical context, the great potential for mindfulness to facilitate psychological wellbeing and

T. Lomas (✉) • I. Ivtzan
Department of Psychology, University of East London, AE.3.29, Stratford Campus, Water Lane, London E15 4LZ, UK
e-mail: t.lomas@uel.ac.uk; i.ivtzan@uel.ac.uk

E. Shonin et al. (eds.), *Mindfulness and Buddhist-Derived Approaches in Mental Health and Addiction*, Advances in Mental Health and Addiction,
DOI 10.1007/978-3-319-22255-4_14

development has been somewhat limited. Of course, that is not to denigrate the pioneering interventions noted above; these have been revolutionary in their impact, improving people's wellbeing in myriad ways. However, these interventions have been constrained by one crucial factor: this clinical context is fundamentally based on a 'deficit' model of human psychology. In their various ways, all these interventions are concerned with treating or alleviating dysfunction or illness—from stress and depression to pain and discomfort. Needless to say, such aims are laudable and necessary. That said, they do not exhaust the vast potential of mindfulness; for example, in its original Buddhist context, mindfulness was the vehicle for radical psycho-spiritual development and the gateway to transcendent states of great import. Sadly, if mindfulness is conceived of narrowly according to a deficit model of wellbeing, such potentials are neglected if not overlooked entirely. This is not an issue that is confined to mindfulness; arguably, much of Western psychology has been founded upon and driven by this deficit model, focussing predominantly on disease, disorder, and dysfunction. Thus, one might argue that mainstream academia generally has failed to appreciate the great potential of people to develop, flourish, and find fulfilment.

However, in recent years, a new branch of psychology has emerged focussing specifically on concepts such as wellbeing and flourishing, namely, positive psychology (PP). It is of course recognised that such phenomena have been studied and analysed for decades, if not centuries. That said, the formulation of an academic field devoted specifically to such 'positive' topics has been valuable in providing a common forum and discursive space where these can be brought together and investigated collectively. And, to return to the topic at hand, PP has brought a fresh perspective to bear on mindfulness, developing interventions that are not focussed on alleviating dysfunction, but on actively promoting positive outcomes, from meaning in life to psychological development. As such, this chapter aims to introduce the contribution that PP has made to our understanding and utilisation of mindfulness in contemporary psychology. It will do so over the course of three parts. Section 1 takes a historical view, exploring the long migration of mindfulness, from its distant Asian roots far back in the Axial age to its transmission to the West over recent centuries. Section 2 then considers the way mindfulness has been embraced by Western psychology and how this was shaped by the clinical context in which early mindfulness-based therapeutic interventions were developed, as noted above. Section 3 then introduces the emergent field of PP and highlights a number of new interventions being developed within the field—including the Positive Mindfulness Programme, created by Dr. Ivtzan—which open up new possibilities for the way in which we might harness mindfulness to promote health and wellbeing.

Transmission of Mindfulness to the West

This first section traces the long journey of mindfulness, from its origins on the Indian subcontinent over 2500 years ago to its current embrace by Western psychology. The practice of mindfulness dates back to Siddhartha Gautama, better known by the honorific *Buddha*, meaning 'Enlightened one'. Although the dates and location of his birth are contested, there is some consensus that he was born in Lumbini in present-day Nepal (Thomas, 2000) and lived from around 480 to 400 BC (Cousins, 1996). The cultural context in which the Buddha was born and lived was suffused by Hinduism, which developed the earliest examples of meditation (excavations of the Indus Valley have uncovered pottery depicting people sitting in the lotus posture dating back to 3000 BC; Varenne, 1977). Hinduism features a comprehensive system of physical, mental, and spiritual disciplines, referred to collectively as yoga (a Sanskrit term derived from the verb *yug*, meaning to bind or to yoke together; thus yoga is interpreted as meaning to 'unite the mind and body in a way that promotes health'; Wren, Wright, Carson, & Keefe, 2011, p. 477). It was in this context that the Buddha developed his own teachings. Having been raised in relative luxury, a series of encounters with illness and mortality aged 19 led to an 'existential crisis', prompting him to pursue a religious existence dedicated to exploring the human condition (Kumar, 2002). However, after spending 5 years engaging in austere yogic practices, he determined that such self-mortification was unhelpful and decided to pursue his own path—leading to the formulation of a unique body of teachings and practices which we now refer to as Buddhism.

Buddhism is a tradition of astonishing depth and breadth, and it is far beyond the scope of the present chapter to provide even a cursory summary of its insights. As such, we can merely hope here to introduce its teachings that pertain to mindfulness (and even then only briefly). That said, mindfulness occupies a central place in the Buddha's teachings, playing a pivotal role in his message of the possibility of psychological development and ultimately of liberation. Arguably, the key teaching of Buddhism is the Four Noble Truths, which acknowledge the ubiquity and universality of suffering, but which also propose a remedy in the form of a medical diagnosis for its alleviation: suffering is universal; it has a cause; cessation is possible, achieved by following the Noble Eightfold Path (Thrangu, 1993). Building on this central insight, much of Buddhism is devoted to elucidating this path, a prescription for 'right living', which involves meditation and other moral recommendations, including right vision, thought, speech, conduct, livelihood, effort, mindfulness, and concentration. As such, in its original context, mindfulness was an integral component of an extensive programme of psycho-spiritual development, which had the radical aim of ending suffering and allowing people to achieve 'enlightenment'. While terms such as enlightenment are hard to operationalise within the ontological and epistemological context of Western psychology, we might view it as the ultimate state of happiness, equanimity, and freedom that a human being is capable of experiencing. Unfortunately, just as the notion of enlightenment is difficult to appreciate within the context of Western science, as mindfulness has been transmitted to the West and conceptualised within psychology, its original potential as a component of psycho-spiritual transformation has to some extent likewise been lost (Van Gordon, Shonin, Griffiths, & Singh, 2014).

So, how did mindfulness reach the West in the form that it did? Buddhism was known to Western cultures as early as the thirteenth century through the accounts of Marco Polo (Abeydeera, 2000). However, it was only in the late nineteenth century that it achieved any degree of cultural prominence, as translations of scriptures became available and religious figures from Asia began to travel abroad. Foremost among the scholars engaged in the exegesis and translation of original Buddhist texts was T. W. Rhys Davids (1881, 1910) who was pivotal in introducing mindfulness to the West. Indeed, it was Rhys Davids who coined the term 'mindfulness' itself, selecting this as a translation of the Pali term *sati* (Gethin, 2011). The notion of *sati* is the basis for *the* foundational teaching on mindfulness in the Buddhist canon, the *Satipaṭṭhāna Sutta* (the 'Discourse on the Establishment of Mindfulness'), in which the Buddha first sets out practical instructions for how to cultivate the desired mental state of *sati*. Now, what is *sati*? Within the Brahmanical tradition of ancient India—the context in which the Buddha lived and taught—the word had connotations of 'remembrance' and 'recollection' (Peacock, 2014, p. 5). However, as used by the Buddha, it does not refer to historical or chronological memory per se, but to a state in which one 'recalls' the activity that 'one is engaged in, in the present moment' (p. 6). This meaning of *sati* is evident in the pre-eminent contemporary definition of mindfulness, proposed by Kabat-Zinn (2003, p. 145)—who explicitly cited *sati* as the origin of his formulation—namely, *the awareness that arises through paying attention on purpose, in the present moment, and nonjudgmentally to the unfolding of experience moment by moment.*

And, it is this particular notion of *sati*—translated and conceptualised by Rhys Davids and subsequently operationalised and defined by Kabat-Zinn—that has fundamentally shaped the way in which mindfulness has been embraced and understood in the West today (alongside the teachings of other influential contemporary masters, such as Thich Nhat Hanh). As we explore in section 2, this harnessing of mindfulness has led to a proliferation of interventions that have helped improve mental health and wellbeing in diverse populations, which is of course hugely welcome. However, this enthusiasm for mindfulness, based on a particular translation of *sati*, has come at a price. There are various issues. Firstly, of all the concepts and practices in Buddhism that could be relevant to wellbeing, *sati* has been emphasised above all others. This means that other potentially equally valuable notions have been overlooked. For example, there are at least two other Buddhist terms which also pertain to awareness (as *sati* does)—and thus which could also be translated as mindfulness—but which possess additional layers of meaning that are largely absent in *sati* (Lomas & Jnanavaca, 2015). These include *appamada*, which can be understood as referring to awareness infused with an ethos of ethical care, and *sampajañña*, which may be thought of as awareness suffused with a sense of spiritual progress. Thus, one consequence of basing our current conception of mindfulness on *sati*, as opposed to *appamada* or *sampajañña*, is that mindfulness has become somewhat detached from considerations around ethics and spirituality that were present in the original teachings.

This latter point brings us to the second issue with the construction of mindfulness in contemporary psychology: it has become largely 'decontextualised' from the Buddhist teachings in which it was originally formulated. That is, mindfulness has tended to be presented in a secular way, without reference to Buddhism (Shapiro, 1994), conceptualised and operationalised using cognitive theories of attention and awareness (Bishop et al., 2004). Now, it is not necessarily the case that constructs such as attention are discordant with the original Buddhist teachings. Moreover, it is likely that this decontextualisation was necessary in order for mindfulness to find a receptive audience in secular Western societies (King, 1999). However, viewing mindfulness as 'just' a form of attention training is somewhat limiting. For example, as noted above, in Buddhist teachings, mindfulness is inextricably linked to ethics, with the ethical quality of one's actions seen as shaping the subjective content of mindfulness itself. Thus, the risk with the current enthusiasm for mindfulness (as a translation of *sati*) is that the precious insights of the original teachings may be overlooked. This danger is recognised by Kabat-Zinn himself, who suggests that 'the rush to define mindfulness within Western psychology may wind up denaturing it in fundamental ways', and thus there is 'the potential for something priceless to be lost' (Williams & Kabat-Zinn, 2011, p. 4).

Indeed, as one analyses the transmission of mindfulness to the West, one can clearly see that the way in which it has been received and interpreted has been shaped and filtered by the values and epistemological contours of Western science. As such, it has been suggested that we are seeing the emergence of a new form of 'Western Buddhism', referred to by sociologists as 'Scientific Buddhism' (McMahan, 2004) or 'Therapised Buddhism' (Obadia, 2008). By way of explanation, critical sociologists have argued that as people in the West have engaged with Buddhism, this engagement has unfolded in three main ways (Lomas, Cartwright, Edginton, & Ridge, 2014): Westerners becoming 'Easternised', Eastern practices being 'Westernised', and the 'intermingling' of East and West. With the first development, Buddhism in the West is seen as retaining its original 'Eastern' form and is valued just for that reason. Here, we see Western Buddhists espousing discourses which Said (1995) identified as being 'Orientalist', featuring the construction of an otherworldly 'mystic East'. For example, Phillips and Aarons (2005) found that Buddhists in a group in Australia had experienced disenchantment with Western society and had consequently sought escape in Eastern ideas and practices.

Conversely, a second movement has seen Buddhism becoming 'Westernised', diverging from traditional forms, eschewing 'ritualized forms and traditional religious affiliations', and being reconstructed to suit secular 'Western sensibilities' (King, 1999, p. 156). From this perspective, even people who meditate in a secular way—as most do (Shapiro, 1994)—might be regarded as 'engaged' with Buddhism, albeit in a form which dis-identifies with its antecedent roots. Finally, a third current has seen the emergence of 'New Religious Movements' which 'intermingle' discourses and practices from various spiritual and therapeutic sources, both East and West, promoting a 'flexible and diffuse version of spiritual identity' (Phillips & Aarons, 2005, p. 217). Here, the practitioner is viewed as a consumer in a 'spiritual marketplace', selecting from interchangeable beliefs and practices—of which Eastern spiritualities are just some of many—to suit their individual needs (Roof, 2001). So, according to the above analysis, clinical and academic engagement with mindfulness can be seen as an example of the second current, 'Eastern' practices becoming 'Westernised'. Such Westernisation is thus reflected in the emergent forms of 'Scientific Buddhism' (McMahan, 2004) or 'Therapised Buddhism' (Obadia, 2008), of which MBSR is just one example, as we explore in section 2.

Clinical and Academic Engagement with Mindfulness

In this second section, we examine the way in which mindfulness has been embraced by clinical practitioners and researchers in the West. Moreover, we consider how such engagement has led to the emergence of new 'Western' forms of Buddhism, in particular, 'Scientific Buddhism' (McMahan, 2004) and 'Therapised Buddhism' (Obadia, 2008). The story here begins over 30 years ago, with Kabat-Zinn's (1982) pioneering MBSR intervention, which played such a pivotal role in introducing mindfulness to the West. Since then, the past few decades have seen an astonishing 'explosion' of interest in mindfulness, in academia and beyond (Brown, Ryan, & Creswell, 2007). This interest encompasses an extensive programme of research across a diverse range of methodological paradigms, from cognitive neuroscience to sociology, as well as a panoply of emergent mindfulness-based interventions aimed at various (mostly clinical) populations. Moreover, this enthusiasm for mindfulness continues to grow and even appears to be accelerating, with over 500 studies published on it in 2012 alone (Shonin, Van Gordon, & Griffiths, 2013). Thus, it can truly be said that mindfulness has entered mainstream academia and clinical practice. As Fortney and Taylor (2010, p. 81) conclude in their review of the use of mindfulness in medical practice, rather than being a 'fringe or marginal concept', it is now widely known and accepted as 'a beneficial mind-body practice by the general public and the scientific community'.

However, as this programme of research and clinical practice has unfolded, it has tended to eschew any overt connection to Buddhism and especially to explicit spiritual or religious ideas or practices (King, 1999). Instead, mindfulness has been filtered through a contemporary scientific understanding, resulting in a number of distinct characteristics. First, as McMahan (2004) has identified, this has produced a form of 'Scientific Buddhism'. This means, for one thing, that mindfulness has generally been 'conceptualized as a nonreligious construct suitable for scientific study', as Baer and Sauer (2009, p. 324) put it, using cognitive theories of attention and awareness rather than the terminology and discourses of Buddhism (Bishop et al., 2004). However, Scientific Buddhism does not just refer to the overarching conceptual approach with which mindfulness has been appraised but also to the type of developments that practitioners themselves are seen as experiencing. That is, rather than emphasising spiritual or ethical progression, for example, research has tended to focus on the development of cognitive skills, such that the practitioner themselves might be seen as cultivating a more 'scientific' mode of thinking and approach to life. This includes the idea that mindfulness enhances emotional intelligence (Lomas, Edginton, Cartwright, & Ridge, 2014), rationality (Lee, 2005), attentional control (Moore, Gruber, Derose, & Malinowski, 2012), brain connectivity (Kilpatrick et al., 2011), and so on.

Perhaps even more significant and dominant than this type of Scientific Buddhism has been the phenomenal development of what Obadia (2008) calls 'Therapised Buddhism'. This encompasses the panoply of mindfulness-based interventions that have emerged over recent decades. Now, as noted above, most such interventions present mindfulness in a secular way, without reference to Buddhism. However, this is exactly Obadia's point—these reflect the way in which mindfulness, and Buddhism more generally, has been 'Westernised' within academia and clinical practice, co-opted into and filtered according to a dominant secular scientific worldview. This worldview places restrictions on the types of outcomes that are considered valid objects of enquiry and, more specifically, tends to denigrate or overlook more nebulous and less quantifiable phenomena, such as spiritual experience and development. Moreover, as highlighted in the introduction, the dominant scientific worldview—evident in contemporary disciplines from psychology to medicine—tends to endorse a somewhat negative 'deficit' model of the person. Generally speaking, this means that humans are regarded as inherently flawed or dysfunctional; as such, any role that therapeutic disciplines such as clinical psychology might play is limited to correcting or ameliorating such deficits, as reflected in Freud's infamous remark (to a hypothetical patient) that psychotherapy could aim no higher than hoping to transform the misery of neurosis into 'common unhappiness' (in Freud & Breuer, 1895, p.351). Of course, there are exceptions, such as humanistic psychology, from Jung's (1939) concept of individuation to Rogers (1961) notion of self-actualisation. Nevertheless, on the whole, a deficit model of human functioning has definitely held sway within psychology and medicine.

And, it was into this context that mindfulness was received and developed. As we shall see, almost without exception, mindfulness-based approaches have been underpinned by this deficit-based approach, seeking to alleviate or correct disease or dysfunction, both mental and physical. It is crucial to emphasise here that this is not a critique of these interventions; these have all played extremely valuable roles in treating the very real issues that people suffer with, from depression and anxiety to pain and discomfort. The pioneer in this regard, as noted above, was Kabat-Zinn's (1982) MBSR intervention. This was designed and intended initially as a treatment for chronic pain and had considerable success in this regard, with half of participants reporting a decrease in perceived pain of 50 %. In the MBSR protocol, an 8–10-week course for groups of between 10 and 40, participants undertake weekly sessions to learn and practise mindfulness, as well as homework activities designed to promote it in everyday life. In essence, these varied activities encourage participants 'to become more aware of, and relate differently to thoughts, feelings and bodily sensations' (Shapiro, Astin, Bishop, & Cordova, 2005, p. 165). This process includes teaching participants to 'decentre' from negative qualia, that is, cultivating the 'ability to observe one's thoughts and feelings as temporary, objective events in the mind, as opposed to reflections of the self that are necessarily true' (Fresco et al., 2007, p. 234). Thus, in the case of chronic pain, rather than resisting or seeking to escape the pain, as patients might normally do, people are encouraged to decentre from it, which helps to lessen its physical and psychological impact.

As the efficacy of MBSR continued to be demonstrated (e.g. Miller, Fletcher, & Kabat-Zinn, 1995), clinicians began exploring its use with other patient populations. Soon, an impressive body of work was accumulating showing that, in clinical trials, MBSR could reduce psychological problems (e.g. anxiety, depression) and even physical issues (e.g. symptomology, pain) across diverse illness groups.

These included people with cancer (Ledesma & Kumano, 2009), HIV (Creswell, Myers, Cole, & Irwin, 2009), migraine (Schmidt et al., 2010), sleep disturbance (Shapiro, Bootzin, Figueredo, Lopez, & Schwartz, 2003), fibromyalgia (Schmidt et al., 2011), irritable bowel syndrome (Kearney, McDermott, Martinez, & Simpson, 2010), rheumatoid arthritis (Pradhan et al., 2007), and coronary disease/cardiac risk symptoms (Olivio, Dodson-Lavelle, Wren, Fang, & Oz, 2009). MBSR was also used successfully with various other groups of people, united by a common deficit or issue, including adolescent psychiatric outpatients (Biegel, Brown, Shapiro, & Schubert, 2009), adolescents with substance abuse problems (Bootzin & Stevens, 2005), transplant patients (Gross et al., 2009), parents/caregivers of children with developmental disabilities (Bazzano et al., 2010), workers in high-stress jobs (Walach et al., 2007), and various groups of healthcare professionals (e.g. to prevent stress-related burnout; see Irving, Dobkin, and Park (2009) for a review). In all these cases, mindfulness was harnessed—very valuably and usefully—to reduce deficits and ameliorate issues, whether psychological (e.g. anxiety) or physical (e.g. pain).

Following the success of the MBSR programme, clinicians and researchers began to develop other mindfulness-based interventions, targeting different clinical issues and populations. Foremost among these was mindfulness-based cognitive therapy (MBCT), designed to prevent relapse or recurrence of major depressive disorder (Segal, Williams, & Teasdale, 2002). Teasdale's (1988) 'differential activation hypothesis' holds that previously depressed individuals are susceptible to relapse because even mildly dysphoric states can reactivate 'depressogenic' thinking patterns (e.g. rumination) associated with previous episodes of depression. Thus, Teasdale, Segal, and Williams (1995) proposed that the attentional training involved in MBSR could be harnessed to prevent such relapse, and so MBCT was developed from the MBSR protocol. Just as MBSR taught patients to decentre from subjective pain, MBCT aimed to help 'recovered recurrently depressed individuals to disengage from dysphoria-activated depressogenic thinking that may meditate recurrence' (Teasdale et al., 2000, p. 615). Corroborating this hypothesis, MBCT was found to significantly reduce relapse rates for people with three or more previous major depressive episodes (Ma & Teasdale, 2004) and as such was included in the National Institute for Health and Care Excellence's (2004) guidelines for prevention of recurrent depression. Subsequent to this success, the MBCT protocol was then used with other patient populations, including people with bipolar disorder (Williams et al., 2008), insomnia (Heidenreich, Tuin, Pflug, Michal, & Michalak, 2006), generalised anxiety disorder (Craigie, Rees, Marsh, & Nathan, 2008), traumatic brain injury (Bedard et al., 2008), panic disorder (Kim et al., 2010), hypochondria (Lovas & Barsky, 2010), and cancer (Foley, Baillie, Huxter, Price, & Sinclair, 2010).

With MBSR and MBCT leading the way in the treatment of psychological and physical issues, clinicians and researchers began to develop new mindfulness-based interventions targeted at a wide range of further conditions and problems, designed specifically to meet the needs of that particular patient population. These include interventions for bipolar disorder (Weber et al., 2010), epilepsy (Thompson et al., 2010), chronic heart failure (Sullivan et al., 2009), age-related cognitive deficits (McHugh, Simpson, & Reed, 2010), multiple sclerosis (Mills & Allen, 2000), irritable bowel syndrome (Ljótsson et al., 2010), maladaptive behaviours in adults with learning disabilities and mental illness (Adkins, Singh, Winton, McKeegan, & Singh, 2010), physical aggression in offenders with learning disabilities (Singh et al., 2008), pain management (Cusens, Duggan, Thorne, & Burch, 2010), post-traumatic stress disorder (Nakamura, Lipschitz, Landward, Kuhn, & West, 2011), obsessive-compulsive disorder (Patel, Carmody, & Simpson, 2007), obesity (Dalen et al., 2010), substance abuse (Bowen et al., 2006), smoking (Bowen & Marlatt, 2009), weight loss (Tapper et al., 2009), and alcohol-dependency relapse (Zgierska et al., 2008). Further unique mindfulness-related interventions—focussed on deficit reduction (e.g. reducing anxiety)—have also been developed for use in a wide variety of clinical and non-clinical groups, including bone marrow transplant patients (Horton-Deutsch, O'Haver Day, Haight, & Babin-Nelson, 2007), people with diabetes (Rungreangkulkij, Wongtakee, & Thongyot, 2011), US marines prior to deployment (Stanley, Schaldach, Kiyonaga, & Jha, 2011), and caregivers of children with developmental disabilities (Singh et al., 2007), as well as for use in therapeutic settings such as couples therapy (Carson, Carson, Gil, & Baucom, 2004) and life-coaching (Collard & Walsh, 2008).

As the previous few paragraphs have demonstrated, there is a burgeoning arsenal of emergent mindfulness-based interventions that is truly extraordinary; the studies featured above—which by no means exhaust the literature in this area—represent a fantastic collective effort among clinicians and researchers to bring mindfulness to people suffering from a wide range of ailments and issues. And, to reiterate a point repeatedly made above, all of these interventions are valuable and to be welcomed. Nevertheless, reading through the list above and the literature generally, it is striking the extent to which almost all the work here takes a deficit-based approach to mindfulness. Almost without exception, all current mindfulness-based interventions are concerned with remedying or ameliorating a deficit of some kind, whether depression (Teasdale et al., 2000), anxiety (Craigie et al., 2008), insomnia (Heidenreich et al., 2006), aggression (Singh et al., 2008), pain (Cusens et al., 2010), substance abuse (Bowen et al., 2006), and so on. As such, there is an almost total absence of interventions, and research more generally, exploring the great 'positive' potential of mindfulness—i.e. not simply as a prophylactic or remedy for dysfunction but as a tool to help people soar and strive for the peaks of human experience and development. However, over the course of the last few years, there has been an effort to augment the deficit-based therapies above with an exploration of the radical positive possibilities offered by mindfulness. At the forefront of this effort has been the emergent field of positive psychology, as the final section explores.

Mindfulness in Positive Psychology

So, we suggested above that most contemporary clinical and academic disciplines have tended to adopt a 'deficit-based' model of the person, focussing on dysfunction and disorder, which has influenced the way mindfulness has been adopted and adapted by these fields. However, in recent years, a new discipline has emerged which has avowedly sought to focus on the assets, capabilities, and potentials of human beings, namely, positive psychology (PP). The field came into being in 1998, when Martin Seligman used his ascension to the presidency of the American Psychological Association to inaugurate this new branch of psychology. His broad intention was to provide a corrective balance to 'psychology as usual'—i.e. to conventional psychology—redressing its 'negative bias' by accentuating the positive (Seligman & Csikszentmihalyi, 2000). That is, in contrast to the deficit model of the person outlined above, PP aimed to focus on all that is 'good' about human beings, their values, strengths, and skills. Above all, PP was concerned with the issue of what makes life worth living; as such, it took a particular interest in valued ends such as meaning and happiness. Of course, prior to the emergence of PP, most of these topics had been studied empirically for years. However, this newly created field offered a conceptual space where all these diverse topics—all of which share the 'family resemblance' (Wittgenstein, 1953) of pertaining to wellbeing in some way—could be analysed collectively. Thus, as a novel branch of academia focussed 'specifically' and entirely on 'the science and practice of improving wellbeing' (Lomas, Hefferon, & Ivtzan, 2014, p. ix), PP was indeed a useful new addition to the broader field of psychology.

Crucially, from the perspective of this chapter's central message—that mindfulness has become detached and decontextualised from its Buddhist origins to its detriment—PP is aligned in various ways with the spirit of Buddhism. For instance, Buddhist teachings contain various prescriptions and exhortations advising practitioners to cultivate particular qualities as a route towards fulfilment (Keown, 2009). In the Theravada tradition, there is an emphasis on the four *brahmaviharas* (divine abidings):*metta* (loving-kindness), *karuṇā* (compassion), *muditā* (sympathetic joy), and *upekkha* (equanimity). Similarly, the Mahayana tradition elucidates six *pāramitās* (perfections): *dāna* (generosity), *sīla* (morality), *khanti* (patience), *viriya* (perseverance), *samādhi* (concentration), and *paññā* (insight). PP not only likewise emphasises many of these qualities as being conducive to wellbeing, but has been at the forefront of developing interventions to help people cultivate such qualities. That is, one of the most important components of PP is the area of 'applied' PP, which is concerned with developing positive psychology interventions (PPIs). As will be outlined further below, PPIs are often modelled on the type of clinical interventions discussed above, but instead of aiming at deficit reduction (e.g. reducing anxiety), they are explicitly focussed on promoting some positive quality or outcome (e.g. increasing compassion). And indeed, there is an emergent body of PPIs which aim to engender the types of qualities encouraged by Buddhism, including interventions based around *metta* (e.g. loving-kindness meditation; Fredrickson, Cohn, Coffey, Pek, & Finkel, 2008), *karuṇā* (e.g. mindful self-compassion; Neff & Germer, 2013), and *dāna* (e.g. charitable giving; Surana & Lomas, 2014).

Such PPIs are quite different in spirit and nature to the type of deficit-based therapies featured above, and as such are valuable additions to the corpus of interventions currently used within psychological and clinical practice. This difference is highlighted in definitions of PPIs provided by scholars within the field. For example, Sin, Della Porta, and Lyubomirsky (2011, p. 469) suggest that a PPI is 'an intervention, therapy, or activity, primarily aimed at increasing positive feelings, positive behaviors, or positive cognitions, as opposed to ameliorating pathology or fixing negative thoughts or maladaptive behavior patterns'. Likewise, Parks and Biswas-Diener (2014) outline a number of rigorous inclusion and exclusion parameters for the classification of PPIs, beginning with the need for the intervention's goal to build a positive variable(s). Now, it is worth stating that, within the field, it is recognised that the concept of 'positive' can be somewhat problematic (Lomas & Ivtzan, 2015; Lomas, Hefferon, & Ivtzan, 2014). Theorists of a critical persuasion have pointed out that qualities or states that might be deemed 'positive' can be detrimental to wellbeing under certain circumstances, while ostensibly 'negative' ones may conversely promote flourishing (Ivtzan, Lomas, Hefferon, & Worth, 2015; Wong, 2011). For example, optimism can be harmful if it becomes unrealistic or 'excessive' (e.g. leading to misperception of risk and subsequently to health risk behaviours; Weinstein, Marcus, & Moser, 2005); likewise, pessimism can be adaptive in certain cases (e.g. if it prompts pre-emptory fault-finding and problem-solving; Norem, 2001). Nevertheless, even while remaining cognisant of such critical caveats, the field has begun to develop an emergent body of PPIs which aim to help individuals flourish.

Crucially—and this is where PP can really be seen as augmenting extant deficit-based therapeutic fields such as clinical psychology—flourishing is not the same as an absence of mental disorder or pathology (Ryff & Singer, 1998). An often used metaphor here is that of a continuum (Ryff et al., 2006), involving a (somewhat arbitrary) scale stretching from minus five (mental illness) through zero (absence of mental illness) and up to plus five (mental health). By eliminating deficits such as anxiety or depression, as interventions such as MBSR and MBCT aim to do, this could be seen as bringing a person from minus five up to zero. However, doing so does not necessarily then mean that a person is thriving and fulfilling their potential, which is represented in this metaphor by the positive integers on the continuum. Thus, PP aims to help people progress beyond zero to reach towards plus five. Thus, in a sense, PP could be seen as complementing fields such as clinical psychology, picking up where they leave off (i.e. once therapies have brought people up to zero, PP can help take them further). It is worth saying that there are issues with this metaphor (Keyes, 2002): mental life is far more multidimensional than implied by a single continuum, and people may have deficits in some aspects of their functioning (and thus be in minus territory) and be flourishing in others (thus being in positive territory). Moreover, recent studies (e.g. Sin & Lyubomirsky, 2009) show that PPIs may also be able to help people while they are still in 'negative territory'—i.e. suffering from mental health issues—as discussed further below. Nevertheless, the metaphor is still a valid way of appreciating the contribution that PP may be able to make in the context of applied psychology (i.e. in terms of where PPIs sit within psychology's diverse array of interventions aimed at improving mental health and wellbeing).

And so, to return to the central topic of this chapter, PP has brought new dimensions to our appreciation of mindfulness by seeking to develop PPIs that harness its 'positive' potential. That is, beyond the deficit reduction of the mindfulness-based interventions highlighted above, these PPIs aim to help people thrive and move towards mental health (which, to reiterate the point above, is not the same as an absence of mental illness). Before we introduce some of these new PPIs, it is worth stating another caveat: despite being ostensibly deficit-focussed, clinical interventions such as the ones detailed above have led to incidental improvements in positive variables, such as positive affect (Geschwind, Peeters, Drukker, van Os, & Wichers, 2011), positive reappraisal of thoughts (Hanley & Garland, 2014), interpersonal interactions (Allen, Bromley, Kuyken, & Sonnenberg, 2009), and quality of life (Godfrin & Van Heeringen, 2010). However, as valuable as such outcomes are, they are not the primary goal of the intervention; rather, they are emerging as beneficial side effects. The central point about PPIs is that there may be much more to be gained if interventions seek to explicitly promote and facilitate such positive outcomes. As outlined below, by specifically designing activities to target such outcomes, it is possible to enhance the efficacy with which these can be facilitated.

Moreover, in a broader sense, having an overarching 'positive' intention for engaging in the intervention—i.e. promoting flourishing rather than correcting deficits—has an impact on the types of outcomes people can experience. Shapiro, Carlson, Astin, and Freedman (2006) suggest that mindfulness comprises three central components: attention ('observing the operations of one's moment-to-moment, internal and external experience'; p. 376), attitude ('a sense of open-hearted, friendly presence and interest'; Kabat-Zinn, 2003, p. 145), and intention (reasons for practising). Shapiro et al. (2006, p. 375) contend that the latter component is often neglected in discussions around mindfulness, which they attribute to the fact that Western psychology has generally sought to 'extract the essence of mindfulness practice from its original religious/cultural roots', a point that is central to this chapter. However, one's intention for practising mindfulness plays a key role in shaping the kinds of outcomes one may experience. As Kabat-Zinn (1990, p. 32) puts it, 'Your intentions set the stage for what is possible. They remind you from moment to moment of why you are practicing in the first place'. The importance of intention is underlined in Shapiro's (1992) study, which showed that the majority of meditators attained effects which were congruent with their original intentions. For example, if they aimed for self-regulation (control over self), they were more likely to achieve greater self-regulation, whereas an intention of self-exploration (knowledge of self) meant that they were more likely to increase self-exploration. Such findings suggest that the intentions of a mindfulness programme—both the stated aim of the intervention itself (whether reducing deficits such as anxiety or promoting flourishing) and the intentions of the practitioner undertaking it—will affect its outcomes.

Given the above considerations, it is encouraging that interventions are being developed within PP which aim to augment existing deficit-based interventions by harnessing some of the positive possibilities offered by mindfulness. Two such PPIs are Mindfulness-Based Strengths Practice (Niemiec, Rashid, & Spinella, 2012), which combines strengths-based approaches with mindfulness, and the Mindful Self-compassion programme (Neff & Germer, 2013), which aims to increase self-compassion and kindness. Both of these have successfully integrated mindfulness and PP variables to good effect. However, these programmes only focus on one quality promoted within PP, i.e. strengths and self-compassion, respectively. As such, a potentially more comprehensive intervention is the Positive Mindfulness

Programme (PMP), created by Dr. Ivtzan, which is currently being validated in a number of independent research studies (e.g. Ivtzan, Young, et al., 2015). The PMP is an online, 8-week programme, which combines mindfulness training with a variety of PPIs and theory. Aimed at the general population, the programme is designed to increase wellbeing by targeting nine positive variables: positive emotions, self-compassion, wellbeing (happiness), autonomy, mindfulness, self-efficacy (strengths), meaning, compassion, and engagement (savouring).

These variables are designed to facilitate different facets of wellbeing; that is, in PP, a distinction is made between 'hedonic' wellbeing (i.e. pleasure, satisfaction) and 'eudaimonic' wellbeing (i.e. fulfilment, psychological development) (Peterson, Park, & Seligman, 2005). Between them, the nine variables were selected to cover both 'types' of wellbeing. For example, engagement and gratitude both increase positive emotions (Adler & Fagley, 2005; McCullough, Emmons, & Tsang, 2002) and as such facilitate hedonic wellbeing (Deci & Ryan, 2008). The remaining seven variables all promote eudaimonic wellbeing, as based on Ryff's (1989) model of 'Psychological Wellbeing', which comprises six dimensions, five of which are targeted in the PMP: self-acceptance (self-compassion), autonomy, environmental mastery (self-efficacy), purpose in life (meaning), and positive relations with others. Finally, mindfulness has been linked to both hedonic and eudaimonic wellbeing (Brown et al., 2007). Early findings from the programme have been promising. For instance, Ivtzan, Young, et al. (2015) offered it to 455 participants in a randomised controlled trial (reduced to 168 in the final analysis due to attrition). Relative to a control group, the experimental group enjoyed significant self-reported post-intervention improvements in all nine positive variables, as well as reductions in depression and stress. Moreover, these gains were also maintained at the 1-month follow-up. Thus, the programme shows good promise as an intervention that harnesses the positive potential of mindfulness, taking it beyond a tool for deficit reduction and helping to actively promote flourishing.

Intriguingly, findings from Ivtzan, Young, et al.'s (2015) study suggest that PPIs such as the PMP may not only be suitable for people who are 'free' of mental health issues but can potentially help people who are currently experiencing such problems. That is, participants who had mild to moderate levels of depression at the beginning of the programme experienced greater benefits—on measures of mindfulness, gratitude, depression, and stress—than those with no depression at baseline. Likewise, participants with lower baseline levels of wellbeing gained more, relative to those with higher baseline levels, in eight variables: mindfulness, wellbeing, depression, stress, gratitude, self-efficacy, and meaning. The researchers suggest that such findings may be due in part to the fact that such participants were in greater initial need of the programme and therefore utilised its tools and benefits more fully. These results are in line with a meta-analysis conducted by Sin and Lyubomirsky (2009), featuring 25 separate studies examining the impact of PPIs on depression, which found that depressed participants gained more from PPIs than nondepressed participants. Such findings suggest that the potential role for PP may be greater than that implied by the continuum metaphor above: rather than PPIs simply assisting people without disorders (i.e. above 'zero') to flourish, they may have a role too in helping treat such disorders. However, such PPIs arguably remain distinct from conventional therapeutic offerings, such as MBSR, as they are still focussed on accentuating positive qualities rather than reducing deficits.

It is important to recognise that PP is still very much a new and emerging field and likewise that PPIs such as the PMP are in the very early stages of development. Nevertheless, hopefully the promise of such interventions is evident. By harnessing the positive potentials of mindfulness, these PPIs may help us further deepen our appreciation of its practice; moreover, they might enable us to capture some of the spirit of the original Buddhist teachings that have to an extent been lost with the deficit-based mindfulness interventions. Indeed, our engagement in the West with mindfulness, and with Buddhism more broadly, is only just beginning. In the context of its long history of evolution and migration, spanning over two and a half millennia, Buddhism has only just begun to make its immense presence felt in the West. Even then, its impact has been remarkable, especially over the past few decades. Thus Western psychology, and academia and society more broadly, has an exciting future ahead exploring the great riches and insights offered by this ancient—and yet still breathtakingly relevant—tradition of wisdom and spiritual practice. To this end, the present chapter, and this book more generally, will hopefully play a useful role in our unfolding appreciation and utilisation of mindfulness and ideally of Buddhism more broadly too.

References

Abeydeera, A. (2000). The travels of Marco Polo in the land of Buddhism. In V. Elisseeff (Ed.), *The silk road: Highways of culture and commerce* (pp. 69–80). Paris: UNESCO.

Adkins, A. D., Singh, A. N., Winton, A. S., McKeegan, G. F., & Singh, J. (2010). Using a mindfulness-based procedure in the community: Translating research to practice. *Journal of Child and Family Studies, 19*(2), 175–183.

Adler, M. G., & Fagley, N. S. (2005). Appreciation: Individual differences in finding value and meaning as a unique predictor of subjective well-being. *Journal of Personality, 73*(1), 79–114.

Allen, M., Bromley, A., Kuyken, W., & Sonnenberg, S. J. (2009). Participants' experiences of mindfulness-based cognitive therapy: "It changed me in just about every way possible". *Behavioural and Cognitive Psychotherapy, 37*(04), 413–430.

Baer, R. A., & Sauer, S. (2009). Mindfulness and cognitive behavioral therapy: A commentary on Harrington and Pickles. *Journal of Cognitive Psychotherapy, 23*(4), 324–332.

Bazzano, A., Wolfe, C., Zylovska, L., Wang, S., Schuster, E., Barrett, C., et al. (2010). Stress-reduction and improved well-being following a pilot community-based participatory mindfulness-based stress-reduction (MBSR) program for parents/caregivers of children with developmental disabilities. *Disability and Health Journal, 3*(2), e6–e7.

Bedard, M., Felteau, M., Marshall, S., Dubois, S., Weaver, B., & Gibbons, C. (2008). Mindfulness-based cognitive therapy reduces depression symptoms in people with a traumatic brain injury: Results from a pilot study. *European Psychiatry, 23*(2), S243–S243.

Biegel, G. M., Brown, K. W., Shapiro, S. L., & Schubert, C. M. (2009). Mindfulness-based stress reduction for the treatment of adolescent psychiatric outpatients: A randomized clinical trial. *Journal of Consulting and Clinical Psychology, 77*(5), 855–866.

Bishop, S. R., Lau, M., Shapiro, S., Carlson, L., Anderson, N. D., Carmody, J., et al. (2004). Mindfulness: A proposed operational definition. *Clinical Psychology: Science and Practice, 11*(3), 230–241.

Bootzin, R. R., & Stevens, S. J. (2005). Adolescents, substance abuse, and the treatment of insomnia and daytime sleepiness. *Clinical Psychology Review, 25*(5), 629–644.
Bowen, S., & Marlatt, A. (2009). Surfing the urge: Brief mindfulness-based intervention for college student smokers. *Psychology of Addictive Behaviors, 23*(4), 666–671.
Bowen, S., Witkiewitz, K., Dillworth, T. M., Chawla, N., Simpson, T. L., Ostafin, B. D., et al. (2006). Mindfulness meditation and substance use in an incarcerated population. *Psychology of Addictive Behaviors, 20*(3), 343–347.
Brown, K. W., Ryan, R. M., & Creswell, J. D. (2007). Mindfulness: Theoretical foundations and evidence for its salutary effects. *Psychological Inquiry, 18*(4), 211–237.
Carson, J. W., Carson, K. M., Gil, K. M., & Baucom, D. H. (2004). Mindfulness-based relationship enhancement. *Behavior Therapy, 35*(3), 471–494.
Collard, P., & Walsh, J. (2008). Sensory awareness mindfulness training in coaching: Accepting life's challenges. *Journal of Rational-Emotive & Cognitive-Behavior Therapy, 26*(1), 30–37.
Cousins, L. S. (1996). The dating of the historical Buddha: A review article. *Journal of the Royal Asiatic Society (Third Series), 6*(1), 57–63.
Craigie, M. A., Rees, C. S., Marsh, A., & Nathan, P. (2008). Mindfulness-based cognitive therapy for generalized anxiety disorder: A preliminary evaluation. *Behavioural and Cognitive Psychotherapy, 36*, 553–568.
Creswell, J. D., Myers, H. F., Cole, S. W., & Irwin, M. R. (2009). Mindfulness meditation training effects on CD4+ T lymphocytes in HIV-1 infected adults: A small randomized controlled trial. *Brain, Behavior, and Immunity, 23*(2), 184–188.
Cusens, B., Duggan, G. B., Thorne, K., & Burch, V. (2010). Evaluation of the breathworks mindfulness-based pain management programme: Effects on well-being and multiple measures of mindfulness. *Clinical Psychology & Psychotherapy, 17*(1), 63–78.
Dalen, J., Smith, B. W., Shelley, B. M., Sloan, A. L., Leahigh, L., & Begay, D. (2010). Pilot study: Mindful eating and living (MEAL): Weight, eating behavior, and psychological outcomes associated with a mindfulness-based intervention for people with obesity. *Complementary Therapies in Medicine, 18*(6), 260–264.
Deci, E., & Ryan, R. (2008). Hedonia, eudaimonia, and well-being: An introduction. *Journal of Happiness Studies, 9*(1), 1–11.
Foley, E., Baillie, A., Huxter, M., Price, M., & Sinclair, E. (2010). Mindfulness-based cognitive therapy for individuals whose lives have been affected by cancer: A randomized controlled trial. *Journal of Consulting and Clinical Psychology, 78*(1), 72–79.
Fortney, L., & Taylor, M. (2010). Meditation in medical practice: A review of the evidence and practice. *Primary Care; Clinics in Office Practice, 37*(1), 81–90.
Fredrickson, B. L., Cohn, M. A., Coffey, K. A., Pek, J., & Finkel, S. M. (2008). Open hearts build lives: Positive emotions, induced through loving-kindness meditation, build consequential personal resources. *Journal of Personality and Social Psychology, 95*(5), 1045–1062.
Fresco, D. M., Moore, M. T., van Dulmen, M. H. M., Segal, Z. V., Ma, S. H., Teasdale, J. D., et al. (2007). Initial psychometric properties of the experiences questionnaire: Validation of a self-report measure of decentering. *Behavior Therapy, 38*(3), 234–246.
Freud, S., & Breuer, J. (1895). *Studies on hysteria, S.E., 2*. London: Hogarth.
Geschwind, N., Peeters, F., Drukker, M., van Os, J., & Wichers, M. (2011). Mindfulness training increases momentary positive emotions and reward experience in adults vulnerable to depression: A randomized controlled trial. *Journal of Consulting and Clinical Psychology, 79*(5), 618–628.
Gethin, R. (2011). On some definitions of mindfulness. *Contemporary Buddhism, 12*(01), 263–279.
Godfrin, K., & Van Heeringen, C. (2010). The effects of mindfulness-based cognitive therapy on recurrence of depressive episodes, mental health and quality of life: A randomized controlled study. *Behaviour Research and Therapy, 48*(8), 738–746.
Gross, C., Cramer-Bornemann, M., Frazier, P., Ibrahim, H., Kreitzer, M. J., Nyman, J., et al. (2009). Results of a double-controlled trial of mindfulness-based stress reduction to reduce symptoms in transplant patients. *Explore: The Journal of Science and Healing, 5*(3), 156–156.

Hanley, A. W., & Garland, E. L. (2014). Dispositional mindfulness co-varies with self-reported positive reappraisal. *Personality and Individual Differences, 66*, 146–152.

Heidenreich, T., Tuin, I., Pflug, B., Michal, M., & Michalak, J. (2006). Mindfulness-based cognitive therapy for persistent insomnia: A pilot study. *Psychotherapy and Psychosomatics, 75*(3), 188–189.

Horton-Deutsch, S., O'Haver Day, P., Haight, R., & Babin-Nelson, M. (2007). Enhancing mental health services to bone marrow transplant recipients through a mindfulness-based therapeutic intervention. *Complementary Therapies in Clinical Practice, 13*(2), 110–115.

Irving, J. A., Dobkin, P. L., & Park, J. (2009). Cultivating mindfulness in health care professionals: A review of empirical studies of mindfulness-based stress reduction (MBSR). *Complementary Therapies in Clinical Practice, 15*(2), 61–66.

Ivtzan, I., Lomas, T., Hefferon, K., & Worth, P. (2015). *Challenging positive psychology: Embracing the dark side of life*. London: Routledge.

Ivtzan, I., Young, T. K., Jeffrey, A. D., Martman, J. L., Hart, R., & Eiroa-Orosa, F. J. (2015). Integrating mindfulness in positive psychology: A randomised controlled trial of an 8-week positive mindfulness programme (PMP). Manuscript submitted for publication.

Jung, C. G. (1939/1963). *The integration of the personality* (S. Dell, Trans.). London: Routledge & Kegan Paul.

Kabat-Zinn, J. (1982). An outpatient program in behavioral medicine for chronic pain patients based on the practice of mindfulness meditation: Theoretical considerations and preliminary results. *General Hospital Psychiatry, 4*(1), 33–47.

Kabat-Zinn, J. (1990). *Full catastrophe living: Using the wisdom of your body and mind to face stress, pain and illness*. New York: Delacorte.

Kabat-Zinn, J. (2003). Mindfulness-based interventions in context: Past, present, and future. *Clinical Psychology: Science and Practice, 10*(2), 144–156.

Kearney, D. J., McDermott, K., Martinez, M., & Simpson, T. (2010). Mindfulness-based stress reduction for irritable bowel syndrome. *Gastroenterology Clinics of North America, 138*(5), S-710.

Keown, D. (2009). *Buddhism: A brief insight*. New York: Sterling Publishing.

Keyes, C. L. M. (2002). The mental health continuum: From languishing to flourishing in life. *Journal of Health and Social Behavior, 43*(2), 207–222.

Kilpatrick, L. A., Suyenobu, B. Y., Smith, S. R., Bueller, J. A., Goodman, T., Creswell, J. D., et al. (2011). Impact of mindfulness-based stress reduction training on intrinsic brain connectivity. *Neuroimage, 56*(1), 290–298.

Kim, B., Lee, S.-H., Kim, Y. W., Choi, T. K., Yook, K., Suh, S. Y., et al. (2010). Effectiveness of a mindfulness-based cognitive therapy program as an adjunct to pharmacotherapy in patients with panic disorder. *Journal of Anxiety Disorders, 24*(6), 590–595.

King, R. (1999). *Orientalism and religion: Post-colonial theory, India and "The Mystic East"*. London: Routledge.

Kumar, S. M. (2002). An introduction to Buddhism for the cognitive-behavioral therapist. *Cognitive and Behavioral Practice, 9*(1), 40–43.

Ledesma, D., & Kumano, H. (2009). Mindfulness-based stress reduction and cancer: A meta-analysis. *Psycho-Oncology, 18*(6), 571–579.

Lee, E.-J. (2005). When placebic information differs from real information cognitive and motivational bases of mindful reactions to informational social influence. *Communication Research, 32*(5), 615–645.

Ljótsson, B., Andréewitch, S., Hedman, E., Rück, C., Andersson, G., & Lindefors, N. (2010). Exposure and mindfulness based therapy for irritable bowel syndrome—An open pilot study. *Journal of Behavior Therapy and Experimental Psychiatry, 41*(3), 185–190.

Lomas, T., Cartwright, T., Edginton, T., & Ridge, D. (2014). A religion of wellbeing? The appeal of Buddhism to men in London, UK. *Psychology of Religion and Spirituality, 6*(3), 198–207.

Lomas, T., Edginton, T., Cartwright, T., & Ridge, D. (2014). Men developing emotional intelligence through meditation? Combining narrative, cognitive, and electroencephalography (EEG) evidence. *Psychology of Men and Masculinity, 15*(2), 213–224.

Lomas, T., Hefferon, K., & Ivtzan, I. (2014). *Applied positive psychology: Integrated positive practice*. London: Sage.
Lomas, T., & Ivtzan, I. (2015). Second wave positive psychology: Exploring the positive-negative dialectics of wellbeing. *Journal of Happiness Studies*. doi: 10.1007/s10902-015-9668-y.
Lomas, T., & Jnanavaca. (2015). Weaving the threads: Types of mindfulness, orders of conditionality, and stages of the spiritual path. In E. Shonin, W. van Gordon, & N. N. Singh (Eds.), *Buddhist foundations of mindfulness*. London: Springer.
Lovas, D. A., & Barsky, A. J. (2010). Mindfulness-based cognitive therapy for hypochondriasis, or severe health anxiety: A pilot study. *Journal of Anxiety Disorders, 24*(8), 931–935.
Ma, S. H., & Teasdale, J. D. (2004). Mindfulness-based cognitive therapy for depression: Replication and exploration of differential relapse prevention effects. *Journal of Consulting and Clinical Psychology, 72*(1), 31–40.
McCullough, M. E., Emmons, R. A., & Tsang, J.-A. (2002). The grateful disposition: A conceptual and empirical topography. *Journal of Personality and Social Psychology, 82*, 112–127.
McHugh, L., Simpson, A., & Reed, P. (2010). Mindfulness as a potential intervention for stimulus over-selectivity in older adults. *Research in Developmental Disabilities, 31*(1), 178–184.
McMahan, D. L. (2004). Modernity and the early discourse of scientific Buddhism. *Journal of the American Academy of Religion, 72*(4), 897–933.
Miller, J. J., Fletcher, K., & Kabat-Zinn, J. (1995). Three-year follow-up and clinical implications of a mindfulness meditation-based stress reduction intervention in the treatment of anxiety disorders. *General Hospital Psychiatry, 17*(3), 192–200.
Mills, N., & Allen, J. (2000). Mindfulness of movement as a coping strategy in multiple sclerosis: A pilot study. *General Hospital Psychiatry, 22*(6), 425–431.
Moore, A., Gruber, T., Derose, J., & Malinowski, P. (2012). Regular, brief mindfulness meditation practice improves electrophysiological markers of attentional control. *Frontiers in Human Neuroscience, 6*, 18.
Nakamura, Y., Lipschitz, D. L., Landward, R., Kuhn, R., & West, G. (2011). Two sessions of sleep-focused mind–body bridging improve self-reported symptoms of sleep and PTSD in veterans: A pilot randomized controlled trial. *Journal of Psychosomatic Research, 70*(4), 335–345.
National Institute for Health and Care Excellence. (2004). Depression: Management of depression in primary and secondary care. *Clinical Guideline, 23*.
Neff, K. D., & Germer, C. K. (2013). A pilot study and randomized controlled trial of the mindful self-compassion program. *Journal of Clinical Psychology, 69*(1), 28–44.
Niemiec, R. M., Rashid, T., & Spinella, M. (2012). Strong mindfulness: Integrating mindfulness and character strengths. *Journal of Mental Health Counseling, 34*(3), 240–253.
Norem, J. K. (2001). *The positive power of negative thinking*. New York: Basic Books.
Obadia, L. (2008). The economies of health in Western Buddhism: A case study of a Tibetan Buddhist group in France. In D. C. Wood (Ed.), *The economics of health and wellness: Anthropological perspectives* (pp. 227–259). Oxford: JAI Press.
Olivio, E., Dodson-Lavelle, B., Wren, A., Fang, Y., & Oz, M. (2009). Feasibility and effectiveness of a brief meditation-based stress management intervention for patients diagnosed with or at risk for coronary artery disease: A pilot study. *Psychology, Health & Medicine, 14*(5), 513–523.
Parks, A. C., & Biswas-Diener, R. (2014). Positive interventions: Past, present and future. In T. Kashdan & J. Ciarrochi (Eds.), *Mindfulness, acceptance, and positive psychology: The seven foundations of well-being* (pp. 140–165). Oakland, CA: New Harbinger.
Patel, S. R., Carmody, J., & Simpson, H. B. (2007). Adapting mindfulness-based stress reduction for the treatment of obsessive-compulsive disorder: A case report. *Cognitive and Behavioral Practice, 14*(4), 375–380.
Peacock, J. (2014). Sati or mindfulness? Bridging the divide. In M. Mazzano (Ed.), *After mindfulness: New perspectives on psychology and meditation* (pp. 3–22). Basingstoke: Palgrave Macmillan.
Peterson, C., Park, N., & Seligman, M. P. (2005). Orientations to happiness and life satisfaction: The full life versus the empty life. *Journal of Happiness Studies, 6*(1), 25–41.

Phillips, T., & Aarons, H. (2005). Choosing Buddhism in Australia: Towards a traditional style of reflexive spiritual engagement. *The British Journal of Sociology, 56*(2), 215–232.

Pradhan, E. K., Baumgarten, M., Langenberg, P., Handwerger, B., Gilpin, A. K., Magyari, T., et al. (2007). Effect of mindfulness-based stress reduction in rheumatoid arthritis patients. *Arthritis Care & Research, 57*(7), 1134–1142.

Rhys Davids, T. W. (1881). *Buddhist suttas*. Oxford: Clarendon.

Rhys Davids, T. W. (1910). *Dialogues of the Buddha* (Vol. 2). London: Henry Frowde.

Rogers, C. R. (1961). *On becoming a person: A therapists view of psychotherapy*. New York: Houghton Mifflin.

Roof, W. (2001). *Spiritual marketplace*. Princeton, NJ: Princeton University Press.

Rungreangkulkij, S., Wongtakee, W., & Thongyot, S. (2011). Buddhist group therapy for diabetes patients with depressive symptoms. *Archives of Psychiatric Nursing, 25*(3), 195–205.

Ryff, C. D. (1989). Happiness is everything, or is it? Explorations on the meaning of psychological well-being. *Journal of Personality and Social Psychology, 57*(6), 1069–1081.

Ryff, C. D., Dienberg Love, G., Urry, H. L., Muller, D., Rosenkranz, M. A., Friedman, E. M., et al. (2006). Psychological well-being and ill-being: Do they have distinct or mirrored biological correlates? *Psychotherapy and Psychosomatics, 75*(2), 85–95.

Ryff, C. D., & Singer, B. (1998). The contours of positive human health. *Psychological Inquiry, 9*(1), 1–28.

Said, E. W. (1995). *Orientalism: Western conceptions of the orient*. London: Penguin.

Schmidt, S., Grossman, P., Schwarzer, B., Jena, S., Naumann, J., & Walach, H. (2011). Treating fibromyalgia with mindfulness-based stress reduction: Results from a 3-armed randomized controlled trial. *Pain and Headache, 152*(2), 361–369.

Schmidt, S., Simshäuser, K., Aickin, M., Lüking, M., Schultz, C., & Kaube, H. (2010). Mindfulness-based stress reduction is an effective intervention for patients suffering from migraine—Results from a controlled trial. *European Journal of Integrative Medicine, 2*(4), 196–196.

Segal, Z. V., Williams, J. M. G., & Teasdale, J. D. (2002). *Mindfulness-based cognitive therapy for depression: A new approach to preventing relapse*. New York: Guilford Press.

Seligman, M. E. P., & Csikszentmihalyi, M. (2000). Positive psychology: An introduction. *American Psychologist, 55*(1), 5–14.

Shapiro, D. H. (1992). A preliminary study of long term meditators: Goals, effects, religious orientation, cognitions. *Journal of Transpersonal Psychology, 24*(1), 23–39.

Shapiro, D. H. (1994). Examining the content and context of meditation: A challenge for psychology in the areas of stress management, psychotherapy, and religion/values. *Journal of Humanistic Psychology, 34*(4), 101–135.

Shapiro, S. L., Astin, J. A., Bishop, S. R., & Cordova, M. (2005). Mindfulness-based stress reduction for health care professionals: Results from a randomized trial. *International Journal of Stress Management, 12*(2), 164–176.

Shapiro, S. L., Bootzin, R. R., Figueredo, A. J., Lopez, A. M., & Schwartz, G. E. (2003). The efficacy of mindfulness-based stress reduction in the treatment of sleep disturbance in women with breast cancer: An exploratory study. *Journal of Psychosomatic Research, 54*(1), 85–91.

Shapiro, S. L., Carlson, L. E., Astin, J. A., & Freedman, B. (2006). Mechanisms of mindfulness. *Journal of Clinical Psychology, 62*(3), 373–386.

Shonin, E., Van Gordon, W., & Griffiths, M. D. (2013). Mindfulness-based interventions: Towards mindful clinical integration. *Frontiers in Psychology, 4*(194). doi:10.3389/fpsyg.2013.00194.

Sin, N. L., Della Porta, M. D., & Lyubomirsky, S. (2011). Tailoring positive psychology interventions to treat depressed individuals. In S. I. Donaldson, M. Csikszentmihalyi, & J. Nakamura (Eds.), *Applied positive psychology: Improving everyday life, health, schools, work, and society* (pp. 79–96). New York: Routledge.

Sin, N. L., & Lyubomirsky, S. (2009). Enhancing well-being and alleviating depressive symptoms with positive psychology interventions: A practice-friendly meta-analysis. *Journal of Clinical Psychology, 65*(5), 467–487.

Singh, N. N., Lancioni, G. E., Winton, A. S., Singh, A. N., Adkins, A. D., & Singh, J. (2008). Clinical and benefit—Cost outcomes of teaching a mindfulness-based procedure to adult offenders with intellectual disabilities. *Behavior Modification, 32*(5), 622–637.

Singh, N. N., Lancioni, G. E., Winton, A. S., Singh, J., Curtis, W. J., Wahler, R. G., et al. (2007). Mindful parenting decreases aggression and increases social behavior in children with developmental disabilities. *Behavior Modification, 31*(6), 749–771.

Stanley, E. A., Schaldach, J. M., Kiyonaga, A., & Jha, A. P. (2011). Mindfulness-based mind fitness training: A case study of a high-stress predeployment military cohort. *Cognitive and Behavioral Practice, 18*(4), 566–576.

Sullivan, M. J., Wood, L., Terry, J., Brantley, J., Charles, A., McGee, V., et al. (2009). The support, education, and research in chronic heart failure study (SEARCH): A mindfulness-based psychoeducational intervention improves depression and clinical symptoms in patients with chronic heart failure. *American Heart Journal, 157*(1), 84–90.

Surana, P. K., & Lomas, T. (2014). The power of charity: Does giving away money improve the wellbeing of the donor? *Indian Journal of Positive Psychology, 5*(3), 223–230.

Tapper, K., Shaw, C., Ilsley, J., Hill, A. J., Bond, F. W., & Moore, L. (2009). Exploratory randomised controlled trial of a mindfulness-based weight loss intervention for women. *Appetite, 52*(2), 396–404.

Teasdale, J. D. (1988). Cognitive vulnerability to persistent depression. *Cognition & Emotion, 2*(3), 247–274.

Teasdale, J. D., Segal, Z., & Williams, J. M. G. (1995). How does cognitive therapy prevent depressive relapse and why should attentional control (mindfulness) training help? *Behaviour Research and Therapy, 33*(1), 25–39.

Teasdale, J. D., Segal, Z. V., Williams, J. M. G., Ridgeway, V. A., Soulsby, J. M., & Lau, M. A. (2000). Prevention of relapse/recurrence in major depression by mindfulness-based cognitive therapy. *Journal of Consulting and Clinical Psychology, 68*(4), 615–623.

Thomas, E. J. (2000). *The life of Buddha as legend and history*. New York: Dover.

Thompson, N. J., Walker, E. R., Obolensky, N., Winning, A., Barmon, C., DiIorio, C., et al. (2010). Distance delivery of mindfulness-based cognitive therapy for depression: Project UPLIFT. *Epilepsy & Behavior, 19*(3), 247–254.

Thrangu, K. (1993). *The practice of tranquility and insight: A guide to Tibetan Buddhist meditation* (R. Roberts, Trans.). Boston: Shambhala Publishing.

Van Gordon, W., Shonin, E., Griffiths, M. D., & Singh, N. N. (2014). There is only one mindfulness: Why science and Buddhism need to work together. *Mindfulness, 6*(1), 49–56.

Varenne, J. (1977). *Yoga and the Hindu tradition*. Chicago: University of Chicago Press.

Walach, H., Nord, E., Zier, C., Dietz-Waschkowski, B., Kersig, S., & Schupbach, H. (2007). Mindfulness-based stress reduction as a method for personnel development: A pilot evaluation. *International Journal of Stress Management, 14*(2), 188–198.

Weber, B., Jermann, F., Gex-Fabry, M., Nallet, A., Bondolfi, G., & Aubry, J.-M. (2010). Mindfulness-based cognitive therapy for bipolar disorder: A feasibility trial. *European Psychiatry, 25*(6), 334–337.

Weinstein, N. D., Marcus, S. E., & Moser, R. P. (2005). Smokers' unrealistic optimism about their risk. *Tobacco Control, 14*(1), 55–59.

Williams, J. M. G., Alatiq, Y., Crane, C., Barnhofer, T., Fennell, M., Duggan, D., et al. (2008). Mindfulness-based cognitive therapy (MBCT) in bipolar disorder: Preliminary evaluation of immediate effects on between-episode functioning. *Journal of Affective Disorders, 107*(1), 275–279.

Williams, J. M. G., & Kabat-Zinn, J. (2011). Mindfulness: Diverse perspectives on its meaning, origins, and multiple applications at the intersection of science and dharma. *Contemporary Buddhism, 12*(01), 1–18.

Wong, P. T. P. (2011). Positive psychology 2.0: Towards a balanced interactive model of the good life. *Canadian Psychology/Psychologie canadienne, 52*(2), 69–81.

Wren, A. A., Wright, M. A., Carson, J. W., & Keefe, F. J. (2011). Yoga for persistent pain: New findings and directions for an ancient practice. *Pain, 152*(3), 477–480.

Wittgenstein, L. (1953). Philosophical Investigations. New York: Macmillan.

Zgierska, A., Rabago, D., Zuelsdorff, M., Coe, C., Miller, M., & Fleming, M. (2008). Mindfulness meditation for alcohol relapse prevention: A feasibility pilot study. *Journal of Addiction Medicine, 2*(3), 165–173.

Part III
Mindfulness in Other Applied Settings

Chapter 15
Mindfulness and Forensic Mental Health

Andrew Day

Introduction

Patients of forensic mental health services are those with diagnosable mental disorders whose behaviour has led, or could lead, them to offend (Mullen, 2000). They include mentally ill inmates of correctional facilities, sex offenders who have a recognised mental disorder, and those who have been judged to be incompetent to stand trial or found guilty but not responsible for their behaviour. Typically, forensic mental health services are offered to those with a 'major mental disorder', a term usually reserved for more serious forms of mental illness such as schizophrenia, major affective disorders, bipolar disorders, and other psychotic conditions but which also encompasses the effects of brain damage, intellectual disability, and serious personality disorder. In practice, this means that forensic mental health patients represent some of the marginalised, troubled, and perhaps difficult-to-treat members of society. The aim of this chapter is to consider the role that mindfulness-based interventions have to play in their effective care and management.

The need to provide effective mental health services for mentally disordered offenders is evident from statistics which show that the prevalence of major mental disorder is particularly high in offending populations, especially prisoners (see Skeem, Manchak, & Peterson, 2011). One of the largest studies in this area, which aggregated the findings of 62 different studies involving a total of almost 23,000 prisoners from 12 different countries, concluded that one in seven inmates experiences either a psychotic illness or major depression (Fazel & Danesh, 2002), with prevalence rates thought to be even higher in female offender populations (Steadman, Osher, Robbins, Case, & Samuels, 2009). Similarly, high rates have

A. Day (✉)
Faculty of Health, School of Psychology, Deakin University,
Geelong Waterfront Campus, Locked Bag 20000, Geelong, VIC, 3220, Australia
e-mail: andrew.day@deakin.edu.au

E. Shonin et al. (eds.), *Mindfulness and Buddhist-Derived Approaches in Mental Health and Addiction*, Advances in Mental Health and Addiction,
DOI 10.1007/978-3-319-22255-4_15

also been reported for those offenders who live in the community (Gunter, Philibert, & Hollenbeck, 2009).

Of course, the notion that mindfulness-based interventions can lead to improvement in mental health is no longer contentious. A large and ever-growing evidence base now exists that demonstrates that mindfulness interventions can benefit those with a wide range of mental health problems, including depressive disorders (Chiesa & Serretti, 2011), bipolar disorders (Perich, Manicavasagar, Mitchell, & Ball, 2013), and anxiety disorders (Hofmann, Sawyer, Witt, & Oh, 2010). The primary focus of this chapter, however, is on understanding the role that mindfulness-based interventions have to play in managing the risk of further offending in forensic patients. In the UK and elsewhere, tragic cases such as those involving Sharon Campbell and Christopher Clunis triggered national enquiries into the way in which the health system identifies and manages risk (Taylor & Gunn, 2008) and led to risk management being identified as of overriding concern for forensic mental health service providers (Duggan, 2008). This has prompted interest in the development of new treatments and interventions which can effectively manage the future risk of offending, particularly violent offending.

Coupled with this are some rather significant changes in how treatment is conceptualised. From times when models of care were firmly entrenched within biological or medical conceptualisations of illness, contemporary forensic mental health services now utilise a range of psychosocial and multidisciplinary approaches to patient care that have opened up a number of possibilities for the development and delivery of new and alternative interventions to support the pharmacological approaches that have long characterised the sector (Soothill, 2008). There is considerable scope for innovation given the (surprisingly) limited evidence base from which to draw any firm conclusions about effectiveness of psychological treatment on reducing aggressive and violent behaviour (McGuire, 2008). In what is still the only published meta-analysis of violent offender treatment programmes, Polaschek and Collie (2004) concluded that although most of the programmes they reviewed showed some level of efficacy, it was difficult to draw any firm conclusions about effectiveness. It is in this context that recent years have seen growing interest in the potential to apply mindfulness-based approaches to risk management and, in particular, to the clinical management of violence. Before discussing the rationale and evidence for using mindfulness interventions in this way, it is first important to consider what is known about those factors that trigger violence and the role of major mental disorder.

Understanding Violence

Violent offenders constitute a group that attract considerable public concern in relation to the risks they present to the community after leaving institutional care. This is understandable given the often catastrophic effects of violence—not only on victims but also on those who are less directly involved, including bystanders, those who know the victims and perpetrators, and children who witness violence (Tolan, 2007). Even for highly aggressive individuals, however, aggressive acts are not random but predictable responses to particular events and situations. Violence that occurs when the perpetrator is in a state of anger, for example, is typically elicited when he or she is blocked from achieving important goals, where expected rewards fail to eventuate, or when events occur that are in some way aversive for the individual. For others, violence can occur in the context of intimate relationships, in the commissioning of other crimes, or sometimes in response to specific mental health symptoms.

Whilst there has been much debate about the nature of the relationship between mental disorder and violence, there now appears to be a broad consensus that the primary predictors of risk are largely the same for mentally disordered offenders as they are for non-disordered offenders (see Andrews & Bonta, 2010). The exception to this is when particular psychotic symptoms such as paranoia (Grossman, Haywood, Cavanaugh, Davis, & Lewis, 1995) and delusions involving personal targets (Nestor, Haycock, Doiron, Kelly, & Kelly, 1995) are present, particularly when these occur in conjunction with substance use (Swanson, Borum, & Swartz, 1996). Ullrich, Keers, and Coid (2014), for example, have recently observed that violence can be precipitated by delusional thinking (such as thoughts about being spied upon, being followed, being plotted against, being under control of a person/force, and having special gifts or powers), particularly when these experiences give rise to angry emotion. In other words, specific symptoms can trigger anger which then motivates aggressive or violent behaviour, at least in some people who experience major mental disorders. Accordingly, when seeking to understand or manage risk in mentally disordered offenders, it becomes important to understand what role, if any, the mental illness plays, particularly in relation to how anger is experienced.

There are also grounds to suspect that negative emotional states more generally are causally related to many types of offending. Zamble and Quinsey's (2001) study of parolees found that over three-quarters of those who reoffended experienced dysphoric emotion in the 30-day period prior to offending, compared with less than half of those who did not reoffend. Two-thirds of the recidivists experienced negative emotion in the 48 h leading up to their offence, compared with only one in ten non-recidivists. This finding, when considered along with Hanson and Harris's (2000) conclusions that recidivist sexual offenders show an increase in negative emotion, anger, and general psychiatric symptoms just prior to offending, identifies negative emotion and anger as key dynamic risk factors. Thus, although effective violence risk management strategies should seek to influence a wide range of risk factors, including antisocial attitudes, substance use, social support, and compliance with treatment (Douglas & Skeem, 2005), the treatment of dysphoric emotion (negative mood, anger) becomes particularly important.

Contemporary theories of aggressive and violent behaviour all highlight the importance of dysphoric emotion. Cognitive-affective theories, for example, focus on the 'instigation' of aggression and the central role that negative emotion, particularly anger, plays in many, though not all, forms of violence (see Novaco, 2011). Self-regulation theories, on the other hand, seek to understand the ways in which aggressive impulses are responded to. The concept of self-regulation has some overlap with the concept of inhibition and also with (low) impulsivity, described by Polaschek (2006) as a lifelong characteristic or pattern of behaviours that is reflected in rule breaking, unstable relationships, poor tolerance of frustration, and an inability to delay gratification. It can also, of course, be a state, induced by factors such as intoxication or stress, which overrides any broad disposition to self-regulate behaviour. Under these conditions, individuals are more likely to experience states characterised by diminished guilt; a focus on immediate, short-term concerns; lessened influence of self-standards; and diminished inhibitions (Baumeister, Heatherton, & Tice, 1994). Other processes are also thought to diminish self-regulation, including desensitisation through repetition of violent acts, escalation as a result of retaliation between perpetrator and victim, or tiredness (see Howells & Day, 2002).

Mindfulness and Negative Emotion

It is in relation to the management of negative emotion that mindfulness-based interventions can perhaps make their most powerful contribution to forensic mental health service delivery. Baer (2003) and Wright, Day, and Howells (2009) have both identified a number of different mechanisms by which mindfulness-based interventions might improve emotional control. For example, they suggest that mindfulness improves an individual's ability to tolerate negative emotional states and the ability to cope with them effectively. They propose that the avoidance that is typically associated with emotional reactivity may be reduced through a process of sustained, non-judgemental observation of emotion-related sensations. Related to this is the idea that mindfulness training interferes with those ruminative patterns that characterise negative emotional episodes (Nolen-Hoeksema, 1991). Teasdale (1999), for example, has suggested that the non-judgemental, decentred view of one's thoughts leads individuals to notice the onset of negative thoughts and redirect their attention to other aspects of the present moment, such as breathing, walking, or sounds in the environment, so avoiding rumination. For Metcalf and Dimidjian (2014), mindfulness is 'a way to help people decrease cognitive reactivity to negative emotion through repeated practice with both neutral and affectively triggering content on a regular basis' (p. 275). To put this another way, the application of mindfulness skills allows the individual to step back from emotional disturbance and to see it clearly as an emotional state that will, in time, pass. Improved self-noticing may thus help the individual to make more informed, wiser, behavioural choices as he or she develops a higher level of tolerance for unpleasant internal states. In addition, the ability of various meditation strategies to induce relaxation has been well documented, and the resulting improved tolerance for provocation may be helpful in its own right. This is illustrated in the work of Gillespie, Mitchell, Fisher and Beech (2012) who have begun to document the neurobiological and cardiorespiratory mechanisms that are associated with controlled breathing (thought to be conducive to a state of mindfulness). They argue that these techniques can be shown to affect the functioning of those neural circuits involved in the regulation of emotional states, including the prefrontal cortex and the amygdala. Several studies utilising brain imaging techniques have shown that mindfulness can alter levels of neural activity in these areas (see the systematic review by Chiesa & Serretti, 2011).

Mindfulness in Forensic Mental Health Practice

It has been suggested so far in this chapter that a strong rationale exists for the application of mindfulness-based interventions with forensic mental health patients. They might reasonably be expected to not only help patients to successfully manage distressing symptoms of mental disorder but also assist in the broader goal of reducing the risk of violence. It might be expected then that mindfulness-based interventions would form a central component of forensic mental health service delivery and yet, despite the growing influence of these approaches in mainstream mental health (Kangas, 2014), their application to the forensic setting seems relatively rare. There are, for example, no references to mindfulness in a well-known handbook of forensic mental health edited by Soothill, Rogers, and Dolan in 2008. Although, it is fair to say that interest has grown substantially since this book first appeared, published accounts of how mindfulness-based interventions are used with forensic populations remain relatively rare. There are, of course, notable exceptions—including the contributions of Singh and colleagues (e.g. Singh et al., 2007, 2008) and the development of mindfulness-based treatment for high-risk patients in a high-security forensic hospital in the UK (e.g. Evershed et al., 2006; Tennant, 2010). Singh, Lancioni, Winton, Singh, and Adkins (2011), for example, describe using the 'soles of the feet' technique and 'mindful observation of thoughts' to reduce deviant sexual arousal in sexual offenders, whereas Tennant and Howells (2010) consider the effects of dialectical behaviour therapy on violent behaviour in a forensic inpatient setting. In addition, there is a growing body of work that has investigated the effects of mindfulness methods on offender and prison populations more broadly. Samuelson, Carmody, Kabat-Zinn, and Bratt (2007), for example, have reported improvements on measures of mood disturbance, hostility, and self-esteem following mindfulness training in a US correctional facility. This body of knowledge has been recently summarised by Shonin, Van Gordon, and Griffiths (2014) and suggests that these methods do have a potentially important role to play with forensic populations.

Some Critical Issues

The rest of this chapter is devoted to a discussion of some of the issues that potentially inhibit the 'scaling up' or wider implementation of mindfulness-based interventions in forensic mental health settings. Perhaps the most obvious of these is the ongoing need to establish that the delivery of these interventions does indeed lead to reductions in violence or reoffending. There are, however, a number of associated issues related to both the diversity and integrity of those mindfulness-based interventions that are currently being delivered. As a consequence, it would seem that service delivery in this area has remained rather fragmented and somewhat dependent on the interests and skills of individual practitioners.

Outcome Evaluation

It is likely that only when direct evidence about the impact of mindfulness-based interventions on reoffending (or at least *risk* of reoffending) can be presented that they will be systematically implemented. Indeed, many of the published reviews of mindfulness-based approaches identify the need for more rigorous evaluation of this type, often linked to calls for a concerted research programme to establish treatment outcomes (e.g. Fix & Fix, 2013; Howells, Tennant, Day, & Elmer, 2010; Shonin, Van Gordon, Slade, & Griffiths, 2013). In short, whilst there is significant early evidence to suggest that mindful meditation represents a viable therapeutic tool to prevent violence, studies which have directly investigated its impact on offending behaviour have yet to be conducted (Shonin et al., 2014). Indeed, current trials fall some way short of providing the type of evidence required to describe mindfulness approaches as 'evidence based', defined by the Washington State Institute for Public Policy in the following way:

> a programme or practice that has been tested in heterogeneous or intended populations with multiple randomised and/or statistically-controlled evaluations, or one large multiple-site randomised or statistically control evaluation, where the weight of evidence from a systematic review demonstrates sustained improvements in recidivism or other outcomes of interest. Further, "evidence-based" means a programme or practice that can be implemented with a set of procedures to allow successful replication… … and, when possible, has been determined to be cost-effective. (Drake, 2013, p. 2)

Random-assignment controlled trial studies are particularly important in establishing an evidence base, primarily because of problems associated with self-selection into treatment groups. There are, however, significant challenges to conducting randomised controlled trials in forensic mental health settings, including the limited number of patients who receive treatment, the heterogeneity of the population, the length of the treatment, the assessment case flow, the occupation of treatment beds by previously assessed patients, and the possibility of dropouts (see Farrington & Jolliffe, 2002). There are additional issues in disentangling the effects of other interventions (e.g. pharmacological) and that arise in relation to the low base rates for reoffending, meaning that very long-term follow-up is required.

Such problems are, of course, not restricted to mindfulness interventions. The National Collaborating Centre for Mental Health (2009) concludes their review of the evidence for the treatment of personality disorder with a number of comments about the limited number of studies that have been conducted, uncertainty about their scientific quality, and problems with small sample sizes, short follow-up periods, and the tendency to focus on community settings. Gilbody, House, and Sheldon (2003) have also noted that psychiatrists 'do not routinely measure outcome (patient-based or otherwise) in the context of their practice' and that 'substantial practical and attitudinal barriers were identified to the collection of standardised outcomes' (p. 87). Such observations are important, as it would be unfair to set different criteria for establishing the effectiveness of mindfulness-based interventions from those used in relation to other treatments.

There are some particular difficulties in establishing the specific effects of mindfulness-based interventions on dynamic risk. As noted above, a wide range of risk factors will inevitably influence the risk of violence including antisocial attitudes, substance use, social support, and compliance with treatment (Douglas & Skeem, 2005). It is suggested in this chapter that the most direct effects of mindfulness-based intervention on risk will be associated with changes to how negative emotion is managed, but clearly change in this area will be influenced by (and influence) change in these other areas. It may also be the case that improved management of dysphoric emotion is a necessary rather than sufficient condition to prevent reoffending for some patients and that treatment success in this area should not be expected, by itself, to lead to observable reductions in future violence.

Finally, there is a need to move beyond group-level outcome studies to examine who these methods work best for (and under what conditions). Teasdale, Segal, and Williams (2003) have emphasised the importance of individualised case formulation before using mindfulness-based methods, arguing that these should not be regarded as generic approaches for coping with distress. In considering how mindfulness might be incorporated into broader approaches to managing risk, it seems important to target interventions to those patients whose offending occurs in response to those issues (such as unregulated dysphoric emotion) that mindfulness-based methods can reasonably be expected to assist with.

Programme Diversity

One of the most significant problems that has inhibited large-scale evaluation of mindfulness-based interventions is the diversity of those interventions that are described as utilising mindfulness techniques. Not only do clear differences exist even between relatively well-articulated approaches such as mindfulness-based stress reduction (Kabat-Zinn, 1990) and mindfulness-based CBT (Kuyken et al., 2008) but forensic mental health services have a tendency to 'import' components of different treatments or to adapt more established treatments to meet the needs of forensic clients or the forensic setting. For example, dialectical behaviour therapy (DBT) has been widely used in the treatment of personality disorder, with over half of all treatment outcome studies for antisocial personal disorder investigating the effects of DBT (see National Collaborating Centre for Mental Health, 2009). DBT does contain elements of mindfulness training but was originally developed by Marsha Linehan to treat individuals with borderline personality disorder (BPD) who were at risk of suicide and self-harm. For Linehan (1993), borderline individuals have problems in regulating some or all of their emotions and these are produced by emotional vulnerability and inadequate emotion regulation strategies. The person is taught to learn to experience and label the emotions before restraining inappropriate behaviour, act in a way that is not dependent on mood, and refocus attention and self-soothe physiological arousal. Treatment thus focuses on changing distressing events and circumstances and learning to tolerate and accept distress. Although DBT is not an intervention designed to manage violence against others or offending, there is a small amount of research that has shown a link between some of the traits associated with BPD and reoffending, particularly in female offender populations (e.g. Hogue, Jones, Talkes, & Tennant, 2007; Nee & Farman, 2005).

There are also a number of other, relatively new, interventions which incorporate aspects of mindfulness and have attracted the interest of forensic mental health practitioners (Woldgabreal, Day, & Ward, 2014). Acceptance and commitment therapy (ACT), for example, is a psychological treatment which has been shown to be particularly useful in decreasing levels of psychological distress. ACT is essentially a behavioural approach that uses acceptance and mindfulness processes to produce psychological flexibility or states in which the person is more consciously aware of the present moment and more willing to engage in values-based actions. Psychological inflexibility is identified as a cause of significant mental ill health and is thought to lead to the adoption of thinking styles commonly associated with offending behaviour (e.g. egocentrism, rumination about past grievances). The approach to treatment is broadly compatible with that used in motivational interviewing (being compassionate, show how to be willing and accepting, no arguing, sarcasm or shaming, some self-disclosure) but involves strategies that aim to actively promote behaviour change. For example, ACT methods focus on the futility of trying to avoid or control unpleasant internal experiences, identifying the differences between a valued direction in life and a more specific goal, and distancing oneself from the feelings and thoughts that motivate antisocial behaviour. Finally, there is an expectation that participants will commit to achieving short-term and long-term goals (see Amrod & Hayes, 2013).

The difficulty here lies in disentangling the effects of the mindfulness components of these treatments with the other techniques that are utilised, many of which draw on behavioural treatment methods. The distinction between therapeutic 'techniques' (systematic actions designed to address or explore client difficulties either within or between sessions), 'strategies' (specific plans for intervention), 'therapeutic processes' (client-therapist interactions), and 'mechanisms of change' (theory-driven reasons that explain why change occurs) made by Petrik and Cronin (2014) is particularly relevant here as it draws attention to the need to be explicit about how specific techniques contribute to a treatment strategy and influence the way in which treatment is delivered. It provides a language to describe what it is that is being delivered, as well as the likely effects of interventions of different levels of depth, intensity, or complexity. In short, there is a need to articulate the underlying programme logic of all mindfulness-based interventions, such that it is clear which components are expected to bring about which type of change.

Programme Integrity

The term programme integrity refers to the extent to which an intervention programme is delivered in practice as intended in theory and design (Hollin, 1995). Waltz, Addis, Koerner, and Jacobsen (1993) suggest that assessing integrity involves two components: therapist adherence to the treatment protocol and therapist competence in delivering the treatment. It is clear that many treatments offered to both forensic patients and offenders have low levels of integrity (Bonta, Rugge, Scott, Bourgon, & Yessine, 2008), leading to moves towards standardised treatment manuals and protocols in an attempt to increase programme integrity. These can be easily translated into checklists of treatment adherence for completion by a clinician and/or patient, although assessing clinical competence is more difficult.

There are grounds to question the integrity of many of those interventions that are described as mindfulness-based but often without sufficient definition. An example of this is a mindfulness intervention reported by McMurran and Jinks (2012) in a study conducted in a secure psychiatric hospital in England for offenders who had been detained under mental health legislation. Participants were personality-disordered men on an assessment ward or who were new to treatment. The intervention was labelled 'self-awareness' and involved 'an experiential exercise, *based upon mindfulness techniques*, in which participants attend to sensations and emotions' (p. 47; emphasis added). Another example is from Suarez et al.'s (2014) prison trial which combines mindfulness with what they refer to as 'compassionate social communication', involving noticing others' behaviours, examining the accompanying feelings, making requests, and acknowledging the needs that have been met/unmet. No information is provided in either of these studies about the integrity of the mindfulness methods or information that might be used to assess this. The concern here is that these interventions may only be approximations of what might be expected in mindfulness training.

The second component of programme integrity concerns the quality of delivery. There are obvious issues around the competence and training of those who deliver mindfulness-based interventions (Shonin et al., 2014), as well as the way in which training occurs. Shonin et al. (2013), for example, note that developing proficiency in meditation and mindfulness practice can often take many years of focused training. None of the published studies of mindfulness-based interventions delivered in forensic mental health settings report the experience or background of treatment providers. Shonin et al. (2013) further note that the interventions that are used in prison settings range from just 10 days to 10 weeks. The low intensity of these interventions may significantly limit their effectiveness, particularly in light of Klainin-Yobas, Cho, and Creedy's (2012) meta-analysis of intervention outcomes for mindfulness-based therapies which reported that effect sizes were significantly associated with the length of intervention.

In summary, there would seem to be a need to develop methods that not only describe what it is that is actually being delivered in forensic mental health services when providers talk about providing mindfulness-based interventions, but also to consider how programme integrity might be routinely monitored.

Conclusion

The aim of this chapter was to provide an overview of how mindfulness-based techniques have been used in forensic mental health settings. It is suggested that a reasonably strong rationale exists for these methods to be used in pursuit of the core goal of risk management, although controlled outcome studies are needed to establish the extent to which mindfulness training does actually lead to meaningful behaviour change. A number of challenges to this type of evaluation are noted, not least of which are those related to the variable diversity and integrity of those treatments offered in forensic mental health that are loosely described as mindfulness-based. There are also significant challenges in determining the impact of those interventions that are delivered as part of a broader approach to treatment and risk management. The conclusion, however, is that the outcomes of mindfulness-based interventions when used with forensic mental health patients do need to be better documented if they are to become more established as part of standard treatment.

As a final note, it is worth raising the broader question of how mindfulness-based interventions sit within institutional efforts to treat or manage patients, often in settings where treatment is coerced. As Singh, Lancioni, Wahler, Winton, and Singh (2008) has argued 'the end point of mindfulness meditation is not in the alleviation of psychological and physical distress' (p. 10) but to gain insight into the nature of one's own mind. It is, in other words, a method by which enlightenment might be pursued, rather than something that might be used instrumentally to meet legal obligations or to reduce the risk of offending. Of course, the goals of forensic mental health services may well be compatible with broader goals relating to social and emotional well-being and it seems evident that greater levels of awareness and compassion are unlikely to be associated with chronic violence or offending. Nonetheless, there is a danger that the integrity of mindfulness-based treatment will be compromised in attempting to realise short-term service-oriented risk management goals. As Howells et al. (2010) comment, 'as utilised in psychological and psychiatric interventions, mindfulness has been largely severed from its fundamental roots and treated in relative isolation from the extensive, deeper and sophisticated philosophical, spiritual and psychological system which generated it' (p. 8). There is, then, a need to ensure that the very real benefits of these methods are not lost in a context in which the management of patients will always be a priority.

References

Amrod, J., & Hayes, S. C. (2013). ACT for the incarcerated. In R. C. Tafrate & D. Mitchell (Eds.), *Forensic CBT: A practitioner's guide* (pp. 377–390). Chichester: Wiley-Blackwell.

Andrews, D. A., & Bonta, J. (2010). *The psychology of criminal conduct* (5th ed.). Cincinnati, OH: Anderson.

Baer, R. (2003). Mindfulness training as a clinical intervention: A conceptual and empirical review. *Clinical Psychology: Science and Practice, 10*, 125–143.

Baumeister, R. F., Heatherton, T. F., & Tice, D. M. (1994). *Losing control: How and why people fail at self-regulation*. San Diego, CA: Academic.

Bonta, J., Rugge, T., Scott, T., Bourgon, G., & Yessine, A. K. (2008). Exploring the black box of community supervision. *Journal of Offender Rehabilitation, 47*, 248–270.

Chiesa, A., & Serretti, A. (2011). Mindfulness based cognitive therapy for psychiatric disorders: A systematic review and meta-analysis. *Psychiatry Research, 187*, 441–453.

Douglas, K. S., & Skeem, J. L. (2005). Violence risk assessment: Getting specific about being dynamic. *Psychology, Public Policy and Law, 11*, 347–383.

Drake, E. (2013). *Inventory of evidence-based and research-based programs for adult corrections*. Olympia: Washington State Institute for Public Policy.

Duggan, C. (2008). Focusing on treatment: The main interventions and their implications. In K. Soothill, P. Rogers, & M. Dolan (Eds.), *Handbook of forensic mental health* (pp. 505–524). Cullompton: Willan publishing.

Evershed, S., Tennant, A., Boomer, D., Rees, A., Barkham, M., & Watson, A. (2006). Practice-based outcomes of dialectical behaviour therapy (DBT) targeting anger and violence, with male forensic patients: A pragmatic and non-contemporaneous comparison. *Criminal Behaviour and Mental Health, 13*, 198–213.

Farrington, D. P., & Jolliffe, D. (2002). *A feasibility study into using a randomised controlled trial to evaluate treatment pilots at HMP Whitemoor* (Home Office Online Report 14/02). Home Office Research, Development and Statistics Directorate.

Fazel, S., & Danesh, J. (2002). Serious mental disorder in 23,000 prisoners: A systematic review of 62 surveys. *The Lancet, 359*, 545–550.

Fix, R. L., & Fix, S. T. (2013). The effects of mindfulness-based treatments for aggression: A critical review. *Aggression and Violent Behavior, 18*, 219–227.

Gilbody, S. M., House, A. O., & Sheldon, T. A. (2003). *Outcome measurement in psychiatry* (CRD Report 24). York: NHS Centre for Reviews in Dissemination.

Gillespie, S. M., Mitchell, I. J., Fisher, D., & Beech, A. R. (2012). Treating disturbed emotional regulation in sexual offenders: The potential applications of mindful self-regulation and controlled breathing techniques. *Aggression and Violent Behavior, 17*, 333–343.

Grossman, L. S., Haywood, T. W., Cavanaugh, J. L., Davis, J. M., & Lewis, D. A. (1995). State hospital patients with past arrests for violent crime. *Psychiatric Services, 46*, 790–795.

Gunter, T. D., Philibert, R., & Hollenbeck, N. (2009). Medical and psychiatric problems among men and women in a community corrections residential setting. *Behavioral Sciences and the Law, 27*, 695–711.

Hanson, R. K., & Harris, A. J. R. (2000). Where should we intervene? Dynamic predictors of sexual offense recidivism. *Criminal Justice and Behavior, 27*, 6–35.

Hofmann, S. G., Sawyer, A. T., Witt, A. A., & Oh, D. (2010). The effect of mindfulness-based therapy on anxiety and depression: A meta-analytic review. *Journal of Consulting and Clinical Psychology, 78*, 169–183.

Hogue, T. E., Jones, L., Talkes, K., & Tennant, A. (2007). The Peaks: A clinical service for those with dangerous and severe personality disorders. *Psychology, Crime and Law, 13*, 57–68.

Hollin, C. R. (1995). The meaning and implications of programme integrity. In J. McGuire (Ed.), *What works: Effective methods to reduce reoffending* (pp. 195–208). Chichester: Wiley.

Howells, K., & Day, A. (2002). Grasping the nettle: Treating and rehabilitating the violent offender. *Australian Psychologist, 37*, 222–228.

Howells, K., Tennant, A., Day, A., & Elmer, R. (2010). Mindfulness in forensic mental health: Does it have a role? *Mindfulness, 1*, 4–9.

Kabat-Zinn, J. (1990). *Full catastrophe living: Using the wisdom of your body and mind in everyday life*. New York: Delacorte.

Kangas, M. (2014). The evolution of mindfulness-based cognitive therapy. *Australian Psychologist, 49*, 280–282.

Klainin-Yobas, P., Cho, M. A., & Creedy, D. (2012). Efficacy of mindfulness-based interventions on depressive symptoms among people with mental disorders: A meta-analysis. *International Journal of Nursing Studies, 49*, 109–21.

Kuyken, W., Byford, S., Taylor, R. S., Watkins, E., Holden, E., White, K., et al. (2008). Mindfulness-based cognitive therapy to prevent relapse in recurrent depression. *Journal of Consulting and Clinical Psychology, 76*, 966–978.

Linehan, M. M. (1993). *Cognitive-behavioral treatment of borderline personality disorder*. New York: Guilford.

McGuire, J. (2008). A review of effective interventions for reducing aggression and violence. *Philosophical Transactions of the Royal Society Bulletin, B,* 1–21.

McMurran, M., & Jinks, M. (2012). Making your emotions work for you: A pilot brief intervention for alexithymia with personality-disordered offenders. *Personality and Mental Health, 6*, 45–49.

Metcalf, C. A., & Dimidjian, S. (2014). Extensions and mechanisms of mindfulness-based cognitive therapy: A review of the evidence. *Australian Psychologist, 49*, 271–279.

Mullen, P. (2000). Forensic mental health. *British Journal of Psychiatry, 176*, 307–311.

National Collaborating Centre for Mental Health. (2009). *Antisocial personality disorder. Treatment, management and preventio*n (Clinical guideline; no. 77). London: National Institute for Health and Clinical Excellence (NICE).

Nee, C., & Farman, S. (2005). Female prisoners with borderline personality disorder: Some promising treatment developments. *Criminal Behaviour and Mental Health, 15*, 2–16.

Nestor, P. G., Haycock, J., Doiron, S., Kelly, J., & Kelly, D. (1995). Lethal violence and psychosis. *Bulletin of the American Academy of Psychiatry and Law, 23*, 331–341.

Nolen-Hoeksema, S. (1991). Responses to depression and their effects on the duration of depressive episodes. *Journal of Abnormal Psychology, 100*, 569–582.

Novaco, R. W. (2011). Anger dysregulation: Driver of violent offending. *Journal of Forensic Psychiatry & Psychology, 22*, 650–668.

Perich, T., Manicavasagar, V., Mitchell, P. B., & Ball, J. R. (2013). The association between meditation practice and treatment outcome in mindfulness-based cognitive therapy for bipolar disorder. *Behaviour Research and Therapy, 51*, 338–343.

Petrik, A. M., & Cronin, M. J. (2014). Defining and measuring mechanisms of change in psychological therapies: The path not taken. *Australian Psychologist, 49*, 283–286.

Polaschek, D. L. L. (2006). Violent offender programmes: Concept, theory and practice. In C. R. Hollin & E. J. Palmer (Eds.), *Offending behaviour programmes: Development, application and controversies*. Chichester: Wiley.

Polaschek, D., & Collie, R. (2004). Rehabilitating serious violent adult offenders: An empirical and theoretical stocktake. *Psychology, Crime and Law, 10*, 321–334.

Samuelson, M., Carmody, J., Kabat-Zinn, J., & Bratt, M. A. (2007). Mindfulness-based stress reduction in Massachusetts correctional facilities. *The Prison Journal, 87*, 254–268.

Shonin, E., Van Gordon, W., & Griffiths, M. D. (2014, March–April). Mindfulness meditation in American correctional facilities: A 'What Works' approach to reducing reoffending. *Corrections Today*, pp. 48–52.

Shonin, E., Van Gordon, W., Slade, K., & Griffiths, M. D. (2013). Mindfulness and other Buddhist-derived interventions in correctional settings: A systematic review. *Aggression and Violent Behavior, 18*, 365–372.

Singh, N. N., Lancionia, G. E., Wahler, R. G., Winton, A. S. W., & Singh, J. (2008). Mindfulness approaches in Cognitive Behavior Therapy. *Behavioural and Cognitive Psychotherapy, 36*, 1–10.

Singh, N. N., Lancioni, G. E., Winton, A. S. W., Adkins, A. D., Wahler, R. G., Sabaawi, M., et al. (2007). Individuals with mental illness can control their aggressive behaviour through mindfulness training. *Behavior Modification, 31*, 313–328.

Singh, N. N., Lancioni, G. E., Winton, A. S. W., Singh, A. N., & Adkins, A. D. (2011). Can adult offenders with intellectual disabilities use mindfulness-based procedures to control their deviant sexual arousal? *Forensic Research in Offenders with Intellectual & Developmental Disabilities, 2*, 165–179.

Singh, N. N., Lancioni, G. E., Winton, A. S. W., Singh, A. N., Adkins, A. D., & Singh, J. (2008). Clinical and benefit-cost outcomes of teaching a mindfulness-based procedure to adult offenders with intellectual disabilities. *Behavior Modification, 32*, 622–637.

Skeem, J., Manchak, S., & Peterson, J. (2011). Correctional policy for offenders with mental disorder: Creating a new paradigm for recidivism reduction. *Law and Human Behavior, 35*, 110–126.

Soothill, K. (2008). Introduction. In K. Soothill, P. Rogers, & M. Dolan (Eds.), *Handbook of forensic mental health* (pp. 85–88). Cullompton: Willan publishing.

Soothill, K., Rogers, P., & Dolan, M. (2008). *Handbook of forensic mental health*. Cullompton: Willan publishing.

Steadman, H. J., Osher, F. C., Robbins, P. C., Case, B., & Samuels, S. (2009). Prevalence of serious mental illness among jail inmates. *Psychiatric Services, 60*, 761–765.

Suarez, A., Dug Y. L., Rowe, C., Alex, A. G., Murowchick, E., & Linn, P. L. (2014). Freedom project: Nonviolent communication and mindfulness training in prison. *Sage Open, 4*. doi:10.1177/2158244013516154.

Swanson, J. W., Borum, R., & Swartz, M. S. (1996). Psychotic symptoms and disorders and the risk of violent behaviour in the community. *Criminal Behaviour and Mental Health, 6*, 309–329.

Taylor, P. J., & Gunn, J. (2008). Diagnosis, medical models and formulations. In K. Soothill, P. Rogers, & M. Dolan (Eds.), *Handbook of forensic mental health* (pp. 227–243). Cullompton: Willan Publishing.

Teasdale, J. D. (1999). Metacognition, mindfulness and the modification of mood disorders. *Clinical Psychology and Psychotherapy, 6*, 146–155.

Teasdale, J. D., Segal, Z. V., & Williams, J. M. G. (2003). Mindfulness training and problem formulation. *Clinical Psychology: Science and Practice, 10*, 157–160.

Tennant, A. (2010). Dialectical behaviour therapy targeting violent behaviour in a male forensic in-patient setting. In A. Tennant & K. Howells (Eds.), *Using time, not doing time: Practitioner perspectives on personality disorder and risk*. Chichester: Wiley.

Tennant, A., & Howells, K. (Eds.). (2010). *Using time, not doing time: Practitioner perspectives on personality disorder and risk*. Chichester: Wiley.

Tolan, P. (2007). Understanding violence. In D. J. Flannery, A. T. Vazsonyi, & I. D. Waldman (Eds.), *The Cambridge handbook of violent behavior and aggression* (pp. 5–18). New York: Cambridge University Press.

Ullrich, S., Keers, R., & Coid, J. W. (2014). Delusions, anger, and serious violence: New findings from the MacArthur violence risk assessment study. *Schizophrenia Bulletin, 40*, 1174–1181. doi:10.1093/schbul/sbt126.

Waltz, J., Addis, M. E., Koerner, K., & Jacobsen, N. S. (1993). Testing the integrity of a psychotherapy protocol: Assessment of adherence and competence. *Journal of Consulting and Clinical Psychology, 61*, 620–30.

Woldgabreal, Y., Day, A., & Ward, T. (2014). The community-based supervision of offenders from a positive psychology perspective. *Aggression and Violent Behavior, 19*, 32–41.

Wright, S., Day, A., & Howells, K. (2009). Mindfulness and the treatment of anger problems. *Aggression and Violent Behavior, 14*, 396–401.

Zamble, E., & Quinsey, V. L. (2001). *The criminal recidivism process*. London: Cambridge University Press.

Chapter 16
Mindfulness and Work-Related Well-Being

Maryanna D. Klatt, Emaline Wise, and Morgan Fish

Introduction to Workplace Stress and Wellness

As employees in first world nations are spending more and more time at work, the impact of stress experienced by employees, no matter what its etiology, has become a central topic of concern voiced at the workplace. Research data supports the hypothesis that chronic stress in society is a contributing factor to the resulting behaviors (including addiction) and physiology that have accelerated the increase in chronic disease. A recent study done by MetLife found that 20 % of those who responded to a survey on stress and work had taken time off due to a stress-related illness in the past 12 months (Crawford, 2014). Even more importantly, 63 % of the respondents to the survey said they "would welcome help and advice from their employer on how to improve their health and well-being" (Crawford, 2014). For employees who are in a delicate balance of home/work obligations, navigating a path out of the chronic stress cycle can be extremely difficult, and employers who miss an opportunity to help employees navigate this cycle may be short-sighted. Low-cost educational mind-body stress reduction programs could be of great assistance in managing this epidemic.

M.D. Klatt, Ph.D. (✉)
The Ohio State University College of Medicine, Suite 250 Northwood-High Building # 261, 2231 North High Street, Columbus, OH, 43201, USA
e-mail: Maryanna.Klatt@osumc.edu

E. Wise, B.S.
Biomedical Science, College of Medicine, The Ohio State University, Columbus, OH, 43201, USA

M. Fish, B.S.B.A.
Economics, Max M. Fisher College of Business, The Ohio State University, Columbus, OH, 43201, USA

E. Shonin et al. (eds.), *Mindfulness and Buddhist-Derived Approaches in Mental Health and Addiction*, Advances in Mental Health and Addiction,
DOI 10.1007/978-3-319-22255-4_16

Financially, decreasing employee stress-related illness is beneficial for employees and employers alike. One study placed the estimated annual cost of stress-related conditions on the American economy at $300 billion, due to absenteeism, turnover, decreased productivity, and other costs (Rosch, 2001). To make this more relevant, this staggering figure compares to about 16 % of the US federal budget and about 3 % of the GDP during the year the estimate was made (Clinton, 2000; World Bank, 2014). Prudent employers are looking for wellness programs to keep employees healthy and insurance costs down, as they purchase much of American health care, spending approximately $13,000 per employee per year on direct and indirect healthcare costs. Interruption of an individual's stress response has implied health consequences, as it has been shown that stress impacts wound healing, immune status, susceptibility to infectious disease, and, among other things, the rate of tumor cell growth (Glaser et al. 1999; Glaser, Sheridan, Malarkey, MacCallum, & Kiecolt-Glaser, 2000; Glaser et al., 2001, 2005; Kiecolt-Glaser & Glaser, 1988, 1999; Kiecolt-Glaser et al., 1995). Chronic conditions such as depression, anxiety, obesity, arthritis, and back/neck pain have been found to be especially linked to productivity loss, with these figures remaining stable across professions, from executives to laborers (Loeppke et al., 2009). In a study of middle-hierarchy managers, who are especially susceptible to high levels of work-related stress, significant improvements in work-related stress, job satisfaction, psychological distress, and employer-related job performance were found and maintained at follow-up of Meditation Awareness Training (Shonin, Van Gordon, Dunn, Singh, & Griffiths, 2014). These findings suggest that MBI's may be useful in combatting some of the serious consequences of workplace stress, even in the most severe cases.

A cultural tipping point has arrived, as the American public has become open to Complementary and Alternative Medicine (CAM) approaches in an unprecedented way, but these approaches must be evidence-based and generalizable to busy adults in order to reap the health benefits. Programs that are pragmatic and are supported at the worksite, via funding, space designations, and with protected time for the mind/body intervention, seem to be the best candidates for success. An example of how powerful stress reduction programs can be in combating chronic disease is highlighted by a recent study that utilized a stress reduction intervention meant for management of emotional factors to prevent recurrent cardiovascular disease (CVD). This intervention showed that the stress reduction group had a 41 % lower rate of fatal and nonfatal first recurrent CVD events, in addition to showing that there was a strong dose–response effect between intervention group attendance and outcome (Gulliksson et al., 2011). Feasible interventions that disrupt a chronic stress response could have huge public health ramifications, including reductions in addictive behaviors, as these are often utilized to cope with stress. The earlier a resiliency technique is learned to combat stress, the greater its potential health impact, both for the health status of the individual and for decreasing escalating healthcare costs.

Mind-Body at Work

Americans already use CAM approaches to manage symptoms of underlying diseases in conjunction with conventional western medicine, as the 2007 National Health Interview Survey showed that more than 38 % of Americans had used some form of CAM in the previous 12 months (Nahin et al., 2009). CAM research evidence has had a huge impact on the public at large. Scientific knowledge about effective workplace mind-body approaches has been critically important in changing behaviors that may impact health care expenditures, and even more importantly, the health and wellness of the individual employee (NIH, 2011).

Mindfulness-Based Stress Reduction

Mind-body approaches, such as Mindfulness-Based Stress Reduction (MBSR), have been shown to modulate stress reactivity. MBSR, traditionally an 8-week, 26-h intervention, is a mind-body approach developed by Jon Kabat-Zinn to reduce pain and stress through mindfulness meditation (Kabat-Zinn, 1982, 2003). More than 30 years of empirical research illustrates the health benefits of this valuable approach. Both controlled and uncontrolled studies of MBSR show effect sizes of approximately 0.5 ($p<0.0001$) with a homogeneity of distribution (Grossman, Niemann, Schmidt, & Walach, 2004). Improvements have been noted in standardized mental health measures including quality of life scales, depression, anxiety, coping style, social functioning, and other affective dimensions of disability, all of which affect one's ability to function (Grossman et al., 2004; Reibel et al., 2001). MBSR is a structured group mind-body program that utilizes mindfulness meditation to help manage stress and to retrain the mind to change its usual responses to stressful situations. Mindfulness is characterized by nonjudgmental, sustained moment-to-moment awareness of physical sensations, perceptions, affective states, thoughts, and imagery. It involves sustained focus of mental phenomena, which arise during waking consciousness. As a form of receptive awareness, mindfulness may create an interval of time where one is able to view one's mental landscape, including one's behavioral options, rather than just reacting to interpersonal events.

The Buddhist tradition of mindfulness is a practice that can aptly be applied in the workplace, as people are focused on pragmatic solutions to pragmatic problems. Kabat-Zinn's conception of vipassana meditation, derived from Burmese Buddhism, is a nonreactive awareness of one's affective response to external events and is an essential key to changing one's internal experience of stress in MBSR. Buddhism teaches followers to move past difficult situations via acceptance in order to experience life as it unfolds, which is widely applicable to the workplace setting as much of our waking moments are spent at work. Mindfulness is an avenue that may encourage individuals to end the cycle of negativity with difficult coworkers and instead foster healthy working relationships. High-stress professions (such as trauma responders) that experience high rates of burnout and depression can potentially be overcome by looking past one's own troubles and instead focusing on encouraging others (Metcalf & Hateley, 2001). Overall, the Buddhist tradition suggests a strategy of "Mind over Matter," which can be applied by using mindfulness interventions to reframe stressful situations at work. These stressful situations may, or may not, be beyond the employee's scope of control, but inviting awareness into one's conscious experience allows an individual to discern the difference.

MBSR has been found useful for a variety of symptoms and illnesses including anxiety, binge-eating disorders, depression, fibromyalgia, cancer, coronary artery disease, chronic pain, psoriasis, and psychiatric disorders, and most recently, attention and brain density (Grossman et al., 2004; Hölzel et al., 2010; Jha et al., 2007). Physical and biological measures were less frequently assessed in the early mindfulness studies, yet improvements were noted in pain control, functional quality of life, psoriatic skin disease, and immune function (Grossman et al., 2004; Davidson et al., 2003). However, those who have the most to benefit from MBSR, stressed individuals who have yet to experience physical symptoms, are deterred by the required time commitment, which negatively influences the applicability of this type of intervention for many working adults.

Workplace Mindfulness

Scientific research in the applicability of workplace mindfulness programming has exploded in the last 5–10 years. It began in 2000 with two papers by Langer and Moldoveanu detailing prior mindfulness research and its application in several settings, including the workplace (Langer & Moldoveanu, 2000a, 2000b). This was soon followed by Riskin's paper on the potential benefits of mindfulness for lawyers and law students (Riskin, 2002). A 2003 study by Richard Davidson et al. implemented MBSR in a high-tech company, yielding biometric differences in response to flu immunization. Participants in the MBSR group had significant increases in antibody titers to the flu vaccine compared to those in the wait-list control group (Davidson et al., 2003). This was a groundbreaking study in two ways: (1) it showed that the worksite was a possible location for MBSR program delivery and (2) it showed evidence-based support of mindfulness meditation's effect on brain and immune function.

The pragmatic applicability of mindfulness to the stress that one associates with work makes the workplace a ripe environment to introduce mindfulness concepts. After a study with employees from The Dow Chemical Company, Aikens et al. (2014) indicated that mindfulness can do more than facilitate stress reduction and coping in the workplace; it can also be used as a tool to increase positive organizational behavior. Increasing the degree to which overall performance can be improved through measurable psychological and administrative advances is advantageous to any company or business as a whole. These advances can be achieved through the implementation of mindfulness in workplace interventions that can help real people apply these concepts toward achieving the life that they want to live. Worksite location of a stress reduction intervention makes sense from both the employer and employee perspective; employers save on productivity and potentially health care costs, while offering the program on-site increases convenience for the employee and likelihood of attendance, which has been shown to impact outcome.

Another pragmatic mindfulness intervention (that is significantly less time intensive) has been successfully implemented with employees in busy intensive care units, yielding 40 % reduction in Salivary α-amylase, reflecting decreased activation of the sympathetic nervous system. Called *Mindfulness in Motion*, (Duchemin, Steinberg, Marks, Vanover, & Klatt, 2015) this program utilizes music for relaxation alongside increased yoga movement as compared to traditional MBSR and has been very well received by a variety of working populations (Duchemin et al., 2015; Malarkey, Jarjoura, & Klatt, 2013).

Research and Demonstrated Outcomes

The amount of mindfulness research being published has increased more than 900 % in the past 10 years (Black, 2014). In just a few decades of mindfulness research, researchers have succeeded in empirically demonstrating that mindfulness, while derived from Buddhism, transcends religion, spirituality, and/or cultural beliefs. The development of various mindfulness scales has also aided the progression of research in this area; scales such as the Kentucky Inventory of Mindfulness Skills (KIMS) (Baer, Smith, & Allen, 2004), Toronto Mindfulness Scale (TMS) (Lau et al., 2006), Cognitive and Affective Mindfulness Scale (CAMS) (Feldman, Hayes, Kumar, Greeson, & Laurenceau, 2007), Five Facet Mindfulness Questionnaire (FFMQ) (Baer, Smith, Hopkins, Krietemeyer, & Toney, 2006), Freiburg Mindfulness Inventory (FMI) (Buchheld, Grossman, & Walach, 2001), and the Philadelphia Mindfulness Scale (PHLMS) (Cardaciotto, Herbert, Forman, Moitra, & Farrow, 2008) have helped increase efficiency in mindfulness research while supporting the concept of mindfulness as scientific and non-mystical (Black, 2010). Each of these scales highlights subtle nuances within mindfulness practice (for example, an increased sense of curiosity and decentering as highlighted in the Toronto Mindfulness Scale).

Exploring the concept of mindfulness as a practice, as well as an outcome, has allowed researchers to supplement the general focus of mindfulness research with various other outcomes of interest. Some of these other scales may be chosen specifically for the population participating in the research study (e.g., scales measuring burnout for populations dealing with victims of trauma or compassion fatigue for those in helping professions), while other outcomes may be applicable across various professions/worksites (e.g., inflammatory biomarkers and/or scales measuring perceived stress).

Health-Related Outcomes

Health and work-life have the potential for a synergistic and antagonistic relationship with each other. When in good health, an individual's productivity at work or job satisfaction might be higher, and vice versa; wellness in one area of an individual's life is beneficial for other areas of life as well. However, when job satisfaction is low, health can suffer/trigger a difficult cycle of stress and illness, including potentially addictive behaviors to cope with either stress or illness. Mindfulness in the workplace, modified for the modern-day employee (while recognizing its traditional Buddhist roots), could provide individuals with tools to prevent the cycle of stress from perpetuating. It can be a means to stop the assumption that our individual perceptions are reality. As discussed below, various health outcomes have been examined to explore the impact of mindfulness programs in the workplace.

Cardiovascular Health

Factors involved in the etiology of cardiovascular disease have been examined in regard to mindfulness. Risk factors for cardiovascular disease include psychosocial conditions, lifestyle habits such as smoking, and preexisting health conditions such as diabetes and hypertension (Younge, Gotink, Baena, Roos-Hesselink, & Hunink, 2014). Correspondingly, mindfulness has demonstrated reductions in conditions related to these factors including anxiety, stress, and depression (Grossman et al., 2004). In one study, a group of individuals reporting high levels of stress participated in an MBSR program and showed significant decreases in overall systolic and diastolic blood pressure after 8 weeks (Nyklíček, Mommersteeg, Van Beugen, Ramakers, & Van Boxtel, 2013). Smoking cessation was also more successful when combined with mindfulness training. These results were sustainable even 17 weeks after the end of mindfulness training (Brewer et al., 2011). Researchers currently believe this is in part due to mindfulness training's emphasis on controlling cravings versus avoiding cues, which has been the focus of traditional smoking cessation programs (Brewer et al., 2011).

Biomarkers

Changes in biomarkers related to stress and immune function can indicate the effectiveness of a workplace mindfulness intervention. Interleukin 6 (IL-6), tumor necrosis factor alpha (TNF-α), C-reactive protein (CRP), and cortisol are immunological and neuroendocrine biomarkers that are commonly used. There are various methods available for collecting information on biomarkers and inflammation in the body, including drawing small samples of blood, collecting saliva through oral swabs, and, to examine cortisol, collecting hair samples.

CRP, a protein made by the liver, indicates inflammation somewhere in the body. A recent study by Malarkey et al. (2013) conducted *Mindfulness in Motion* at the workplace for university faculty and staff employees with elevated CRP levels. Participants significantly benefited from the 8-week mindfulness intervention designed specifically for the workplace, and nonobese subjects (BMI < 30) experienced a clinically significant decrease in CRP (Malarkey et al., 2013). Trait mindfulness has been associated with lower levels of IL-6, a pro-inflammatory cytokine that is secreted by T cells and macrophages to promote an immune response in healthy adults. Two subscales of the Five Facet Mindfulness Questionnaire, *observing* and *nonreacting*, were implicated in this change. However, increased *observing* was only correlated with decreased IL-6 when *nonreacting* was also high (Tomfohr, Pung, Mills, & Edwards, 2014). TNF-α is an adipokine mainly secreted by macrophages that is implicated in systemic inflammation as well as cell differentiation and apoptosis. Rosenkranz et al. (2013) showed that an MBSR intervention reduced TNF-α levels in participants significantly more than an active control program.

Cortisol, a steroid hormone released during the stress response, can also be affected by mindfulness practice. One study showed that participants in a 3-month meditation program demonstrated decreased P.M. cortisol levels as mindfulness increased (Jacobs et al., 2013). More conclusive work on cortisol has been done with cancer survivors and caregivers, but more data is needed on the healthy, working population (Lengacher, Kip, & Barta, 2013).

As additional research emerges, especially using randomized, controlled trials (RCTs), there is a strengthened indication that mindfulness can affect immune and stress response pathways in the body. Employers may be more likely to adopt evidenced-based programs where the research has both biologic and work-related outcomes. Pragmatic workplace mindfulness interventions could be utilized for both decreasing inflammation and increasing levels of mindfulness and work engagement in employee populations. Scientific research identifying changes in biomarkers in response to worksite mindfulness programming is building as employers become open to the idea of trying mind/body interventions at the workplace to help their employees with stresses, inside and out of work.

Quality of Life

Quality of life may also increase as a result of participation in a workplace mindfulness intervention. The World Health Organization (WHO) defines quality of life as the following:

> Quality of Life [is] individuals' perception of their position in life in the context of the culture and value systems in which they live and in relation to their goals, expectations, standards and concerns. It is a broad ranging concept affected in a complex way by the person's physical health, psychological state, level of independence, social relationships, personal beliefs and their relationship to salient features of their environment. (WHO, 1997)

There may be variations in the interpretation and quantification of quality of life, but it is commonly described in a similar fashion to the WHO's definition. Some scales used to quantify quality of life through self-report are the Quality of Life Scale (QOLS) (Burckhardt & Anderson, 2003), Professional Quality of Life Scale (ProQOL) (Stamm, 2005), and World Health Organization Quality of Life (WHOQOL)-BREF (Skevington, Lotfy, O'Connell, & WHOQOL Group, 2004). Questions on these scales often speak to the user's satisfaction with various aspects of their lives, including home, health, work, relationships, self-understanding, expression, socializing, and independence. Completion of these scales allows for a quantification of quality of life that allows for quantitative analysis and comparison across studies. However, qualitative research involving focus groups and participant interviews is also a common technique used to document changes in quality of life, yet they are often supplemented with data from validated and reliable scales.

An example of use of such a scale was done with Mayo Clinic employees. A yoga-based program that incorporated mindfulness and meditation practice found that linear analog self-assessment (LASA) scores among Mayo Clinic employees increased significantly over the course of 6 weeks (Thomley, Ray, Cha, & Bauer, 2011). Increased LASA scores indicated that participants were experiencing increased physical, emotional, and spiritual well-being. Quantitative values describing a qualitative construct such as quality of life may appeal to an employer's sensibility when investigating the efficacy of programs for employees. And, one could certainly argue that such outcomes may be correlated with less need for coping mechanisms that lead to addictive ways of dealing with uncontrollable feelings of stress.

Stress

Mindfulness does in fact contribute to employees' perceptions of stress and their abilities to cope with stressors in their lives. A widely used measure of perceived stress amongst researchers is the Perceived Stress Scale (PSS), but the Stress Appraisal Measure (SAM) and Impact of Event Scale (IES) are also popular (Andreou et al., 2011). These scales incorporate questions and statements such as "In the last month, how often have you found that you could not cope with all the things that you had to do?"; "How threatening is this situation?"; and "I got waves or pangs of intense or deep feelings about [a particular event]," respectively (Cohen, Kamarck, & Mermelstein, 1983; Peacock & Wong, 1990; Horowitz, Wilner, & Alvarez, 1979). These questions are a starting point for employees to begin to recognize the source of what they experience as "stress."

MBSR was originally created with the purpose of training individuals to practice yoga and meditation to increase their health and decrease their stress (Brantley, 2005). Since then, the original program has been modified and adapted for various companies and populations and to address a variety of concerns, including stress, pain, illness, and disease (Brantley, 2005). One example of this is "Mindfulness at Work," a 12-week stress management program. Participants in Mindfulness at Work showed significant decreases in Perceived Stress Scale (PSS) scores (Wolever et al., 2012). The results of this program are particularly of interest, because employees who participated in the class online and those who participated in-person achieved nearly identical results (Wolever et al., 2012). This supports the effectiveness of an online mindfulness intervention for the workplace, which, for many businesses and employees, could be more feasible than an extensive class conducted outside the workday hours.

Sleep Quality

Sleep can have both direct and indirect effects on work engagement and performance. Self-report instruments such as the Pittsburgh Sleep Quality Index (PSQI) can be helpful in understanding an individual's perception of his or her sleep habits and quality of sleep. This instrument categorizes questions into subcategories of sleep quality, including sleep latency, sleep duration, sleep disturbances, day dysfunction due to sleepiness, habitual sleep efficiency, use of sleep medication, and subjective sleep quality (Buysse, Reynolds, Monk, Berman, & Kupfer, 1989). Researchers may also employ clinical tests such as polysomnography (PSG) (Krystal & Edinger, 2008). Most useful in sleep research may be the combination of self-report measures such as PSQI and qualitative information obtained from a sleep diary along with results from a PSG.

Results from previous research show that poor sleep quality can drastically affect employees' work. Kessler et al. (2011) found that work-related insomnia, which correlates to decreased productivity, costs US businesses approximately $63.2 billion each year. An inability to detach from work can increase insomnia, which prevents employees from experiencing the restorative effects of a good night's sleep (Hülsheger et al., 2014). Mindfulness in the workplace can facilitate recovery from work stressors and help prevent burnout by increasing psychological detachment after work as well as encouraging sleep quality (Hülsheger et al., 2014). A restful night of sleep may be the most valuable outcome experienced by participants in a worksite mindfulness program.

Work-Specific Outcomes

Significant improvements in work-related outcomes are critical in developing MBIs for the workplace. Successful demonstration of positive changes in absenteeism and/or productivity creates a much higher incentive (and perhaps more tangible result) for employers to support the implementation and sustainability of any MBI in the workplace. The prevalence of chronic disease has increased 25 % in working-age adults in the past 10 years, a startling change that increases the overall number of sick days and time on disability (Hoffman & Schwartz, 2008). A Rand Report published in 2013, established to investigate workplace wellness programs, emphasized that an earlier onset of chronic disease contributes to the cost of chronic disease through absence from work and decreased productivity and performance at work due to illness (Mattke et al., 2013). Stress, therefore, is a multi-headed beast, affecting physical health, work, mental well-being, and economics. Prioritizing stress reduction at work via MBIs could, in other words, have an impact throughout the infrastructure of society and business, from the organizational level to the individual. Identifying sources of stress through an MBI delivered at the worksite may be a first step in accomplishing this.

Absenteeism and Mental Health

When employees are suffering from stress, anxiety, or depression, their work tends to suffer as well. A study by McCraty, Atkinson, and Tomasino (2003) shows that these employees struggling with mental health issues take 10 more days of sick leave than their healthy coworkers. This places a heavy burden on both employers, who suffer from a loss of productivity, and employees, who fall farther behind in their work the more often they are absent. Mindfulness can be a mediator in this cycle. MBIs are correlated positively with sleep quality, which is also strongly linked to absenteeism (Winbush, Gross, & Kreitzer, 2007). A study by Godet-Cayré et al. (2006) shows that people who suffer from severe sleep disturbances are absent for longer stretches of time and are absent twice as frequently as those with better sleep hygiene.

Presenteeism

A factor that rarely enters into discussions on worksite wellness is presenteeism. This refers to the concept that employees who are stressed or sick, even though they come to work, experience a decline in productivity and in the quality of the work they are able to accomplish. Research shows that a loss of productivity due to presenteeism is 2.3 times more costly than medical costs for those who are absent (Loeppke et al., 2009). One study shows that in a breakdown of annual health costs for an employee of Dow Chemical Company, only \$2278 went directly to health care; \$661 was lost to absenteeism versus a staggering \$6721 to work impairment as a result of presenteeism (Collins et al., 2005). The demands made of an employee who, while still coming to work, is too stressed or sick to do their job can create even more stress for the workplace. The Rand Report made the following overall conclusions concerning implementation of worksite wellness programs:

> Our own review of the most recent scientific literature evaluating the impact of workplace wellness programs on health-related behavior and medical cost outcomes identified 33 peer-reviewed publications that met our standards for methodological rigor. We found, consistent with previous reviews, evidence for positive effects on diet, exercise, smoking, alcohol use, physiologic markers, and health care costs, but limited evidence for effects on absenteeism and mental health. We could not conclusively determine whether or not program intensity was positively correlated with impact. (Mattke et al., 2013)

Before implementing a program at the worksite, it is important to explore what facets would make it most valuable to both employee and employer. A pre-assessment of the stresses of the particular worksite culture is recommended (Klatt, Steinberg, & Duchemin, 2015), but there are general guidelines to successful implementation of worksite wellness programs. Based on an investigation into 10 different companies with successful worksite wellness programs, Berry, Mirabito, and Baun (2010) proposed 6 commonalities between the programs that they thought exemplified success of worksite wellness programming. These commonalities included multilevel leadership and cooperation, alignment with each business's identity, comprehensive, relevant, and engaging program material, ease of accessibility, partnerships with internal and external entities, and effective communication between administration and workers about the mission or importance of the program.

Mindfulness Applied in the Working World

The deleterious effects of chronically high-stress work environments have been investigated, but interventions to mediate this stress have been more recent as the impact of stress on personal physical and mental health has become more clearly established (Duchemin et al., 2015; Klatt et al., 2015; Wolever et al., 2012). Effects of chronically high-stress work environments also extend to the institutions that have to incur the costs of dealing with employee absenteeism and high turnover of expert personnel, such as highly trained nurses (Li & Jones, 2013). Interventions at the level of the organization (including mindfulness interventions) have been effective at reducing stress for personnel in various work environments, such as fire fighters, police officers, and prison guards (Chopko & Schwartz, 2009; Oginska-Bulik, 2005; Williams, Ciarrochi, & Deane, 2010). But the actuality and severity of the situation for nurses in particular have been recognized by many as shown by the number of publications on the topic of nursing stress in recent years (Bazarko, Cate, Azocar, & Kreitzer, 2013; Foureur et al., 2013; Hulsheger et al., 2013; McGibbon, Peter, & Gallop, 2010; Moody et al., 2013; Orly, Rivka, Rivka, & Dorit, 2012; Pipe et al., 2009; Shapiro, Astin, Bishop, & Cordova, 2005; Smith et al., 2011). However, there are very few reports of pragmatic MBI's that have been successfully implemented during the workday, on-site, as part of an institutional initiative to combat stress and its impact in an attempt to transform organizational culture.

Nurses

Mindfulness has a history of effectiveness for health care professionals. An early randomized trial indicated that health care professionals who participate in MBSR benefited from decreases in perceived stress, job burnout, and distress, while nurse participants increased in self-compassion and satisfaction with life (Shapiro et al.,

2005). Researchers in this study believed that, "*stress may harm professional effectiveness: It decreases attention, reduces concentration, impinges on decision-making skills, and reduces providers' abilities to establish strong relationships with patients*" (Shapiro et al., 2005). Nurses, who have cited fiscal responsibilities, inadequate human resources, emotional distress, competing priorities, burden of responsibility, negotiating hierarchical power, and engaging in bodily care as some of their workplace stressors, have been the subject of many studies on stress and coping in the workplace (McGibbon et al., 2010; Udod & Care, 2013). Cognitive-behavioral interventions have demonstrated a positive impact on nurses' sense of coherence, vigor, perceived stress, and fatigue (Orly et al., 2012). Mindfulness-based interventions in particular have exhibited an ability to provide nurses with the tools they require to be more satisfied with their work, worry less about what they are not able to accomplish during the work day, and lessen the amount of catastrophizing they do at home or work (Fortney, Luchterhand, Zakletskaia, Zgierska, & Rakel, 2013). This indicates that the completion of a cognitive-behavioral intervention may provide nurses with techniques to increase their coping skills, which could prevent burnout and compassion fatigue.

In a very recent study (Duchemin et al., 2015), utilizing the mindfulness intervention, *Mindfulness in Motion*, designed specifically for the workplace, surgical intensive care unit (SICU) personnel ($n=32$), was randomized to the MBI ($n=16$) or a wait-list control group ($n=16$). The 8-week program included mindfulness, gentle yoga, and music. The yoga movement was emphasized in the protocol to facilitate a quieting of the mind. The music was included for participants to associate the relaxed state experienced in the group session with their individual practice (the same music was included in the daily practice recordings). ICUs represent a high-stress work environment where personnel experience chronic exposure to catastrophic situations as they care for seriously injured/ill patients. Despite high levels of work-related stress, few interventions have been developed and delivered on-site for such environments. The intervention was delivered on-site in the ICU, during work hours, with participants receiving time release (institutional coverage) to attend sessions.

The intervention was well received with a 97 % retention rate. Work satisfaction and resiliency increase significantly in the intervention group, compared to the control group, while participant respiration rates decrease significantly pre–post in 6/8 of the weekly sessions. Participants valued institutional support, relaxing music, and the CD as pivotal to program success. This provides evidence that a pragmatic MBI is feasible, well accepted, and beneficial and can be effectively implemented in a chronically high-stress work environment (Duchemin et al., 2015; Klatt et al., 2015). Psychological and biological markers of stress were measured 1 week before and 1 week after the intervention. The mindfulness intervention was delivered on the unit, in a conference room, with nursing coverage provided by the hospital. Nurses did not need to take time off work to participate in *Mindfulness in Motion* and expressed that they felt supported by their employer. The large hospital employer had sought out a worksite wellness program for employees to increase their sense of well-being at work, recognizing the high-stress environment of an intensive care unit. Salivary α-amylase levels, an index of sympathetic activation, were significantly decreased by 40 %. Most significant was that there was a positive correlation between reductions in salivary α-amylase levels and burnout scores. These data suggest that this type of intervention could not only decrease reactivity to stress but also decrease the risk of burnout, which has been cited as a precursor to addictive behavior (Montero-Marín & García-Campayo, 2010). The hospital recognized that the high-stress nature of working in an intensive care unit required an intervention to provide employees additional tools to navigate such stresses.

Physicians

Physicians have been shown to benefit from mindfulness interventions as well. A study by Krasner et al. (2009) showed that primary care physicians who participated in a mindful communication program experienced a stronger sense of personal well-being and improvements in empathy, a step toward practicing patient-centered care, a desired focus of their work. More recent research confirmed that mindfulness is an evidence-based innovation that can improve both healthcare professionals' well-being, job burnout, depression, anxiety, and stress, while increasing patient-centered communication and satisfaction (Beach et al., 2013; Fortney et al., 2013). Programs for physicians are most effective if they include an opportunity for individuals to share and discuss professional stories, learn mindfulness skills in the context of patient care, and provide time for personal reflection and growth (Beckman et al., 2012). Mindfulness is an educational intervention of internal change appropriate for both patient and provider, as it can improve both the care process (by offering additional coping skills to the provider) and patient outcomes (Fang et al., 2010; Gulliksson et al., 2011), as has been shown in many studies. It is an educational innovation that has great potential to enhance the work of caring for patients.

Police Officers

Mindfulness interventions have been used as a tool to combat the harmful effects associated with working in law enforcement. Officers are exposed to violence, death, and other environmental influences on a daily basis, which leave them at a higher risk for cardiovascular disease, cancer, chemical intoxication, and posttraumatic stress disorder (Violanti, 2014). A study on the North Wales police indicated an increase in mental health problems and depression upon entering the police force (Williams et al., 2010). Mindfulness was found to be an accurate predictor of depression, with higher levels of mindfulness correlating with smaller increases in depression. When compared to a similar demographic, it was found that as a group, police officers show significantly less emotion regulation, consistent with reported difficulties dealing with negative emotions (Berking, Meier, & Wupperman, 2010). An emotion-regulation intervention focusing on awareness and mindfulness significantly enhanced participants' ability to deal with negative emotions, which may arise as a result of working in a stressful, and oft times, adversarial environment. Furthermore, in a study of 183 frontline police officers, findings indicated that spiritual growth and acceptance were predictive of growth after incidents causing traumatic stress (Chopko & Schwartz, 2009). One quarter of police officers were found to be alcohol dependent, a behavior that is strongly correlated with stress, suggesting that law enforcement officers are in need of additional methods/approaches of coping with job-related hazards (Violanti, 2014). Mindfulness interventions may be a prime candidate to interrupt addictive coping mechanisms employed by police officers.

Firefighters

Similar to police officers, firefighters experience a high level of job stress due to the risky and hazardous work environment. A 6-week intervention involving 108 firefighters indicated that yoga conducted during work shifts significantly reduced perceived stress (Cowen, 2010). Accordingly, high levels of mindfulness among firefighter correlated with fewer symptoms of PTSD, depression, physical malaise, and alcohol problems. Mindfulness interventions have important implications for improving resilience in firefighters and helping to decrease some of the job-related side effects (Smith et al., 2011).

Teachers

Frequently struggling to maintain balance of students' needs and educational directives, teachers could benefit from the implementation of a mindfulness-based intervention. Good teachers face many daily demands, including attention, flexibility, and, unfortunately, often a lack of support from an administrative level (Roeser et al., 2012). One recent study examined a mindfulness program for teachers that focussed on improving resilience, stress, and the facilitation of teaching and learning in the schools. In this 8-week, 36-h intervention that focussed on supporting teachers' self-compassion and resilience through mindfulness instruction, group discussion, and yoga practice, Roeser et al. (2013) found that teachers experienced higher levels of mindfulness and self-compassion while benefiting from decreased occupational stress and burnout. Currently there are some programs for teachers looking to limit stress and increase mindfulness. These include Cultivating Awareness and Resilience in Education (CARE for Teachers), Stress Management and Relaxation Techniques (SMART-in Education), Inner Resilience, Mindfulness, Courage, and Reflection for Educators, Mindful Schools, and Passageworks Soul of

Education Course for Teachers. These programs are all mindfulness-based and are aimed at strengthening certain skill-sets and supporting emotional engagement. Some are in-person and some online, and they range from short workshops to 36-h long programs spread out over days or weeks (Roeser et al., 2012). Increasing mindfulness in teachers has the potential to impact a much larger group of individuals as each teacher interacts with a multitude of students each day. Similar to the way in which physicians' mindfulness can improve the physician–patient relationship, teachers' mindfulness can foster relationship-building with students (Frank et al., 2013). This is a different approach to classroom dynamics than has been explored in the past but could further increase teachers' job satisfaction while bettering the educational environment for students.

Lawyers

Lawyers are subject to a work environment with a culture of distrust and anger, as well as high levels of stress to perform high-detail work in a tight time frame (Keeva, 2005). Additionally, lawyers' preparation via law school does not train attorneys concerning strategies to be resilient (James, 2011) and may even encourage maladaptive coping behaviors. Accordingly, high levels of clinical depression and substance abuse are prevalent in this group of professionals (Benjamin et al., 1990). Alternately, practicing mindfulness in this highly charged environment allows lawyers to manage their emotions, leading to increased empathy and patience with clients and better relationships both at work and at home (Orenstein, 2014). Mindfulness has also been shown to be useful in the trial setting, helping lawyers to actually listen to what is currently happening in the courtroom and respond appropriately, rather than clinging to their notes (Zlotnick, 2011), being fully present in the moment. Robert Zeglovitch, a litigation partner who teaches a meditation course at a Minneapolis law firm, attributes the success of his program, which is based on the MBSR model, to the fact that it was held in the law firm setting. Zeglovitch explains that practicing mindfulness in the workplace, where it is difficult to be yourself, promotes self-healing and relief (Keeva, 2004). The location of mindfulness program delivery at the worksite is a common theme of successful worksite wellness programming across professions.

Value Added

Organizations are increasingly burdened with employee healthcare costs, most of which can be attributed to a short list of controllable risk factors and many of which are associated with eventual cause of death (Katz, 2014). A 2012 study based on 92,486 employees across 7 different employers found high blood pressure, obesity, physical inactivity, and depression to be significantly predictive of rising healthcare costs. Psychosocial risks, including depression and inability to manage stress, were associated with an especially large increase in expenditures. Compared to individuals who were not at risk, health care costs were found to be 48.0 % ($2184) higher in those with depression and 8.6 % ($413) more expensive for those reporting high levels of stress (Goetzel et al., 2012). These findings suggest a need for health promotion programs within organizations to help reduce or prevent some of these risk factors, in turn increasing employee value and lessening health care costs. The study performed by Aikens et al. (2014) administered a modified MBSR program for the workplace to a group of 44 employees, which was compared to a control group of 45 employees. The intervention group showed significant decreases in burnout and high-stress days, which could potentially lead to an increase in employee productivity and a decrease in absenteeism, resulting in savings for the employer. Additionally, the group showed a significant decrease in fast-food meals consumed, as well as a significant increase in servings of fruits and vegetables consumed per week (Aikens et al., 2014). A mindfulness health promotion program implemented in the workplace could serve to reduce psychosocial risk factors as well as those related to dietary patterns. Reducing these individual risk factors has implications for overall reduction of chronic physiological and psychological diseases that cost organizations money. Individual reduction of risk factors is likely to lead to enhancement of employee well-being at the workplace as well. Hence, value is added at both the individual and organizational levels.

There has been a growth in pragmatic mindfulness programs for the workplace in the past decade, including many that utilize the MBSR model. An example of such programming is Mindfulness at Work, a 12-week stress management program created by Drs. Elisha Goldstein and Michael Baine. Mindfulness at Work teaches mindfulness while tailoring the content of the didactic portion of the program as well as practices to fit the specific needs of the working population. The practices are also shorter than traditional MBSR, 5–10 min compared to 20 min, so that they may be done while at work by the employee. Research with Mindfulness at Work showed that it can significantly improve perceived stress and sleep quality, as well as marginally improve breathing rate and autonomic balance. Mood and work productivity also improved, but not significantly. Currently, Mindfulness at Work is contracted for use by Aetna health insurance because of the demonstrated effects it showed on participants' health and well-being. One unique feature of this study was its indication that an online version of the class demonstrated a much higher adherence rate than the classes done at the worksite (Wolever et al., 2012). This is promising for the ease of accessibility for employees and ease of distribution for employers and health insurance companies as the practice of utilizing mindfulness programs for employee well-being expands.

Another promising mindfulness-based worksite wellness program is telephonic MBSR (tMBSR) geared toward supporting positive lifestyle, workplace, and mental health well-being in nurses (Bazarko et al., 2013). In this particular program, 2 out of the 8 weekly sessions are still conducted in-person. This program shows significant effects on health, stress, burnout, self-compassion, serenity, and empathy.

Similar to Mindfulness at Work, tMBSR is more cost-effective and feasible than traditional MBSR because it does not require extensive travel time commitment for the participant. Yet, tMBSR demonstrated significant sustainability up to 4 months after the program for individuals who continued their practice, particularly in burnout and subscales of self-compassion, including self-kindness, common humanity, and overall self-compassion (Bazarko et al., 2013). This is very significant in regard to both the effectiveness and cost-effectiveness related to the implementation of one of these programs in a workplace setting.

Mindfulness in Motion (research results detailed under the section on mindfulness programs delivered to nurse employees) is an 8-week series to improve resiliency and reduce daily stress and is a final example of a pragmatic worksite wellness program with foundations in MBSR. It differs from MBSR in that it is done at work, lasts only 1 h instead of 2.5 h, and incorporates yoga that can be done from a chair in professional attire or whatever the individual typically wears to work (in the study with surgical intensive care nurses they wore scrubs). This makes the class more accessible to busy participants who are unable to commit to extra time outside of their working hours. The impact of *Mindfulness in Motion* has been researched across various high-stress populations, including personnel at a large urban university. Successful completion of the 8-week program has led to significant decreases in perceived stress and inflammation, significant reductions in salivary amylase, enhanced neuroplasticity in older adults, increased sleep quality and work engagement, and correlated changes in mRNA between high and low reported levels of stress (Duchemin et al., 2015; Klatt, Buckworth, & Malarkey, 2009; Prakash, De Leon, Klatt, Malarkey, & Patterson, 2013). Similarly to Mindfulness at Work and tMBSR, the overall goals of *Mindfulness in Motion* are to help individuals identify stressors, respond to stress in a resilient manner, be more aware and focussed at work, and set the intention to live with purpose, clarity, and commitment to the life they want to lead. End of program participant responses reflect an enhanced well-being not only at work but in home life as well (Klatt et al., 2015). Program delivery may be most prudent at the worksite, but the impact of various worksite mindfulness programming extends well beyond the hours the employee spends at work. The skills learned through mindfulness programming enlarge the skill set of the employee to deal with various stresses—inside and outside of the workday.

Current Programs and Coverage

Due to the significant findings of the effectiveness of the MBSR program, a multitude of universities nationwide offer programs to students and employees, as well as the general public. In the American higher education environment, there are currently 14 universities that offer cost-recovery supplement to students and employees who participate in the university mindfulness program. Coverage ranges from 15 % to full reimbursement, with tuition assistance, scholarships, and payment plans

Table 16.1 American employers offering MBIs

Institution/company	Allowed research with employees	Fully covered employee benefit	Partially covered employee benefit
University of California—San Diego			X
University of California—San Francisco			X
Duke University			X
Harvard University			X
Howard University			X
University of Iowa		X	
University of Massachusetts			X
University of Miami			X
University of Minnesota		X[a]	X
University of Missouri			X
Thomas Jefferson University			X
Tufts University			X
University of Wisconsin			X
The Dow Chemical Company	X		
The Ohio State University	X		X
The Children's Hospital at Montefiore NYC	X		
Aetna International	X	X	
General Mills Inc	X	X	
AOL Time Warner Inc		X	
Medtronic		X	
AstraZeneca Pharmaceuticals		X	
Green Mountain Coffee Roasters		X	
Google Inc		X	

[a]*Mindfulness in Motion* covered 100 %, MBSR covered 50 %

available to help reduce the burden of cost. The University of Minnesota offers partial coverage for a traditional MBSR program (approximately 26 h) and full coverage for *Mindfulness in Motion* (8 h). In addition, there are several universities that offer tuition assistance, scholarships, and payment plans to help reduce the burden of cost for MBIs meant to impact well-being.

In an attempt to change the culture of the work environment to support employee well-being, an increasing amount of companies have begun the transition to a mindful work environment. Companies such as General Mills and AOL Time Warner Inc., among others, have incorporated mindfulness classes for employees, resulting in increased focus, motivation, and overall productivity (Adams, 2011; General Mills, 2010) (See Table 16.1).

Conclusion: Well-Being and Mental Health

The outlook for chronic disease may not be promising as chronic stress continues to rise, but MBIs are increasingly being utilized by both private and public employers at the workplace to address the effects of chronic stress. There are various forms of these workplace mindfulness programs including, telephonic delivery and internet delivery and those programs that include increased yoga with music added in the background (Duchemin et al., 2015). The benefits of mindfulness programs delivered at work are multifaceted. In the interests of the employer, mindfulness in the workplace could increase productivity, limit absenteeism, and decrease the cost of health insurance as employees' overall health increases. For employees, mindfulness at work can improve mental health, quality of life, and job satisfaction, as well as decrease stress, burnout, and inflammation in the body. Having mindfulness as an available tool for lifestyle behavior change could be crucial in circumventing specific types of burnout, such as the frenetic profile of burnout that may lead to addiction, as well as, providing individuals with an alternative to substances to cope with the stressors of work and daily life (Montero-Marín & García-Campayo, 2010). However, to incorporate mindfulness interventions and workplace wellness, employees and employers need to work together to reap the benefits. Researchers believe that to really effect change, the entire way the workforce looks at health must change, that *"what is needed is a transformational system if organizations desire to create a healthy workplace and workforce"* (Edington, Pitts, & Schultz, 2014). Worksite mindfulness programming to increase well-being is a prudent delivery location and use of resources, both human and financial, for employer and employee alike as we introduce ways to remain resilient, encouraging both individual and organizational well-being.

References

Adams, J. (2011). *The business case for mindfulness part 1: Companies who have adopted mindfulness practices.* Retrieved from http://www.mindfulnet.org/The%20business%20case%20for%20Mindfulness%20in%20the%20workplace%20Part%201a.pdf

Aikens, K. A., Astin, J., Pelletier, K. R., Levanovich, K., Baase, C. M., Park, Y. Y., et al. (2014). Mindfulness goes to work: Impact of an online workplace intervention. *Journal of Occupational and Environmental Medicine, 56*(7), 721–731.

Andreou, E., Alexopoulos, E. C., Lionis, C., Varvogli, L., Gnardellis, C., Chrousos, G. P., et al. (2011). Perceived stress scale: Reliability and validity study in Greece. *International Journal of Environmental Resources and Public Health, 8*(8), 3287–3298.

Baer, R. A., Smith, G. T., Hopkins, J., Krietemeyer, J., & Toney, L. (2006). Using self-report assessment methods to explore facets of mindfulness. *Assessment, 13*(1), 27–45.

Baer, R. A., Smith, G. T., & Allen, K. B. (2004). Assessment of mindfulness by self-report: The Kentucky inventory of mindfulness skills. *Assessment, 11*(3), 191–206.

Bazarko, D., Cate, R. A., Azocar, F., & Kreitzer, M. J. (2013). The impact of an innovative mindfulness-based stress reduction program on the health and well-being of nurses employed in a corporate setting. *Journal of Workplace Behavioral Health, 28*(2), 107–133.

Beach, M. C., Roter, D., Korthuis, P. T., Epstein, R. M., Sharp, V., Ratanawongsa, N., et al. (2013). A multicenter study of physician mindfulness and health care quality. *Annals of Family Medicine, 11*(5), 421–428.

Beckman, H. B., Wendland, M., Mooney, C., Krasner, M. S., Quill, T. E., Suchman, A. L., & Epstein, R. M. (2012). The impact of a program in mindful communication on primary care physicians. *Academic Medicine, 87*(6), 815–819.

Benjamin, G. A. H., Darling, E. J., & Sales, B. (1990). The prevalence of depression, alcohol abuse, and cocaine abuse among United States lawyers. *International Journal of Law and Psychiatry, 13*(3), 233–246.

Berking, M., Meier, C., & Wupperman, P. (2010). Enhancing emotion-regulation skills in police officers: Results of a pilot controlled study. *Behavior Therapy, 41*(3), 329–339.

Berry, L. L., Mirabito, A. M., & Baun, W. B. (2010). What's the hard return on employee wellness programs? *Harvard Business Review, 88*(12), 104–112.

Black, D. S. (2010). Defining mindfulness. *Mindfulness Research Guide*. Retrieved from http://www.mindfulexperience.org/

Black, D. S. (2014). Mindfulness-based interventions: an antidote to suffering in the context of substance use, misuse, and addiction. *Substance use & misuse, 49*(5), 487–491.

Brantley, J. (2005). Mindfulness-based stress reduction. In S. M. Orsillo & L. Roemer (Eds.), *Acceptance and mindfulness-based approaches to anxiety: Conceptualization and treatment* (pp. 131–145). New York: Springer.

Brewer, J. A., Mllik, S., Babuscio, T., Nich, C., Johnson, H., Deleone, C., et al. (2011). Mindfulness training for smoking cessation: Results from a randomized controlled trial. *Drug and Alcohol Dependence, 119*(1–2), 72–80.

Buchheld, N., Grossman, P., & Walach, H. (2001). Measuring mindfulness in insight meditation (Vipassana) and meditation-based psychotherapy: The development of the Freiburg Mindfulness Inventory (FMI). *Journal for Meditation and Meditation Research, 1*(1), 11–34.

Burckhardt, C. S., & Anderson, K. L. (2003). The quality of life scale (QOLS): Reliability, validity, and utilization. *Health and Quality of Life Outcomes, 1*, 60.

Buysse, D. J., Reynolds, C. F., Monk, T. H., Berman, S. R., & Kupfer, D. J. (1989). The Pittsburgh sleep quality index: A new instrument for psychiatric practice and research. *Psychiatry Research, 28*(2), 193–213.

Cardaciotto, L., Herbert, J. D., Forman, E. M., Moitra, E., & Farrow, V. (2008). The assessment of present-moment awareness and acceptance: The Philadelphia mindfulness scale. *Assessment, 15*(2), 204.

Chopko, B. A., & Schwartz, R. C. (2009). The relation between mindfulness and posttraumatic growth: A study of first responders to trauma-inducing incidents. *Journal of Mental Health Counseling, 31*(4), 363–376.

Clinton, W. J. (2000). *A citizen's guide to the federal budget*. Retrieved from http://www.gpo.gov/fdsys/pkg/BUDGET-2001-CITIZENSGUIDE/pdf/BUDGET-2001-CITIZENSGUIDE.pdf

Cohen, S., Kamarck, T., & Mermelstein, R. (1983). A global measure of perceived stress. *Journal of Health and Social Behavior, 24*, 386–396.

Collins, J. J., Baase, C., Sharda, C., Orzminkowski, R., Nicholson, S., Billotti, G., et al. (2005). The assessment of chronic health conditions on work performance, absence, and total economic impact for employers. *Journal of Occupational and Environmental Medicine, 47*(6), 547–557.

Cowen, V. S. (2010). Functional fitness improvements after a worksite-based yoga initiative. *Journal of Bodywork & Movement Therapies, 14*(1), 50–54.

Crawford, R. (2014). 20% take time off work due to stress. *Employee Benefits, 3*.

Davidson, R. J., Kabat-Zinn, J., Schumacher, J., Rosenkranz, M., Muller, D., Santorelli, S. F., et al. (2003). Alterations in brain and immune function produced by mindfulness meditation. *Psychosomatic Medicine, 65*(4), 564–570.

Duchemin, A. M., Steinberg, B., Marks, D., Vanover, K., & Klatt, M. (2015). A small randomized pilot study of workplace mindfulness-based intervention for surgical intensive care unit personnel: Effects on self-reported stress and salivary α-amylase levels. *Journal of Occupational and Environmental Medicine, 57*(4), 393–399.

Edington, D. W., Pitts, J. S., & Schultz, A. B. (2014). Health as an economic strategy special emphasis on the workplace. *American Journal of Lifestyle Medicine, 8*(5), 330–335.
Fang, C. Y., Reibel, D. K., Longacre, M. L., Rosenzweig, S., Campbell, D. E., & Douglas, S. D. (2010). Enhanced psychosocial well-being following participation in a mindfulness-based stress reduction program is associated with increased natural killer cell activity. *Journal of Alternative and Complementary Medicine, 16*(5), 531–538.
Feldman, G., Hayes, A., Kumar, S., Greeson, J., & Laurenceau, J. P. (2007). Mindfulness and emotion regulation: The development and initial validation of the cognitive and affective mindfulness scale-revised (CAMS-R). *Journal of Psychopathology and Behavioral Assessment, 29*(3), 177–190.
Fortney, L., Luchterhand, C., Zakletskaia, L., Zgierska, A., & Rakel, D. (2013). Abbreviated mindfulness intervention for job satisfaction, quality of life, and compassion in primary care clinicians: A pilot study. *Annals of Family Medicine, 11*(5), 412–420.
Foureur, M., Besley, K., Burton, G., Yu, N., & Crisp, J. (2013). Enhancing the resilience of nurses and midwives: Pilot of a mindfulnessbased program for increased health, sense of coherence and decreased depression, anxiety and stress. *Contemporary nurse, 45*(1), 114–125.
Frank, J. L., Reibel, D., Broderick, P., Cantrell, T., & Metz, S. (2013). The effectiveness of mindfulness-based stress reduction on educator stress and well-being: Results from a pilot study. *Mindfulness, 6*(2), 208–216.
Glaser, R., Kiecolt-Glaser, J. K., Marucha, P. T., MacCallum, R. C., Laskowski, B. F., & Malarkey, W. B. (1999). Stress-related changes in proinflammatory cytokine production in wounds. *Archive of General Psychiatry, 56*(5), 450–456.
Glaser, R., MacCallum, R., Laskowski, B., Malarkey, W., Sheridan, J., & Kiecolt-Glaser, J. (2001). Evidence for a shift in the Th-1 to Th-2 cytokine response associated with chronic stress and aging. *Journals of Gerontology Series A: Biological Sciences and Medical Sciences, 56*(8), M477–M482.
Glaser, R., Padgett, D., Litsky, M., Baiocchi, R., Yang, E., Chen, M., et al. (2005). Stress-associated changes in the steady-state expression of latent Epstein-Barr virus: Implications for chronic fatigue syndrome and cancer. *Brain, Behavior, and Immunity, 19*(2), 91–103.
Glaser, R., Sheridan, J., Malarkey, W. B., MacCallum, R. C., & Kiecolt-Glaser, J. K. (2000). Chronic stress modulates the immune response to a pneumococcal pneumonia vaccine. *Psychosomatic Medicine, 62*(6), 804–807.
Godet-Cayré, V., Pelletier-Fleury, N., Le Vaillant, M., Dinet, J., Massuel, M., & Léger, D. (2006). Insomnia and absenteeism at work. Who pays the cost? *Sleep, 29*(2), 179–184.
Goetzel, R. Z., Pei, X., Tabrizi, M. J., Henke, R. M., Kowlessar, N., Nelson, C. F., et al. (2012). Ten modifiable health risk factors are linked to more than one-fifth of employer-employee health care spending. *Health Affairs, 31*(11), 2474–2484.
Grossman, P., Niemann, L., Schmidt, S., & Walach, H. (2004). Mindfulness-based stress reduction and health benefits. A meta-analysis. *Journal of Psychosomatic Research, 57*(1), 35–43.
Gulliksson, M., Burell, G., Vessby, B., Lundin, L., Toss, H., & Svardsudd, K. (2011). Randomized controlled trial of cognitive behavioral therapy vs standard treatment to prevent recurrent cardiovascular events in patients with coronary heart disease: Secondary prevention in Uppsala primary health care project (SUPRIM). *Archives of Internal Medicine, 171*(2), 134–140.
Hoffman, C., & Schwartz, K. (2008). Eroding access among nonelderly U.S. adults with chronic conditions: Ten years of change. *Health Affairs, 27*(5), w340–w348.
Hölzel, B. K., Carmody, J., Evans, K. C., Hoge, E. A., Dusek, J. A., Morgan, L., et al. (2010). Stress reduction correlates with structural changes in the amygdala. *Social Cognitive and Affective Neuroscience, 5*(1), 11–17.
Horowitz, M., Wilner, N., & Alvarez, W. (1979). Impact of event scale: A measure of subjective stress. *Psychosomatic Medicine, 41*(3), 209–218.
Hülsheger, U. R., Alberts, H. J., Feinholdt, A., & Lang, J. W. (2013). Benefits of mindfulness at work: The role of mindfulness in emotion regulation, emotional exhaustion, and job satisfaction. *Journal of Applied Psychology, 98*(2), 310.
Hülsheger, U. R., Lang, J. W. B., Depenbrock, F., Fehrmann, C., Zijlstra, F. R. H., & Alberts, H. J. E. M. (2014). The power of presence: The role of mindfulness at work for daily levels and

change trajectories of psychological detachment and sleep quality. *Journal of Applied Psychology*. Advance online publication. Retrieved from http://psycnet.apa.org/psycarticles/2014-36699-001.pdf
Jacobs, T. L., Shaver, P. R., Epel, E. S., Zanesco, A. P., Aichele, S. R., Bridwell, D. A., et al. (2013). Self-reported mindfulness and cortisol during a Shamatha meditation retreat. *Health Psychology, 32*(10), 1104.
James, C. (2011). Law student wellbeing: Benefits of promoting psychological literacy and self-awareness using mindfulness, strengths theory and emotional intelligence. *Legal Education Review, 21*(1/2), 217.
Jha, A. P., Krompinger, J., & Baime, M. J. (2007). Mindfulness training modifies subsystems of attention. *Cognitive, Affective, & Behavioral Neuroscience, 7*(2), 109–119.
Kabat-Zinn, J. (1982). An outpatient program in behavioral medicine for chronic pain patients based on the practice of mindfulness meditation: Theoretical considerations and preliminary results. *General Hospital Psychiatry, 4*(1), 33–47.
Kabat-Zinn, J. (2003). Mindfulness-based interventions in context: Past, present and future. *Clinical Psychology: Science and Practice, 10*, 144–156.
Katz, D. L. (2014). Lifestyle is the medicine, culture is the spoon: The covariance of proposition and preposition. *American Journal of Lifestyle Medicine, 8*(5), 301–305.
Keeva, S. (2004). A mindful law practice: Lawyers stay calm and focused with the help of a meditation technique. *ABA Journal, 90*(3), 78–79.
Keeva, S. (2005). A meditative perspective. *ABA Journal, 91*(3), 76.
Kessler, R. C., Berglund, P. A., Coulouvrat, C., Hajak, G., Roth, T., Shahly, V., et al. (2011). Insomnia and the performance of U.S. workers: Results from the America insomnia survey. *Sleep, 34*(9), 1161–1171.
Kiecolt-Glaser, J., & Glaser, R. (1988). Major life changes, chronic stress, and immunity. *Advances in Biochemical Psychopharmacology, 44*, 217–224.
Kiecolt-Glaser, J. K., & Glaser, R. (1999). Chronic stress and mortality among older adults. *JAMA, 282*(23), 2259–2260.
Kiecolt-Glaser, J. K., Marucha, P. T., Malarkey, W. B., Mercado, A. M., & Glaser, R. (1995). Slowing the wound healing by psychological stress. *Lancet, 346*, 1194–1196.
Klatt, M., Buckworth, J., & Malarkey, W. B. (2009). Effects of low-dose mindfulness-based stress reduction (MBSR-ld) on working adults. *Health Education and Behavior, 36*(3), 601–614.
Klatt, M., Steinberg, B., & Duchemin, A. M. (2015). Development of an on-site mindfulness based intervention (MBI) for chronically high stress work environments to increase resilience and work engagement. *Journal of Visualized Experiments*.
Krasner, M. S., Epstein, R. M., Beckman, H., Suchman, A. L., Chapman, B., Mooney, C. J., et al. (2009). Association of an educational program in mindful communication with burnout, empathy, and attitudes among primary care physicians. *JAMA, 302*(12), 1284–1293.
Krystal, A. D., & Edinger, J. D. (2008). Measuring sleep quality. *Sleep Medicine, 9*(Supp 1), S10–S17.
Langer, E. J., & Moldoveanu, M. (2000a). Mindfulness research and the future. *Journal of Social Issues, 56*(1), 129–139.
Langer, E. J., & Moldoveanu, M. (2000b). The construct of mindfulness. *Journal of Social Issues, 56*(1), 1–9.
Lau, M. A., Bishop, S. R., Segal, Z. V., Buis, T., Anderson, N. D., Carlson, L., et al. (2006). The Toronto mindfulness scale: Development and validation. *Journal of Clinical Psychology, 62*(12), 1445–1467.
Lengacher, C. A., Kip, K. E., & Barta, M. (2013). A pilot study evaluating the effect of mindfulness-based stress reduction on psychological status, physical status, salivary cortisol, and interleukin-6 among advanced stage cancer patients and their caregivers. *Journal of Holistic Nursing, 30*(3), 170–185.
Li, Y., & Jones, C. B. (2013). A literature review of nursing turnover costs. *Journal of nursing management, 21*(3), 405–418.

Loeppke, R., Taitel, M., Haufle, V., Parry, T., Kessler, R., & Jinnett, K. (2009). Health and productivity as a business strategy: A multiemployer study. *Journal of Occupational Environmental Medicine, 51*(4), 411–428.

Malarkey, W. B., Jarjoura, D., & Klatt, M. (2013). Workplace based mindfulness practice and inflammation: A randomized trial. *Brain, Behavior, and Immunity, 27*(1), 145–154.

Mattke, S., Liu, H., Caloyeras, J. P., Huang, C. Y., Van Busum, K. R., Khodyakov, D., et al. (2013). *Workplace wellness programs study: Final report*. Retrieved from http://www.rand.org/content/dam/rand/pubs/research_reports/RR200/RR254/RAND_RR254.pdf

McCraty, R., Atkinson, M., & Tomasino, D. (2003). Impact of a workplace stress reduction program on blood pressure and emotional health in hypertensive employees. *Journal of Alternative and Complementary Medicine, 9*(3), 355–369.

McGibbon, E., Peter, E., & Gallop, R. (2010). An institutional ethnography of nurses' stress. *Qualitative Health Research, 20*(10), 1353–1378.

Metcalf, F., & Hateley, B. J. G. (2001). *What would Buddha do at work?: 101 answers to workplace dilemmas*. San Francisco, CA: Berrett-Koehler.

Moody, K., Kramer, D., Santizo, R. O., Magro, L., Wyshogrod, D., Ambrosio, J., ... & Stein, J. (2013). Helping the Helpers Mindfulness Training for Burnout in Pediatric Oncology—A Pilot Program. *Journal of Pediatric Oncology Nursing, 30*(5), 275–284.

Montero-Marín, J., & García-Campayo, J. (2010). A newer and broader definition of burnout: Validation of the. *BMC Public Health, 10*(1), 302.

General Mills. (2010). *Inside general mills: Leadership program helps train the mind.* Retrieved from http://www.generalmills.com/en/ChannelG/Inside_General_Mills_archive/leadership_6_8_2010.aspx

Nahin RL, Barnes PM, Stussman BJ, & Bloom B. (2009). *Costs of complementary and alternative medicine (CAM) and frequency of visits to CAM practitioners: United States, 2007.* National health statistics reports; no: 18. Hyattsville, MD: National Center for Health Statistics.

National Institutes of Health. (2011). The national center for complementary and alternative medicine's (NCCAM) third strategic plan, U.S. department of health and human services. *NIH Publication, 11*, 7643.

Nyklíček, I., Mommersteeg, P. M. C., Van Beugen, S., Ramakers, C., & Van Boxtel, G. J. (2013). Mindfulness-based stress reduction and physiological activity during acute stress: A randomized controlled trial. *Health Psychology, 32*(10), 1110–1113.

Oginska-Bulik, N. (2005). The role of personal and social resources in preventing adverse health outcomes in employees of uniformed professions. *International Journal of Occupational Medicine and Environmental Health, 18*(3), 233–240.

Orenstein, J. (2014). Mindfulness and the law-a different approach to sustainable and effective lawyering. *QUT Law Review, 14*(1), 106.

Orly, S., Rivka, B., Rivka, E., & Dorit, S. E. (2012). Are cognitive-behavioral interventions effective in reducing occupational stress among nurses? *Applied Nursing Research, 25*(3), 152–157.

Peacock, E. J., & Wong, P. T. P. (1990). The stress appraisal measure (SAM): A multidimensional approach to cognitive appraisal. *Stress Medicine, 6*(3), 227–236.

Pipe, T. B., Bortz, J. J., Dueck, A., Pendergast, D., Buchda, V., & Summers, J. (2009). Nurse leader mindfulness meditation program for stress management: A randomized controlled trial. *Journal of Nursing Administration, 39*(3), 130–137.

Prakash, R., De Leon, A., Klatt, M., Malarkey, W., & Patterson, B. (2013). Mindfulness disposition and default-mode network connectivity: Implications for preservative cognition. *Social Cognitive and Affective Neuroscience, 1*, 112–117.

Reibel, D. K., Greeson, J. M., Brainard, G. C., & Rosenzweig, S. (2001). Mindfulness-based stress reduction and health-related quality of life in a heterogeneous patient population. *General Hospital Psychiatry, 23*, 183–192.

Riskin, L. L. (2002). Contemplative lawyer: On the potential contributions of mindfulness meditation to law students, lawyers, and their clients. *The Harvard Negotiation Law Review, 7*, 1.

Roeser, R. W., Skinner, E., Beers, J., & Jennings, P. A. (2012). Mindfulness training and teachers' professional development: An emerging area of research and practice. *Child Development Perspectives, 6*(2), 167–173.

Roeser, R. W., Schonert-Reichl, K. A., Jha, A., Cullen, M., Wallace, L., Wilensky, R., ... & Harrison, J. (2013). Mindfulness training and reductions in teacher stress and burnout: Results

from two randomized, waitlist-control field trials. *Journal of Educational Psychology, 105*(3), 787.
Rosch, P. J. (2001). The quandary of job stress compensation. *Health & Stress, 3*(1), 1.
Rosenkranz, M. A., Davidson, R. J., MacCoon, D. G., Sheridan, J. F., Kalin, N. H., & Lutz, A. (2013). A comparison of mindfulness-based stress reduction and an active control in modulation of neurogenic inflammation. *Brain, Behavior, and Immunity, 27*, 174–184.
Shapiro, S. L., Astin, J. A., Bishop, S. R., & Cordova, M. (2005). Mindfulness-based stress reduction for health care professionals: Results from a randomized trial. *International Journal of Stress Management, 12*(2), 164–176.
Shonin, E., Van Gordon, W., Dunn, T. J., Singh, N. N., & Griffiths, M. D. (2014). Meditation awareness training (MAT) for work-related wellbeing and job performance: A randomized controlled trial. *International Journal of Mental Health and Addiction, 12*(6), 806–823.
Skevington, S. M., Lotfy, M., O'Connell, K. A., & WHOQOL Group. (2004). The World Health Organization's WHOQOL-BREF quality of life assessment: Psychometric properties and results of the international field trial. A report from the WHOQOL group. *Quality of Life Research, 13*(2), 299–310.
Smith, B. W., Oritz, J. A., Steffen, L. E., Tooley, E. M., Wiggins, K. T., Yeater, E. A., et al. (2011). Mindfulness is associated with fewer PTSD symptoms, depressive symptoms, physical symptoms, and alcohol problems in urban firefighters. *Journal of Consulting and Clinical Psychology, 79*(5), 613–617.
Stamm, B. H. (2005). *The ProQOL manual: The professional quality of life scale: Compassion satisfaction, burnout & compassion fatigue/secondary trauma scales*. Baltimore, MD: Sidran.
Thomley, B. S., Ray, S. H., Cha, S. S., & Bauer, B. A. (2011). Effects of a brief, comprehensive, yoga-based program on quality of life and biometric measures in an employee population: A pilot study. *Explore, 7*(1), 27–29.
Tomfohr, L. M., Pung, M. A., Mills, P. J., & Edwards, K. (2014). Trait mindfulness is associated with blood pressure and interleukin-6: Exploring interactions among subscales of the Five Facet Mindfulness Questionnaire to better understand relationships between mindfulness and health. *Journal of Behavioral Medicine*. Advance online publication. Retrieved from http://download.springer.com/static/pdf/563/art%253A10.1007%252Fs10865-014-9575-4.pdf?auth66=1416406883_d955aa4347974ad88187f1af83b65e4f&ext=.pdf
Udod, S. A., & Care, W. D. (2013). 'Walking a tight rope': An investigation of nurse managers' work stressors and coping experiences. *Journal of Research in Nursing, 18*(1), 67–79.
Violanti, J. M. (2014). *Dying for the job: Police work exposure and health*. Springfield, IL: Charles C. Thomas.
Williams, V., Ciarrochi, J., & Deane, F. P. (2010). On being mindful, emotionally aware, and more resilient: Longitudinal pilot study of police recruits. *Australian Psychologist, 45*(4), 274–282.
Winbush, N. Y., Gross, C. R., & Kreitzer, M. J. (2007). The effects of mindfulness-based stress reduction on sleep disturbance: A systematic review. *Explore, 3*(6), 585–591.
Wolever, R. Q., Bobinet, K. J., McCabe, K., Mackenzie, E. R., Fekete, E., Kusnick, C. A., et al. (2012). Effective and viable mind-body stress reduction in the workplace: A randomized controlled trial. *Journal of Occupational Health Psychology, 17*(2), 246–258.
World Bank. (2014). Table of each country's GDP from 1980–2013. *Data: GDP (Current US$)*. Retrieved from http://data.worldbank.org/indicator/NY.GDP.MKTP.CD
World Health Organization. (1997). *WHOQOL: Measuring quality of life*. Retrieved from http://www.who.int/mental_health/media/68.pdf
Younge, J. O., Gotink, R. A., Baena, C. P., Roos-Hesselink, J. W., & Hunink, M. G. M. (2014). Mind-body practices for patients with cardiac disease: A systematic review and meta-analysis. *European Journal of Preventative Cardiology*. Advance online publication. Retrieved from http://cpr.sagepub.com/content/early/2014/09/15/2047487314549927.full.pdf
Zlotnick, D. M. (2011). Integrating mindfulness theory and practice into trial advocacy. *Journal of Legal Education, 61*(4), 654–664.

Chapter 17
Is Aging a Disease? Mental Health Issues and Approaches for Elders and Caregivers

Lucia McBee and Patricia Bloom

The real adventure is, and always has been, your whole life.

Kabat-Zinn, 2013, p. xxix

Introduction

We are all aging, moment by moment. How we perceive aging creates our experience of it. Do we regard our aging as part of the natural trajectory of life, as an adventure, as a tragedy, or as a pathological medical condition? Ageism, as described by Robert Butler (1980), is the stereotyping of and prejudicial attitude toward older adults. Similar to other "isms," ageism includes external bias and discrimination and the internalization of the stereotypes. If we have internalized bias, we may regard our aging as a tragedy or ailment to be remedied. Mindfulness, the nonjudgmental awareness of the present moment (Kabat-Zinn, 2013), offers new perspectives, reacquainting us with the adventure of our lives. The practices of mindfulness hold a wide range of promise for the aging, including new viewpoints, holistic connection, and empowerment.

Complex psychosocial factors such as loss, pain, and loneliness impact elders more frequently and routinely than other age groups. In addition, we are living longer, but with more disabilities. Currently, 62 % of US citizens over 65 have two or more chronic conditions, and this number is expected to rise significantly (Vogeli et al., 2007). Mindfulness is a 2500-year-old Buddhist practice and is one of many mind/body approaches to health and healing that view and treat the mind, body, and spirit holistically. A small but significant study by Creswell et al. (2012) nicely

L. McBee (✉)
Columbia University School of Social Work, 207 West 106 St., Apt. 12C,
New York, NY 10025, USA
e-mail: lucia@luciamcbee.com

P. Bloom
Mt. Sinai School of Medicine, 145 Euclid Avenue, Hastings on Hudson,
New York, NY 10705, USA
e-mail: Patriciaabloom@gmail.com

E. Shonin et al. (eds.), *Mindfulness and Buddhist-Derived Approaches in Mental Health and Addiction*, Advances in Mental Health and Addiction,
DOI 10.1007/978-3-319-22255-4_17

illustrates the multifaceted nature of issues facing elders and the benefits of holistic, wellness-centered programs such as mindfulness-based stress reduction (MBSR) and other mindfulness-based interventions (MBIs). Following an MBSR class with non-frail elders, these researchers found that participants self-reported less loneliness (an emotional state elders often face and that is associated with health problems) and also had reduced pro-inflammatory gene expression (inflammation is increasingly associated with chronic conditions, including Alzheimer's, heart diseases, and stress).

Conventional medical approaches treat individual diagnoses separately, often with specialists. For elders, this approach has increased the likelihood of polypharmacy and even potentially inappropriate medicine use especially for elders with cognitive loss (Lau et al., 2010). In addition, conventional medicine tends to focus on pathology, while MBIs focus on abilities, not disabilities.

Mental health conditions in elders are also complex and multifaceted. Physical illness may systemically impact mental and emotional health. Distressing symptoms, such as pain, may lead to mental and emotional suffering. Chronic conditions are associated with an increased risk of major depression and substantial disability (Moussavi et al., 2007). Healthcare professionals routinely screen elders for depression before a diagnosis of dementia because depression is common among elders and may cause confusion and memory loss (Rodda, Walker, & Carter, 2011). In one scenario, an elder admitted to the emergency room for confusion became increasingly verbally and physically agitated. She was temporarily restrained, sedatives were administered, and she was scheduled for admission to the psychiatric unit when her caregiver arrived with her hearing aids. Once she could hear, this elder's agitation vanished, and she was able to communicate her complaints and needs (McBee, 2008, p. 74).

Frail elders experience multiple losses, and the loss of meaning and control in life has profound effects (Krause, 2004). Mindfulness practice can be adapted and taught to elders and provides tools to cope with these challenges. While frail elders may be dependent on others for their basic needs, they may realize they have choices in how they respond to dependency. Mindfulness practice also reminds us of our basic interconnectedness and that we all have meaning in the web of life.

In this chapter, we will describe the most common mental health problems for elders and adaptations to MBIs to provide relief. We will also describe why caregivers are an integral component of mental health for elders, the common emotional suffering and mental health problems experienced by family and professional caregivers, and how MBIs can be best offered to this population.

Despite the complexities of conditions, mindfulness holds a promise of preventing the major ailments facing elders and caregivers, as well as treating distressing symptoms and improving quality of life. A primary tenet of mindfulness-based approaches is health, rather than disease. Or, as Jon Kabat-Zinn writes in *Full Catastrophe Living*, "as long as you are breathing, there is more right with you than there is wrong with you" (2013, p. xxvii).

Reflection

Step back and consider how aging is viewed in the media and culture. How have I internalized these views?

Practice

Start with yourself. Contemplate your body. How has it changed over time? How might it change more as you age? What thoughts and feelings arise? How might you cope with limitations to your life and lifestyle? Can you accept that it is challenging, but perhaps the ultimate practice of our life?

Mindfulness as a Prescription for Preventing and the Ameliorating of Age-Associated Diseases

> Old age is not a diagnosis.
>
> Gawande (2014, p. 27)

Many adults over 65 are healthy, and their mental health/addiction problems are similar to those of their younger peers. In this chapter, we will include the spectrum of aging, with a particular focus on frail elders and adaptations of MBIs for this underserved population. More than 75 % of US adults over age 65 suffer from at least one chronic medical condition that requires ongoing care and management (Institute of Medicine (IOM) of the National Academies, 2008). Pain and disability clearly impact mental as well as physical health. Older adults who adopt the proactive stance of preventing, or at least delaying, the onset of age-associated diseases may find mindfulness practice beneficial in either avoiding or reducing the symptom burden of the major categories of age-associated diseases and mental health conditions.

Older adults are at particular risk of stress-related illness. The top three causes of mortality with aging are heart disease, cancer, and stroke (Sahyoun, Lentzner, Hoyert, & Robinson, 2001). Heart disease and stroke are clearly stress-related while the role of stress is less clear with regard to cancer (Sapolsky, 2004). A recent review by Carlson (2012) illustrated strong evidence in multiple studies for the emotional and mental, as well as physical benefits of MBIs for mixed-age adults with medical conditions. A meta-analysis by Goyal et al. (2014) found that meditation programs can reduce multiple negative dimensions of psychological stress with no reported harm. Given the strong evidence that meditation programs and MBIs reduce both physical and psychological suffering, as well as offer preventative value, clinicians need to make their patients aware of mindfulness and meditation in an array of recommended best practices. The challenge for clinicians working with frail older adults is identifying methods of teaching or conveying the essence of mindfulness practice to this population.

Mental Health

> Some people feel the rain. Others just get wet.
>
> Miller, R. (January 1, 1973)

Mental health problems in older adults reflect the general population and are specific to aging. According to a review (Goodwin, 1983), the four most prevalent psychiatric disorders specific to elderly persons are dementia, depression, alcoholism, and paranoia. The sections below will review the first three of these in detail, and the forth – paranoia – will be encompassed in the section on dementia.

Ageism, the stereotyping and discrimination toward older adults, was first labeled in 1980 by Robert Butler and continues to negatively impact elders. While the negative impact of discrimination is clear, internalization of the ageist stereotype has been linked to detrimental physical and cognitive outcomes (Levy, 2009). Mindfulness teaches us how much our perceptions of life impact our emotions and understanding. A holistic perception of well-being would include a true sense of mental wellness, not simply an absence of mental health problems. For elders, this perception itself may be empowering.

Reflection

How do I view/perceive aging? Do I focus on illness or the worst case scenario? When I look at frail elders, do I see the whole person behind the frailty?

Practice

Practice taking slow, long, deep belly breaths. When you do this exercise, feel your breath filling your torso, your whole body. After you feel comfortable with this practice, teach it to an elder. If the elder cannot follow your instructions, just practice the deep breathing in their presence. Notice what happens.

Cognitive Decline

> The mind can go in a thousand directions, but on this beautiful path, I walk in peace. With each step, a gentle wind blows. With each step, a flower blooms.
>
> Thich Nhat Hanh (1990, p. 376)

Loss of cognitive function is one of the most feared experiences of aging. Alzheimer's disease (AD), the most common cause of chronic dementia, is the sixth leading cause of mortality in the United States; a recent article in a leading neurology journal gives evidence suggesting that it is actually the third leading cause of death (James et al., 2014). Lesser manifestations of cognitive dysfunction with aging include mild cognitive impairment (MCI) and age-associated memory impairment (AAMI). And, as the population ages worldwide, the prevalence of Alzheimer's disease and other dementias increases exponentially (James et al., 2014).

In view of the projected epidemic of Alzheimer's disease and other forms of age-related cognitive impairment, as well as the as yet lack of a good pharmacological intervention, a technique that has been shown to be feasible and acceptable to older adults and possibly efficacious in altering the course of cognitive changes with aging is of major interest. Even a small shift in the inexorable trajectory of the Alzheimer's disease process would manifest major economic and social benefits.

In recent studies, mindfulness and MBIs demonstrate a moderate to strong effect in improving brain elasticity and function, while reducing emotional stress and disability. A review article by Newberg and colleagues (2014) found that meditation can change both brain structure and function, improve cognitive function, enhance memory, and protect against age-related and high stress-related cognitive decline. One of the highest profile articles in this area of inquiry demonstrated that the traditional MBSR 8-week course in healthy, meditation-naïve, mixed-age adults resulted in significant increases in the density of the brain in areas related to learning and memory (Holzel et al., 2011). An analysis of the link between aging and cerebral gray matter suggested a slower decline in gray matter with aging among long-term meditators (Luders, Cherbuin, & Kurth, 2015). A systematic review of meditation on cognition and age-related cognitive decline found meditation both feasible and effective for older adults (Gard, Holzel, & Lazar, 2014). An article in the Spanish medical literature attributed stabilization of global cognitive function, functional status, and behavioral symptoms to a mindfulness intervention involving 127 probable Alzheimer's patients over a two-year follow-up period, compared with progressive muscle relaxation and cognitive stimulation experimental groups (Quintana Hernandez et al., 2014). Recent small studies demonstrate promising evidence for teaching elders in supportive housing/assisted living. Elders were able to participate in MBSR groups and reported decreased anxiety and stress (Sasi, Ramesh, & Anice, 2014; Moss et al., 2014)

Often, behavioral problems accompany dementia, resulting in frustration, anger, and disinhibition regardless of the person's previous nature and customs (Cohen-Mansfield, 1997). Dementia can produce behaviors ranging from mild agitation to spitting, hitting, kicking, biting, cursing, and elopement. (Cohen-Mansfield, 1997). These behaviors lead to suffering and injury for both the care receiver and care provider and are a leading cause of institutionalization or hospitalization (Phillips & Diwan, 2003). Here, also, mindfulness may benefit by addressing these painful and often escalating behaviors. With modifications, mindfulness can be taught in groups or individually to those with cognitive loss. While carryover benefits are limited and quantitative research difficult, anecdotally, elders with dementia are able to benefit from simplified meditation and mindfulness (Lantz, Buchalter, & McBee, 1997, McBee, 2008). Environmental and, specifically, caregiver interactions may also serve to escalate or de-escalate challenging situations. For this reason, this chapter will include information on working with both family and paid caregivers, describing research on mindfulness interventions and offering general tips on teaching mindfulness to caregivers.

Reflection

How do I identify myself? Am I my body? My history? My material or scholarly acquisitions? What if I lost the ability to access memory?

Practice

Consider the image of ourselves as a wave. We believe we are the wave, but often forget the wave is only a temporary manifestation of the ocean. Do you view your thinking mind as "you?" Is there a bigger "you?" Without expecting answers, walk with this question. Feel the ground, smell the wind, taste your life.

Depression

> Above all, I have been a sentient being, a thinking animal, on this beautiful planet, and that in itself has been an enormous privilege and adventure.
>
> Oliver Sacks, The New York Times Opinion Page, 2/19/2015, My Own Life: On learning he has terminal cancer

Depression in older adults is associated with medical illness, disability, and death, and medical illness and disability are associated with higher levels of concomitant depression (Murrell, Himmelfarb, & Wright, 1983). Incidence of depression in persons with Alzheimer's disease may be as high as 86 %, indicating the importance of this issue (Rodda et al., 2011). Mindfulness-based cognitive therapy (MBCT), an offshoot of MBSR formulated by Segal, Williams, and Teasdale (2002) as an intervention for recurrent depression, has demonstrated significant positive results. A meta-analysis commissioned by the US Agency for Healthcare Research and Quality (AHRQ) on the efficacy of programs for psychological stress and well-being concluded that mindfulness meditation had moderate evidence of both short- and long-term improvement in depression (Goyal et al., 2014). A few studies have targeted MBCT and MBIs specifically for older adults with depression. Results included improvements in anxiety, depression, and "purpose in life" and no relapse after 6 months (Meeten, Whiting, & Williams, 2014; O'Connor, Piet, & Hougaard, 2013; Smith, Graham, & Senthinathan, 2007). A retrospective review of 141 older adults who had taken MBSR found a >50 % reduction in the number reporting clinically significant depression and anxiety (Young & Baime, 2010). MBIs appear to be acceptable and efficacious in treating elders for both the symptoms of depression and the root causes.

While MBIs may clearly translate for an older population with minimal disability, many elders suffer from multiple disabilities, including those that require modification in teaching mindfulness practices. In institutional or other group settings, one author (LM) taught mindfulness skills to elders with a wide range of physical and cognitive disabilities, described in greater detail below in: Teaching Mindfulness. MBI groups for elders served to connect an often disconnected population and also to empower a disempowered population. Elders reported benefiting from the group connection and significantly improved in their sense of well-being. Or as one group participant observed, "(Mindfulness) makes me feel at peace with the world. It helps my whole body and spirit. I forgot all my troubles" (McBee, 2008).

Reflection

How do I respond to challenges? Physically, emotionally, mentally? Can I step back and observe?

Practice

A fellow teacher and friend describes how he works with frail elders. "You enter a space with people who are in that way of being in the world and work from there." When you are with an elder, can you step into their space?

Alcoholism and Substance Abuse

But I would not feel so all alone, everybody must get stoned.

Dylan (1966)

Alcoholism and substance abuse are largely undiagnosed and studied in older adults (Benshoff, Harrawood, & Koch, 2003). Alcohol abuse is often associated with self-treatment of depression, sadness, loneliness, and dysphoric moods, conditions disproportionately impacting elders (Gupta & Warner, 2008; Goodwin, 1983). Diagnosing alcohol and other substance abuse in elders is challenging, partly due to age bias but also due to the different metabolism of alcohol in aging bodies and its effects on the aging brain. Alcohol-related dementia may not be appropriately diagnosed, leading to treatment error (Ridley, Draper, & Withall, 2013). Ultimately, the complicated medical and social etiology and diagnosis of older adult alcoholism may lead to poor or no treatment. The legalization of marijuana and growing acceptance of it as a treatment for disease and end-of-life suffering will also present potential areas for discussion. In addition, certain pain medications carry risk for addiction and misuse, compounded by elders with confusion (Malec & Shega, 2014).

Unfortunately, there are few studies to recommend specific treatment for elders with a substance abuse problem. The aging population is increasing, and older addicted adults are unlikely to decrease usage or become abstinent (Patterson & Jeste, 1999). Problematic substance abuse in elders is predicted to increase considerably in the near future, creating an urgent need for treatment models specific to this population. One study projects a 70 % increase in US older adults needing treatment for substance abuse by 2020 (Gfroerer, Penne, Pemberton, & Folsom, 2003). Mindfulness-Based Relapse Prevention (MBRP), an MBI targeting substance abuse in the general population, has proved promising (Witkiewitz, Marlatt, & Walker, 2005). With modifications for elders such as those described elsewhere in this chapter, this treatment may offer one model for addressing the upcoming epidemic and warrants further study. For the frail elders unable to participate in the cognitive/behavioral aspects of MBIs, mindfulness treatments for distressing behaviors may offer relief.

Family caregivers are at risk for substance abuse as a maladaptive response to stress and substance abuse often leads to elder abuse (Homer & Gilleard, 1990; Gordon & Brill, 2001). Healthcare workers are also at risk for substance abuse problems. In a 2001 review of the literature, Bennett and O'Donovan (2001) describe the risk of substance misuse in healthcare workers related to the high-stress environments and relative ease of access to pharmaceuticals. This report also reviewed the personal and professional negative effects of substance abuse in this population. As above, both MBRP and other MBIs may offer partial solutions to substance abuse in caregivers, with possible adaptations of time and locations as described elsewhere in this chapter.

Reflection
Do I use behaviors or substances to find relief from suffering?
Practice
Sit. Practice. Stay with whatever comes up: pleasant, unpleasant, boring, painful, distressing, no matter how strong the call, sit. Notice where you wish to go, what you wish to do. Is it habitual? Is it an addictive response?

Quality of Life: Pain, Insomnia and End of Life

As previously described, elders face complex and interdependent issues. While pain, insomnia, and end of life are not considered mental health problems, problems in these areas are common to elders and in the clinical experience of the authors often lead to mental and emotional distress.

> Your suffering is not you.
>
> Kabat-Zinn (2013, p. 411)

Pain

Pain is one of the biggest causes of reduced quality of life for older adults. Up to 50 % of community-dwelling older adults and 85 % of nursing home residents experience persistent pain (Cavalieri, 2007). Pain is often untreated or undertreated in older adults for a variety of reasons, from mythologies concerning pain being a part of the aging process to lack of expertise on the part of healthcare professionals. Undertreatment of pain has numerous mental health consequences, including anxiety, depression, cognitive impairment, insomnia, loss of mobility, and social isolation (Zeidan, Grant, Brown, McHaffie, & Coghill, 2012).

Much pain, especially if it is chronic, has an element of "secondary pain." This secondary pain is a reaction to the perception of pain and may include anxiety, fear, anger, and frustration, resulting in a physiologic response that can exacerbate the perception of pain, including muscle contraction and other "fight-or-flight" reactions (Kabat-Zinn, 1982; Kabat-Zinn, Lipworth, & Burney, 1985). In addition, chronic pain is increasingly being recognized as a phenomenon of the central nervous system, in which previously inadequately treated pain may cause the imbedding of the neural circuitry of pain perception in the brain, which is subsequently initiated by minimal stimuli, a sort of broken record repeating itself. It is thought that mindfulness practice, by strengthening certain regions of the brain, overrides and creates new circuits that diminish the prominence of the pain circuitry (Grant, 2014; Zeidan et al., 2012). Goyal et al. (2014), in a meta-analysis commissioned by the AHRQ, found that meditation reduced pain by one third in the general population. Two large recent meta-analyses found that mindfulness did not statistically significantly diminish pain but did positively impact mental health and quality of life in a general population of those who suffer from pain (Rajguru et al., 2014; Song, Lu, Chen, Geng, & Wang, 2014). Studies of mindfulness for chronic low back pain in older adults reported improved disability, pain, and psychological function (Morone, Rollman, & Moore, 2009) and improved pain acceptance and physical function (Morone, Greco, & Weiner, 2008). These findings are consistent with the author's own small study with older nursing home adults (McBee, 2008). In this group, frail elders reported a trend toward less pain and a statistically significant reduction in feelings of sadness, or as one member reported: "I feel uplifted. I realize we all have pain." These findings clearly reflect that perception of an experience is the experience.

Insomnia

Sleep-related disorders are common in older adults; 25 % of American adults 50 and older self-report a sleep "problem" (Gallup Poll, 2005). This high level of sleep disruption, contrary to popular myth, is not an inevitable concomitant of aging but reflects the prevalence of medical and psychological morbidities in this population. There is a bidirectionality involved: older individuals with sleep disorders are more likely to develop multiple medical problems, and those with medical problems are more likely to develop sleep disturbances. Increased morbidity and mortality accompany all manifestations of these interrelated problems (Bloom et al., 2009).

Mindfulness for sleep problems has not been adequately studied in older adults, but it has been shown in studies to benefit other patient groups with insomnia (Carlson, Speca, Patel, & Goodey, 2003; Gross et al., 2010). Black and colleagues (2015) recently reported a randomized clinical trial of mindful awareness practices for older adults with sleep disturbances which found improvements in sleep quality superior to results in the control sleep hygiene education group (Black, O'Reilly, Olmstead, Breen, & Irwin, 2015).

A Good Death

> Everything is changeable, everything appears and disappears; there is no blissful peace until one passes beyond the agony of life and death.
>
> Kyokai (2006, p. 123)

While mindfulness and meditation are often taught without reference to their spiritual roots, the essence of these practices is grounded in the teachings of the Buddha. At times, it is helpful to reflect on these core teachings, which some view as philosophical and could align with most religions.

The practice of being "with dying" is considered the most important of practices. The natural affiliation of mindfulness practice and dying and end-of-life care has been embraced by ancient texts (Coleman & Thupten, 2006) as well as by modern meditation teachers (Levine & Levine, 1989, Rosenberg & Guy, 2000). Although the usage of mindfulness and meditation practices at the end of life is increasing, scientific research evidence concerning the use of mindfulness and dying is limited. Ball and Vernon (2014) elucidate these limitations and suggest areas to be researched. At the end of life, mindfulness can benefit the dying and also their caregivers (Mackenzie & Poulin, 2006). Currently, many hospice and palliative care movements, such as the New York Zen Center for Contemplative Care, teach mindful presence to end-of-life care doctors, nurses, chaplains, medical students, and other healthcare professionals (www.zencare.org). As one 93-year-old MBSR participant reported in a group run by one of the present authors (PB), "I have come to understand and embrace the concept of impermanence."

Reflection

How comfortable am I with death? Could I allow the idea of my own death to be a mindfulness practice?

Considerations for elders and caregivers

Remember that hearing is the last sense to leave us. Be mindful of what is said around the dying person. Even if there is no response, offer comforting words, music, prayers. If no words come, use the breath as a teaching. How is the dying person breathing?What does this tell us about her/him? Can we sync our breathing to him/her as a way of relating?

Caregivers may be suffering more than the dying patient. How can mindfulness practice offer relief?

Suggestions for Teaching Mindfulness to Frail Elders

> We are always the same age inside.
>
> Stein (1955, p. 946)

Mindfulness practices may be helpful for all of the above mental health problems and physical symptoms. Elders with few or no physical and cognitive limitations would be appropriate for mixed-age groups of MBSR and MBCT. Mindfulness may also be taught to elders with a range of limitations, with teaching modifications addressing communication, physical, and cognitive frailties. The teacher's authentic respect and conviction will convey the essential qualities of mindfulness – awareness and compassion – for all sentient beings. If we as teachers accept that there is more right with us than wrong with us, how do we convey this essential "rightness and intrinsic wisdom" to elders?

The authors have taught mindfulness to elders with a range of abilities and disabilities, in a variety of environments. The grounding of all adaptations and training of both teachers is in Mindfulness-Based Stress Reduction, the 8-week, 2–2 ½-hour class with homework and an all-day retreat, developed by Kabat-Zinn (2013). This class includes the formal practices of meditation, yoga, mindful walking, and loving-kindness, as well as informal inquiry and awareness of everyday events. These practices are based on, but not limited to, the stricter interpretations of mindfulness. For example, deep breathing is included in MBSR, while more traditional mindfulness might instruct participants to only observe, rather than direct the breath. Also, guided imagery could be viewed as distancing oneself from the present. In MBSR, guided imagery, such as the mountain meditation, is used as a metaphor to assist in deepening practice (Kabat-Zinn, 2013). In working with frail elders and caregivers, the authors taught the formal and informal practices listed above with some adaptations. For example, the all-day retreat and homework expectations would be shortened or eliminated. For the mindfulness-based elder care program developed by McBee, these modifications also included use of music and aromatherapy as a way of creating a calming milieu in a sometimes chaotic institutional environment (2008). Other adaptations for frail elders included mindful hand massage as one way of connecting with elders with cognitive loss (2008).

Guidelines below describe some teaching modifications. While these methods include adaptations from traditional mindfulness teaching, the core teaching of awareness and compassion remains. As mindfulness teaching expands, there have been, and will continue to be, discussions on the integrity of teaching. The teacher emerges as a key component of teaching, or "The work ultimately depends on you, on who you are as a person" (McCown, Reibel, & Micozzi, 2010, p. 91). What the teacher ideally conveys is authenticity, compassion and presence, and teaching via embodiment as well as words. In working with frail elders, mindfulness teachers are encouraged to be especially aware of conveying these qualities nonverbally, communicating through body language, facial expression, hand gestures, hands-on guidance as well as tone and cadence of voice.

It is impossible to offer detailed guidelines here for teaching mindfulness to frail elders due to the wide range of abilities and disabilities. Some common themes include:

Communication

Elders often experience communication limitations including hearing and vision loss. Identifying this in advance is helpful. In a group, teachers can sit near those with more profound hearing or vision loss to repeat or communicate the instructions or feedback. Demonstrating instructions through dramatic gestures or hands-on instruction in the case of mindful movement is another suggestion. Elders with cognitive limitations will benefit from repeated, simple, concrete instructions, with nonverbal cuing.

Adapting Formal Practices

Meditation times may be shorter, and instructions repeated more frequently. Allow time for participants to settle in and understand the instructions. Physical exercises can be adapted for seated or prone participants. For example, if a group member could only lift one arm, she was encouraged to do so, focusing on remaining abilities rather than disabilities. Mindful walking may become mindful wheeling (in wheelchairs). Some group members may be passive participants and yet still may benefit from the experience of participating in a mindfulness group.

Adapting Informal Practice and Group Discussion

Group discussion may focus on complaints about physical ailments or care providers. This can be an excellent opportunity to encourage group members to use mindfulness skills during challenging moments. For example, if a participant is upset about having to wait for a caregiver, they can practice deep breathing or mindful movement. If concerned about pain, a breath awareness meditation can be suggested.

Caregivers and Mental Health

> Three things in human life are important: the first is to be kind; the second is to be kind; and the third is to be kind.
>
> James (in Edel, ed.) (1972)

Caregivers are integral to the frail elders' physical and mental well-being, and healthier elders may stay well longer with the support of an involved caregiver. Absence of a family caregiver has been linked to hospital readmissions, and caregiver stress is linked to institutionalization of frail elders, demonstrating the overall importance of the caregiver role (Schwartz & Elman, 2003; Spillman & Long, 2009).

The complex and multifaceted medical conditions of elders present challenges for caregivers, especially when combined with cognitive decline, impaired judgment, and even combative behavior. Caregiving is provided by family, friends, volunteers (informal or unpaid), and professionals (formal or paid), often a combination of them. Each of these caregiving groups has unique benefits and stresses associated with the caregiving experience. The sections below will review the research on informal and formal caregivers as well as benefits and options for MBIs. While caregiving can be stressful and lead to physical and emotional challenges for the caregiver, 83 % of caregivers report that the experience is positive (National Opinion

Research Center, 2014). And, perceiving the benefits of caregiving is correlated with lower levels of reported depression (Haley, LaMonde, Han, Burton, & Schonwetter, 2003).

Informal Caregivers

> As desire abates, generosity is born. When we are connected and present, what else is there to do but give?
>
> Kornfield (2015)

Overview

Informal caregivers, unpaid family and friends, provide the majority of assistance for frail elders. Exact numbers are varied, but most estimates are in the tens of millions. The survey "Caregiving in the US" (2009) found that 65 million individuals, or approximately 29 % of the US population, were providing informal care for a disabled friend or family member (National Alliance for Caregiving &AARP, 2009). The majority of care recipients are elders, and their main problems, as reported by their caregivers, are "old age" and dementia. In addition, the average age of both those who give and receive care is increasing, and caregivers may have their own age-related conditions. While all figures cited here are from a US study, they reflect global trends, where developed and less-developed countries also face the complex problems of an aging population.

Engaged informal caregivers have a critical effect on those they care for. Caregiver involvement has been shown to improve outcomes in dementia (Mittelman, Haley, Clay, & Roth, 2006; Vickrey et al., 2006) and to postpone institutionalization (Miller & Weissert, 2000). Caregiver duties may be as basic as a daily phone call but ultimately are unpredictable and may become continuous round-the-clock care. Caregivers may be unable to leave the recipient alone and often neglect their own physical illness or impairments to provide assistance. This situation may affect the caregiver in various ways, including disrupted sleep, emotional and financial difficulties, and physical strain (Wolff, Dy, Frick, & Kasper, 2007). The impact of caregiver stress is so pervasive that a recent article in the Journal of the American Medical Association cautioned physicians to assess caregivers for their level of "caregiver burden" when providing care for frail elders (Adelman, Tmanova, Delgado, Dion, & Lachs, 2014). While not a diagnosis, caregiver burden is defined as the perceived negative effect of caregiving on the caregiver's life and ability to function (Zarit, Todd, & Zarit, 1986). Approximately 30 % of caregivers report that caregiving is highly stressful (National Alliance for Caregiving & AARP, 2009). Supporting this, research strongly correlates links between informal caregiving and elevated stress hormones (Kiecolt-Glaser et al., 2003; Vitaliano, Zhang, & Scanlan, 2003).

Caregivers are also more susceptible to physical illness and psychological distress (Emanuel, Fairclough, Slutsman, & Emanuel, 2000; Pinquart & Sorensen, 2006; Sörensen, Duberstein, Gill, & Pinquart, 2006) and even elevated mortality rates (Christakis & Allison, 2006; Schulz & Beach, 1999). Multiple studies have found that long-term informal caregiving is associated with increasing depression (Burton, Zdaniuk, Schulz, Jackson, & Hirsch, 2003; Cannuscio et al., 2002).

Caregiver mental and physical illness will have obvious tangible effects on their ability to assist care recipients. Less tangible, but equally potent, are the emotional contagions of stress and depression (Goodman & Shippy, 2002; Joiner & Katz, 1999). No matter how frail, cognitively impaired, and/or noncommunicative they are, elders receiving care may perceive the emotional distress of their caregiver and may become distressed as a result. In a French study of 100 community-dwelling informal caregivers and care receivers diagnosed with Alzheimer's disease (AD), Thomas et al. (2006) found that the caregiver's depressive symptoms and quality of life correlated with the care receiver's depressive symptoms, quality of life, and behavior problems.

MBIs for Informal Caregivers

In a meta-analysis of evidence-based practices for caregiver distress, Gallagher-Thompson and Coon (2007) identified key elements of successful interventions as skill building, education, and support. MBSR and MBIs more generally include these elements and show strong evidence in reducing caregiver stress. Pilot studies have demonstrated that teaching MBSR, or modified MBIs, benefitted AD caregivers. Following an 8-week MBSR course one author (LM) offered for informal caregivers at a nursing home, participants reported decreased stress, anxiety, grief, and caregiver burden. After a 4-week follow-up, they reported further reduction in all measures except depression. Participants also expressed greater satisfaction in the caregiving role and found the group discussions focused on reducing stress while caregiving (Epstein-Lubow, McBee, Darling, Armey, & Miller, 2011). Other pilot studies have found that AD caregivers participating in mindfulness training improved psychological symptoms compared to control participants (Franco, Sola Mdel, & Justo, 2010; Ho et al., 2011; Norouzi, Golzari, & Sohrabi, 2013; Oken et al., 2010). In two randomized controlled studies for family AD caregivers, an MBSR group was compared with a matched control support group. Participants in both groups showed reduced stress and depression (Coogle, Brown, Hellerstein, & Rudolph, 2011; Whitebird et al., 2012).

MBSR and MBIs more generally hold significant potential for mitigating caregiver stress and increasing a sense of self-efficacy. Unfortunately, while caregivers are at high risk for stress and stress-related problems, there are realistic practical and emotional obstacles to providing needed self-care. The majority of caregivers are also employed, and many report juggling work schedules as well as sacrificing time with friends and other family members for caregiving (National Alliance for

Caregiving & AARP, 2009). There may also be underlying resistance to self-care or to viewing oneself as vulnerable. Moreover, a frequent symptom of depression is a lack of motivation, decreasing the likelihood of seeking support. Modifications of mindfulness teaching may increase participation in either brief MBI programs or traditional MBSR for this busy and stressed population. To begin, it may be helpful to consider adapting time commitment expectations for meeting and practice, accessibility of location of classes, and highlighting applicability to caregiving. Dosage and effect of mindfulness teaching and practice is a focus of current and ongoing studies, with some targeting caregivers. Carmody and Baer (2009) reviewed published standard and shortened MBSR programs and found no significant correlation between mean effect size and number of in-class hours. In one study for caregivers, a yogic form of meditation, Kirtan Kriya, was assigned for 12 minutes per day for 8 weeks. Participants in the experimental Kirtan Kriya group improved in mental health and cognitive functioning, psychological distress, and telomerase activity as compared to controls (Lavretsky et al., 2013). Another study found that a 4-hour mindfulness training offered to caregivers increased acceptance, presence, peace, and hope, as well as decreased reactivity and caregiver burden (Hoppes, Bryce, Hellman, & Finlay, 2012).

Research conducted with caregivers and populations with intellectual disabilities (ID) and developmental disabilities (DD) holds implications for AD caregivers, since both cope regularly with behavioral challenges. Singh et al. (2004) found that when ID caregivers received mindfulness training, their patients were happier. In another study, he and colleagues found that when ID parents received mindfulness training, their children showed greater positive and less aggressive behaviors (Singh et al., 2007). Research increasingly points to the benefits of learning stress reduction skills for both caregivers and care receivers. Harmell, Chattillion, Roepke, and Mausbach, (2011) analyzed key characteristics of resilience in caregivers for persons with dementia and found higher levels of personal mastery and self-efficacy and increased use of positive coping strategies appear to have a protective effect on various health outcomes. In addition, Lewallen and Neece (2015) found family caregiver stress was reduced following participation in an MBSR class and that this was also associated with improved behavior and social skills for their developmentally delayed children with DD.

Reflection

How do I feel about caregiving? Do I view it as a burden? Am I bringing a light heart to the experience? How would I feel if I were dependent on others for my basic needs?

Practice

Can I find ways to bring lightness and joy to caregiving? Remember, "we don't stop playing because we grow old; we grow old because we stop playing."- George Bernard Shaw

How am I cared for in less obvious ways by others? How would I feel if my needs increased?

Smile, fake it if you have to. Laugh. Smile and laugh with the person(s) you care for.

Paraprofessional and Professional Caregivers

We cannot cure the world of sorrows, but we can choose to live in joy.

Campbell (2011)

Medical professionals working with frail elders are under increasing pressure due to changing reimbursement systems, managed care, challenging end-of-life decision-making, and treating simultaneous chronic conditions, many of which are drug resistant. Job stress directly impacts patient care. Doctors experiencing burnout, a result of long-term stress, report giving less than optimal patient care (Shanafelt, Bradley, Wipf, & Back, 2002). Geriatric healthcare workers may be especially vulnerable to "burnout," the emotional exhaustion experienced by those who work with people (Freudenberger, 1974). Both nurses and nursing assistants studied in a long-term care facility linked a significant correlation between stress and inadequate preparation to meet the emotional needs of clients and perform job duties (Kennedy, 2005).

Professionals, such as doctors, social workers, nurses, and therapists, all deliver care to frail elders, but paraprofessionals, or nursing assistants, provide 70–80 % of the basic, life-sustaining personal care. This direct-care workforce is currently the largest US occupational group and the fastest growing (Paraprofessional Healthcare Institute (PHI), 2013, Bureau of Labor Statistics (BLS), 2007). The aging population with multiple chronic conditions will require exactly the personal care provided by paraprofessionals, over longer and longer periods. US paraprofessionals are overwhelmingly female; many are of ethnic minority and/or foreign born, and most have a high school diploma or less (Figueiredo, 2010). They are at physical risk due to disease exposure and the physical demands of direct care with often confused and combative patients (Bureau of Labor Statistics (BLS), 2008). The work is high risk, yet poorly paying, leading to significant job stress (Figueiredo, 2010). Unsurprisingly, more than one in ten paraprofessionals have reported depression lasting 2 weeks or longer, the highest rates of any occupation (Mental Health Services Administration & Office of Applied Studies (October 11, 2007)). Paraprofessional stress results in high job turnover and unsatisfactory communication (DHHS and DOL U.S. Department of Health and Human Services and U.S. Department of Labor (DHHS and DOL), 2003).

MBIs for Formal Caregivers

A recent study found that burnout was significantly associated with suboptimal self-reported patient care (Shanafelt et al., 2002). In 2009, the *Journal of the American Medical Association* published a study by Krasner and colleagues (2009) reporting reductions in burnout and improvements in mood and professional behavior following an 8-week MBSR course with 10-month follow-up for physicians. Additional studies also demonstrate that mindfulness-based programs for healthcare professionals are feasible and effective for reducing burnout and improving patient care (Beckman et al., 2012; Irving, Dobkin, & Park, 2009; Schenstrom, Ronnberg, &

Bolund, 2006). In addition, a doctoral study found that professional dementia caregivers who participated in an 8-week mindfulness class that included information on dementia and challenging behaviors showed improvements in staff well-being and adaptive attitudes toward people with dementia (Clague, 2010). One author (LM) experimented with a wide range of formats, locations, timing, and other teaching adaptations of mindfulness for staff at a large nursing home. All models were found to have some success and created a broader facility awareness of the personal and professional benefits of mindfulness for self-care [see below and McBee, 2008]. Finding time to attend stress reduction classes, either by taking time on or off the job, was the most challenging obstacle. In a shortened (4-week) class based on MBSR and MBCT offered to nurses and nursing assistants in a geriatric hospital, researchers found that participants demonstrated significant improvements in symptoms of burnout and increased relaxation and life satisfaction when compared to a similar wait-listed group (Mackenzie, Poulin, & Seidman-Carlson, 2006).

Cognitive problems, including dementia and intellectual disability, often lead to challenging behaviors as a result of frustration and lack of inhibition, causing distress and injury to both patient and staff (Ozga, M. (November 3, 2011); Rymer et al., 2002). Pilot studies offering mindfulness-based programs to staff caring for people with intellectual disabilities(ID) report promising results, including increased awareness of stress and reductions in psychological distress as well as improvements in self-care and interactions with peers and clients (Bethay, Wilson, Schnetzer, Nassar, & Bordieri, 2012; Brooker et al., 2012; Noone & Hastings, 2010). Studies have also shown a correlation between mindfulness programs for staff and improved patient/client care (Singh et al., 2004). One meta-analysis reviewed 11 studies and found mindfulness programs offered to persons with ID improved behaviors, and that mindfulness programs offered to family and professional caregivers improved relationships and job satisfaction (Chapman et al., 2013). Following a 7-day intensive training of mindfulness-based positive behavior support (MBPBS) for staff caring for those with developmental disabilities (DD) in three residential group homes, staff stress level improved, resident restraints were discontinued, and staff and peer injuries ceased (Singh et al., 2014). Byron, Ziedonis, McGrath, Frazier, and Fulwiler (2014) also found that residential staff caring for adolescents with DD reported an MBI program provided an environmental shift that increased focus and increased cohesion on the unit.

Suggestions for Teaching Mindfulness to Informal and Formal Caregivers

> It is relationality above all else... that is at the heart of mindfulness.
>
> Kabat-Zinn (2013, p. 265)

The range of those who receive care and those who give care, as well as their environments, additional support or lack thereof, financial resources, and other essential factors, are as varied as the general population. Despite some differences, the overwhelming majority of caregivers readily assert a need for stress reduction in the experience of these authors. The major obstacles for caregivers are time limitations; inability to leave care receiver and/or find backup care; and resistance to, or postponement of, self-care. Thus, the primary challenge to teaching mindfulness to caregivers may be to get them in the room.

Educating caregivers on the causes and effects of chronic long-term stress on their emotional and physical well-being may be an incentive. One author (LM) offered a one hour in-service for all nursing home staff that included this information followed by mindful meditation and gentle stretching. Family and professional caregivers may also benefit from a discussion on the contagious nature of emotions (see description above under Caregiver/Overview). Family caregivers for noninstitutionalized elders may need respite arrangements and even transportation to attend mindfulness groups. Groups held in nursing homes or hospitals could include both caregivers and care receivers, modifying instructions and programs as appropriate. Holding classes in locations convenient for caregivers is also helpful.

Once recruited, groups or individual classes for caregivers may need to be briefer. One author (LM) visited nursing units during times when not providing direct care (charting time) and offered simple skills training on breath awareness or mindful movement. Both family and professional caregivers anecdotally report benefiting from skills that they could use in the midst of their busy lives (Author LM). Caregivers used diaphragmatic/deep breathing when in challenging situations and practiced standing or seated mountain pose throughout the day. In addition to teaching these practices, suggesting practical applications helps. For example, caregivers can be encouraged to stop and take a deep breath before encountering a challenging situation or to stand in mountain pose while waiting in line. These pauses with intentional awareness on physical sensation lead to more habitual poses and perhaps an ability to respond, rather than react, to stressful situations.

Teacher presence is also an important factor. Caregivers may miss classes or spend class time complaining about the challenges of caregiving. If classes are missed, the teacher can call the absent participants with encouragement and support. When caregivers complain, the teacher may find this an excellent teaching opportunity. With curiosity and compassion, the discussion can reframe the conversation as inquiry. Inquiry into the caregivers' subjective experience, as described by McCown, Reibel, and Micozzi (2010), is "'cultivating observation' and 'moving towards acceptance'" (p. 127) that honors the individual wisdom held by all.

Conclusion: Cultivating Equanimity

In 2008, the Institution of Medicine described the "impending crisis" in healthcare provision for older adults. Aside from workforce shortages, recommendations for fundamental changes include promoting new models of care, increased training and support for family and professional caregivers, and a comprehensive view of health for older adults and inclusion of patients and families in decision-making. Mindfulness practices might offer key benefits for this aging population and their caregivers. Cultivating awareness and compassion may provide frail elders and caregivers with equanimity in the face of mortality, illness, loss, and frailty. Equanimity, an attitude of openness and acceptance, has not previously been regarded as a quantifiable outcome in mindfulness research, but a leading group of scientific mindfulness researchers has reviewed the psychological, physiological, and neuroimaging assessments that have been applied in measuring equanimity and also endorses this outcome measure as potentially the most important element in reflecting the ability of mindfulness to improve overall well-being (Desbordes et al., 2014).

Mindfulness practices promote our ability to view aging holistically, not pathologically. Increasing evidence supports the preventative benefits of mindfulness on our brain and body. Recent studies also link mindfulness and measures of psychological well-being, including self-reported depressive symptoms, quality of life, and stress profile (Fiocco & Mallya, 2015). Anecdotally, and through various studies, both authors (LM and PB) have found mindfulness not only teachable to elders and caregivers but also overwhelmingly well received and profoundly informative for the challenges of aging. One author (LM) found in groups in the nursing home that included residents, staff, and family/friend caregivers, the lines between teacher and taught diminish, and all learned from one another. Following many mindfulness groups, elders report increased acceptance, quiet, and peace. One informal caregiver found: "I feel less anxious about stresses than I formerly did. I think about 'riding the waves' instead of getting anxious about them or 'fighting' the waves. I feel less responsible for my husband's well-being." Both formal and informal caregivers report increased self-efficacy as well as a deeper understanding described by this formal caregiver, "I remember thinking many times during the class that this work has a way of bringing us all to a common denominator. We all have bodies, breath, and thoughts." One family caregiver even stated "she no longer felt she ever had to be alone again" (McBee, 2008).

Ultimately, the true practice for teachers and clinicians is to work with our own perceptions and beliefs on aging, limitations, dependency, and dying. Embodiment of the practice of awareness and compassion is conveyed verbally and nonverbally by the teacher. As mindfulness teachers, practitioners, and clinicians, we can teach mindfulness practices with adaptations to frail elders and caregivers. However, the most important skill/intervention/knowledge we bring to frail elders and their caregivers is our presence, who we are in each moment.

> Within each health care practitioner lives the Wounded One; in every patient, every sick and suffering human being, abides a powerful Inner Healer.
>
> Santorelli (1990, p. 15)

References

Adelman, R. D., Tmanova, L. L., Delgado, D., Dion, S., & Lachs, M. S. (2014). Caregiver burden: A clinical review. *JAMA, 311*, 1052–1060.

Ball, M. S., & Vernon, B. (2014). A review on how meditation could be used to comfort the terminally ill. *Palliative Support Care, 30*, 1–4.

Beckman, H. B., Wendland, M., Mooney, C., Krasner, M. S., Quill, T. E., Suchman, A. L., et al. (2012). The impact of a program in mindful communication on primary care physicians. *Academy of Medicine, 87*, 815–819.
Bennett, J., & O'Donovan, D. (2001). Substance misuse by doctors, nurses and other healthcare workers. *Current Opinion in Psychiatry, 14*, 195–199.
Benshoff, J. J., Harrawood, L. K., & Koch, D. S. (2003). Substance abuse and the elderly: Unique issues and concerns. *Journal of Rehabilitation, 69*, 43–48.
Bethay, J. S., Wilson, K. G., Schnetzer, L. W., Nassar, S. L., & Bordieri, M. J. (2012). A controlled pilot evaluation of acceptance and commitment training for intellectual disability staff. April 2012. Retrieved online 3/24/13 from *Mindfulness.*http://link.springer.com/article/10.1007%2Fs12671-012-0103-8?LI=true#
Black, D. S., O'Reilly, G. A., Olmstead, R., Breen, E. C., & Irwin, M. R. (2015). Mindfulness meditation and improvement in sleep quality and daytime impairment among older adults with sleep disturbances: A randomized clinical trial. *JAMA Internal Medicine*. doi:10.1001/jamainternmed.2014.8081. Published online February 16, 2015.
Bloom, H. G., Ahmed, I., Alessi, C. A., Ancoli-Israel, S., Buyesse, D. J., Kryger, M. H., et al. (2009). Evidence-based recommendations for the assessment and management of sleep disorders in older persons. *Journal of the American Geriatric Society, 57*, 761–789.
Brooker, J., Julian, J., Webber, L., Chan, J., Shawyer, F., & Meadows, G. (2012). Evaluation of an occupational mindfulness program for staff employed in the disability sector in Australia. Published online, May 2012, retrieved 3/23/13 from *Mindfulness*. http://link.springer.com/article/10.1007%2Fs12671-012-0112-7?LI=true#
Bureau of Labor Statistics (BLS). (2007). *The 0 fastest-growing occupations, 00–0*. http://www.bls.gov/news release/ecopro.t06.htm. Accessed December 26, 2007.
Bureau of Labor Statistics (BLS). (2008). *Household data annual averages*. http://www.bls.gov/cps/cpsa2007.pdf. Accessed February 24, 2008. (BLS. 2008b)
Burton, L. C., Zdaniuk, B., Schulz, R., Jackson, S., & Hirsch, C. (2003). Transitions in spousal caregiving. *Gerontologist, 43*, 230–241.
Butler, R. N. (1980). Ageism: A foreword. *Journal of Social Issues, 36*, 8–11. doi:10.1111/j.1540-4560.1980.tb02018.x.
Byron, G., Ziedonis, D. M., McGrath, C., Frazier, J. A., & Fulwiler, C. (2014). Implementation of mindfulness training for mental health staff: Organizational context and stakeholder perspectives. *Mindfulness, 1–12*.
Campbell, J. (2011). *In the Field*. In R. Walker, & D. Kudler (Eds.), *A Joseph Campbell companion: Reflections on the art of living* [E-book by Stillpoint Digital Press for Kindle]. ISBN: 9781611780062.
Cannuscio, C. C., Jones, C., Kawachi, I., Colditz, G. A., Berkman, L., & Rimm, E. (2002). Reverberations of family illness: A longitudinal assessment of informal caregiving and mental health status in the nurses' health study. *American Journal of Public Health, 92*, 1305–1311.
Carlson, L. E. (2012). Mindfulness-based interventions for physical conditions. *ISRN Psychiatry*. Article ID: 651583. doi:10.5402/2012/651583
Carlson, L. E., Speca, M., Patel, K. D., & Goodey, E. (2003). Mindfulness-based stress reduction in relation to quality of life, mood, symptoms of stress, and immune parameters in breast and prostate cancer outpatients. *Psychosomatic Medicine, 65*, 571–581.
Carmody, J., & Baer, R. A. (2009). How long does a mindfulness-based stress reduction program need to be? A review of class contact hours and effect sizes for psychological distress. *Journal of Clinical Psychology, 65*, 627–638.
Cavalieri, T. A. (2007). Management of pain in older adults. *Journal of the American OsteopathicAssociation, 107*(6 suppl), ES10–ES16.
Chapman, M. J., Hare, D. J., Caton, S., Donalds, D., McInnis, E., & Mitchell, D. (2013). The use of mindfulness with people with intellectual disabilities: A systematic review and narrative analysis. *Mindfulness, 4*, 179–189.
Christakis, N. A., & Allison, P. D. (2006). Mortality after the hospitalization of a spouse. *New England Journal of Medicine, 354*, 719–730.

Clague, F. (2010). Doctoral thesis: The impact of mindfulness training on reflective thinking and attitudes towards patients in dementia care. Retrieved 7/29/13 from www.ed.ac.uk/polopoly_fs/1.70576!/fileManager/abstracts2010.pdf

Cohen-Mansfield, J. (1997). Conceptualization of agitation: Results based on the Cohen-Mansfield agitation inventory and the agitation behavior mapping instrument. *International Psychogeriatrics, 8*, 309–315.

Coleman, G., & Thupten, J. (Eds.). (2006). *The Tibetan book of the dead*. New York: Penguin Group.

Coogle, C. L., Brown, K. W., Hellerstein, J. M., & Rudolph, A. (2011). *Mindfulness-based Alzheimer's caregiving: A randomized controlled trial, a replication report*. Retrieved 2/3/13 at www.sahp.vcu.edu/vcoa/program/reports/pdfs/aoa_reporting.pdf

Creswell, J. D., Irwin, M. R., Burklund, L. J., Lieberman, M. D., Arevalo, J. M., Ma, J., et al. (2012). Mindfulness-based stress reduction training reduces loneliness and pro-inflammatory gene expression in older adults: A small randomized controlled trial. *Brain, Behavior, and Immunity, 26*, 1095–1101.

Desbordes, G., Gard, T., Hoge, E. A., Holzel, B., Kerr, C., Lazar, S., et al. (2014). Moving beyond mindfulness: Defining equanimity as an outcome measure in meditation and contemplative research. *Mindfulness*. doi:10.1007/s12671-013-0269-8.

DHHS and DOL U.S. Department of Health and Human Services and U.S. Department of Labor (DHHS and DOL). (2003). *The future supply of long-term care workers in relation to the aging baby boom generation*. Washington, DC: U.S. Department of Health and Human Services.

Dylan, B. (1966). Rainy day women #12 & 35, from *Blonde on Blonde,* Dwarf Music.

Edel, L. (1972). *Henry James: A life* (The Master 1901–1916, Vol. V). Philadelphia, PA: Lippincott.

Emanuel, E. J., Fairclough, D. L., Slutsman, J., & Emanuel, L. L. (2000). Understanding economic and other burdens of terminal illness: The experience of patients and their caregivers. *Annals of Internal Medicine, 132*, 451–459.

Epstein-Lubow, G., McBee, L., Darling, E., Armey, M., & Miller, I. W. (2011). A pilot investigation of mindfulness-based stress reduction for caregivers of frail elderly. *Mindfulness, 2*, 95–102.

Figueiredo, C. (2010). PHI analysis of U.S. census Bureau, current population survey, 2010 *Annual Social & Economic (ASEC) Supplement,* Retrieved from http://phinational.org/direct-care-workers-glance. May 20, 2015.

Fiocco, A. J., & Mallya, S. (2015). The importance of cultivating mindfulness for cognitive and emotional well-being in late life. *Journal of Evidence-Based Complementary & Alternative Medicine, 20*, 35–40.

Franco, C., Sola Mdel, M., & Justo, E. (2010). Reducing psychological discomfort and overload in Alzheimer's family caregivers through a mindfulness meditation program. *Revista Española de Geriatría y Gerontología, 45*, 252–258.

Freudenberger, H. J. (1974). Staff burn-out. *Journal of Social Issues, 30*, 159–165.

Gallagher-Thompson, D., & Coon, D. W. (2007). Evidence-based psychological treatments for distress in family caregivers of older adults. *Psychology and Aging, 22*, 37–51.

Gallup Poll. (2005). Sleep and healthy aging. *The Gallup Organization.* Published online July 21, 2008. Available at http://www.gallup.com/poll/20323/Older-Americans-Dream-Good-Nights-Sleep.aspx

Gard, T., Holzel, B. K., & Lazar, S. W. (2014). The potential effects of meditation on age-related cognitive decline: A systematic review. *Annals of the New York Academy of Sciences, 1307*, 89–103. doi:10.1111/nyas.12348.

Gawande, A. (2014). *Being mortal: Medicine and what matters in the end*. New York: Metropolitan Books, Henry Holt and Company, LLC.

Gfroerer, J., Penne, M., Pemberton, M., & Folsom, R. (2003). Substance abuse treatment need among older adults in 2020: The impact of the aging baby-boom cohort. *Drug and Alcohol Dependence, 69*, 127–135.

Goodman, C. R., & Shippy, R. A. (2002). Is it contagious? Affect similarity among spouses. *Aging & Mental Health, 6*, 266–274.

Goodwin, J. (1983). Common psychiatric disorders in elderly persons. *Western Journal of Medicine, 139*, 502–506.

Gordon, R. M., & Brill, D. (2001). The abuse and neglect of the elderly. *International Journal of Law and Psychiatry, 24*, 183–197.

Goyal, M., Singh, S., Sibinga, E. M., Gould, N. F., Rowland-Seymoore, A., Shama, R., et al. (2014). Meditation programs for psychological stress and well-being: A systematic review and meta-analysis. *JAMA Internal Medicine., 174*(3), 357–368. doi:10.1001/jamainternmed.2013.13018.

Grant, J. (2014). Meditative analgesia: The current state of the field. *Annals of the New York Academy of Sciences, 1307*, 55–63.

Gross, C. R., Kreitzer, M. J., Thomas, W., Reilly-Spong, M., Cramer-Bernemann, M., Nyman, J. A., et al. (2010). Mindfulness-based stress reduction for solid organ transplant recipients: A randomized controlled trial. *Alternative Therapy Health Medicine, 16*, 30–38.

Gupta, S., & Warner, J. (2008). Alcohol-related dementia: A 21st-century silent epidemic? *The British Journal of Psychiatry, 193*, 351–353.

Haley, W. E., LaMonde, L. A., Han, B., Burton, A. M., & Schonwetter, R. (2003). Predictors of depression and life satisfaction among spousal caregivers in hospice: Application of a stress process model. *Journal of Palliative Medicine, 6*, 215–224.

Harmell, A. L., Chattillion, E. A., Roepke, S. K., & Mausbach, B. T. (2011). A review of the psychobiology of dementia caregiving: A focus on resilience factors. *Current Psychiatry Reports, 13*, 219–224.

Ho, L., Bloom, P., Vega, J., Yemul, S., Zhao, W., & Pasinetti, G. (2011). Mindfulness-based stress reduction for caregivers of patients with Alzheimer's disease. *Alzheimer's & Dementia*, 7(Supplement), S431.

Holzel, B. K., Carmody, J., Vangel, M., Congleton, C., Yerramsetti, S. M., Gard, T., et al. (2011). Mindfulness practice leads to increases in regional brain gray matter density. *Psychiatry Research: Neuroimaging, 191*, 36–43. doi:10.1016/j.psychresns.2010.08.006.

Homer, A. C., & Gilleard, C. (1990). Abuse of elderly people by their carers. *British Medical Journal, 301*(6765), 1359–1362.

Hoppes, S., Bryce, H., Hellman, C., & Finlay, E. (2012). The effects of brief mindfulness training on caregivers' well-being. *Activities, Adaptation, & Aging, 36*, 147–166.

Institute of Medicine (IOM) of the National Academies. (2008). *Retooling for an aging America: Building the health care workforce*. Washington, DC: The National Academies. Retrieved March 8, 2015, from http://www.iom.edu/agingamerica.

Irving, J. A., Dobkin, P. L., & Park, J. (2009). Cultivating mindfulness in health care professionals: A review of empirical studies of mindfulness-based stress reduction (MBSR). *Complementary Therapies in Clinical Practice, 15*, 61–66.

James, B. D., Leurgans, S. E., Hebert, L. E., Scherr, P. A., Yaffe, K., & Bennett, D. A. (2014). Contribution of Alzheimer disease to mortality in the United States. *Neurology*. doi:10.1212/WNL.0000000000000240. Published online December 11, 2013.

Joiner, T. E., Jr., & Katz, J. (1999). Contagion of depressive symptoms and mood: Meta-analytic review and explanations from cognitive, behavioral, and interpersonal viewpoints. *Clinical Psychology: Science and Practice, 6*(2), 149–164.

Kabat-Zinn, J. (1982). An out-patient program in behavioral medicine for chronic pain patients based on the practice of mindfulness meditation: Theoretical considerations and preliminary results. *General Hospital Psychiatry, 4*, 33–47.

Kabat-Zinn, J. (2013). *Full catastrophe living, revised edition*. New York: Bantam Books.

Kabat-Zinn, J., Lipworth, L., & Burney, R. (1985). The clinical use of mindfulness meditation for the self-regulation of chronic pain. *Journal of Behavioral Medicine, 8*, 163–190.

Kennedy, B. R. (2005). Stress and burnout of nursing staff working with geriatric clients in long-term care. *Journal of Nursing Scholarship, 37*, 381–382.

Kiecolt-Glaser, J. K., Preacher, K. J., MacCallum, R. C., Atkinson, C., Malarkey, W. B., & Glaser, R. (2003). Chronic stress and age-related increases in the proinflammatory cytokine IL-6. *Proceedings of the National Academy of Sciences of the United States of America, 100*, 9090–9095.

Kornfield, J. (2015). *You will survive*. Retrieved May 15, 2015 from http://www.jackkornfield.com/you-will-survive/

Krasner, M. S., Epstein, R. M., Beckman, H., Suchman, A. L., Chapman, B., Mooney, C. J., et al. (2009). Association of an educational program in mindful communication with burnout, empathy, and attitudes among primary care physicians. *Journal of the American Medical Association, 302*, 1284–1293.

Krause, N. (2004). Stressors arising in highly valued roles, meaning in life, and the physical health status of older adults. *The Journals of Gerontology Series B: Psychological Sciences and Social Sciences, 59*, S287–S297.

Kyokai, B. D. (2006). *The teachings of Buddha*. New Delhi: Sterling.

Lantz, M. S., Buchalter, E. N., & McBee, L. (1997). The wellness group: A novel intervention for coping with disruptive behavior in elderly nursing home residents. *The Gerontologist, 37*, 551–557.

Lau, D. T., Mercaldo, N. D., Harris, A. T., Trittschuh, E., Shega, J., & Weintraub, S. (2010). Polypharmacy and potentially inappropriate medication use among community-dwelling elders with dementia. *Alzheimer Disease and Associated Disorders, 24*, 56–63. doi:10.1097/WAD.0b013e31819d6ec9.

Lavretsky, H. H., Epel, E. S., Siddarth, P., Nazarian, N., Saint-Cyr, N., Khalsa, D. S., et al. (2013). A pilot study of yogic meditation for family dementia caregivers with depressive symptoms: Effects on mental health, cognition, and telomerase activity Yogic meditation for stress reduction in dementia caregivers. *International Journal of Geriatric Psychiatry, 28*, 57–65.

Levine, S., & Levine, O. (1989). *Who dies? An investigation of conscious living and conscious dying*. New York: Anchor Books, a Division of Random House, Inc.

Levy, B. (2009). Stereotype embodiment a psychosocial approach to aging. *Current Directions in Psychological Science, 18*, 332–336.

Lewallen, A. C., & Neece, C. L. (2015). Improved social skills in children with developmental delays after parent participation in MBSR: The role of parent–child relational factors. *Journal of Child and Family Studies*. Retrieved 5/5/15 from: http://link.springer.com/article/10.1007/s10826-015-0116-8#page-1

Luders, E., Cherbuin, N., & Kurth, F. (2015). Forever young(er): Potential age-defying effects of long-term meditation on gray matter atrophy. *Frontiers in Psychology*. doi:10.3389/fpsyg.2014.01551.

Mackenzie, C. S., & Poulin, P. A. (2006). Living with the dying: Using the wisdom of mindfulness to support caregivers of older adults with dementia. *International Journal of Health Promotion and Education, 44*, 43–47.

Mackenzie, C. S., Poulin, P. A., & Seidman-Carlson, R. (2006). A brief mindfulness-based stress reduction intervention for nurses and nurse aides. *Applied Nursing Research, 19*, 105–109.

Malec, M., & Shega, J. W. (2014). Pain management in the elderly. *Medical Clinics of North America, 99*, 337–50.

McBee, L. (2008). *Mindfulness-based elder care: A CAM model for frail elders and their caregivers*. New York: Springer.

McCown, D., Reibel, D., & Micozzi, M. S. (2010). *Teaching mindfulness: A practical guide for clinicians and educators*. New York: Springer.

Meeten, F., Whiting, S., & Williams, C. M. (2014). An exploratory study of group mindfulness-based cognitive therapy for older people with depression. *Mindfulness*. doi:10.1007/s12671-014-0279-1.

Miller, R. (January 1, 1973). *Roger Miller with his friends and his music*. ABC television http://quoteinvestigator.com/2012/09/21/get-wet/

Miller, E. A., & Weissert, W. G. (2000). Predicting elderly people's risk for nursing home placement, hospitalization, functional impairment, and mortality: A synthesis. *Medical Care Research and Review, 57*, 259–297.

Mittelman, M. S., Haley, W. E., Clay, O. J., & Roth, D. L. (2006). Improving caregiver well-being delays nursing home placement of patients with Alzheimer Disease. *Neurology, 67*, 1592–1599.

Morone, N. E., Greco, C. M., & Weiner, D. K. (2008). Mindfulness meditation for the treatment of chronic low back pain in older adults: A randomized controlled pilot study. *Pain, 134*, 310–319.

Morone, N. E., Rollman, B. L., & Moore, C. G. (2009). A mind-body program for older adults with chronic low back pain: Results of a pilot study. *Pain Medicine, 10*, 1395–1407.

Moss, A. S., Reibel, D. K., Greeson, J. M., Thapar, A., Bubb, R., Salmon, J. et al. (2014). An adapted mindfulness-based stress reduction program for elders in a continuing care retirement community: Quantitative and qualitative results from a pilot randomized controlled trial. *Journal of Applied Gerontology*. pii: 0733464814559411. [Epub ahead of print]

Moussavi, S., Chatterji, S., Verdes, E., Tandon, A., Patel, V., & Ustun, B. (2007). Depression, chronic diseases, and decrements in health: Results from the World Health Surveys. *The Lancet, 370*(9590), 851–858.

Murrell, S. A., Himmelfarb, S., & Wright, K. (1983). Prevalence of depression and its correlates in older adults. *American Journal of Epidemiology, 117*, 173–185.

National Alliance for Caregiving &AARP. (2009). *Caregiving in the US*. Retrieved from www.caregiving.org/data/Caregiving_in_the_US_2009_full_report.pdf. Accessed on May 22, 2015.

National Opinion Research Center. (2014, May). *Long term care in America: Expectations and realities*. Retrieved from http://www.longtermcarepoll.org/PDFs/LTC%202014/AP-NORC-Long-Term%20Care%20in%20America_FINAL%20WEB.pdf

Newberg, A. B., Serruya, M., Wintering, N., Moss, A. S., Reibel, D., & Monti, D. A. (2014). Meditation and neurodegenerative diseases. *Annals of the New York Academy of Sciences, 1307*, 112–123.

Nhat Hanh, T. (1990). *Present moment wonderful moment: Mindfulness verses for daily living*. Berkeley, CA: Parallax.

Noone, S. J., & Hastings, R. P. (2010). Using acceptance and mindfulness-based workshops with support staff caring for adults with intellectual disabilities. *Mindfulness, 1*, 67–73.

Norouzi, M., Golzari, M., & Sohrabi, F. (2013). Effectiveness of mindfulness based cognitive therapy on the quality of life, depression and burden of Alzheimer's women caregivers. *Journal of Research in Medical Sciences*. Retrieved 3/22/13 from http://www.zjrms.ir/browse.php?a_code=A-10-1770-2&slc_lang=en&sid=en

O'Connor, M., Piet, J., & Hougaard, E. (2013). The effects of mindfulness-based cognitive therapy on depressive symptoms in elderly bereaved people with loss-related distress: A controlled pilot study. *Mindfulness*. doi:10.1007/s12671-013-0194-x.

Oken, B. S., Fonareva, I., Haas, M., Wahbeh, H., Lane, J. B., Zajdel, D., et al. (2010). Pilot controlled trial of mindfulness meditation and education for dementia caregivers. *The Journal of Alternative and Complementary Medicine, 16*, 1031–1038.

Ozga, M. (November 3, 2011). *Nursing and residential care workers suffer highest occupational injury rates*. Retrieved from http://phinational.org/blogs/nursing-and-residential-care-workers-suffer-highest-occupational-injury-rates. Accessed on May 20, 2015.

Paraprofessional Healthcare Institute (PHI). (2013). *PHI facts*. Retrieved from http://phinational.org/fact-sheets/facts-3-americas-direct-care-workforce. Accessed on May 20, 2015.

Patterson, T. L., & Jeste, D. V. (1999). The potential impact of the baby-boom generation of substance abuse among elderly persons. *Psychiatric Services: Special Section on Mental Health and Aging, 50*, 1184–1188. doi:10.1176/ps.50.9.1184.

Phillips, V. L., & Diwan, S. (2003). The incremental effect of dementia-related problem behaviors on the time to nursing home placement in poor, frail, demented older people. *Journal of the American Geriatrics Society, 51*, 188–193.

Pinquart, M., & Sorensen, S. (2006). Helping caregivers of persons with dementia: Which interventions work and how large are their effects? *International Psychogeriatrics, 18*, 577–595.

Quintana Hernandez, D. J., Miro Barrachina, M. T., Ibanez Fernandez, I., Del Pino, A. S., Garcia Rodriguez, J. R., & Hernandez, J. R. (2014). Effects of a neuropsychology program based on mindfulness on Alzheimer's disease: Randomized double-blind clinical study. *Revista española de geriatría y gerontología*. pii: S0211-139X(14)00056-0. doi:10.1016/j.regg.2014.03.002

Rajguru, P., Kolber, M. J., Garcia, A. N., Smith, M. T., Patel, C. K., & Hanney, W. J. (2014). Use of mindfulness meditation in the management of chronic pain: A systematic review of randomized controlled trials. *American Journal of Lifestyle Medicine*. doi:10.1177/1559827614522580.

Ridley, N. J., Draper, B., & Withall, A. (2013). Alcohol-related dementia: An update of the evidence. *Alzheimer's Research & Therapy*. doi:10.1186/alzrt157. Published online January 25, 2013.

Rodda, J., Walker, Z., & Carter, J. (2011). Depression in older adults. *British Medical Journal*. doi:10.1136/bmj.d5219. Published online July 28, 2011.

Rosenberg, L., & Guy, D. (2000). *Living in the light of death: On the art of being truly alive*. Boston, MA: Shambala.

Rymer, S., Salloway, S., Norton, L., Malloy, P., Correia, S., & Monast, D. (2002). Impaired awareness, behavior disturbance, and caregiver burden in Alzheimer disease. *Alzheimer Disease & Associated Disorders, 16*(4), 248–253.

Sacks, O. (2015, February 19). *My own life*. The New York Times. Retrieved from http://www.nytimes.com/2015/02/19/opinion/oliver-sacks-on-learning-he-has-terminal-cancer.html?_r=3

Sahyoun, N. R., Lentzner, H., Hoyert, D., & Robinson, K. N. (2001).Trends in causes of death among the elderly. *Aging Trends*, 1, Hyattsville, Maryland: National Center for Health Statistics.

Santorelli, S. (1990). *Heal thyself: Lessons on mindfulness in medicine*. New York: Bell Tower.

Sapolsky, R. M. (2004). *Why Zebras don't get ulcers*. New York: Henry Holt.

Sasi, K., Ramesh, A. K., & Anice, G. (2014). Effectiveness of mindfulness based stress reduction (MBSR) on stress and anxiety among elderly residing in residential homes. *International Journal of Nursing Care, 2*(2), 81–85. doi:10.5958/2320-8651.2014.01276.9.

Schenstrom, A., Ronnberg, S., & Bolund, O. (2006). Mindfulness-based cognitive attitude training for primary care staff: A pilot study. *Complementary Health Practice Review, 11*, 144–152.

Schulz, R., & Beach, S. R. (1999). Caregiving as a risk factor for mortality. *Journal of the American Medical Association, 282*, 2215–2219.

Schwartz, K., & Elman, C. (2003). Identification of factors predictive of hospital readmissions for patients with heart failure. *Heart and Lung, 32*, 88–99.

Segal, Z. V., Williams, J. M. G., & Teasdale, J. D. (2002). *Mindfulness-based cognitive therapy for depression: A new approach to preventing relapse*. New York: Guildford.

Shanafelt, T. D., Bradley, K. A., Wipf, J. E., & Back, A. L. (2002). Burnout and self-reported patient care in an internal medicine residency program. *Annals of Internal Medicine, 136*, 358–367.

Singh, N. N., Lancioni, G. E., Karazsia, B. T., Myers, R. E., Winton, A. S., Latham, L. L., et al. (2014). Effects of training staff in MBPBS on the use of physical restraints, staff stress and turnover, staff and peer injuries, and cost effectiveness in developmental disabilities. *Mindfulness, 1–12*.

Singh, N. N., Lancioni, G. E., Winton, A. S. W., Singh, J., Curtis, W. J., Wahler, R. G., et al. (2007). Mindful parenting decreases aggression and increases social behavior in children with developmental disabilities. *Behavior Modification, 3*, 1–6.

Singh, N. N., Lancioni, G. E., Winton, A. S. W., Wahler, R. G., Singh, J., & Sage, M. (2004). Mindful caregiving increases happiness among individuals with profound multiple disabilities. *Research in Developmental Disabilities: A Multidisciplinary Journal, 25*, 207–218.

Smith, A., Graham, L., & Senthinathan, S. (2007). Mindfulness-based cognitive therapy for recurring depression in older people: A qualitative study. *Aging & Mental Health, 11*, 346–357.

Song, Y., Lu, H., Chen, H., Geng, G., & Wang, J. (2014). Mindfulness intervention in the management of chronic pain and psychological comorbidity: A meta-analysis. *International Journal of Nursing Science*. doi:10.1016/j.ijnss.2014.05.014.

Sörensen, S., Duberstein, P., Gill, D., & Pinquart, M. (2006). Dementia care: Mental health effects, intervention strategies, and clinical implications. *Lancet Neurology, 5*, 961–973.

Spillman, B. C., & Long, S. K. (2009). Does high caregiver stress predict nursing home entry? *Inquiry, 46*, 140–161.

Stein, G. (1955). In C. Fadiman, & C. Van Doren, (Eds.), *The American treasury, 1455–1955*. New York: Joanna Cotler Books.

Substance Abuse and Mental Health Services Administration, Office of Applied Studies. (October 11, 2007). *The NSDUH report: Depression among adults employed full-time, by occupational category*. Rockville, MD. Available at. http://oas.samhsa.gov/2k7/depression/occupation.htm

Thomas, P., Lalloue, F., Preux, P. M., Hazif-Thomas, C., Pariel, S., Inscale, R., et al. (2006). Dementia patients' caregivers quality of life: The PIXEL study. *International Journal of Geriatric Psychiatry, 21*, 50–56.

Vickrey, B. G., Mittman, B. S., Connor, K. I., Pearson, M. L., Della Penna, R. D., Ganiats, T. G., et al. (2006). The effect of a disease management intervention on quality and outcomes of dementia care: A randomized, controlled trial. *Annals of Internal Medicine, 145*(10), 713–726.

Vitaliano, P. P., Zhang, J., & Scanlan, J. M. (2003). Is caregiving hazardous to one's physical health? A meta-analysis. *Psychological Bulletin, 129*, 946–972.

Vogeli, C., Shields, A. E., Lee, T. A., Gibson, T. B., Marder, W. D., Weiss, K. B., et al. (2007). Multiple chronic conditions: Prevalence, health consequences, and implications for quality, care management, and costs. *Journal of General Internal Medicine, 22*(3), 391–395.

Whitebird, R. R., Kreitzer, M., Crain, A. L., Lewis, B. A., Hanson, L. R., & Enstad, C. J. (2012). Mindfulness-based stress reduction for family caregivers: A randomized controlled trial. *Gerontologist, 53*, 676–686.

Witkiewitz, K., Marlatt, G. A., & Walker, D. (2005). Mindfulness-based relapse prevention for alcohol and substance use disorders. *Journal of Cognitive Psychotherapy, 19*, 211–228.

Wolff, J. L., Dy, S. M., Frick, K. D., & Kasper, J. D. (2007). End of life care: Findings from a national survey of family caregivers. *Archives of Internal Medicine, 167*, 40–46.

Young, L. A., & Baime, M. J. (2010). Mindfulness-based stress reduction: Effect on emotional distress in older adults. *Journal of Evidence-Based Complementary & Alternative Medicine, 15*, 59–64.

Zarit, S. H., Todd, P. A., & Zarit, J. M. (1986). Subjective burden of husbands and wives as caregivers: A longitudinal study. *Gerontologist, 26*, 260–266.

Zeidan, F., Grant, J. A., Brown, C. A., McHaffie, J. G., & Coghill, R. C. (2012). Mindfulness meditation-related pain relief: Evidence for unique brain mechanisms in the regulation of pain. *Neuroscience Letters, 520*, 165–173.

Chapter 18
Mindfulness and Transformative Parenting

Koa Whittingham

Mindfulness and Parenting

The quality of parenting that an individual child receives will influence many and varied aspects of that child's life. Parenting impacts upon a child's physical health, emotional competence, intelligence, verbal abilities, behavioural competence, social abilities, educational aptitude and, indeed, a child's very happiness (Ainsworth, Blehar, Waters, & Wall, 1978; Bowlby, 1988; Eshel, Daelmans, Cabral de Mello, & Martines, 2006; Gottman, Katz, & Hooven, 1997; Hart & Risley, 1995). In fact, the relationship between parenting and child outcomes is so clear that if we as a society care about our children, and wish to optimise the abilities, health and happiness of the next generation Keywords Frail elders Keywords Frail elders, then we also must, by necessity, care about parents and the quality of parenting that they are providing.

With the recent explosion of interest in mindfulness, there has also been growing interest in the application of mindfulness to parenting. Within the scientific literature, multiple researchers have highlighted an urgent need for research into mindfulness and parenting (Cohen & Semple, 2010; Dumas, 2005; Duncan, Coatsworth, & Greenberg, 2009; Greco & Eifert, 2004; Whittingham, 2014a). Parenting interventions, incorporating mindfulness, have been developed and tested. Mindfulness may make unique contributions to parenting interventions by addressing parenting behaviour that has become automatic (Dumas, 2005), targeting the psychological functions of parenting behaviour for the parent (Coyne & Wilson, 2004) and supporting

K. Whittingham (✉)
Queensland Cerebral Palsy and Rehabilitation Research Centre, School of Medicine, The University of Queensland, Brisbane, Australia

School of Psychology, The University of Queensland, Brisbane, Australia
e-mail: koawhittingham@uq.edu.au

E. Shonin et al. (eds.), *Mindfulness and Buddhist-Derived Approaches in Mental Health and Addiction*, Advances in Mental Health and Addiction,
DOI 10.1007/978-3-319-22255-4_18

flexible parenting (Whittingham, 2014a). As with the explosion of interest in mindfulness more generally, this growing interest in the application of mindfulness to parenting has not been limited to academic circles. When entered into Google, "mindfulness AND parenting" produces over 21,300,000 results and "mindful parenting" over 1,840,000 results (Google search January 2015). Results include books on mindful parenting, websites for mindful parenting workshops and blogs discussing the use of mindfulness by parents. This demonstrates the level of interest amongst ordinary parents.

Mindfulness has multiple definitions and there is not a clear consensus on the exact meaning of the term within either the psychological or the Buddhist literature (Fletcher & Hayes, 2005; Kang & Whittingham, 2010; Kostanski & Hassed, 2008; Shonin, Gordon, & Griffiths, 2014). This chapter is written to be inclusive to the multiple nuances in the way the term mindfulness may be used particularly within the psychological literature but also within wider philosophical and Buddhist literature. Widely agreed upon key features of mindfulness include: (1) awareness of the present moment; (2) psychological contact with your own unfolding experiences, including physical sensations, cognitions and emotions; and (3) a nonjudgemental or open or kind quality to awareness. The concept of mindfulness overlaps with the concept of experiential acceptance within the acceptance and commitment therapy (ACT) literature. Experiential acceptance is the acceptance of your own experiences, including thoughts, feelings and memories as they arise within the present moment (Hayes, Luoma, Bond, Masuda, & Lillis, 2006). Due to the extensive overlap between the concepts of mindfulness and acceptance, research on the relationship between experiential acceptance and parenting will also be considered.

Mindful Parenting

Just as there is no exact consensus on the definition of mindfulness, there is no exact consensus on the definition of mindful parenting (Bogels, Lehtonen, & Restifo, 2010; Duncan et al., 2009; Harnett & Dawe, 2012; Kabat-Zinn & Kabat-Zinn, 1997). As a broad definition, mindful parenting involves bringing mindful awareness to parent–child interactions (Kabat-Zinn & Kabat-Zinn, 1997). Mindful parenting includes parenting with a nonjudgemental, open awareness of the present moment, of your own unfolding experiences in the present moment and of the experiences of your child in the present moment. Some models, definitions and interventions also include self-compassion, as well as compassion for your child.

Duncan's (2009) conceptual model of mindful parenting provides a theoretical basis for some of the existing interventions and research and includes the following components: (1) listening with full attention to your child, (2) nonjudgemental acceptance of both self and child, (3) emotional awareness of self and child, (4) self-regulation in parenting and (5) compassion for self and child. Further, Bogels et al. (2010) propose that there are six potential mechanisms by which parental mindfulness improves outcomes for children: (1) reducing parental reactivity and stress, (2) reducing parental preoccupation, ruminative thinking and negative biases, (3) improving executive functioning and reducing impulsive parenting, (4) breaking the cycle of intergenerational transmission of attachment patterns, schemas and dysfunctional parenting, (5) increasing parental self-compassion or self-nourishing attention and (6) improving the couple relationship and co-parenting.

Models of mindful parenting such as that by Duncan (2009) and Bogels (2010) are important to guiding further research and intervention development and should be further tested empirically. It is also important to consider the application of mindfulness to parenting by using existing, empirically supported theoretical frames (Harnett & Dawe, 2012), including attachment theory and relational frame theory. Mindful parenting can be understood as foundational to both parental responsiveness and parental flexibility.

Interpersonal Mindfulness and Responsive Parenting

Development Is Interpersonal

Infant and child development is fundamentally an interpersonal process (Bowlby, 1988). A human infant can only develop into full personhood, as a verbal and self-aware human being, if that infant develops within the context of interpersonal relationships. Further, the quality of the interpersonal relationships experienced by an individual child has ramifications for that child's development. A systematic review of the literature on parental responsiveness and child outcomes across both developed and developing countries showed that parent-child relationships with high parental responsiveness—prompt, child-directed, contingent and developmentally appropriate parenting— are associated with improved cognitive, emotional, behavioural and social outcomes (Eshel et al., 2006).

In order to fully understand the importance of parental responsiveness and the interpersonal nature of child development, it is necessary to view human parenting from an evolutionary context. Parental care is a key characteristic of mammalian behaviour and mammals fall into one of two types: altricial and precocial (Ball, 2009). Altricial mammals are born developmentally immature and in litters (e.g. mice). The parental care strategy is to keep the litter in a nest for warmth and security. Altricial mothers typically produce high-fat milk and thus the infants can space out feeds allowing the mother to leave the nest in order to search for food. Precocial mammals are born developmentally mature and as singletons or in pairs (e.g. horses). Precocial mammals are mobile shortly after birth. The parental care strategy for precocial mammals is for the infant to maintain close proximity to the mother through its own efforts and volition. Precocial mothers typically produce low-fat, high-lactose milk providing easily digestible calories to a mobile infant who is able to follow the mother, feeding frequently and at will. Humans evolved from precocial ancestors; however, human infants are secondarily altricial (Ball, 2009). Although humans show some characteristics of precocial mammals, including high-lactose milk and typically singleton birth, human infants are born developmentally immature and with poor neuromuscular control. In fact, humans are born with only a quarter of their total brain volume (chimpanzees are born with half). A newborn human infant, unlike a newborn horse, is incapable of maintaining close proximity to the parent; instead, the parent must respond to the infant's signals for proximity and care.

Neurodevelopmentally immature human birth has another consequence: human infants undergo much neurodevelopment within a stimulating, verbal and interpersonal context. Without such a context, development into a self-aware, verbal adult is impossible. Stimulation is crucial to early neurodevelopment (Douglas & Hill, 2011), and yet a newborn infant, with poor neuromuscular control, has little control over their environment. It is not surprising then to find that parental responsiveness predicts cognitive development (Eshel et al., 2006): parental responsiveness to infant cues serves as a dose-control system for stimulation, ensuring that an infant's stimulation exposure is kept in the 'just right' zone for learning and neurodevelopment. From birth, human infants seek interpersonal stimulation, and when parents respond to their infant's signals with interaction, they naturally expose their child to language and other uniquely human cognitive processes. This early language exposure, occurring naturally within every day interactions, is crucial to later cognitive and verbal development (Hart & Risley, 1995).

Towards the end of the first year of life, humans reach the neurodevelopmental maturity and mobility that precocial mammals show at birth. Infants are now able to maintain proximity to their caregivers, through their own efforts and volition, and as a result pre-attachment behaviours consolidate into attachment behaviours at this time (Bowlby, 1988). The attachment behavioural system is activated when the child experiences a threat and includes any behaviour aimed at seeking proximity to and nurturance from caregivers (Bowlby, 1988). Parental caregiving behaviour, particularly parental responsiveness, is key to determining the pattern of attachment behaviours displayed by any particular child (Ainsworth et al., 1978; Sroufe, 2005). Further, patterns of attachment are related to later psychological health and success in relationships (Ainsworth et al., 1978; Sroufe, 2005). Children who experienced responsive parenting, and subsequently developed a secure attachment style, fare better in terms of mental health and relational success. Parental responsiveness continues to be important to the parent-child relationship as children develop (Biringen, Derscheid, Vliegen, Closson, & Easterbrooks, 2014).

What Is Parental Responsiveness?

Parental responsiveness to child cues is then the bedrock of human parental care, and parental responsiveness predicts diverse child outcomes including social, psychological, cognitive, emotional and relational outcomes (Ainsworth et al., 1978; Bowlby, 1988; Eshel et al., 2006; Sroufe, 2005). But what are the crucial ingredients to parental responsiveness? Responsiveness involves three key features: (1) the parent must be aware of their child's cues or signals; (2) the parent must accurately interpret their child's cues, correctly deducing the needs of their child; and (3) the parent must promptly and consistently act in response to cues, in a manner that meets the needs of the child (Ainsworth et al., 1978; Eshel et al., 2006). Importantly, a responsive parent is warm and caring but is not merely warm and caring. A responsive parent is also parenting 'on cue'; their caregiving behaviour is under the contextual control of their child's signals (Whittingham, 2014b; Whittingham & Douglas, 2014). This is not to say that responsiveness requires perfection. In fact, parental responsiveness includes ordinary human error. What is crucial, however, is that there is an 'intention' to respond, coupled with a continual returning of awareness to the child in the present moment and a continual taking of the child's perspective in order to accurately deduce the child's needs.

Mindfulness Is Crucial to Responsiveness

In breaking down the components of parental responsiveness, the relevance of mindfulness to parenting is immediately apparent (Synder, Shapiro, & Treleaven, 2012). In order for a parent to respond to their child's cue, the parent must, necessarily, be aware of their child's cue. For a parent to engage in a responsive pattern of care over time, the parent must be aware of their child's cues as they unfold in the present moment. That is, the parent must be able to keep their attention within the present moment and focussed upon their child. Although the parent's attention may be drawn to other things, including their own thoughts or emotions, other people, specific tasks or simply distractions, a responsive parent must return their attention again and again to their child. In other words, the parent must practise interpersonal or relational mindfulness: mindfulness of another person and of the relationship between self and other (Surrey, 2005).

Proximity is a key feature of the attachment bond, the ongoing dance between the attachment behavioural pattern of the child and the caregiving behavioural pattern of the parent (Bowlby, 1988), not only in the sense that the evolutionary purpose of infant attachment behaviour is to maintain proximity to the parent but also because proximity is required for responsive parenting and secure attachment. In fact, increased physical proximity (through babywearing with a soft infant carrier) has been shown to increase the responsiveness of mothers to their infants at three and a half months of age in an experimental study (Ainsfeld, Capser, Nozyce, & Cunningham, 1990). Further, rates of secure attachment in their infants at 13 months of age were also improved.

In human relationships we can distinguish not just physical proximity but also psychological proximity. In order to flourish psychologically, our children require us to be not just physically available to them, but also emotionally available (Biringen et al., 2014). Emotional availability includes awareness of emotions and emotional signalling within a relationship as well as an awareness and responsiveness to the needs and goals of the other. That is, emotional availability requires relational mindfulness.

The non-judgemental, open aspect of mindfulness means holding reflexive judgements of objects, people and situations lightly and, instead, maintaining psychological contact with reality as it is (Duncan et al., 2009). Such openness enables a clear understanding of your immediate experience without distortions caused by desires, biases and opinions and may better enable parents to appreciate the legitimate needs behind their child's cues, even when the cues are inconvenient, distressing or at odds with the parent's own needs. The increased emotional awareness that comes with mindfulness, and the ability to accept the ebb and flow of your own emotional life, may enhance parental willingness to experience intense emotions while continuing to be psychologically present with their child and while continuing to respond, as best they can, to their child's cues (Duncan et al., 2009).

Mindfulness, Parental Flexibility and Resilience

Parental Flexibility

Psychological flexibility, the ability to adapt to specific situations, to flexibly shift attention and perspective and to balance competing needs, desires and domains of life, is a key underpinning of psychological health (Kashdan & Rotteberg, 2012). Psychological flexibility includes an openness to learning from direct experience and a willingness to either persist or change, according to what is workable (Hayes, 2004). Parental flexibility refers to parenting with psychological flexibility (Whittingham, 2014a). It involves approaching parenting with flexible, relaxed experimentation and openness to learning from your own direct moment by moment experiences interacting with your child. It includes shifting attention easily and flexibly between your child and other competing demands, shifting perspective to imagine the needs, emotions and desires of your child and balancing the competing needs of self and child or the competing needs of multiple children as well as balancing parenting with other life domains. Through flexible parenting, the parent is able to respond to the unique needs of his or her unique child in the unique circumstances in which they find themselves. As psychological flexibility broadly underpins psychological resilience (Kashdan & Rotteberg, 2012), parental flexibility is crucial to parental resilience (Whittingham & Douglas, 2014). Yet, parental flexibility can be undermined by key features of human language and cognition: cognitive fusion and experiential avoidance (Coyne & Wilson, 2004).

Parental Flexibility and Cognitive Fusion

The concept of cognitive fusion is informed by relational frame theory (RFT), a contextual theory of language and cognition suggesting that the language and complex cognitive skills of humans are underpinned by our ability to learn to relate stimuli 'arbitrarily' (Coyne, McHugh, & Martinez, 2011; Hayes, Strosal, & Wilson, 2003). Humans can learn that the sound 'dog' is equivalent to (i.e. means) dog, even though the sound 'dog' and dogs are not physically related. In addition to learning to relate stimuli arbitrarily, humans also learn behavioural responses through 'derived' relations, not merely through direct experience (Coyne et al., 2011; Coyne & Wilson, 2004; Hayes et al., 2003). So, if a human learns that the sound 'dog' is equivalent to an actual dog and that human also learns that the sound 'cane' is equivalent to an actual dog, the human will 'derive' that 'dog' is equivalent to (i.e. means) 'cane'. Humans can learn that stimuli are related not just in terms of equivalence but in terms of multiple relational frames including opposition, hierarchy or temporal relations.

An important property of this phenomenon is the transformation of stimulus functions (Coyne et al., 2011; Coyne & Wilson, 2004; Hayes et al., 2003). The psychologically relevant features of a stimulus are transformed according to the derived relations applicable in a specific context. For example, both humans and animals can be trained to fear dogs through direct experience with actual dogs. But only an English-speaking human will then exhibit fear if someone says, 'Look, a dog!' Further, if that same person goes on holiday to Italy and learns that the sound 'cane' means 'dog' in Italian, they will also exhibit fear upon hearing, 'Guarda un cane!' even though they have never learnt, through direct experience, to become fearful when hearing the sound 'cane'.

Although derived relational responding makes human language and complex cognition possible, it comes with a cost. We have a tendency to treat our own internal experiences as if they were real phenomena (Coyne & Wilson, 2004). Through derived relations, neutral or even positive stimuli may be experienced as aversive (Murrell, Wilson, LaBorde, Drake, & Rogers, 2009). For example, a parent experiencing significant parenting stress may come to experience their child themselves as aversive, even in the absence of problem behaviour. In addition, human behaviour may come under the control of verbal processes or rules. When a person's behaviour is under the control of verbal processes, and this is unworkable, this is termed cognitive fusion (Coyne & Wilson, 2004; Hayes et al., 2003).

Two kinds of rule-governed behaviour are particularly likely to be problematic: pliance and incorrect, unworkable or untestable tracks (Hayes et al., 2003). Pliance refers to when a person's behaviour is under the control of socially mediated consequences identified in the rule. For example, a parent may follow the rule, 'good parents teach their children to sleep in their own bed', in order to be recognised by others as a 'good parent'. The socially mediated consequence is the approval that the parent anticipates receiving from others for their successful compliance with the rule. Pliance may be problematic when the course of action specified in the rule is not the most useful behaviour for that individual in that context. A parent fused with the rule 'good parents teach their children to sleep in their own bed' may fail to notice salient aspects of their specific situation, for example, that their own sleep is not disturbed by bed sharing or that their child's desire to sleep in the parent's bed is related to specific emotional needs.

Tracks, in contrast, are verbal rules describing naturally occurring consequences within the world (Hayes et al., 2003). When tracks are factually accurate and workable, they can be incredibly useful, for example, 'if your baby is under 3 months of age and has a fever then take your baby to the doctor because medical treatment may be needed'. Parents don't need to learn every aspect of caregiving through their own experience; instead, they can follow verbal rules and hence learn from other parents as well as from professionals. However, tracks may also be inaccurate, unworkable or untestable. For example, 'spare the rod and spoil the child'. When fused with tracks, a parent may fail to notice salient aspects of their individual situation. For example, a parent may fail to notice that since they began using corporal punishment, their child's behaviour has gotten worse and their relationship with their child has deteriorated. Behaviours under the control of verbal rules are less sensitive to context. When rule-following, it is more difficult to learn from our direct experiences (Coyne & Wilson, 2004). Derived relations that are salient in the current context and have a strong learning history dominate making it difficult to respond in new and creative ways (Murrell et al., 2009).

Parental Flexibility and Experiential Avoidance

Cognitive fusion makes experiential avoidance (the opposite of experiential acceptance) possible. Experiential avoidance is an unwillingness to experience painful cognitions, emotions and memories and includes deliberate efforts to avoid, minimise or control our own experiences (Hayes et al., 2003). It is a direct consequence of the fact that we treat our internal experiences like real phenomena (Coyne & Wilson, 2004). When our internal experiences are unwanted, we try to eliminate or escape them, just as we would do with real phenomena. In small doses, experiential avoidance is not necessarily problematic, for example, the use of distraction during a brief medical procedure. However, internal experiences are not the same as real phenomena and experiential avoidance attempts may, paradoxically, increase suffering (Hayes et al., 2003). For example, attempts to suppress specific cognitions may create a rebound effect in which the suppressed cognition is experienced more frequently. In addition, experiential avoidance may have other consequences that increase suffering. A parent may find that it decreases their own distress in the immediate future to avoid having an open discussion with their child about a recent conflict. But there is a cost paid in the long-term for such avoidance in terms of greater connection and intimacy within the parent-child relationship.

Some parenting choices and strategies, such as harsh discipline, intrusive parenting, lax parenting or simply tuning out, may serve the function of experiential avoidance for the parent (Coyne et al., 2011; Coyne & Murrell, 2009; Shea & Coyne, 2011; Tiwari et al., 2008). Parents may attempt to control their children's behaviour or even their children's cognitions and emotions in order to control their own internal experiences. With parental attention narrowed to unwanted thoughts and emotions, and the avoidance of such thoughts and emotions, parents may be unable to access and choose from the full array of parenting options they may have (Shea & Coyne, 2011).

Mindfulness as the Antidote

Mindfulness involves deliberately re-establishing psychological contact with the world as it is in the present moment, including the unique aspects of your own experience. It involves bringing an open and non-judgemental awareness to cognitions, memories and emotions. In fact, mindfulness as it is understood within the ACT literature includes 'defused' awareness or cognitive defusion (instead of cognitive fusion). Defused awareness refers to psychological contact with cognitions, memories and emotions, as experientially distinct from self and the world (Fletcher & Hayes, 2005). This defused aspect of mindfulness involves the liberation of a person's behaviour from the control of verbal rules which may be centred on obtaining approval from others, unworkable in the specific circumstances in which the individual finds themselves or simply inaccurate (Hayes et al., 2003). Mindful parenting involves letting go of firm and fixed views about how things should be (Kabat-Zinn & Kabat-Zinn, 1997) and, instead, opening up to flexible experimentation.

Mindfulness and Parenting: The Evidence So Far

Mindfulness, Responsiveness and Attachment

Cross-sectional research has demonstrated a link between mindfulness and attachment style in adults, with dispositional mindfulness predicting attachment security within romantic relationships (Goodall, Trejnowska, & Darling, 2012; Hertz, Laurent, & Laurent, 2014; Walsh et al., 2009). Mindfulness predicts both decreased avoidance (Hertz et al., 2014) and decreased anxiety (Hertz et al., 2014; Walsh et al., 2009) within romantic relationships. This, in turn, buffers stress response during and after conflict, as measured by cortisol levels and negative affect (Hertz et al., 2014). These relational benefits of mindfulness would be expected to also impact on parent-child relationships as well, and the available evidence suggests they do.

Within the high-risk population of mothers of infants born preterm (<37 weeks of gestation), experiential acceptance was found to be a significant predictor of self-reported bonding and parental responsiveness ($n = 127$) (Evans, Whittingham, & Boyd, 2012). In another study, the relationship between maternal attachment patterns to her own mother and child quality of life was mediated by maternal self-compassion and parenting stress within 171 mother-child (8–18 years of age) dyads (Moreira, Gouveia, Carona, Silva, & Canavarro, 2014). Higher attachment related anxiety and avoidance predicted lower self-compassion and higher parenting stress, which in turn predicted lower child quality of life.

Mindfulness and Parenting

Mindfulness and experiential acceptance predict parental adjustment including parenting stress, parental anxiety, parental depressive symptoms, parental grieving and the experienced burden of parenting, including in high-risk populations.

Parental dispositional mindfulness was significantly associated with parental stress above and beyond child behaviour problems in both mothers of children with autism spectrum disorders ($n = 67$) and mothers of typically developing children ($n = 87$) (Conner & White, 2014). In a cross-sectional study with parents of children with autism spectrum disorders ($n = 28$), mindful parenting was correlated with parental stress and depressive symptoms, although it was not found to mediate the relationship between child behaviour problems and parental stress and depressive symptoms (Beer, Ward, & Moar, 2013). However, another study did find a mediational relationship. Parental dispositional mindfulness and mindful parenting were both found to be significant mediators of the relationship between child behaviour problems and maternal anxiety, stress and depressive symptoms in parents of children with autism (71 mothers, 39 fathers) (Jones, Hastings, Totsika, Keane, & Rhule, 2014).

Acceptance, too, is important. In mothers of Head Start pre-schoolers (3–5 years of age; $n = 144$), experiential acceptance was found to mediate the relationship between maternal depressive symptoms and parenting-related stress, with lower levels of acceptance linked to higher parenting-related stress (Shea & Coyne, 2011). Experiential acceptance has been found to mediate the relationship between child behaviour problems and maternal anxiety, stress and depressive symptoms as well as the relationship between child behaviour problems and paternal depressive symptoms in parents of children with autism (71 mothers, 39 fathers) (Jones et al., 2014). Within the high-risk group of parents of infants born preterm, experiential acceptance predicts parental psychological adjustment (Evans et al., 2012; Greco et al., 2005). Experiential acceptance partially mediates the relationship between stress related to their infant's early hospitalisation within the neonatal intensive care unit and both parenting-related stress and parental posttraumatic stress (Greco et al., 2005). Experiential acceptance predicted parental adjustment, as well as the current intensity grief symptoms and the experienced burden of parenting in parents of children with cerebral palsy ($n = 94$) (Whittingham, Wee, Sanders, & Boyd, 2013). Parents with greater experiential acceptance reported that parenting was less burdensome and reported fewer current grief symptoms related to their child's diagnosis.

Mindfulness, Parenting and Child Outcomes

In mothers of Head Start pre-schoolers (3–5 years old; $n = 144$), lower levels of experiential acceptance were linked to higher parenting-related stress, and parenting stress, in turn, was a unique predictor of inconsistent and harsh parenting (Shea &

Coyne, 2011). Within a sample of clinic-referred mother-child dyads, mothers with higher dispositional mindfulness rated their parenting style as more authoritative and less authoritarian, and this, in turn, predicted lower parent-reported internalising and externalising behaviour in their children (Williams & Wahler, 2010). In another study, parental non-judgemental self-acceptance significantly predicted decreased depressive and anxious symptoms in their adolescent children ($n=901$) (Geurtzen, Scholte, Engels, Tak, & van Zundert, 2014). Other aspects of mindful parenting outlined in Duncan's model (2009) were not significant predictors. Dispositional mindfulness has also been found to relate to experienced parenting effort in mothers of pre-schoolers and adolescents ($n=50$, $n=118$) (Bluth & Wahler, 2011a, 2011b). Parents with high levels of mindfulness found parenting less burdensome and found it less effortful to make moment to moment parenting decisions.

Mindfulness in the Transition to Parenthood

The transition to parenthood demands significant personal change and is a steep learning curve. In addition, for most women, it is a uniquely embodied time of life, including pregnancy, childbirth and breastfeeding. As such, it is an excellent opportunity for mindfulness practice (Kabat-Zinn & Kabat-Zinn, 1997). Mindfulness during the transition to parenthood may prove beneficial in the management of pain during pregnancy and childbirth, in reducing risk of postnatal depression and anxiety, in increasing parental well-being and in improving parental responsiveness to the baby (Hughes et al., 2009; Whittingham, 2013).

Multiple mindfulness interventions for the transition to parenting have been developed and the research to date is promising. The Mindfulness-Based Childbirth and Parenting Programme (MBCP) adapts mindfulness-based stress reduction (MBSR) practices to pregnancy, birth and early parenting including breastfeeding (Bardacke, 2012). Alongside familiar MBSR practices such as body scan meditation, participants practice mindfulness of their baby and explore the use of mindfulness during childbirth and breastfeeding. For example, participants practice sounding, that is, concentrative focus upon making specific vocalisations such as "ah" or "aum" as a mindfulness practice for childbirth. It is suggested that participants practice mindfulness during breastfeeding as the calm, peaceful mental state may support oxytocin release and the milk ejection reflex (Bardacke, 2012). MBCP is delivered in nine 3-h group sessions. MBCP was found to be associated with significant gains in positive affect and mindfulness, as well as significant reductions in negative affect and depressive and anxious symptoms in a pilot study with pregnant women participating in the third trimester of pregnancy ($n=27$) (Bardacke, 2012).

The Mindful Motherhood intervention was developed drawing from MBSR, mindfulness-based cognitive therapy (MBCT) and ACT (Vieten & Astin, 2008). Within the Mindful Motherhood programme, the cultivation of bodily awareness includes awareness of the developing foetus. Familiar mindfulness practices such as mindful movements with yoga, mindfulness of thoughts and emotions and the cultivation of acceptance are also practised. In a small pilot randomised controlled trial ($n=31$), the Mindful Motherhood programme delivered antenatally (between 12 and 30 weeks at the beginning of the intervention) was associated with reductions in anxiety and negative affect during pregnancy for the mindfulness group compared to a waitlist control. Differences were not significant at 3-month follow-up; however, the small sample size may explain this null result.

A 6-week antenatal mindfulness-based intervention including mindfulness of the body, emotions and cognitions was tested in a pilot randomised controlled trial ($n=47$) (Guardino, Schetter, Bower, Lue, & Smalley, 2014). Participants were randomly assigned to the mindfulness condition or to a reading control condition and were between 10 and 25 weeks of gestation at commencement. The mindfulness group showed reductions in pregnancy-specific and pregnancy-related anxiety during the intervention as compared to the control group, but this was not sustained at follow-up 6 weeks post-intervention. Further, both groups showed increased mindfulness and reductions in anxious symptoms and stress. The finding that the control group also demonstrated increases in mindfulness is intriguing. The effects of pregnancy, childbirth and breastfeeding themselves on mindfulness have not, to my knowledge, been investigated. It is plausible that this uniquely embodied time of life, with dramatic physical changes, frequent foetal movements and great physical challenges, may, in and of itself, precipitate increased mindfulness in some women.

An 8-week antenatal MBCT intervention was piloted with women between 12 and 28 weeks of gestation at commencement ($n=10$) (Dunn, Hanieh, Roberts, & Powrie, 2012). Participants showed reductions in depressive and anxious symptoms as well as stress. In addition, participants showed gains in mindfulness and self-compassion. Results were sustained at follow-up 6 weeks postpartum.

Mindfulness to Prevent Postnatal Depression and Anxiety

Mindfulness has also been tested with women at risk of postnatal depression and anxiety, with the evidence so far suggesting that mindfulness could play an important role in the prevention of postnatal depression and anxiety disorders.

A mindfulness yoga class, conducted in groups for 90 min a week for 10 weeks, was tested in a pilot study with women ($n=22$) recruited through a perinatal psychiatry clinic all with a score on the Edinburgh Postnatal Depression Scale of nine or over (Muzik, Hamilton, Rosenblum, Waxler, & Hadi, 2012). Participants showed significant reductions in depressive symptoms, as well as significant gains in mindfulness and maternal-foetal attachment. Antenatal MBCT has been piloted in women with a history of depression ($n=49$) (Dimidjian et al., 2014). The participants demonstrated significant reductions in depressive symptoms throughout the intervention, with these reductions sustained during pregnancy and postpartum. Across pregnancy and through to 6 months postpartum, relapse/recurrence rates for this high-risk group were 18 %, as compared to rates of 30 % with standard care found in naturalistic studies.

Mindfulness may also be useful in preventing perinatal and postnatal anxiety, as well as depression. The Coping with Anxiety through Living Mindfully (CALM) Pregnancy programme is an adaptation of MBCT for perinatal anxiety (Goodman et al., 2014). CALM Pregnancy includes familiar MCBT practices such as mindfulness with thoughts and mindfulness of baby practices. The CALM Pregnancy intervention was piloted in women with generalised anxiety disorder (GAD) or subclinical features of GAD ($n=24$). Participants reported significant reductions in anxiety and depressive symptoms and significant gains in mindfulness and self-compassion. Of the 24 participants, 17 met full criteria for GAD at baseline and only one continued to meet criteria at post-intervention.

Mindfulness Postpartum

Mindfulness can be built, not just into antenatal care, but into postnatal care. ACT has been adapted for use during the antenatal and the postnatal period. This approach includes familiar mindfulness practices such as mindfulness of breathing, along with mindfulness of baby and acceptance of baby practices (Whittingham, 2013). In addition, it includes the identification of parenting values, exercises to develop compassion for baby and for self, behavioural activation and strategies to increase social support. This full approach has not yet been tested empirically. An ACT approach to postnatal care has been integrated with an interdisciplinary lens including complexity science, evolutionary anthropology, neuroscience, clinical lactation science and developmental theory in the Possums Sleep Intervention (Whittingham & Douglas, 2014). The Possums Sleep Intervention is a new paradigm in parent-infant sleep that integrates lifestyle advice drawn from understanding the biological regulation of sleep with cued care, safe sleep advice, and parental mindfulness, cognitive defusion and acceptance practices. The Possums Sleep Intervention is currently being evaluated. It is a good example of the role mindfulness can play, within a larger interdisciplinary framework, in generating novel solutions to everyday problems.

Mindfulness Interventions with Parents

Mindfulness-based interventions can bolster parental adjustment, decreasing parental stress and anxious and depressive symptoms and increasing parental well-being. Further, increased parental mindfulness may also improve child functioning.

An adapted MBSR intervention, including 8 weekly 2 h sessions and a 4 h silent retreat, was piloted with parents and caregivers of children with developmental disabilities ($n=76$) (Bazzano et al., 2013). Participants reported significant reductions in stress and parenting stress, as well as significant increases in mindfulness, self-compassion and well-being. Reductions in stress continued at follow-up

2 months after programme completion. In a within-subject repeated-measures design study with a within-group waitlist, a mindfulness intervention for both parents and children was tested with families of children with ADHD ($n=22$) (Van der Oord, Bogels, & Pejnenberg, 2012). The intervention was grounded in both MBSR and MBCT practices. Parents reported significant reductions in parenting stress and gains in child adjustment were reported both by parents and by teachers.

Mindfulness has been shown to decrease parental stress, child aggression and child non-compliance and to increase child social behaviour in families of children with autism spectrum disorders and developmental disabilities in multiple-baseline across-subjects designs (Singh et al., 2006, 2007). Strengths of these studies include a lengthy post-intervention practice period with a 1-year follow-up. The intervention combined familiar mindfulness practices, such as mindfulness of breathing, with mindfulness of child, non-judgemental acceptance and loving-kindness practices. In another study with a multiple-baseline design, the effects of an 8-week mindfulness programme focussing on occupational mindfulness as a caregiver for individuals with physical and intellectual disabilities was found to generalise to parent–child interactions for three mothers (Singh et al., 2011). Child non-compliance was found to decrease during the mindfulness intervention and to decrease further during the practice period, even though the intervention focussed on occupational, not parental, mindfulness.

In a randomised controlled trial of MBSR for parents of children (2.5–5 years of age) with developmental delays ($n=46$), MBSR showed beneficial effects (Neece, 2014). Parents who received MBSR reported significantly less stress and depressive symptoms, as well as greater life satisfaction, than the control group at post-intervention. In addition, they reported fewer behavioural problems in their children, particularly decreases in attentional difficulties and hyperactivity. Given the decreases in child attentional difficulties and hyperactivity in particular, this study suggests that increased parental mindfulness may, through relational mindfulness in parent–child interactions, increase the regulatory capacity of children.

In a randomised controlled trial of a 5-week mindfulness intervention for parents ($n=32$) and teachers ($n=38$) of children with special needs, participants receiving the mindfulness intervention showed significant reductions in stress and anxiety as well as gains in mindfulness, self-compassion and empathic concern (Benn, Akiva, Arel, & Roeser, 2012). Results were sustained at follow-up 2 months later and the outcomes at follow-up were mediated by changes in mindfulness. A small pilot randomised controlled trial compared an 8-week mindfulness programme to an 8-week parenting skills programme for families of children with autism ($n=15$) (Ferraioli & Harris, 2013). Families were randomised to the intervention groups after being matched on parenting stress. Only the participants receiving mindfulness reported significant improvements in parental stress and global health outcomes.

The Mindful Parenting Programme combines familiar mindfulness practices such as mindfulness of breathing, with strategies to increase the frequency of connection-promoting parent–child interactions, for example, listening to your child. The Mindful Parenting Programme was piloted in group sessions over 12 weeks ($n=12$) (Altmaier & Maloney, 2007). Parents reported significant gains in mindfulness during the intervention; however, parenting stress and parent-child connectedness (as measured by a home observation) remained unchanged.

The Mindful Parenting intervention includes mindfulness practices drawn from MBSR and MBCT such as body scan meditation. In addition, Mindful Parenting includes compassion and loving-kindness exercises and practices intended to bring greater mindful awareness to parenting interactions. The Mindful Parenting intervention was piloted with families recruited from referrals to a child and youth secondary mental health centre ($n=86$) (Bogels, Hellemans, van Duersen, Romer, & van der Meulen, 2014; Bogels & Restifo, 2014). The children experienced a variety of neurodevelopmental and/or psychological disorders including ADHD (47 %), autism spectrum disorder (21 %) and an anxiety disorder (7 %). All families received the Mindful Parenting intervention in 8 weekly 3 h group sessions. Following participation in the Mindful Parenting course, parents reported reductions in parental psychological symptoms and parenting stress, as well as reductions in their child's internalising and externalising behaviour problems. In addition, parents reported gains in their ability to co-parent.

In a second study of the Mindful Parenting intervention, families were again recruited from referrals at child mental health centres ($n=74$) (Bogels & Restifo, 2014). The children experienced a variety of neurodevelopmental and/or psychological disorders including ADHD (19 %), autism spectrum disorder (23 %) and an anxiety disorder (3 %). Parents reported gains in mindful parenting, parental dispositional mindfulness and parental experiential acceptance. In addition, parents reported reductions in parenting stress at follow-up 8 weeks after completion of the programme. In a third study of the Mindful Parenting intervention, improvements in mindful parenting, dispositional mindfulness and experiential acceptance, as well as reductions in parental stress, parental psychological symptoms and child internalising and externalising behaviour, were again noted ($n=14$) (Bogels & Restifo, 2014). In addition, parents reported reductions in parental over-reactivity.

ACT has also been adapted for parents. A 14 h ACT workshop was tested with parents of children with autism spectrum disorders in a within-subject repeated-measures design ($n=20$) (Blackledge & Hayes, 2006). Parents reported significant reductions in stress and depressive symptoms at post-intervention and at 3-month follow-up. In addition, gains were reported in experiential acceptance.

Parenting Interventions Incorporating Mindfulness

Mindfulness has also been integrated into existing, well-established parenting interventions and has been shown to make an additional contribution. In a multiple-baseline design study, three mothers of adolescents with autism spectrum disorder received an 8-week mindfulness programme as well as behaviour support on the application of behavioural parenting strategies in the context of mindful parenting (Singh et al., 2014). All three mothers reported challenging behaviours in their children at intake. The mindfulness intervention tested was a second-generation mindfulness approach, an overtly spiritual intervention, aiming at both personal and transpersonal transformation and not merely improved health and decreased stress. The intervention content drew upon Mahayana Buddhism. In addition to mindfulness practices, the programme included practices for each of the four immeasurables: loving-kindness, compassion, equanimity and sympathetic joy. Participants reported reductions in parental stress as well as reductions in their child's challenging behaviour and increases in child compliance.

The mindfulness-enhanced Strengthening Families Programme was compared to the Strengthening Families Programme and to a waitlist control group in a pilot randomised controlled trial with three arms, recruiting families of children aged 10–14 ($n=65$) (Coatsworth, Duncan, Greenberg, & Nix, 2010). The mindfulness-enhanced programme included familiar mindfulness practices such as mindfulness of breathing, as well as loving-kindness practices, and reflections intended to increase mindful parenting. The programme is grounded within Duncan's (2009) conceptual model of mindful parenting. Overall, the mindfulness-enhanced Strengthening Families Programme showed similar effects to the original programme for parenting style, with families in both groups showing benefits relative to waitlist control for parent-reported rules communication. For parent-reported discipline consistency, however, the original programme showed greater benefit. This may reflect the adoption of a more flexible parenting style in the parents practising mindfulness. The mindfulness-enhanced version showed stronger effects for mindful parenting, as measured by parent-report, and parent-child relationship quality measured by parent and youth report as compared to both the waitlist control group and the original programme. Further, the changes found in parent-child relationship quality were mediated by changes in mindful parenting.

The mindfulness-enhanced Strengthening Families Programme has been further refined and tested in comparison to the Strengthening Families Programme and a minimal-treatment control condition in a randomised controlled trial with three arms recruiting families of children aged 10–14 ($n=432$) (Coatsworth et al., 2014). A significant strength of this study is the inclusion of mother, father and youth reports. Both the Strengthening Families Programme and the mindfulness-enhanced Strengthening Families Programme were clearly effective interventions, with significant differences in interpersonal mindfulness, parent-child relationship quality, parenting style and parental well-being as compared to the waitlist control condition apparent at either post-intervention to 1-year follow-up or both. However, the pattern of the results was complex. Some effects were apparent at post-intervention but not at follow-up, some were sustained and some apparent only at follow-up. In addition, there were differences in the patterns of outcomes between mothers and fathers and differences between parent and youth report. Given this level of complexity, it is difficult to distil overall conclusions about the additive effects of mindfulness to the Strengthening Families Programme. Overall, fathers made greater gains than mothers in the mindfulness-enhanced version. For mothers, gains in interpersonal mindfulness, as compared to the waitlist control, were not made until 1-year follow-up, and the mindfulness-enhanced Strengthening Families group was never significantly different to the group receiving the original programme.

In contrast, for fathers, gains in interpersonal mindfulness were made by the mindfulness-enhanced Strengthening Families group as compared to the waitlist control group and the Strengthening Families group, at post-intervention and 1-year follow-up, and these gains were evident by both parent and youth reports. Further, fathers reported clear benefits in terms of their own well-being at 1-year follow-up. The differences in outcomes for mothers and fathers are not explained by baseline differences. It is possible that the programme presents mindfulness in a manner better suited to the typical experiences of fathers rather than mothers. Further investigation is required. However, the ability for the mindfulness-enhanced Strengthening Families Programme to enhance the interpersonal mindfulness of fathers is itself not trivial as the improvement of father-child relationships is an important end goal in itself.

The Parents under Pressure (PUP) programme is grounded in the ecological model of child development, targets multiple domains of family functioning and includes mindfulness training (Dawe & Harnett, 2007; Dawe, Harnett, Rendalls, & Staiger, 2003). Mindfulness practices, once learnt, are applied directly to child-directed play and to discipline situations (reducing impulsive, emotive discipline practices). In addition, PUP includes information on behavioural parenting strategies, extending social support, building a stronger spousal relationship and improving health behaviours like diet and exercise. PUP was piloted with parents participating in a methadone programme ($n=12$) (Dawe et al., 2003). Parents reported reductions in parenting stress, child abuse potential and child externalising behaviour. Later, PUP was trialled in a three arm randomised controlled trial with parents on methadone maintenance and with a child between the ages of two and eight ($n=64$) (Dawe & Harnett, 2007). Parents were randomly assigned to either PUP, standard care or a brief parenting skills intervention. PUP was delivered over 10–12 weeks in the family's own home. Both parents receiving PUP and parents receiving the brief parenting intervention reported significant reductions in child abuse potential compared to standard care. The parents receiving PUP also reported reductions in child internalising and externalising behaviour, parenting stress, parental methadone dose and parental rigidity.

ACT has been tested in conjunction with the behavioural parenting intervention Stepping Stones Triple P (Positive Parenting Programme) for families of children with acquired brain injury (Brown, Whittingham, McKinlay, Boyd, & Sofronoff, 2013; Brown, Whittingham, Boyd, McKinlay, & Sofronoff, 2014) and cerebral palsy (Whittingham, Sanders, McKinlay, & Boyd, 2013, 2014). Stepping Stones Triple P is a variant of Triple P tailored specifically for families of children with developmental disabilities. Within both studies ACT for parents was a brief (4 h) group intervention that combined familiar mindfulness practices, such as mindfulness of breathing, with cognitive defusion techniques, experiential acceptance exercises and reflections on parenting values.

The combination of Stepping Stones Triple P and ACT was tested in a randomised controlled trial with families of children (2–12 years of age) with acquired brain injury ($n=59$) (Brown et al., 2014). Parents receiving Stepping Stones Triple P combined with ACT reported reductions in child externalising and internalising behaviour, as well as reductions in dysfunctional parenting style of laxness and over-reactivity.

The combination of Stepping Stones Triple P and ACT was also tested in a three arm randomised controlled trial with families of children (2–12 years of age) with cerebral palsy ($n=67$) (Whittingham et al., 2014). Families were randomly assigned to one of three groups: waitlist control, Stepping Stones Triple P alone or Stepping Stones Triple P combined with ACT. Parents receiving Stepping Stones Triple P alone reported decreases in internalising behaviour and in the number of externalising behaviour problems as compared to the waitlist control group. Parents receiving Stepping Stones Triple P combined with ACT reported decreases in the number and intensity of externalising behaviour problems, decreases in child hyperactivity and reductions in dysfunctional parenting styles of over-reactivity and verbosity as compared to the waitlist control group. Parents who received the combined Stepping Stones Triple P and ACT intervention reported reductions in child hyperactivity and the dysfunctional parenting styles of laxness and verbosity at 6-month follow-up, compared to parents who received Stepping Stones Triple P alone.

The fact that parents who received Stepping Stones Triple P reported a reduction in child internalising behaviour but the parents receiving ACT in addition to Stepping Stones Triple P did not is surprising, as it is difficult to explain how the addition of ACT could undermine the intervention effect of Stepping Stones Triple P. It may be the case that ACT increased parental capacity to recognise child affect and hence to recognise and report child internalising symptoms. Overall, this study suggests that ACT has an additive contribution to make, above and beyond established behavioural parenting interventions.

Mindful Parenting as Relational Mindfulness

Relational or interpersonal mindfulness involves not solitary mindfulness practices, but practising mindfulness 'during' interpersonal interactions (Falb & Pargament, 2012; Surrey & Jordan, 2012; Wilson & Dufrene, 2008). That is, interpersonal connection itself is the object of mindfulness practice. The practitioner of relational mindfulness brings mindful awareness to the moment to moment changes within themselves, the moment to moment changes within the behaviour of the other person and the moment to moment changes in the flow of the relationship between the two. In particular, the practitioner is aware of moments of connection and disconnection and of the emotional aspects of the ongoing interaction. In terms of communication, interpersonal mindfulness involves listening fully to the other without judgement and speaking honestly and genuinely. There is a compassionate, kind and open aspect to the interaction. Further, the practitioner trusts in emergence within the interaction, that is, the practitioner trusts in the process of co-creation rather than controlling the interaction (Surrey & Jordan, 2012). Interpersonal mindfulness forms an integral part of existing models of mindful parenting (Bogels et al., 2010; Duncan et al., 2009) and relational mindfulness practices have been incorporated into mindfulness interventions for parents (Altmaier & Maloney, 2007; Bogels et al., 2014; Bogels & Restifo, 2014; Coatsworth et al., 2010; Dawe & Harnett, 2007; Dawe et al., 2003; Singh et al., 2006, 2007). Relational mindfulness practices may not be as familiar to the reader. To aid familiarity, and to see how relational mindfulness may be applied to parenting, the following is a script of a relational mindfulness practice for parent–child interaction. The script is written to be inclusive to parents of children of all ages and flexible to individual family circumstances.

Mindfulness of a Parent–Child Interaction

- Your mindfulness practice begins when your child next desires interaction. Your child will call you to practise and your child's call may sound like a cry or a question or it may feel like a small hand grasping at your leg. Wait for the call and, when it comes, respond to it as you might to chimes or bells or the gentle urgings of a kind, wise teacher calling you to wakefulness.
- Allow your child's call to wake you up completely.
- Allow distracting thoughts to simply drift away. Let go of whatever you were thinking or doing and bring your attention to focus on your child.
- Bring your full awareness into your physical body, as it is in the here and now as you respond to your child.
- Ground yourself in your breathing, steady and deep, as you respond to your child.
- Be aware of the preciousness of the moments you are about to spend with your child. Relish them in full awareness and wakefulness.
- As your interaction begins, follow your child's lead. If your child wishes to play then let your child lead the play. If your child wishes to talk, then let your child lead the conversation. If your child is asking for comfort, either in words or cries, then comfort them.
- Notice your own physical sensations, in the here and now, as you interact.
- If thoughts arise, notice them and bring your attention back to your child.
- If emotions arise, make room for them, and expand your awareness to include your child's emotions too.
- Savour the interaction.
- Notice your child as if you were meeting him or her, again, for the very first time. Children change so fast. Notice your child exactly as he or she is right now, at this stage of his or her life.
- When your child talks or babbles or cries, listen to your child without judgement. Let go of your own beliefs and your own agenda and just understand who your child is in this moment.
- Allow yourself to grow open and spacious for your child.
- Find within yourself kindness for your child.
- Be the open, accepting space that your child needs.
- Be the open, accepting space that you need.

- Interact with your child, person to person, in this very moment, without judging your child and without judging yourself.
- Let connection emerge from open awareness. Don't force it. Let it come: in the spontaneous creativity of child-led play, in the joyous laughter of shared fun, in the empathic connection of suffering heard and understood or in the sweetness of spontaneous affection. Let connection come.
- Your mindfulness session ends when your child signals, through words or non-verbally, that he or she is ready to end the interaction. Wait for the signal, and when it comes, treat it as you might chimes or bells or the compassionate words of a wise teacher, gently ending your mindfulness session and urging you to remain awake in your day to day life.

Transformative Parenting

Mindfulness and Personal Transformation

Second-generation mindfulness approaches aim not merely at improved physical and psychological health and decreased stress, but also at both personal and transpersonal transformation (Singh et al., 2014; Shonin & Gordon, 2014). As such, these approaches can be described as explicitly spiritual with a goal of liberation. Second-generation mindfulness approaches include mindfulness, and they also draw more broadly upon other aspects of Buddhist philosophy and practices including wisdom and ethics. For example, the second-generation mindfulness approach used by Singh et al. (2014) is grounded in Mahayana Buddhism more broadly. In addition to mindfulness, the intervention contains practices for developing the four immeasurables: loving-kindness, compassion, equanimity and sympathetic joy.

The Buddhist path contains three pillars: meditation (including mindfulness), wisdom and ethics (Shonin et al., 2014). Of the complete Buddhist path, mindfulness has enjoyed considerable uptake and attention within the scientific literature and within clinical practice. Practices aimed at the cultivation of compassion have also received significant attention and are incorporated into many of the existing mindfulness interventions for parents. However, Buddhist concepts and practices from the wisdom pillar, such as the realisation that there is no inherently existing self, that all phenomena are impermanent or that all phenomena are interconnected, have received little attention. Such concepts may prove useful to parents in a number of ways. The realisation that there is no inherently existing self may assist parents in navigating the identity crisis that the transition to parenthood may bring (Napthali, 2003). The interconnected state of pregnancy and life as a primary caregiver may be better understood and lived when seen as an example of the interconnectedness of all phenomena. The concept of impermanence puts into perspective current parenting challenges and calls parents to enjoy their child's current developmental stage. Ethical practices beyond compassion, such as the practice of generosity or speaking truthfully, have also been given little attention and yet are highly relevant to parenting. For example, parents could practice these ethical principles by giving parental attention generously and by communicating truthfully and genuinely with their children.

Arguably, ACT is already a second-generation mindfulness intervention. Although ACT does not explicitly draw from Buddhist philosophy and practices, in common with second-generation approaches, ACT situates mindfulness within the context of a wider intervention (Hayes, 2002). Within ACT mindfulness is practised alongside exercises to increase acceptance or willingness, strategies to increase cognitive defusion, practices aimed at undermining a conceptualised self in favour of a transcendent self (self-as-context) and purposeful, values-based action. Also similarly to the Buddhist path, ACT is grounded in a universally applicable understanding of suffering. With an overarching goal of promoting psychological flexibility, the ability to act flexibly in accordance with your own chosen values, rather than on reducing stress or depressive or anxious symptoms, ACT is also primarily concerned with personal transformation.

Situating mindfulness within a broader intervention, grounded within a universally applicable understanding of suffering and aiming at personal transformation, is key to truly addressing the full human condition. We need to develop a mindful parenting culture, not just to reduce the distress of parents or even to optimise parenting behaviour, but to empower parents, to enable parents to be more fulfilled, authentic and complete human beings, to enable them to find meaning within parenting and to empower them in the raising of fulfilled and empowered children.

Parenting as Fertile Soil

The Buddha himself ordained women and recognised both male and female lay practitioners within the early Buddhist community as attaining advanced states of spiritual awareness, virtue and wisdom (Harvey, 1990; Thera & Hecker, 2003; Hecker, 2003). This clear early recognition of the capacity for women and lay practitioners to achieve enlightenment has been inconsistently preserved. Although there are accounts of lay practitioners and women achieving enlightenment, in many Buddhist communities, the 'complete' Buddhist path, including mindfulness practices, has historically been the domain of the ordained Sangha: the celibate and childless monastic (Harvey, 1990). In some Buddhist countries, the 'complete' Buddhist path has been the domain of an exclusively male class of celibate and childless monastics (in some countries the tradition of ordaining women has been lost and in others ordained women have a lower status and less access to complete practice opportunities). In cultures where taking robes is a common life stage within a life inclusive of parenthood (e.g. a rite of passage in early adulthood or retirement), it is nevertheless understood as a separate life stage. The contemporary uptake of Buddhism in the West, along with the renewed interest in mindfulness practices amongst lay Buddhist practitioners in traditional Buddhist countries and the growing interest in mindfulness and related practices from outside the Buddhist community itself, offers a unique opportunity. It is possible to explore fully the opportunities for mindfulness, wisdom and ethical development that exist within the life of a committed parent. Arguably, parenting is rich in opportunities for personal development (Kabat-Zinn & Kabat-Zinn, 1997). Becoming a parent may be associated with personal growth, flourishing and transpersonal experiences (Athan, 2011; Galliano Desai, 2012). Instead of simply bringing mindfulness to parents, we should also ask: what unique possibilities for transformation exist within the path of parenthood itself?

Parenting offers rich opportunities for relational or interpersonal mindfulness practices, that is, mindfulness practised during an interpersonal interaction focussing on mindfulness of self, others and the ongoing interaction (Bogels et al., 2010; Duncan et al., 2009). Interpersonal mindfulness practice, by its very nature, includes wisdom and ethics. Done fully, it is a whole-of-path practice, requiring flexible attending to your own unfolding experience and the perspective of another, with wisdom guiding ongoing interaction within a compassionate, generous and open space. The transformative potential of rich interpersonal mindfulness practices, developed to specifically suit life as a parent, needs to be more fully explored. Relational mindfulness practices have been incorporated into mindfulness interventions for parents (Altmaier & Maloney, 2007; Bogels et al., 2014; Bogels & Restifo, 2014; Coatsworth et al., 2010; Dawe & Harnett, 2007; Dawe et al., 2003; Singh et al., 2006, 2007), and interpersonal mindfulness is key to existing models of mindful parenting (Bogels et al., 2010; Duncan et al., 2009); however, solitary mindfulness practices, such as mindfulness of breathing performed in the absence of the child, still form the bulk of mindful parenting interventions. A creative diversity of interpersonal mindfulness practices need to be developed. We need language and practices specifically suited to the transformative possibilities found within life as a parent.

Embodiment refers to our psychological grounding within bodily states (Michalak, Burg, & Heidenreich, 2012). Many mindfulness practices, such as mindfulness of breathing, body scan meditation and mindfulness of walking, bring mindful awareness to the body and bodily sensations. With increased awareness of the physical body comes increased awareness of emotional and mental states (Bogels et al., 2014; Michalak et al., 2012).

The antenatal and postnatal period is a uniquely embodied time of life for women, and there is a paucity of exploration of the practice opportunities that exist within this time of life for women within traditional Buddhist teachings. The dramatic physical changes of pregnancy, the physical challenge of childbirth and the interconnectedness of early parenting, including feeding, bring the physical body and bodily sensations into sharp focus. Further, at this time of life, women are 'interconnectedly embodied'; their very physical space is also occupied by another. The antenatal and postnatal period may be associated with transpersonal experiences, personal growth and flourishing (Athan, 2011; Galliano Desai, 2012; Kabat-Zinn & Kabat-Zinn, 1997). To give one specific example, the embodied experience of feeling the moment to moment movements of another being, within your own physical body, is an experience as profound and potentially transformative as viewing the Earth from space, and its potential transformative power should not be underestimated merely because it is more common.

The finding that participants in a reading control condition also showed increases in mindfulness in a randomised controlled trial (n=47) of a 6-week antenatal mindfulness-based intervention suggests that increases in mindfulness may be a natural aspect of the antenatal period for some women (Guardino et al., 2014). The potential for mindfulness, wisdom and compassion, within the embodied experiences of the antenatal and postnatal period, needs exploration. The development of mindfulness exercises specifically for the antenatal period, including mindfulness of the developing foetus (Bardacke, 2012; Goodman et al., 2014; Whittingham, 2013) and mindfulness for childbirth through sounding, mindful awareness of your own vocalisations (Bardacke, 2012), is an encouraging beginning.

Looking Forward: Future Research

Overall, the existing literature is promising. This area of research is coming of age, and the next several decades will be crucial to its development. We need more carefully constructed empirical studies, including multiple-baseline design research, and, crucially, randomised controlled trials. We also need to recontextualise mindfulness, to embed mindfulness within a larger intervention, such as a second-generation mindfulness intervention or ACT. These interventions should be, as relevant, specifically tailored to the embodied experiences of the antenatal and postnatal period, as well as to the unique opportunities for interpersonal mindfulness practice that exist within life as a parent. Much of this development and clinical research is already happening within the literature, which is deeply encouraging.

In addition to well-constructed clinical research, we also need basic research to inform further clinical developments. A better understanding of the potential for mindfulness that naturally exists within the antenatal period and within life as a parent needs to be developed. Is there a natural trajectory towards increased mindfulness during pregnancy? Can a solely interpersonal mindfulness practice, in the absence of more familiar mindfulness exercises, lead to personal transformation? We also need to explore the impact of parental mindfulness on the children that they are raising, as well as the parenting practices that foster the development of mindfulness, acceptance and compassion in children. Does parenting with mindfulness and compassion, in and of itself, increase the mindfulness and compassion of children? Are particular parenting practices associated with increased acceptance, compassion and mindfulness in children? Can mindful parenting improve the parent child relationship?

Mindful parenting needs to be linked, at a theoretical level, to basic science and to wider theoretical frames and concepts such as parental responsiveness and attachment theory as well as psychological flexibility and relational frame theory. Mindfulness, in conjunction with an interdisciplinary perspective, can form an important part of innovative solutions to the everyday problems that parents face.

Conclusion

The research on the application of mindfulness to parenting is beginning to come of age, and the existing literature is encouraging. Mindfulness-based interventions may soon form a key aspect of services to parents, from pregnancy and beyond. Parenting, as a near-universal experience with inbuilt transformative potential and a vast ability to influence the next generation, is an ideal target for efforts to build a wiser, accepting, mindful and compassionate society.

References

Ainsfeld, E., Capser, V., Nozyce, M., & Cunningham, N. (1990). Does infant carrying promote attachment? An experimental study of the effects of increased physical contact on the development of attachment. *Child Development, 61*(5), 1617–1627.

Ainsworth, M. D. S., Blehar, M. C., Waters, E., & Wall, S. (1978). *Patterns of attachment: A psychological study of the strange situation*. Hillsdale, NJ: Erlbaum.

Altmaier, E., & Maloney, R. (2007). An initial evaluation of a mindful parenting program. *Journal of Clinical Psychology, 63*(12), 1231–1238.

Athan, A. M. (2011). *Postpartum flourishing: Motherhood as opportunity for positive growth and self-development.* Ph.D., Columbia University, New York (3451512).

Ball, H. (2009). Bed-sharing and co-sleeping: Research overview. *NCT New Digest, 48*, 22–27.

Bardacke, N. (2012). *Mindful birthing training the mind body and heart for childbirth and beyond.* New York: Harper One.

Bazzano, A., Wolfe, C., Zylowska, L., Wang, S., Shuster, E., Barrett, C., et al. (2013). Mindfulness Based Stress Reduction (MBSR) for parents and caregivers of individuals with developmental disabilities: A community-based approach. *Journal of Child and Family Studies, 24*, 298–308.

Beer, M., Ward, L., & Moar, K. (2013). The relationship between mindful parenting and distress in parents of children with an autism spectrum disorder. *Mindfulness, 4*, 102–112.

Benn, R., Akiva, T., Arel, S., & Roeser, R. W. (2012). Mindfulness training effects for parents and educators of children with special needs. *Developmental Psychology, 48*(5), 1476–1487.

Biringen, Z., Derscheid, D., Vliegen, N., Closson, L., & Easterbrooks, M. A. (2014). Emotional availability (EA): Theoretical background, empirical research using the EA Scales and clinical applications. *Developmental Review, 34*, 114–167.

Blackledge, J. T., & Hayes, S. C. (2006). Using acceptance and commitment training in the support of parents of children diagnosed with autism. *Child and Family Behavior Therapy, 28*(1), 1–18.

Bluth, K., & Wahler, R. G. (2011a). Does effort matter in mindful parenting? *Mindfulness, 2*, 175–178.

Bluth, K., & Wahler, R. G. (2011b). Parenting preschoolers: Can mindfulness help? *Mindfulness, 2*, 282–285.

Bogels, S. M., Hellemans, J., van Duersen, S., Romer, M., & van der Meulen, R. (2014). Mindful parenting in mental health care: Effects on parental and child psychopathology, parental stress, parenting, coparenting, and marital functioning. *Mindfulness, 5*, 536–551.

Bogels, S. M., Lehtonen, A., & Restifo, K. (2010). Mindful parenting in mental health care. *Mindfulness, 1*, 107–120.

Bogels, S. M., & Restifo, K. (2014). *Mindful parenting a guide for mental health practitioners.* New York: Springer.

Bowlby, J. (1988). *A secure base: Parent-child attachment and healthy human development.* New York: Basic Books.

Brown, F. L., Whittingham, K., Boyd, R. N., McKinlay, L., & Sofronoff, K. (2014). Improving child and parenting outcomes following paediatric acquired brain injury: A randomised controlled trial of stepping stones triple P plus acceptance and commitment therapy. *Journal of Child Psychology and Psychiatry, and Allied Disciplines, 55*(10), 1172–1183.

Brown, F., Whittingham, K., McKinlay, L., Boyd, R. N., & Sofronoff, K. (2013). Efficacy of stepping stones triple P plus a stress management adjunct for parents of children with acquired brain injury: The protocol of a randomised controlled trial. *Brain Impairment, 14*(2), 253–269.

Coatsworth, D. J., Duncan, L. G., Greenberg, M. T., & Nix, R. L. (2010). Changing parent's mindfulness, child management skills and relationship quality with their youth: Results from a randomised pilot intervention trial. *Journal of Child and Family Studies, 19*, 203–217.

Coatsworth, D. J., Duncan, L. G., Nix, R. L., Greenberg, M. T., Gayles, J. G., Bamberger, K. T., et al. (2014). Integrating mindfulness with parent training: Effects of the mindfulness-enhanced strengthening families program. *Developmental Psychology, 51*, 26–35.

Cohen, J. A. S., & Semple, R. J. (2010). Mindful parenting: A call for research. *Journal of Child and Family Studies, 19*(2), 145–151.

Conner, C. M., & White, S. W. (2014). Stress in mothers of children with autism: Trait mindfulness as a protective factor. *Research in Autism Spectrum Disorders, 8*, 617–624.

Coyne, L. W., McHugh, L., & Martinez, E. R. (2011). Acceptance and commitment therapy (ACT): Advances and applications with children, adolescents and families. *Child and Adolescent Psychiatric Clinics of North America, 20*(2), 379–399.

Coyne, L. W., & Murrell, A. R. (2009). *The joy of parenting an acceptance and commitment therapy guide to effective parenting in the early years*. Oakland: New Harbinger.

Coyne, L. W., & Wilson, K. G. (2004). The role of cognitive fusion in impaired parenting: An RFT analysis. *International Journal of Psychology and Psychological Therapy, 4*(3), 469–486.

Dawe, S., & Harnett, P. H. (2007). Reducing potential for child abuse among methadone-maintained parents: Results from a randomized control trial. *Journal of Substance Abuse Treatment, 32*, 381–390.

Dawe, S., Harnett, P. H., Rendalls, V., & Staiger, P. (2003). Improving family functioning and child outcome in methadone maintained families: The parents under pressure programme. *Drug and Alcohol Review, 22*, 299–307.

Dimidjian, S., Goodman, S. H., Felder, J. N., Gallop, R., Brown, A. P., & Beck, A. (2014). An open trial of mindfulness-based cognitive therapy for the prevention of perinatal depressive relapse/recurrence. *Archives of Women's Mental Health, Epub ahead of print., 18*, 85–94.

Douglas, P. S., & Hill, P. S. (2011). The crying baby: What approach? *Current Opinion in Pediatrics, 23*, 523–529.

Dumas, J. E. (2005). Mindfulness-based parent training: Strategies to lessen the grip of automaticity in families with disruptive children. *Journal of Clinical Child & Adolescent Psychology, 34*(4), 779–791.

Duncan, L. G., Coatsworth, J. D., & Greenberg, M. T. (2009). A model of mindful parenting: Implications for parent-child relationships and prevention research. *Clinical Child and Family Psychology Review, 12*(3), 255–270.

Dunn, C., Hanieh, E., Roberts, R., & Powrie, R. (2012). Mindful pregnancy and childbirth: Effects of a mindfulness-based intervention on women's psychological distress and well-being in the perinatal period. *Archives of Women's Mental Health, 15*, 139–143.

Eshel, N., Daelmans, B., Cabral de Mello, M., & Martines, J. (2006). Responsive parenting: Interventions and outcomes. *Bulletin of the World Health Organisation, 84*(12), 991–998.

Evans, T., Whittingham, K., & Boyd, R. (2012). What helps the mother of a preterm infant become securely attached, responsive and well-adjusted? *Infant Behavior and Development, 35*(1), 1–11.

Falb, M. D., & Pargament, K. I. (2012). Relational mindfulness, spirituality, and the therapeutic bond. *Asian Journal of Psychiatry, 2012*, 351–354.

Ferraioli, S. J., & Harris, S. L. (2013). Comparative effects of mindfulness and skills-based parent training programs for parents of children with autism: Feasibility and preliminary outcome data. *Mindfulness, 4*, 89–101.

Fletcher, L., & Hayes, S. C. (2005). Relational frame theory, acceptance and commitment therapy and a functional analytic definition of mindfulness. *Journal of Rational-Emotive and Cognitive-Behavior Therapy, 23*(4), 315–336.

Galliano Desai, F. (2012). *Transpersonal experiences and the emergence of transpersonal motherhood.* PhD, Institute of Transpersonal Psychology, California.

Geurtzen, N., Scholte, R. H. J., Engels, R. C. M. E., Tak, Y. T., & van Zundert, R. M. P. (2014). Association between mindful parenting and adolescents' internalizing problems: Nonjudgmental acceptance of parenting as core element. *Journal of Child and Family Studies, 24*, 1117–1128.

Goodall, K., Trejnowska, A., & Darling, S. (2012). The relationship between dispositional mindfulness, attachment security and emotion regulation. *Personality and Individual Differences, 52*, 622–626.

Goodman, J. H., Guarino, A., Chenausky, K., Klein, L., Prager, J., Peterson, R., et al. (2014). CALM pregnancy: Results of a pilot study of mindfulness-based cognitive therapy for perinatal anxiety. *Archives of Women's Mental Health, 17*, 373–387.

Gottman, J. M., Katz, L. F., & Hooven, C. (1997). *Meta-emotion: How families communicate emotionally*. Mahwah, NJ: Lawrence Erlbaum.

Greco, L. A., & Eifert, G. H. (2004). Treating parent-adolescent conflict: Is acceptance the missing link for an integrative family therapy? *Cognitive and Behavioral Practice, 11*(3), 305–314.

Greco, L., Heffner, M., Poe, S., Ritchie, S., Polak, M., & Lynch, S. (2005). Maternal adjustment following preterm birth: Contributions of experiential avoidance. *Behaviour Therapy, 36*, 177–184.

Guardino, C. M., Schetter, C. D., Bower, J. E., Lue, M. C., & Smalley, S. L. (2014). Randomised controlled pilot trial of mindfulness training for stress reduction during pregnancy. *Psychology and Health, 29*(3), 334–349.

Harnett, P. H., & Dawe, S. (2012). Review: The contribution of mindfulness-based therapies for children and families and proposed conceptual integration. *Child and Adolescent Mental Health, 17*(4), 195–208.

Hart, B., & Risley, T. R. (1995). *Meaningful differences in the everyday experience of young American children*. Baltimore: Paul H Brookes.

Harvey, P. (1990). *An introduction to Buddhism teachings, history and practices*. Melbourne: Cambridge University Press.

Hayes, S. C. (2002). Buddhism and acceptance and commitment therapy. *Cognitive and Behavioral Practice, 9*(1), 58–66.

Hayes, S. C. (2004). Acceptance and commitment therapy and the new behavior therapies. In S. C. Hayes, V. M. Follette, & M. M. Linehan (Eds.), *Mindfulness and acceptance expanding the cognitive-behavioral tradition*. New York: The Guilford Press.

Hayes, S. C., Luoma, J. B., Bond, F. W., Masuda, A., & Lillis, J. (2006). Acceptance and commitment therapy: Model, processes and outcomes. *Behaviour Research and Therapy, 44*, 1–25.

Hayes, S. C., Strosal, K. D., & Wilson, K. G. (2003). *Acceptance and commitment therapy: An experiential approach to behavior change*. New York: Guilford Press.

Hecker, H. (2003). Great women disciplines of the Buddha. In N. Thera & H. Hecker (Eds.), *Great disciplines of the Buddha their lives their works their legacy* (pp. 254–310). Massachusetts: Buddhist Publication Society.

Hertz, R. M., Laurent, H. K., & Laurent, S. M. (2014). Attachment mediates effects of trait mindfulness on stress responses to conflict. *Mindfulness, 6*, 483–489.

Hughes, A., Williams, M., Bardacke, N., Duncan, L. G., Dimidjian, S., & Goodman, S. H. (2009). Mindfulness approaches to childbirth and parenting. *British Journal of Midwifery, 17*(10), 630–635.

Jones, L., Hastings, R. P., Totsika, V., Keane, L., & Rhule, N. (2014). Child behavior problems and parental well-being in families of children with autism: The mediating role of mindfulness and acceptance. *American Journal on Intellectual and Developmental Disabilities, 119*(2), 171–185.

Kabat-Zinn, M., & Kabat-Zinn, J. (1997). *Everyday blessings the inner work of mindful parenting*. New York: Hyperion.

Kang, C., & Whittingham, K. (2010). Mindfulness: A dialogue between Buddhism and clinical psychology. *Mindfulness, 1*(3), 161–173.

Kashdan, T. B., & Rotteberg, J. (2012). Psychological flexibility as a fundamental aspect of health. *Clinical Psychology Review, 30*, 865–878.

Kostanski, M., & Hassed, C. (2008). Mindfulness as a concept and a process. *Australian Psychologist, 43*(1), 15–21.

Michalak, J., Burg, J., & Heidenreich, T. (2012). Don't forget your body: Mindfulness, embodiment, and the treatment of depression. *Mindfulness, 3*, 190–199.

Moreira, H., Gouveia, M. J., Carona, C., Silva, N., & Canavarro, M. C. (2014). Maternal attachment and children's quality of life: The mediating role of self-compassion and parenting stress. *Journal of Child and Family Studies*. doi:10.1007/s10826-014-0036-z.

Murrell, A. R., Wilson, K. G., LaBorde, C., Drake, C. E., & Rogers, L. J. (2009). Relational responding in parents. *Behavior Analyst Today, 9*, 196–214.

Muzik, M., Hamilton, S. E., Rosenblum, L., Waxler, E., & Hadi, Z. (2012). Mindfulness yoga improve scores on depression scales and fosters maternal-fetal attachment. *Complementary Therapy and Clinical Practice, 18*(4), 235–240.

Napthali, S. (2003). *Buddhism for mothers*. Crows Nest: Allen & Unwin.

Neece, C. L. (2014). Mindfulness-based stress reduction for parents of young children with developmental delays: Implications for parental mental health and child behavior problems. *Journal of Applied Research in Intellectual Disabilities, 27*, 174–186.

Shea, S. E., & Coyne, L. W. (2011). Maternal dysphoric mood, stress and parenting practices in mothers of head start preschoolers: The role of experiential avoidance. *Child and Family Behavior Therapy, 33*, 231–247.

Shonin, E., & Gordon, W. V. (2014). Manager's experiences of meditation awareness training. *Mindfulness*. doi:10.1007/s12671-014-0334-y.

Shonin, E., Gordon, W. V., & Griffiths, M. D. (2014). The emerging role of Buddhism in clinical psychology: Toward effective integration. *Psychology of Religion and Spirituality, 6*(2), 122–137.

Singh, N. N., Lancioni, G. E., Winton, A. S. W., Fisher, B. C., Wahler, R. G., McAleaney, K. M., et al. (2006). Mindful parenting decreases aggression, non-compliance and self-injury in children with Autism. *Journal of Emotional and Behavioural Disorders, 14*(3), 169–177.

Singh, N. N., Lancioni, G. E., Winton, A. S. W., Karazsia, B. T., Myers, R. E., Latham, L. L., et al. (2014). Mindfulness-based positive behavior support (MBPBS) for mothers of adolescents with autism spectrum disorder: Effects on adolescents' behavior and parental stress. *Mindfulness, 5*, 646–657.

Singh, N. N., Lancioni, G. E., Winton, A. S. W., Singh, J., Curtis, W. J., Wahler, R. G., et al. (2007). Mindful parenting decreases aggression and increase social behaviour in children with developmental disabilities. *Behaviour Modification, 31*(6), 749–771.

Singh, N. N., Lancioni, G. E., Winton, A. S. W., Singh, J., Singh, A. N., Adkins, A. D., et al. (2011). Training in mindful care giving transfers to parent-child interactions. *Journal of Child and Family Studies, 19*, 167–174.

Sroufe, A. L. (2005). Attachment and development: A prospective, longitudinal study from birth to adulthood. *Attachment and Human Development, 7*(4), 349–367.

Surrey, J. L. (2005). Relational psychotherapy, relational mindfulness. In C. K. Germer, R. D. Siegel, & P. R. Fulton (Eds.), *Mindfulness and psychotherapy* (pp. 91–110). New York: The Guilford Press.

Surrey, J., & Jordan, J. V. (2012). The wisdom of connection. In C. K. Germer & R. D. Siegel (Eds.), *Wisdom and compassion in psychotherapy deepening mindfulness in clinical practice*. New York: The Guilford Press.

Synder, R., Shapiro, S., & Treleaven, D. (2012). Attachment theory and mindfulness. *Journal of Child and Family Studies, 21*, 709–717.

Thera, N., & Hecker, H. (2003). Shorter lives of the disciplines. In N. Thera & H. Hecker (Eds.), *Great disciplines of the Buddha their lives their works their legacy* (pp. 254–310). Massachusetts: Buddhist Publication Society.

Tiwari, S., Podell, J. C., Martin, E. D., Mychailysezyn, M. P., Furr, J. M., & Kendall, P. C. (2008). Experiential avoidance in the parenting of anxious youth: Theory, research and future directions. *Cognition and Emotion, 22*(3), 480–496.

Van der Oord, S., Bogels, S. M., & Pejnenberg, D. (2012). The effectiveness of mindfulness training for children with ADHD and mindful parenting for their parents. *Journal of Child and Family Studies, 21*(1), 139–147.

Vieten, C., & Astin, J. (2008). Effects of a mindfulness-based intervention during pregnancy on prenatal stress and mood: Results of a pilot study. *Archives of Women's Mental Health, 11*, 67–74.

Walsh, J. J., Balint, M. G., David, R., Smolira, S. J., Fredericksen, L. K., & Madsen, S. (2009). Predicting individual differences in mindfulness: The role of trait anxiety, attachment anxiety and attentional control. *Personality and Individual Differences, 46*, 94–99.

Whittingham, K. (2013). *Becoming mum*. Brisbane: Pivotal.

Whittingham, K. (2014a). Parents of children with disabilities, mindfulness and acceptance: A review and a call for research. *Mindfulness, 5*(6), 704–709.

Whittingham, K. (2014b). Parenting in context. *Journal of Contextual Behavioral Science, 3*, 212–215.

Whittingham, K., & Douglas, P. (2014). Optimising parent-infant sleep from birth to six months: A new paradigm. *Infant Mental Health Journal, 35*, 614–623.

Whittingham, K., Sanders, M. R., McKinlay, L., & Boyd, R. N. (2013). Stepping stones triple p and acceptance and commitment therapy for parents of children with cerebral palsy: Trial protocol. *Brain Impairment, 14*(2), 270–280.

Whittingham, K., Sanders, M., McKinlay, L., & Boyd, R. N. (2014). Interventions to reduce behavioral problems in children with cerebral palsy: An RCT. *Pediatrics, 133*, e1249–e1257.

Whittingham, K., Wee, D., Sanders, M., & Boyd, R. (2013). Predictors of psychological adjustment, experienced parenting burden and chronic sorrow symptoms in parents of children with cerebral palsy. *Child: Care, Health and Development, 39*(3), 366–373.

Williams, K. L., & Wahler, R. G. (2010). Are mindful parents more authoritative and less authoritarian? an analysis of clinic-referred mothers. *Journal of Child and Family Studies, 19*, 230–235.

Wilson, K. G., & Dufrene, T. (2008). *Mindfulness for two an acceptance and commitment therapy approach to mindfulness in psychotherapy*. Oakland: New Harbinger.

Chapter 19
Mindfulness and Couple Relationships

Christopher A. Pepping and W. Kim Halford

Introduction

Alex and Jo have been in a committed romantic relationship for 5 years. Despite both expressing a strong desire to spend their lives together, they often feel unhappy in their relationship, which frequently escalates into conflict between them. Both Alex and Jo have busy careers and very active social lives and report it can be difficult to ensure they have time together as a couple. When Alex and Jo do spend time together, they both find that they are often preoccupied with thoughts about work. Alex also complains that Jo is often texting and calling friends when he tries to talk with her and that "we never can just be there and talk". For example, he reported she spent nearly 45 min on the telephone to a friend when they were out to dinner as a couple recently. Jo complains that Alex is preoccupied with his work and is often distracted by a call or message when they speak. She mentioned how they were talking about coming to therapy when Alex dashed off to respond to an incoming message alert on his mobile telephone. These patterns make it very difficult to fully engage in positive shared activities together. They both report wanting to make their relationship work but are feeling increasingly unsure of how to improve things.

The above case illustrates an increasingly common complaint of couples that distraction, particularly around social media, work responsibilities, and online

C.A. Pepping (✉)
La Trobe University, Melbourne, VIC, Australia
e-mail: c.pepping@latrobe.edu.au

W.K. Halford
University of Queensland, Brisbane, QLD, Australia

E. Shonin et al. (eds.), *Mindfulness and Buddhist-Derived Approaches in Mental Health and Addiction*, Advances in Mental Health and Addiction,
DOI 10.1007/978-3-319-22255-4_19

activity, prevents full engagement in the couple relationship. In the present chapter, we review the potential contribution that mindfulness can have on understanding and enhancing couple relationships.

Couple Relationships

Being in a satisfying romantic relationship is one of the strongest predictors of life satisfaction and well-being (Diener, Eunkook, Lucas, & Smith, 1999; Schmaling & Sher, 2000; Wade & Pevalin, 2004) and is associated with greater physical health (Dupre & Meadows, 2007; Waite & Gallagher, 2002) and increased life expectancy (Waite & Gallagher, 2002). Individuals in distressed relationships, however, experience lower well-being (Diener et al., 1999) and are at greater risk for the development of mood and anxiety disorders and substance misuse (Overbeek et al., 2006; Whisman, Uebelacker, & Bruce, 2006). Importantly, much evidence indicates that relationship quality influences mental health; relationship quality is not simply an outcome of mental health. Firstly, relationship distress prospectively predicts mental health problems. For example, national surveys in the USA and the Netherlands demonstrate that relationship dissatisfaction predicts the onset of adults' first episode of depression (Overbeek et al., 2006; Whisman & Bruce, 1999. Further, relationship distress predicts future alcohol abuse, even when controlling for prior history of alcohol abuse (Whisman et al., 2006).

With regard to treatment of psychological disorders, when disorders are treated with individual evidence-based treatments, relationship distress predicts poor outcome in depression (Denton et al., 2010; Whisman, 2001), alcohol abuse (Fals-Stewart, O'Farrell, & Lam, 2009), and a range of anxiety disorders (Dewey & Hunsley, 1990; Durham, Allan, & Hackett, 1997). Further, enhancing couple relationships via clinical interventions improves the mental health of individual partners. Specifically, couple interventions enhance both the couple relationship and individual adjustment when treating substance abuse (Powers, Vedel, & Emmelkamp, 2008), depression (Barbato & D'Avanzo, 2008), and possibly eating disorders, obsessive-compulsive disorder (Baucom, Whisman, & Paprocki, 2012), and post-traumatic stress disorder (PTSD) (Monson et al., 2012). In addition, couple relationship education (CRE) (a relatively brief educational intervention) assists couples to sustain high relationship satisfaction (Halford & Bodenmann, 2013), and this promotes the individual spouse's mental health (Wadsworth & Markman, 2012).

Here, we examine the possibility that mindfulness may be beneficial to romantic relationships. To date, most of the scientific literature has examined whether mindfulness enhances individual well-being and functioning or reduces individual distress (Keng, Smoski, & Robins, 2011). However, more recently, there has been increasing focus on the potential benefits of mindfulness for interpersonal outcomes. We begin by reviewing the available theoretical and empirical evidence pertaining to the influence of dispositional mindfulness on relationship outcomes and then discuss the use of mindfulness-based interventions to enhance couple relationships. We conclude with a discussion of the clinical utility of mindfulness for use with distressed couples and outline directions for future research.

Mindfulness

Mindfulness is commonly defined as the process of "paying attention in a particular way: on purpose, in the present moment, non-judgementally" (Kabat-Zinn, 1994, p. 4). Almost all individuals are capable of mindfulness, but there are individual differences in naturally occurring levels of mindfulness (Brown & Ryan, 2003; Kabat-Zinn, 2003). As such, dispositional mindfulness refers to an individual's capacity and "tendency to abide in mindful states over time" (Brown, Ryan, & Creswell, 2007a, p. 218). The enhanced awareness to the present moment that characterises high dispositional mindfulness is said to facilitate cognitive and behavioural flexibility, which allows for more adaptive responses to situations as opposed to responding in a habitual or impulsive manner to situations (Baer, 2003; Bishop et al., 2004; Brown et al., 2007a, 2007b; Brown, Ryan, & Creswell, 2007a). Much evidence converges as to the beneficial effects of dispositional mindfulness (Keng et al., 2011). Individuals higher in dispositional mindfulness fare better on a variety of psychosocial outcomes than their less mindful counterparts (Brown & Ryan, 2003; Brown et al., 2007a; Keng et al., 2011), many of which are likely to contribute to satisfying romantic relationships.

Dispositional Mindfulness and Relationship Outcomes

Theoretically, dispositional mindfulness should facilitate a relationally focussed, non-judgemental, and experientially non-avoidant stance towards difficult emotions that can arise in interactions with others and in relationships (Wachs & Cordova, 2007). This non-judgemental and accepting stance towards difficult emotions in relationships may allow appropriate, constructive responses in relationships rather than reactive, impulsive responses. Consistent with this proposition, high dispositional mindfulness is associated with increased romantic relationship satisfaction (Barnes, Brown, Krusemark, Campbell, & Rogee, 2007; Wachs & Cordova, 2007) and satisfaction with interpersonal relationships more broadly (Pepping, O'Donovan, Zimmer-Gembeck, & Hanish, 2014). Here, we review six broad reasons as to why dispositional mindfulness may enhance couple relationships, namely, (1) enhanced individual adjustment, (2) greater emotion regulation capacity, (3) increased acceptance of one's own experiences and acceptance of one's partner, (4) enhanced capacity for self-reflection and relationship self-regulation, (5) increased empathy and support-giving skills, and (6) greater capacity to engage in shared enjoyable couple activities.

Individual Adjustment

High dispositional mindfulness is associated with less psychopathology and enhanced psychological adjustment (Keng et al., 2011). Much evidence indicates that psychopathology in one or both partners is a strong predictor of couple relationship distress (Whisman & Baucom, 2012; Whisman, Uebelacker, & Weinstock, 2004). For example, in a sample of 774 married couples, Whisman and colleagues (2004) found that anxiety and depression predicted one's own relationship distress and that depression also predicted partner distress. Mindfulness is associated with lower levels of depression (Brown & Ryan, 2003), anxiety (Brown & Ryan, 2003; Dekeyser, Raes, Leijssen, Leysen, & Dewulf, 2008), eating pathology (Pepping, O'Donovan, Zimmer-Gembeck, & Hanisch, 2015), and substance misuse (Bowen & Enkema, 2014). Further, mindfulness-based clinical interventions, such as mindfulness-based stress reduction, have been effective for the treatment of depression (Grossman et al., 2010; Shapiro, Schwartz, & Bonner, 1998; Vollestad, Sivertsen, & Nielsen, 2011) and anxiety disorders (Anderson, Lau, Segal, & Bishop, 2007; Shapiro et al., 1998; Vollestad et al., 2011). Further, dialectical behaviour therapy, which incorporates mindfulness skills, is effective for the treatment of borderline personality disorder (Kliem, Kroger, & Kosfelder, 2010). In brief, there is clear evidence that mindfulness is protective against psychopathology. Thus, one plausible mechanism by which mindfulness might enhance romantic relationships is that it moderates the risk of psychopathology.

High dispositional mindfulness is also associated with a wide range of positive psychological outcomes likely to affect individual well-being and, in turn, romantic relationship functioning. Of particular relevance to couple relationship processes, low dispositional mindfulness is associated with insecure attachment (specifically, attachment anxiety and avoidance; Pepping, O'Donovan, & Davis, 2014). Attachment anxiety refers to the tendency to be fearful of abandonment and rejection in romantic relationships, whereas attachment avoidance reflects discomfort with emotional intimacy and closeness (Mikulincer & Shaver, 2007). Both forms of attachment insecurity are associated with poor relationship outcomes, including maladaptive communication, low relationship satisfaction, and negative partner attributions (Mikulincer & Shaver, 2007). Moreover, in a sample of 104 married adults, Jones, Welton, Oliver, and Thoburn (2011) found that mindfulness was associated with increased relationship satisfaction, and this association was mediated by low attachment avoidance. Thus, mindfulness may, over time, impact upon relationships via attachment processes and, in particular, by reducing avoidant attachment. However, it is important to note that the established association between low mindfulness and attachment insecurity is cross-sectional (Pepping, Davis, & O'Donovan, 2015), and further longitudinal work is needed to eliminate competing explanations for the associations. For example, low avoidant attachment might enable mindful engagement with relationships. Alternatively, a third variable, such as low neuroticism or quality of parenting received in childhood, might lead to both high mindfulness and low avoidant attachment.

Attachment insecurity is a risk factor for relationship break-up (Mikulincer & Shaver, 2007) as well as low relationship satisfaction. Saavedra, Chapman, and Rogge (2010) found that mindfulness attenuated the negative effects of attachment anxiety on risk of relationship break-up. This finding combined with the Jones and colleagues' (2011) findings that attachment avoidance mediated effects of mindfulness on relationship satisfaction suggests a possible reciprocal influence between insecure attachment and mindfulness. That is, high mindfulness might promote low insecure attachment and vice versa.

In summary, mindfulness is associated with a wide range of positive individual qualities, including low risk of psychopathology and secure attachment. It seems likely that the association between mindfulness and greater relationship satisfaction is, at least in part, due to the association between mindfulness and individual adjustment.

Emotion Regulation

High unregulated negative affect is one of the characteristic features of couple relationship distress (Cordova, Gee, & Warren, 2005; Gottman, 2014; Gottman, Coan, Carrere, & Swanson, 1998; Greenberg & Johnson, 1988), which often prevents the successful resolution of relationship conflicts (Gottman, 2014). On the other hand, the ability to effectively identify and communicate emotion is associated with high romantic relationship satisfaction (Cordova et al., 2005). High negative emotion can lead to negative cycles of couple interaction (Christensen & Heavey, 1993; Gottman, 2014; Greenberg & Johnson, 1988). For example, couples often engage in mutual blaming and escalating conflict, which predicts deteriorating relationship satisfaction and risk of separation (Gottman, 2014). Sometimes the demand-withdraw pattern of interaction develops when one partner exerts pressure for change through criticism or complaints and the spouse responds with defensiveness and emotional withdrawal (Christensen & Heavey, 1990, 1993).

Emotion-focussed couple therapy (Greenberg & Johnson, 1988; Johnson, 1999) is an empirically supported approach to couple therapy that aims to modify distressed couples' negative cycles of interaction (such as the demand-withdraw pattern described earlier). A critical component of emotion-focussed couple therapy is the identification and expression of previously unacknowledged primary emotions such as fear, hurt, or sadness. It is suggested people often express secondary emotions, notably anger, as a response to unacknowledged primary emotions. In other words, individuals are often most aware of, and express most freely, the secondary emotions such as anger. Emotion-focussed therapy facilitates the expression of the vulnerable primary emotions between partners in an effort to de-escalate the negative cycle of interaction (Johnson & Greenberg, 1987; Johnson, 1999).

Individuals higher in dispositional mindfulness may be better able to identify emotion and, in particular, more vulnerable primary emotions and may also have greater capacity to tolerate, cope with, and respond to difficult emotion that can occur in couple relationships. Much evidence indicates that mindfulness is associated with enhanced ability to recognise and tolerate difficult emotion (Baer, Smith, & Allen, 2004; Brown & Ryan, 2003; Liu, Wang, Chang, Chen, & Si, 2013) and regulate emotion effectively (e.g. Arch & Craske, 2006; Broderick, 2005; Campbell-Sills, Barlow, Brown, & Hofmann, 2006). Further, Wachs and Cordova (2007) found that individuals higher in mindfulness rated themselves as better able to respond adaptively to intense emotion (Wachs & Cordova, 2007). Wachs and Cordova (2007) proposed that dispositional mindfulness should assist individuals to maintain openness and receptiveness to difficult emotions that can arise in romantic relationships. The authors also posited that mindfulness should prevent experiential avoidance in response to emotion in relationships, for example, by not withdrawing.

A non-judgmental accepting stance towards emotion in relationships should facilitate the open expression of emotion and enhance each partner's ability to respond in a constructive way to intense emotion. For example, mindful acceptance of strong emotion arising in response to difficult relationship experiences should enable an individual to respond in a constructive manner that will enhance the relationship (Gambrel & Keeling, 2010; Wachs & Cordova, 2007). On the other hand, low capacity to tolerate negative affect might lead to unhelpful behaviours to terminate the interaction (e.g. yelling to shut the other person up) or attempts to experientially avoid difficult emotion arising through emotional withdrawal and distancing.

Consistent with the above-mentioned possibilities of mindfulness enhancing emotion regulation in the context of couple relationships, in a sample of 33 couples, Wachs and Cordova (2007) found that high dispositional mindfulness was associated with low emotional distress, ability to identify and communicate emotion, and effective regulation of anger and impulsivity. Importantly, identifying and communicating emotion, and anger regulation, fully mediated the association between mindfulness and relationship satisfaction. Barnes and colleagues (2007) investigated the impact of dispositional mindfulness on communication behaviours during couple conflict discussion and found that individuals' own mindfulness predicted lower anger and hostility following the conflict discussion and female mindfulness also predicted less anger and hostility in men following the discussion. In brief, high dispositional mindfulness may enhance couple relationships via the capacity to identify, accept, tolerate, and respond to difficult emotions that can arise in romantic relationships.

Acceptance

A defining feature of mindfulness is the concept of acceptance (Baer, 2003; Keng et al., 2011). Mindfulness-based interventions include a strong focus on acceptance of experiences as they are, without engaging in efforts to avoid or escape from these experiences (Kabat-Zinn, 1994; Baer, 2003). Individuals who are dispositionally high in mindfulness may be able to accept their internal experiences of relationship challenges. Being able to accept these experiences could reduce the felt need to reduce these experiences, whereas desperation to modify distressing internal experience can sometimes induce impulsive responses like aggression or substance abuse (Peterson, Eifert, Feingold, & Davidson, 2009). It is also likely that high dispositional mindfulness facilitates acceptance of one's partner's qualities that may be challenging (Christensen, Sevier, Simpson, & Gattis, 2004; Peterson et al., 2009). The question of whether acceptance of internal reactions and one's partner is responsible for the association between mindfulness and relationship satisfaction is yet to be investigated empirically.

Enhanced Self-reflection and Self-regulation

Mindfulness may enhance an individual's ability to reflect on their own behaviour and implement self-change to enhance the relationship (Carson, Carson, Gil, & Baucom, 2006). High dispositional mindfulness is cross-sectionally associated with greater self-reflection and insight into one's own thoughts, emotions, and behaviours (Harrington, Loffredo, & Perz, 2014). Further, this insight mediates the relationship between dispositional mindfulness and psychological well-being (Harrington et al., 2014). Although this research is cross-sectional, it does provide some preliminary evidence that the mechanism underlying the mindfulness-well-being association may, at least in part, be due to enhanced insight. Mindfulness is also associated with insight problem-solving abilities, which refers to the process of restructuring a problem (Ostafin & Kassman, 2012). For example, a person who becomes resentful that their partner is not keen to attend their favourite sporting event might mindfully note that the desire to attend the sporting event reflects two desires: to spend time with the partner and to attend the sporting event. That mindfulness might lead to the insight that these two desires need not be met simultaneously, they could go to the sporting event with someone else and plan a mutually enjoyable activity with their partner. Perhaps the greater insight, personal reflection, and creative problem-solving abilities associated with mindfulness contribute not only to individual well-being but also to relationship outcomes. Individuals high in dispositional mindfulness may be able to reflect on their own behaviour in relationships and engage in efforts to modify or adapt their behaviour to enhance the relationship.

The concept of relationship self-regulation refers to the extent to which partners work at their relationship and engage in relationship-enhancing behaviours (Wilson, Charker, Lizzio, Halford, & Kimlin, 2005). Specifically, it involves self-appraisal of the impact of one's own behaviour on the quality of the relationship and identifying aspects of one's behaviour that may be modified in order to enhance the quality of the relationship. Relationship self-regulation is associated with relationship satisfaction in newlywed and long-term married couples (Wilson et al., 2005) and also longitudinally predicts relationship satisfaction (Halford & Wilson, 2009). It seems likely that individuals high in dispositional mindfulness may be able to non-judgementally reflect on their relationship, identify aspects of their behaviour they wish to modify, and subsequently engage in a process of self-change directed towards building the relationship they desire.

Finally, distressed couples tend to attribute negative relationship behaviours or relationship difficulties to their partner's behaviour and internal qualities of the partner (Bradbury & Fincham, 1990; Durtschi, Fincham, Cui, Lorenz, & Conger, 2011). Further, these negative partner attributions tend to be global (i.e. reflecting a personal quality of the partner rather than being situationally specific) and stable (i.e. the belief that one's partner always acts in this manner). Negative partner attributions predict poor relationship quality longitudinally, and importantly, this effect is mediated by negative partner behaviour (Durtschi et al., 2011). Given that mindfulness is characterised by a non-judgemental and nonreactive stance towards the present moment and internal experiences, it is possible that individuals higher in mindfulness may be less likely to form negative partner attributions in the first place. However, even when mindful individuals do experience negative partner attributions, they may be better able to remain nonreactive to these thoughts, as opposed to engaging in partner blaming or criticism of one's partner in response. Although this possibility seems theoretically plausible, research is needed to address this proposition empirically.

Empathy and Support

Mindfulness involves a non-judgemental stance towards, and non-elaborative processing of, thoughts, emotions, and experiences (Kabat-Zinn, 1990; Baer, 2003). Individuals high in dispositional mindfulness are likely to have capacity to suspend judgement in the context of difficult experiences in relationships and engage constructively with their relationship partner. The capacity to feel empathic concern for the other person may be facilitated by the awareness of experiences associated with mindfulness and thus enhance relationship outcomes (Block-Lerner, Adair, Plumb, Rhatigan, & Orsillo, 2007; Kozlowski, 2013). Wachs and Cordova (2007) found associations between dispositional mindfulness and self-reported empathy and perspective taking in a sample of married couples. Further, Shapiro and colleagues (1998) investigated the effects of an 8-week mindfulness intervention and found that increased mindfulness was associated with increased empathy. It therefore seems likely that individuals high in dispositional mindfulness enjoy enhanced romantic relationships because they have greater capacity for empathy and perspective taking.

Related to the concept of empathy is the provision of mutual support by partners during times of stress. There is now a wealth of evidence that major life stress can impact negatively on couple relationship satisfaction, but that these negative effects can be attenuated if the couples are effective in coping with these stresses together (Bodenmann, 2005). The term dyadic coping is used by Bodenmann and Shantinath (2004) to describe a process whereby partners communicate with each other empathically to develop a shared understanding of the effect of particular stresses on each partner and then develop an agreed-upon conjoint approach to manage these stresses. Dyadic coping is strongly associated with relationship satisfaction in couples confronting both major life stresses such as a cancer diagnosis (Kuijer et al., 2000), as well as couples managing more common daily life hassles (Dehle, Larsen, & Landers, 2001).

To date, very little empirical research has examined the association between mindfulness and dyadic coping in couples. However, in a sample of 51 couples in which one partner was suffering chronic pain, Williams and Cano (2014) found that chronic pain patients who were better able to remain nonreactive to fluctuating internal pain experiences perceived their partners as being more supportive. For example, individuals who are suffering from chronic pain can experience substantial negative emotion, physical pain, and disturbing thoughts about the condition. Those high in mindfulness are able to accept these experiences and not react in unhelpful ways (e.g. trying to avoid these experiences by substance abuse or becoming angry at their spouse). The mindful acceptance of pain experiences likely allows them to accept and perceive support from their partner more readily, despite these difficult internal experiences.

In addition, partners' who scored high on the acting with awareness subscale of mindfulness were rated by the pain patients as being high in emotional and instrumental support (Williams & Cano, 2014). That is, partners who were more aware were perceived by chronic pain sufferers as more emotionally and instrumentally supportive. This makes theoretical sense, as the supporting partner who is high in mindful awareness is likely to be better able to detect the needs of their partner and their pain. In brief, this study provides some preliminary evidence that aspects of mindfulness play a role in couple support and dyadic coping, which may be an additional mechanism by which mindfulness influences relationship processes.

Engagement in Positive Couple Activities

The final mechanism by which mindfulness might enhance romantic relationship functioning is via increased engagement within the relationship. As mentioned earlier, mindfulness is associated with increased positive affect and lower negative affect (Brown & Ryan, 2003). It seems plausible that mindfulness may enhance engagement in, and enjoyment of, positive couple interactions. The couple described at the start of the chapter were low in mindfulness of the couple relationship, with both partners being preoccupied with thoughts of work and distracted by social media. Perhaps cultivating mindfulness would enhance their ability to be fully present with each other and engage more completely in activities they do as a couple. Research from a clinical trial of a mindfulness-based relationship enhancement programme supports this contention. Carson, Carson, Gil, and Baucom (2007) found that the beneficial effects of a mindfulness-based relationship enhancement programme were mediated largely by couples reporting they increased engagement in exciting and absorbing activities.

In summary, there are numerous potential mechanisms by which high mindfulness may enhance romantic relationship functioning. Individuals high in mindfulness enjoy more positive romantic relationships (Barnes et al., 2007; Wachs & Cordova, 2007), which may be because of enhanced individual adjustment, emotion regulation capacity, self-regulation, acceptance of self and partner, heightened empathy, and increased engagement in positive couple activities. We now turn to the use of mindfulness-based clinical interventions to enhance relationship functioning in couples.

Mindfulness-Based Interventions to Enhance Couple Relationships

There are two broad approaches to enhancing couple relationships: couple relationship education and couple therapy. Couple relationship education (RE) was developed to enrich couples' relationships and help couples to sustain a healthy, mutually satisfying, and stable relationship (Halford, Markman, Kling, & Stanley, 2003). RE usually works with couples who are currently satisfied in their relationship and are committed to that relationship. Evidence-based RE usually is brief, typically consisting of a 12–15 h curriculum that introduces key relationship knowledge (e.g. the importance of commitment, developing shared and realistic relationship expectations) and skills (e.g. couple communication, problem-solving, coping) (Halford, Markman, & Stanley, 2008). Here, RE builds upon the high level of positive emotion typical of currently satisfied couples and has a strong emphasis on building the positive foundations for a mutually satisfying life together.

Couple therapy is usually addressed to couples who are distressed in their relationship. In contrast to the typically fixed curriculum of RE, evidence-based couple therapy typically involves developing a couple specific conceptualisation of distress and an individually tailored treatment programme (Snyder & Halford, 2012). Couple therapists usually are trained mental health professionals who have the skills to deliver this specialised treatment and to manage the high levels of negative affect many distressed couples feel (Halford & Snyder, 2012).

There are well replicated short-term benefits of RE, particularly if the programmes are of sufficient duration. A meta-analysis of 117 studies of curriculum-based RE reported medium effect size improvements in couple communication, $d=0.44$, and small increases in relationship satisfaction, $d=0.36$, immediately after RE (Hawkins, Blanchard, Baldwin, & Fawcett, 2008). Programmes with moderate dosage (9–20 h) had substantially larger effect sizes than low-dose programmes (1–8 h) on satisfaction, with limited variability in pre-RE means across studies.

The modest magnitude of short-term effects of RE has been a source of debate in the literature. Bradbury and Lavner (2012) argued that the effect of existing forms of RE on relationship satisfaction was variable across studies, with a mixture of null and small (possibly trivial) effects. The overall null findings of the recent large, multisite Building Strong Families (BSF) study (Wood, McConnell, Moore, Clarkwest, & Hsueh, 2012) and the very small effects observed in the large multisite

Supporting Healthy Marriage (SHM) study (Hsueh et al., 2012) might seem to support the view of Bradbury and Lavner. However, both BSF and SHM involved extensive contact hours for couples, and there was a lot of attrition from the programmes. Nonetheless there have been calls to seek to be more innovative in the content of RE in an attempt to enhance its effects (e.g. Bradbury & Lavner, 2012).

There are over 30 randomised controlled trials of couple therapy for distressed couples, most of which have examined efficacy of behavioural couple therapy (BCT) or emotion-focussed couple therapy (Snyder & Halford, 2012). Meta-analyses demonstrate a large effect size gain in couple adjustment for couple therapy compared to control conditions (Shadish & Baldwin, 2003) and pre-therapy to post-therapy in couple adjustment (Baucom, Hahlweg, & Kuschel, 2003). There is little evidence of systematic differences in the efficacy of different approaches to couple therapy (Shadish & Baldwin, 2003; Snyder & Halford, 2012). However, although couple therapy is beneficial for many distressed couples, only approximately 50 % of couples who end treatment are no longer distressed, 25–30 % increase in satisfaction but remain distressed following therapy, and 20 % do not significantly benefit from treatment (Snyder & Halford, 2012). Although to date no new approach has been replicated as being more efficacious than pre-existing approaches (Snyder, Castellani, & Whisman, 2006), researchers are continuing to develop new approaches to couple therapy, or refine existing approaches, in attempts to enhance efficacy of couple therapy.

The evidence reviewed earlier clearly indicates that mindfulness is associated with many outcomes related to satisfying romantic relationships. It therefore seems likely that enhancing mindfulness via mindfulness-based clinical interventions may have beneficial effects on couple relationships. Specifically, mindfulness- and acceptance-based interventions may be useful for the treatment of couple relationship distress but may also be beneficial for relationship enhancement. In this section, we describe mindfulness-based relationship enhancement (Carson, Carson, Gil, & Baucom, 2004, 2006; Carson et al., 2006) and integrative behavioural couple therapy (Jacobson, Christensen, Prince, Cordova, & Eldridge, 2000; Christensen et al., 2004) which incorporates acceptance-based strategies for treatment of couple relationship distress.

Mindfulness-Based Relationship Education

Carson and colleagues (2004) developed and evaluated mindfulness-based relationship education for non-distressed couples. The intervention was closely modelled on mindfulness-based stress reduction programmes (Kabat-Zinn, 1990), modified to be appropriate for couple relationships. Consistent with mindfulness-based approaches (Kabat-Zinn, 1990), the intervention focussed on the cultivation and development of mindful attention and awareness. Further, a non-striving stance was encouraged, and couples were not encouraged to strive for the development of particular outcomes or behaviours as their primary goal (Carson et al., 2004).

The intervention consisted of eight 2.5-h weekly sessions and a full day mindfulness retreat. Several important modifications to the standard mindfulness-based stress reduction protocol were made in order to be more suitable for the purposes of enhancing couple relationships. For example, participants were encouraged to meditate upon and cultivate loving-kindness towards their partners (Carson et al., 2004). Couples were "asked to recall the days when they first fell in love and decided to be together, and observe whether they could actually 'feel' again in the present moment the sense of discovery, closeness, trust, sweetness, or fun that they had at the time" (Carson et al., 2006, p. 318).

Couples also completed yoga exercises as a couple and physically supported each other in various yoga postures. In addition, there were mindful touch exercises completed by the couples (e.g. giving each other a mindful back massage and discussing any implications of this activity for sexuality). The authors also described an eye-gazing exercise in which the two partners gaze into each other's eyes while focussing on the inherent goodness in each other. Couples were encouraged to develop enhanced awareness of shared pleasant activities, as well as unpleasant or challenging situations, and to reflect on what each individual learned from such situations.

Carson and colleagues (2004) also reviewed the use of mindfulness skills for managing life stressors and relationship difficulties, focussing on the use of mindfulness to promote emotion and problem-focussed coping. In addition, a key focus was on the cultivation of mindful attention and awareness to relationship processes and activities. For example, the authors emphasised the importance of cultivation of mindfulness skills during shared positive and enjoyable activities, as well as during difficult or stressful situations or activities. Importantly, mindfulness skills were practised within each session, and regular practice of mindfulness skills was encouraged as homework activities.

Carson and colleagues (2004) evaluated the efficacy of the above-mentioned mindfulness-based relationship enhancement intervention in a sample of 44 non-distressed couples relative to a wait-list control condition. Couples assigned to the mindfulness-based relationship enhancement programme evidenced higher relationship satisfaction, acceptance of partner, autonomy, relatedness, closeness, and less relationship distress compared to the wait-list control group. In addition, partners in the intervention condition displayed enhanced optimism, spirituality, daily coping and relaxation, relative to the control condition, and less psychological distress. Importantly, those in the mindfulness group who practised mindfulness meditation more frequently evidenced greater relationship satisfaction and coping with stress.

Couple Therapy

Emotion-focussed couple therapy has a very strong empirical base for its efficacy (see Halford & Snyder, 2012 for a recent review of the evidence). The emotion-focussed approach has as its central tenet that emotional reactions to the partner are at the heart of couple distress and that enhancing distressed relationships requires a focus on those emotional reactions (Greenberg & Goldman, 2008; Johnson, 2007). More specifically, emotion-focussed couple therapists seek to help the couple become more aware of their emotional reactions, how these emotional reactions influence couple interaction, and how to modify these reactions. Central ideas in the emotion-focussed approach overlap considerably with mindfulness concepts. For example, Johnson (2007, p. 47) suggests that emotion-focussed couple therapy is about helping individuals be *"open to experience"* and that *"problems arise then from lack of or denial of awareness, constriction in processing ongoing experience so that this experience cannot be understood and trusted"*.

The attempt to facilitate emotional awareness in emotion-focussed couple therapy is done by increasing mindfulness of the experienced emotion. For example, Johnson and Greenberg (1987) describe the process of tracking the emotional cycle of a couple's interactions in terms of the therapist being empathic by reflecting back emotional statements, having the partners amplify emotions through repeating statements and gestures, having the partners focus on their subjective experiences of feelings, and the therapist making tentative interpretations of partially expressed emotions. Greenberg and Goldman (2008) refer to this process as emotional coaching, by which they mean teaching the individual to better tune in to their own emotional experience and using that emotional mindfulness constructively within their relationship. Three studies of emotion-focussed couple therapy show that couples make the predicted increase in emotional expression, particularly revealing more primary and vulnerable emotions across the course of therapy (Bradley & Furrow, 2004; Greenberg, Ford, Alden, & Johnson, 1993; Makinen & Johnson, 2006).

Integrative behavioural couple therapy (IBCT) is an acceptance-based intervention for the treatment of relationship distress (Jacobson et al., 2000). Whereas traditional behavioural couple therapy (TBCT) is focussed on assisting partners to change their behaviour to enhance the relationship and alleviate distress, IBCT emphasises the importance of emotional acceptance of aspects of their partner and relationship that may have been considered problematic and may not be able to be changed (Jacobson et al., 2000). Specifically, IBCT facilitates acceptance of the emotional responses, the conditions that elicit them, and the outcomes of such responses, for each partner (Christensen et al., 2004; Jacobson et al., 2000). Importantly, however, acceptance does not refer to passive resignation to relationship challenges and should not be encouraged for abusive behaviour or addictive behaviour (Christensen et al., 2004). Rather, it recognises that there are often aspects of a partner that are not able to be changed and problems in relationships that do not have solutions to them, and thus acceptance is often warranted (Christensen et al., 2004; Jacobson et al., 2000). However, the authors note that acceptance can often paradoxically lead to change.

IBCT uses three specific strategies to facilitate acceptance in couple relationships: empathic joining, unified detachment, and tolerance building (Christensen et al., 2004; Jacobson et al., 2000). With regard to empathic joining, therapists engage in strategies to elicit emotion associated with the couple's challenges that the partner's may not typically express. Often partners may not be fully aware of these emotions until a therapist conjectures as to what a client may be experiencing. However, at other times, partners may be aware of the emotion but may avoid expressing these softer, more vulnerable emotions because of fear or embarrassment (Christensen et al., 2004; Jacobson et al., 2000). The therapist therefore aims to facilitate an empathic connection between the partners about the emotionally charged difficulties the couple is experiencing (Christensen et al., 2004). These strategies seem to overlap considerably with emotion-focussed couple therapy approaches to tracking the cycle.

Unified detachment refers to the process of generating an objective stance to the relationship difficulties and obtaining some distance from these problems (Christensen et al., 2004). That is, the therapist encourages the partner's to view their ongoing relationship difficulties from a distance and engage in a descriptive analysis of the problematic behavioural patterns and the sequence of events. Therapists may also make use of metaphors, humour, and labelling the problem with names to generate distance from the problems, in a similar way to defusion exercises in acceptance and commitment therapy (Hayes, Strosahl, & Wilson, 2012) or decentring (Shapiro, Carlson, Astin, & Freedman, 2006). One goal of unified detachment is to view the actual relationship difficulties as the problem, as opposed to blaming any one partner. Importantly, both emotional exploration of the problem (empathic joining) and unified detachment serve to develop mindfulness of their relationship and non-judgemental awareness of relationship patterns and sequences of interactions (Christensen et al., 2004; Jacobson et al., 2000).

Finally, tolerance building recognises that relationship challenges stemming from differences between partners are likely to always exist. These differences between partners are unlikely to be completely removed. However, it is possible to reduce the intensity of the emotional impact of these differences. Building tolerance and acceptance of these differences can take many forms during therapy. For example, a therapist might review the benefits of differences between partners. A therapist may also ask a client to enact problematic behaviours in session when both partners are "not" feeling highly emotionally charged at the time so that the couple experiences these behaviours differently (Christensen et al., 2004). Because the typical sequence of negative events is unlikely to occur in the absence of intense emotional arousal, partner's can experience these behavioural patterns and respond in ways that differ from their usual pattern of responding, and thus gain tolerance of these usually distressing behaviours, and more adaptive ways to respond (Christensen et al., 2004; Jacobson et al., 2000).

The focus of IBCT is emotional acceptance. However, when it becomes apparent that a couple may benefit from direct skills training to rectify a skill deficit, the IBCT therapist may engage in direct change strategies (Christensen et al., 2004; Jacobson et al., 2000). For example, a couple may benefit from communication skills training or problem-solving training, and thus these change skills can be incorporated into the couple therapy in addition to the key acceptance-based strategies. Christensen and colleagues (2004) note that these change strategies are, however, generally taught in an individualised manner and applied to the specific sequences of problematic behaviour occurring in the couple. Further, when strong emotions appear in the context of change-based strategies, the IBCT therapist reverts back to acceptance-based strategies of emotional acceptance (e.g. empathic joining).

Evidence indicates that the acceptance-based IBCT is at least as efficacious as traditional behavioural couple therapy (TBCT; Christensen et al., 2004; Christensen, Atkins, Baucom, & Yi, 2010). Christensen and colleagues (2004) compared IBCT with TBCT in a sample of significantly and chronically distressed married couples. Results revealed that couples in both intervention conditions improved in satisfaction. Although there were somewhat different trajectories of change between the two conditions, with TBCT evidencing more rapid improvement early in therapy and IBCT displaying steady improvement over therapy, both conditions were similar in regard to clinically significant improvement at post-therapy. These results held at 5-year follow-up (Christensen et al., 2010). Interestingly, with regard to observed couple communication at 2-year follow-up, Baucom, Sevier, Eldridge, Doss, and Christensen (2011) found that couples in the acceptance-based IBCT evidenced more positive communication compared to those in the TBCT. Thus, IBCT is at least as efficacious as existing evidence-based couple therapies, and there is some evidence that it may be more beneficial on communication behaviours.

Conclusions and Future Directions

In this chapter, we have outlined how mindfulness may be beneficial to romantic relationship functioning and the utility of mindfulness-based clinical interventions to enhance romantic relationships and alleviate relationship distress. Evidence clearly indicates that high mindfulness is associated with enhanced relationship satisfaction (Barnes et al., 2007; Wachs & Cordova, 2007). This may be because high mindfulness is associated with less psychopathology, secure attachment, enhanced emotion regulation and self-regulation, increased acceptance of self and partner, and greater capacity to be empathic and enjoy positive couple activities. The challenge for future research is to examine the relative importance of these and other potential mechanisms underlying the association between mindfulness and relationship outcomes. Further, it would be useful to examine not only cognitive and emotional mechanisms but also behavioural mediators. In other words, it is important that we begin to understand what individuals higher in mindfulness actually "do" that enhances the relationship for themselves and their partner.

With regard to the use of mindfulness-based interventions to enhance couple relationships and reduce relationship distress, the evidence to date is promising. Specifically, one randomised controlled trial demonstrates that mindfulness-based relationship enhancement is beneficial for non-distressed couples and found larger effect size improvements than existing evidence-based relationship enhancement programmes on satisfied couples (Carson et al., 2004). It is important, however, to directly compare the efficacy of mindfulness-based relationship enhancement with existing evidence-based programmes. Emotion-focussed couple therapy seems to do things that are closely associated with mindfulness. Acceptance-based integrative behavioural couple therapy also seems to promote mindfulness.

In summary, much evidence indicates that mindfulness and mindfulness-based clinical interventions produce beneficial outcomes on a wide range of psychological factors (Keng et al., 2011). It is encouraging that research is beginning to examine not only the individual benefits of mindfulness but also the interpersonal and relational outcomes of mindfulness and mindfulness-based interventions. Although there is further work to be done to elucidate the mechanisms underlying the beneficial effects of mindfulness on relationship outcomes, the available evidence pertaining to the benefits of mindfulness on romantic relationships is promising.

References

Anderson, N. D., Lau, M. A., Segal, Z. V., & Bishop, S. R. (2007). Mindfulness-based stress reduction and attentional control. *Clinical Psychology and Psychotherapy, 14*(6), 449–463. doi:10.1002/cpp.544.

Arch, J. J., & Craske, M. G. (2006). Mechanisms of mindfulness: Emotion regulation following a focused breathing induction. *Behaviour Research and Therapy, 44*(12), 1849–1858. doi:10.1016/j.brat.2005.12.007.

Baer, R. A. (2003). Mindfulness training as a clinical intervention: A conceptual and empirical review. *Clinical Psychology: Science and Practice, 10*(2), 125–143. doi:10.1093/clipsy.bpg015.

Baer, R. A., Smith, G. T., & Allen, K. B. (2004). Assessment of mindfulness by self-report: The Kentucky inventory of mindfulness skills. *Assessment, 11*(3), 191–206. doi:10.1177/1073191104268029.

Barbato, A., & D'Avanzo, B. (2008). Efficacy of couple therapy as a treatment for depression: A meta-analysis. *Psychiatric Quarterly, 79*(2), 121–132. doi:10.1007/s11126-008-9068-0.

Barnes, S., Brown, K. W., Krusemark, E., Campbell, W. K., & Rogee, R. D. (2007). The role of mindfulness in romantic relationship satisfaction and responses to relationship stress. *Journal of Marital and Family Therapy, 33*(4), 482–500. doi:10.1111/j.1752-0606.2007.00033.x.

Baucom, D. H., Hahlweg, K., & Kuschel, A. (2003). Are waiting-list control groups needed in future marital therapy outcome research? *Behavior Therapy, 34*(2), 179–188. doi:10.1016/S0005-7894(03)80012-6.

Baucom, K. J., Sevier, M., Eldridge, K. A., Doss, B. D., & Christensen, A. (2011). Observed communication in couples two years after integrative and traditional behavioral couple therapy: outcome and link with five-year follow-up. *Journal of Consulting and Clinical Psychology, 79*(5), 565. doi:10.1037/a0025121.

Baucom, D. H., Whisman, M. A., & Paprocki, C. (2012). Couple-based interventions for psychopathology. *Journal of Family Therapy, 34*(3), 250–270. doi:10.1111/j.1467-6427.2012.00600.x.

Bishop, S. R., Lau, M., Shapiro, S., Carlson, L., Anderson, N. D., Carmody, J., et al. (2004). Mindfulness: A proposed operational definition. *Clinical Psychology: Science and Practice, 11*(3), 230–241. doi:10.1093/clipsy.bph077.

Block-Lerner, J., Adair, C., Plumb, J. C., Rhatigan, D. L., & Orsillo, S. M. (2007). The case for mindfulness-based approaches in the cultivation of empathy: Does nonjudgmental, present-moment awareness increase capacity for perspective-taking and empathic concern? *Journal of Marital and Family Therapy, 33*(4), 501–516. doi:10.1111/j.1752-0606.2007.00034.x.

Bodenmann, G. (2005). Dyadic coping and its significance for marital functioning. In T. A. Revenson, K. Kayser, & G. Bodenmann (Eds.), *Couples coping with stress: Emerging perspectives on dyadic coping* (pp. 33–50). Washington, DC: American Psychological Association.

Bodenmann, G., & Shantinath, S. D. (2004). The Couples Coping Enhancement Training (CCET): A new approach to prevention of marital distress based upon stress and coping. *Family Relations, 53*(5), 477–484. doi:10.1111/j.0197-6664.2004.00056.x.

Bowen, S., & Enkema, M. C. (2014). Relationship between dispositional mindfulness and substance use: Findings from a clinical sample. *Addictive Behaviors, 39*(3), 532–537. doi:10.1016/j.addbeh.2013.10.026.

Bradbury, T. N., & Fincham, F. D. (1990). Attributions in marriage: Review and critique. *Psychological Bulletin, 107*(1), 3–33. doi:10.1037/0033-2909.107.1.3.

Bradbury, T. N., & Lavner, J. A. (2012). How can we improve preventive and educational interventions for intimate relationships? *Behavior Therapy, 43*(1), 113–122. doi:10.1016/j.beth.2011.02.008.

Bradley, B., & Furrow, J. L. (2004). Toward a mini-theory of the blamer softening event: Tracking the moment-by-moment process. *Journal of Marital and Family Therapy, 30*(2), 233–246. doi:10.1111/j.1752-0606.2004.tb01236.x.

Broderick, P. C. (2005). Mindfulness and coping with dysphoric mood: Contrasts with rumination and distraction. *Cognitive Therapy and Research, 29*(5), 501–510. doi:10.1007/s10608-005-3888-0.

Brown, K. W., & Ryan, R. M. (2003). The benefits of being present: Mindfulness and its role in psychological well-being. *Journal of Personality and Social Psychology, 84*(4), 822–848. doi:10.1037/0022-3514.84.4.822.

Brown, K. W., Ryan, R. M., & Creswell, J. D. (2007a). Mindfulness: Theoretical foundations and evidence for its salutary effects. *Psychological Inquiry, 18*(4), 211–237. doi:10.1080/10478400701598298.

Brown, K. W., Ryan, R. M., & Creswell, J. D. (2007b). Addressing fundamental questions about mindfulness. *Psychological Inquiry, 18*(4), 272–281. doi:10.1080/10478400701703344.

Campbell-Sills, L., Barlow, D. H., Brown, T. A., & Hofmann, S. G. (2006). Effects of suppression and acceptance on emotional responses of individuals with anxiety and mood disorders. *Behaviour Research and Therapy, 44*(9), 1251–1263. doi:10.1016/j.brat.2005.10.001.

Carson, J. W., Carson, K. M., Gil, K. M., & Baucom, D. H. (2004). Mindfulness-based relationship enhancement. *Behavior Therapy, 35*(3), 471–494. doi:10.1016/S0005-7894(04)80028-5.

Carson, J. W., Carson, K. M., Gil, K. M., & Baucom, D. H. (2006). Mindfulness-based relationship enhancement (MBRE) in couples. In R. A. Baer (Ed.), *Mindfulness-based treatment approaches: Clinician's guide to evidence base and applications* (pp. 309–331). Amsterdam: Elsevier.

Carson, J. W., Carson, K. M., Gil, K. M., & Baucom, D. H. (2007). Self-expansion as a mediator of relationship improvements in a mindfulness intervention. *Journal of Marital and Family Therapy, 33*(4), 517–528. doi:10.1111/j.1752-0606.2007.00035.x.

Christensen, A., Atkins, D. C., Baucom, B., & Yi, J. (2010). Marital status and satisfaction five years following a randomized clinical trial comparing traditional versus integrative behavioral couple therapy. *Journal of Consulting and Clinical Psychology, 78*(2), 225. doi:10.1037/a0018132.

Christensen, A., & Heavey, C. L. (1990). Gender and social structure in the demand/withdraw pattern of marital conflict. *Journal of Personality and Social Psychology, 59*(1), 73. doi:10.1037/0022-3514.59.1.73.

Christensen, A., & Heavey, C. L. (1993). *Gender differences in marital conflict: The demand/withdraw interaction pattern*. Thousand Oaks, CA: Sage.

Christensen, A., Sevier, M., Simpson, L. E., & Gattis, K. S. (2004). Acceptance, mindfulness, and change in couple therapy. In S. Hayes, V. Follette, & M. Linehan (Eds.), *Mindfulness and acceptance: Expanding the cognitive-behavioral tradition* (pp. 288–309). New York: Guilford.

Cordova, J. V., Gee, C. B., & Warren, L. Z. (2005). Emotional skillfulness in marriage: Intimacy as a mediator of the relationship between emotional skillfulness and marital satisfaction. *Journal of Social and Clinical Psychology, 24*(2), 218–235. doi:10.1521/jscp.24.2.218.62270.

Dehle, C., Larsen, D., & Landers, J. E. (2001). Social support in marriage. *American Journal of Family Therapy, 29*(4), 307–324. doi:10.1080/01926180126500.

Dekeyser, M., Raes, F., Leijssen, M., Leysen, S., & Dewulf, D. (2008). Mindfulness skills and interpersonal behaviour. *Personality and Individual Differences, 44*(5), 1235–1245. doi:10.1016/j.paid.2007.11.018.

Denton, W. H., Carmody, T. J., Rush, A. J., Thase, M. E., Trivedi, M. H., Arnow, B. A., et al. (2010). Dyadic discord at baseline is associated with lack of remission in the acute treatment of chronic depression. *Psychological Medicine, 40*(3), 415–424. doi:10.1017/S0033291709990535.

Dewey, D., & Hunsley, J. (1990). The effects of marital adjustment and spouse involvement on the behavioral treatment of agoraphobia: A meta-analytic review. *Anxiety Research, 2*(2), 69–83. doi:10.1080/08917779008249327.

Diener, E., Eunkook, M. S., Lucas, R. E., & Smith, H. L. (1999). Subjective well-being: Three decades of progress. *Psychological Bulletin, 125*, 276–302. doi:10.1037/0033-2909.125.2.276.

Dupre, M. E., & Meadows, S. O. (2007). Disaggregating the effects of marital trajectories on health. *Journal of Family Issues, 28*(5), 623–652. doi:10.1177/0192513X06296296.

Durham, R. C., Allan, T., & Hackett, C. A. (1997). On predicting improvement and relapse in generalized anxiety disorder following psychotherapy. *British Journal of Clinical Psychology, 36*(1), 101–119. doi:10.1111/j.2044-8260.1997.tb01234.x.

Durtschi, J. A., Fincham, F. D., Cui, M., Lorenz, F. O., & Conger, R. D. (2011). Dyadic processes in early marriage: Attributions, behavior, and marital quality. *Family Relations, 60*(4), 421–434. doi:10.1111/j.1741-3729.2011.00655.x.

Fals-Stewart, W., O'Farrell, T. J., & Lam, W. K. K. (2009). Behavioral couple therapy for gay and lesbian couples with alcohol use disorders. *Journal of Substance Abuse Treatment, 37*(4), 379–387. doi:10.1016/j.jsat.2009.05.001.

Gambrel, L. E., & Keeling, M. L. (2010). Relational aspects of mindfulness: Implications for the practice of marriage and family therapy. *Contemporary Family Therapy, 32*(4), 412–426. doi:10.1007/s10591-010-9129-z.

Gottman, J. M. (2014). *What predicts divorce?: The relationship between marital processes and marital outcomes*. New York: Psychology Press.

Gottman, J. M., Coan, J., Carrere, S., & Swanson, C. (1998). Predicting marital happiness and stability from newlywed interactions. *Journal of Marriage and the Family, 5–22*.

Greenberg, L. S., Ford, C. L., Alden, L. S., & Johnson, S. M. (1993). In-session change in emotionally focused therapy. *Journal of Consulting and Clinical Psychology, 61*(1), 78. doi:10.1037/0022-006X.61.1.78.

Greenberg, L. S., & Goldman, R. N. (2008). *Emotion-focused couples therapy: The dynamics of emotion, love, and power*. Washington DC: American Psychological Association.

Greenberg, L. S., & Johnson, S. M. (1988). *Emotionally focused therapy for couples*. New York: Guilford Press.

Grossman, P., Kappos, L., Gensicke, H., D'Souza, M., Mohr, D. C., Penner, I. K., et al. (2010). MS quality of life, depression, and fatigue improve after mindfulness training: A randomized trial. *Neurology, 75*(13), 1141–1149. doi:10.1212/WNL.0b013e3181f4d80d.

Halford, W. K., & Bodenmann, G. (2013). Effects of relationship education on maintenance of couple relationship satisfaction. *Clinical Psychology Review, 33*, 512–525. doi:10.1016/j.cpr.2013.02.001.

Halford, W. K., Markman, H. J., Kling, G. H., & Stanley, S. M. (2003). Best practice in couple relationship education. *Journal of Marital and Family Therapy, 29*(3), 385–406. doi:10.1111/j.1752-0606.2003.tb01214.x.

Halford, W. K., Markman, H. J., & Stanley, S. (2008). Strengthening couples' relationships with education: Social policy and public health perspectives. *Journal of Family Psychology, 22*(4), 497. doi:10.1037/a0012789.

Halford, W. K., & Snyder, D. K. (2012). Universal processes and common factors in couple therapy and relationship education. *Behavior Therapy, 43*(1), 1–12. doi:10.1016/j.beth.2011.01.007.

Halford, W. K., & Wilson, K. L. (2009). Predictors of relationship satisfaction four years after completing flexible delivery couple relationship education. *Journal of Couple & Relationship Therapy, 8*(2), 143–161.

Harrington, R., Loffredo, D. A., & Perz, C. A. (2014). Dispositional mindfulness as a positive predictor of psychological well-being and the role of the private self-consciousness insight factor. *Personality and Individual Differences, 71*, 15–18. doi:10.1016/j.paid.2014.06.050.
Hawkins, A. J., Blanchard, V. L., Baldwin, S. A., & Fawcett, E. B. (2008). Does marriage and relationship education work? A meta-analytic study. *Journal of Consulting and Clinical Psychology, 76*(5), 723. doi:10.1037/a0012584.
Hayes, S. C., Strosahl, K. D., & Wilson, K. G. (2012). *Acceptance and commitment therapy: The process and practice of mindful change*. New York: Guilford Press.
Hsueh, J., Alderson, D. P., Lundquist, E., Michalopoulos, C., Gubits, D., Fein, D., et al. (2012). *The supporting healthy marriage evaluation: Early impacts on low-income families*. Office of Planning, Research and Evaluation Report 2012–11. Office of Planning, Research and Evaluation, Administration for Children and Families, United States Department of Health and Human Services, Washington, DC.
Jacobson, N. S., Christensen, A., Prince, S. E., Cordova, J., & Eldridge, K. (2000). Integrative behavioral couple therapy: An acceptance-based, promising new treatment for couple discord. *Journal of Consulting and Clinical Psychology, 68*(2), 351. doi:10.1037/0022-006X.68.2.351.
Johnson, S. M. (1999). Emotionally focused couple therapy. In J. M. Donovan (Ed.), *Short-term couple therapy* (pp. 13–41). New York: Guilford.
Johnson, S. M. (2007). The contribution of emotionally focused couples therapy. *Journal of Contemporary Psychotherapy, 37*(1), 47–52. doi:10.1007/s10879-006-9034-9.
Johnson, S. M., & Greenberg, L. S. (1987). Emotionally focused marital therapy: An overview. *Psychotherapy: Theory, Research, Practice, Training, 24*, 552–560. doi:10.1037/h0085753.
Jones, K. C., Welton, S. R., Oliver, T. C., & Thoburn, J. W. (2011). Mindfulness, spousal attachment, and marital satisfaction: A mediated model. *The Family Journal, 19*(4), 357–361. doi:10.1177/1066480711417234.
Kabat-Zinn, J. (1990). *Full catastrophe living: Using the wisdom of your body and mind to face stress, pain and illness*. New York: Delacorte.
Kabat-Zinn, J. (1994). *Wherever you go, there you are: Mindfulness meditation in everyday life*. New York: Hyperion.
Kabat-Zinn, J. (2003). Mindfulness-based interventions in context: Past, present, and future. *Clinical Psychology: Science and Practice Summer, 10*(2), 144–156. doi:10.1093/clipsy.bpg016.
Keng, S.-L., Smoski, M. J., & Robins, C. J. (2011). Effects of mindfulness on psychological health: A review of empirical studies. *Clinical Psychology Review, 31*(6), 1041–1056. doi:10.1016/j.cpr.2011.04.006.
Kliem, S., Kroger, C., & Kosfelder, J. (2010). Dialectical behavior therapy for borderline personality disorder: A meta-analysis using mixed-effects modeling. *Journal of Consulting and Clinical Psychology, 78*(6), 936–951. doi:10.1037/a0021015.
Kozlowski, A. (2013). Mindful mating: exploring the connection between mindfulness and relationship satisfaction. *Sexual and Relationship Therapy, 28*(1–2), 92–104. doi:10.1080/14681994.2012.748889.
Kuijer, R. G., Ybema, J. F., Buunk, B. P., De Jong, G. M., Thijs-Boer, F., & Sanderman, R. (2000). Active engagement, protective buffering, and overprotection: Three ways of giving support by intimate partners of patients with cancer. *Journal of Social and Clinical Psychology, 19*(2), 256–275. doi:10.1521/jscp.2000.19.2.256.
Liu, X., Wang, S., Chang, S., Chen, W., & Si, M. (2013). Effect of a brief mindfulness intervention on tolerance and distress of pain induced by cold-pressor task. *Stress and Health, 29*(3), 199–204. doi:10.1002/smi.2446.
Makinen, J. A., & Johnson, S. M. (2006). Resolving attachment injuries in couples using emotionally focused therapy: Steps toward forgiveness and reconciliation. *Journal of Consulting and Clinical Psychology, 74*(6), 1055–1064. doi:10.1037/0022-006X.74.6.1055.
Mikulincer, M., & Shaver, P. R. (2007). *Attachment in adulthood: Structure, dynamics, and change*. New York: Guilford.

Monson, C. M., Fredman, S. J., Macdonald, A., Pukay-Martin, N. D., Resick, P. A., & Schnurr, P. P. (2012). Effect of cognitive-behavioral couple therapy for PTSD: A randomized controlled trial. *JAMA, 308*(7), 700–709. doi:10.1001/jama.2012.9307.

Ostafin, B. D., & Kassman, K. T. (2012). Stepping out of history: Mindfulness improves insight problem solving. *Consciousness and Cognition, 21*(2), 1031–1036. doi:10.1016/j.concog.2012.02.014.

Overbeek, G., Vollebergh, W., de Graaf, R., Scholte, R., de Kemp, R., & Engels, R. (2006). Longitudinal associations of marital quality and marital dissolution with the incidence of DSM-III-R disorders. *Journal of Family Psychology, 20*(2), 284–291. doi:10.1037/0893-3200.20.2.284.

Pepping, C. A., Davis, P. J., & O'Donovan, A. (2015). The association between state attachment security and state mindfulness. *PLoS ONE, 10*(3), e0116779. doi:10.1371/journal.pone.0116779.

Pepping, C. A., O'Donovan, A., Zimmer-Gembeck, M. J., & Hanisch, M. (2015). Individual differences in attachment and eating pathology: The mediating role of mindfulness. *Personality and Individual Differences, 75*, 24–29. doi:10.1016/j.paid.2014.10.040.

Pepping, C. A., O'Donovan, A., Zimmer-Gembeck, M. J., & Hanish, M. (2014). Is emotion regulation the process underlying the relationship between low mindfulness and psychosocial distress? *Australian Journal of Psychology, 66*, 130–138. doi:10.1111/ajpy.12050.

Pepping, C. A., O'Donovan, A., & Davis, P. J. (2014). The differential relationship between mindfulness and attachment in experienced and inexperienced meditators. *Mindfulness, 5*, 392–399. doi:10.1007/s12671-012-0193-3.

Peterson, B. D., Eifert, G. H., Feingold, T., & Davidson, S. (2009). Using acceptance and commitment therapy to treat distressed couples: A case study with two couples. *Cognitive and Behavioral Practice, 16*(4), 430–442. doi:10.1016/j.cbpra.2008.12.009.

Powers, M. B., Vedel, E., & Emmelkamp, P. M. (2008). Behavioral couples therapy (BCT) for alcohol and drug use disorders: A meta-analysis. *Clinical Psychology Review, 28*(6), 952–962. doi:10.1016/j.cpr.2008.02.002.

Saavedra, M. C., Chapman, K. E., & Rogge, R. D. (2010). Clarifying links between attachment and relationship quality: Hostile conflict and mindfulness as moderators. *Journal of Family Psychology, 24*(4), 380–390. doi:10.1037/a0019872.

Schmaling, K. B., & Sher, T. G. E. (2000). *The psychology of couples and illness: Theory, research, & practice*. Washington, DC: American Psychological Association.

Shadish, W. R., & Baldwin, S. A. (2003). Meta-analysis of marriage and family therapy interventions. *Journal of Marital and Family Therapy, 29*(4), 547–570. doi:10.1111/j.1752-0606.2003.tb01694.x.

Shapiro, S. L., Carlson, L. E., Astin, J. A., & Freedman, B. (2006). Mechanisms of mindfulness. *Journal of Clinical Psychology, 62*(3), 373–386. doi:10.1002/jclp.20237.

Shapiro, S. L., Schwartz, G. E., & Bonner, G. (1998). Effects of mindfulness-based stress reduction on medical and premedical students. *Journal of Behavioral Medicine, 21*(6), 581–599. doi:10.1023/A:1018700829825.

Snyder, D. K., Castellani, A. M., & Whisman, M. A. (2006). Current status and future directions in couple therapy. *Annual Review of Psychology, 57*, 317–344. doi:10.1146/annurev.psych.56.091103.070154.

Snyder, D. K., & Halford, W. K. (2012). Evidence-based couple therapy: Current status and future directions. *Journal of Family Therapy, 34*(3), 229–249. doi:10.1111/j.1467-6427.2012.00599.x.

Vollestad, J., Sivertsen, B., & Nielsen, G. H. (2011). Mindfulness-based stress reduction for patients with anxiety disorders: Evaluation in a randomized controlled trial. *Behaviour Research and Therapy, 49*(4), 281–288. doi:10.1016/j.brat.2011.01.007.

Wachs, K., & Cordova, J. V. (2007). Mindful relating: Exploring mindfulness and emotion repertoires in intimate relationships. *Journal of Marital and Family Therapy, 33*(4), 464–481. doi:10.1111/j.1752[--]0606.2007.00032.x.

Wade, T. J., & Pevalin, D. J. (2004). Marital transitions and mental health. *Journal of Health and Social Behavior, 45*, 155–170. doi:10.1177/002214650404500203.

Wadsworth, M. E., & Markman, H. J. (2012). Where's the Action? Understanding what works and why in relationship education. *Behavior Therapy, 43*(1), 99–112. doi:10.1016/j.beth.2011.01.006.

Waite, L., & Gallagher, M. (2002). *The case for marriage: Why married people are happier, healthier and better off financially*. New York: Random House.

Whisman, M. A. (2001). Marital adjustment and outcome following treatments for depression. *Journal of Consulting and Clinical Psychology, 69*(1), 125–129. doi:10.1037/0022-006X.69.1.125.

Whisman, M. A., & Baucom, D. H. (2012). Intimate relationships and psychopathology. *Clinical Child and Family Psychology Review, 15*(1), 4–13. doi:10.1007/s10567-011-0107-2.

Whisman, M. A., & Bruce, M. L. (1999). Marital dissatisfaction and incidence of major depressive episode in a community sample. *Journal of Abnormal Psychology, 108*(4), 674–678. doi:10.1037/0021-843X.108.4.674.

Whisman, M. A., Uebelacker, L. A., & Bruce, M. L. (2006). Longitudinal association between marital dissatisfaction and alcohol use disorders in a community sample. *Journal of Family Psychology, 20*(1), 164–167. doi:10.1037/0893-3200.20.1.164.

Whisman, M. A., Uebelacker, L. A., & Weinstock, L. M. (2004). Psychopathology and marital satisfaction: The importance of evaluating both partners. *Journal of Consulting and Clinical Psychology, 72*(5), 830. doi:10.1037/0022-006X.72.5.830.

Williams, A. M., & Cano, A. (2014). Spousal mindfulness and social support in couples with chronic pain. *The Clinical Journal of Pain, 30*(6), 528–535. doi:10.1097/AJP.0000000000000009.

Wilson, K. L., Charker, J., Lizzio, A., Halford, K., & Kimlin, S. (2005). Assessing how much couples work at their relationship: The behavioral self-regulation for effective relationships scale. *Journal of Family Psychology, 19*(3), 385. doi:10.1037/0893-3200.19.3.385.

Wood, R. G., McConnell, S., Moore, Q., Clarkwest, A., & Hsueh, J. (2012). The effects of building strong families: A healthy marriage and relationship skills education program for unmarried parents. *Journal of Policy Analysis and Management, 31*(2), 228–252. doi:10.1002/pam.21608.

Index

E. Shonin et al. (eds.), *Mindfulness and Buddhist-Derived Approaches in Mental Health and Addiction*, Advances in Mental Health and Addiction,
DOI 10.1007/978-3-319-22255-4

N

O

P